KU-489-452

Target Organ Pathology

A Basic Text

Target Organ Pathology

A Basic Text

Edited by

J. TURTON
Department of Toxicology, The School of Pharmacy, University of London
and
J. HOOSON
ITR Laboratories Inc., Montréal

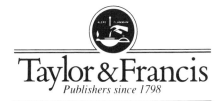

Taylor & Francis
Publishers since 1798

UK   Taylor & Francis Ltd, 1 Gunpowder Square, London EC4A 3DE
USA   Taylor & Francis Inc., 1900 Frost Road, Suite 101, Bristol, PA 19007

Copyright © Taylor & Francis Ltd 1998

All rights reserved. No part of this publication may be reproduced, stored in a retrieval system, or transmitted, in any form or by any means, electronic, electrostatic, magnetic tape, mechanical, photocopying, recording or otherwise, without the prior permission of the copyright owner.

British Library Cataloguing in Publication Data

A catalogue record for this book is available from the British Library

ISBN 0-7484-0156-3 (cased)
ISBN 0-7484-0157-1 (paperback)

Library of Congress Cataloguing in Publication data are available

Cover design by Jim Wilkie

Typeset in Times 10/12pt by Mathematical Composition Setters Ltd, Salisbury, UK

Printed by T. J. International Ltd, Padstow, UK

Contents

Foreword   *page* vii

Preface   ix

Contributors   xi

1 The Integumentary System   1
Andrew J. Ingram

**2 The Digestive System I: The Gastrointestinal Tract and
Exocrine Pancreas**   29
Graham R. Betton

3 The Digestive System II: The Hepatobiliary System   61
John G. Evans and Brian G. Lake

4 The Urinary System   99
Peter Greaves

5 The Cardiovascular System   141
Kevin R. Isaacs
    Section A   The Heart   141
    Section B   The Vascular System   158

6 The Haematopoietic System   177
C. Michael Andrews

7 The Immune System   207
Joseph G. Vos, Ian Kimber, C. Frieke Kuper,
Henk van Loveren and Henk-Jan Schuurman

v

Contents

8   The Musculoskeletal System   239
Ruth M. Lightfoot
   Section A   Skeletal Muscle   239
   Section B   Bone, Cartilage and Joints   254

9   The Nervous System   273
Peter Buckley

10   The Endocrine System   311
Mary J. Tucker

11   The Respiratory System   335
John R. Foster

12   The Male Reproductive System   371
Dianne M. Creasy

13   The Female Reproductive System   407
David J. Lewis and Chirukandath Gopinath

14   The Mammary Gland   429
Jean Hooson

15   Organs of Special Sense I: The Eye   451
Mervyn Robinson

16   Organs of Special Sense II: The Ear   467
Ernest S. Harpur

Index   483

Foreword

This comprehensive text and reference comprises sixteen chapters dedicated to the main organ systems of the body and their responses to toxic injury. The authors are all practising toxicological pathologists from academia and research laboratories with an international reputation in their field. The adoption of the classical approach to target organ toxicity was influenced by the specific, and sometimes unique, manner in which compounds manifest toxic injury. Each chapter therefore addresses the normal anatomy and physiology of the given organ system before detailing the morphological and pathophysiological events leading to toxic injury. It is this integration of altered form and function that defines the processes of target organ toxicity, the cornerstone of understanding hazard and hence risk and safety assessment. The practising toxicologist needs to receive from the pathologist a lucid appreciation of the likely clinical impact of the toxic changes observed; first in the test species and then, by extrapolation, to man. The information provided in each chapter is directed at understanding the underlying processes of toxicity involved. An appreciation of the significant species differences in the toxic manifestations to these processes is an essential factor in the effective extrapolation of animal test data to the human clinical environment.

This synthesis of normality and toxicity states is illustrated by a diverse array of toxic changes induced by natural substances, industrial chemicals, pesticides and pharmaceuticals. Each of these examples illustrates the links between the primarily biochemical approach of classic texts of toxicology and the morphological descriptions of textbooks of pathology. The intended readership – both toxicologists and toxicological pathologists – is given a comprehensive and systematic review of target organ pathology, delivering both basic principles for those in training and learning points as part of the continuous professional development of those working in the field. These concepts are extensively supported by illustrations and key references. These lead the reader into more advanced details, as appropriate, to the practitioner working in academic research, health and safety, chemical and biomedical R&D and contract research. On behalf of the Council of the British

Society of Toxicological Pathologists, I can commend this work to both toxicologists and pathologists engaged in all these fields.

Dr Graham R. Betton,
Senior Vice-President,
British Society of Toxicological Pathologists

Preface

Toxicology is the study of the adverse effects of chemical substances on living systems. It is a relatively new but increasingly important science. Forty or fifty years ago, toxicology was barely recognised as a scientific discipline. However, over the last twenty to thirty years the subject has developed rapidly and there has been a dramatic increase in the number of books and publications on toxicology, the number of learned societies devoted to the subject, and the number of establishments, departments and units involved in toxicological investigations. Similarly, there has been a great expansion in the number of courses teaching toxicology and in the number of individuals describing themselves as toxicologists.

This volume is intended as an introductory text. It covers the essentials of target organ pathology that all toxicologists should know. The book is aimed at undergraduate and postgraduate students of toxicology and its allied sciences, and at toxicologists, particularly those in non-pathological branches of the subject, in the early stages of their careers. The objective is to provide a basic understanding of the pathological reactions of the various organs of the body in response to toxic injury induced by chemical substances. Furthermore, the text should help all toxicologists understand the language of toxicological pathology.

There is a lack of student texts in the area of target organ pathology. The concept for the book arose from the involvement of both editors in teaching on various courses in toxicology at the undergraduate and postgraduate level. Although there are several volumes now available on the subject of toxicological pathology which include coverage of target organ effects, these books are generally specialist and comprehensive reference texts aimed at the trained pathologist. There are no suitable books to recommend to students, or to the toxicologist who does not have an extensive background in pathology. For these reasons this book is intended primarily as a teaching and basic reference text which will allow the reader to progress, when necessary, to the more specialised volumes of toxicological pathology which are currently available, for example, *Toxicologic Pathology*, edited by W.M. Haschek and C.G. Rousseau, 1991, Academic Press, San Diego.

We have attempted to make this book comprehensive and user friendly. All the major organ systems of the body are covered, with each chapter written by an eminent authority in the field. A systematic approach has been taken for each organ system, with each of the sixteen chapters having a similar outline, including, Introduction; Anatomy, Histology and Physiology; Biochemical and Cellular Mechanisms of Toxicity; Morphological Responses to Injury; Testing for Toxicity; Conclusions. Chapter length is weighted according to the toxicological importance of each organ system. This repeatable format allows the reader to move from chapter to chapter and find the contents organised in a similar way. This arrangement also permits the reader to progress through the book in a systematic way, or consult each chapter, or part of a chapter, in isolation.

It goes without saying that we are deeply indebted to our twenty-one authors, without whom this book would not exist. We would also like to take the opportunity of acknowledging the many students we have taught, both at the undergraduate and postgraduate level. These students were unknowingly the stimulus for the concept of the book, and for defining the approach and direction of the editorial policy. We also wish to thank Mary Fagg who has dealt with the very large amount of correspondence and word processing necessary in the editing of such a volume; it is her diligent work which made the book possible. Finally we wish to thank the members of staff at Taylor and Francis who have been involved with the publication. Their professionalism, advice, guidance and encouragement, ensured that the book saw the light of day.

The editors wish to thank Astra Charnwood, Unilever Environmental Safety Laboratory, and Shell Research Limited for assistance towards the editorial costs of this book.

John Turton, London
Jean Hooson, Montréal

Contributors

C. Michael Andrews
Glaxo Wellcome Research and Development, Park Road, Ware, Hertfordshire, SG12 0DP, UK

Graham R. Betton
Zeneca Pharmaceuticals, Mereside, Alderley Park, Macclesfield, Cheshire, SK10 4TG, UK

Peter Buckley
Unilever Research, Environmental Safety Laboratory, Colworth House, Sharnbrook, Bedfordshire, MK44 1LQ, UK

Dianne M. Creasy
Huntingdon Life Sciences, Eye, Suffolk, IP23 7BR, UK

John G. Evans
Astra Charnwood, Bakewell Road, Loughborough, Leicestershire, LE11 0RH, UK

John R. Foster
Zeneca Central Toxicology Laboratory, Mereside, Alderley Park, Macclesfield, Cheshire, SK10 4TJ, UK

Chirukandath Gopinath
Huntingdon Life Sciences, PO Box 2, Huntingdon, Cambridgeshire, PE18 6ES, UK

Peter Greaves
Zeneca Pharmaceuticals, Mereside, Alderley Park, Macclesfield, Cheshire, SK10 4TG, UK

Contributors

Ernest S. Harpur
Sanofi Research Division, Alnwick Research Centre, Willowburn Avenue, Alnwick, Northumberland, NE66 2JH, UK

Jean Hooson
ITR Laboratories Canada Inc., 19601 Boul. Clark Graham, Baie d'Urfé (Montréal), Québec, Canada, H9X 3T1

Andrew J. Ingram
Ingram Pathology and Toxicology Services (IPTS), 31 Esher Avenue, Walton-on-Thames, Surrey, KT12 2SZ, UK

Kevin R. Isaacs
14 Rossett Park Road, Harrogate, North Yorkshire, HG2 9NP, UK

Ian Kimber
Zeneca Central Toxicology Laboratory, Mereside, Alderley Park, Macclesfield, Cheshire, SK10 4TJ, UK

C. Frieke Kuper
TNO Toxicology and Nutrition Institute, PO Box 360, 3700 AJ Zeist, The Netherlands

Brian G. Lake
BIBRA International, Woodmansterne Road, Carshalton, Surrey, SM5 4DS, UK

David J. Lewis
Huntingdon Life Sciences, PO Box 2, Huntingdon, Cambridgeshire, PE18 6ES, UK

Ruth M. Lightfoot
Glaxo Wellcome Research and Development, Five Moore Drive, Box 13398, Research Triangle Park, North Carolina 27709, USA

Mervyn Robinson
Zeneca Central Toxicology Laboratory, Mereside, Alderley Park, Macclesfield, Cheshire, SK10 4TJ, UK

Henk-Jan Schuurman
Novartis Ltd, Preclinical Research, CH-4002, Basel, Switzerland

Mary J. Tucker
Zeneca Pharmaceuticals, Mereside, Alderley Park, Macclesfield, Cheshire, SK10 4TG, UK

John Turton
Department of Toxicology, The School of Pharmacy, University of London, 29/39 Brunswick Square, London, WC1N 1AX, UK

Henk van Loveren
Laboratory of Pathology and Immunobiology, National Institute of Public Health and the Environment (RIVM), PO Box 1, 3720 BA Bilthoven, The Netherlands

Joseph G. Vos
Laboratory of Pathology and Immunobiology, National Institute of Public Health and the Environment (RIVM), PO Box 1, 3720 BA Bilthoven, The Netherlands

1

The Integumentary System

ANDREW J. INGRAM

1.1 Introduction

The skin is often described as being the largest organ of the body and it is frequently exposed to a wide variety of xenobiotics. It is also, from time to time, exposed to various grades of physical trauma and attack by a variety of organisms (including bacteria, viruses, fungi and parasites). In man, it is one of the most frequent sites of adverse drug reactions, however, there is no good animal model for this.

The functions performed by the skin include protection, temperature regulation, sensory perception, excretion, synthesis and storage.

1   Protection is one of the main functions. This includes prevention of water loss (or gain) and protection from UV light, heat, cold, trauma, chemical insult or microbial attack.

2   Temperature regulation is also an important function and this includes prevention of heat loss by subcutaneous fat and hair as well as heat dissipation by sweat evaporation and radiation.

3   Sensory perception is also a vital function of the skin and receptors are present for heat, cold, touch, pressure and pain.

4   Excretion is a relatively minor function with sweat, sebum, cerumen (ear wax) and salts being released onto the skin surface.

5   Vitamin D synthesis takes place in the skin in the presence of light, though this is only of importance when insufficient is available from the diet.

6   Storage functions include energy storage in the form of subcutaneous fat and storage of blood, water, electrolytes and vitamins.

To maintain these functions, the skin has a well-developed capacity to contain and repair any damage. This is achieved by inflammatory and regenerative processes. The inflammatory processes block up any breaks in the barrier layer, fight infection, break down damaged tissues and generally prepare the way for tissue replacement. Immune responses form an important part of the inflammatory processes and these include both humoral (antibody) and cell-mediated responses. Contact sensitization is a cell-mediated response. The regenerative processes involve cell migration and multiplication in adjacent tissues to replace the damaged tissues and restore the barrier and other functions.

1.2 Anatomy, Histology and Physiology

The skin arises from two principal embryonic layers, the ectoderm and the mesoderm. The ectoderm forms the thin outer layer or epidermis and the various skin appendages and glands, whereas the mesoderm gives rise to the underlying supporting tissues (the dermis and hypodermis) (see Figure 1.1).

Although the ectodermal and mesodermal components of the skin are closely associated they are separated by a basement membrane which consists of a thin amorphous layer containing glycoproteins supported by reticular fibres. This is best seen by the electron microscope, but it can be seen as a thin line if stained with periodic acid Schiff (PAS) for glycoprotein or with a silver stain for reticulin.

The epidermis and the structures derived from it are composed mainly of cells, whereas the dermis is composed mainly of an extracellular matrix forming a fibrous

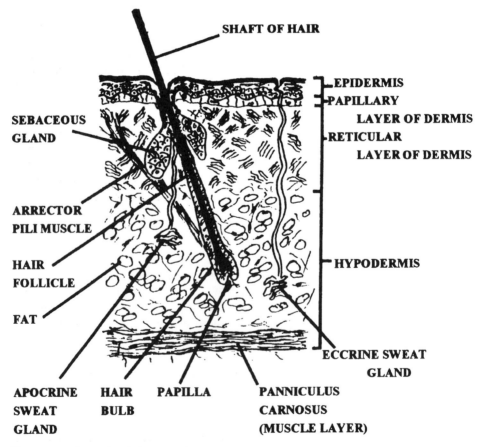

Figure 1.1 Generalized diagram of mammalian skin showing main structures.

network with relatively few cells. The hypodermis (subcutaneous tissue) is also composed largely of extracellular material but the network of fibres is looser and contains many fat cells (subcutaneous fat), which in normally stained preparations appear empty. The hypodermis is bounded on the inside by a thin layer of muscle, the panniculus carnosus, which in rodents and many other mammals is only loosely bound to the body wall, allowing considerable free movement. In man it is fused to the body wall.

1.2.1 *Epidermis*

The epidermis is a stratified squamous epithelium composed of cells called keratinocytes. These cells synthesize internally a protein, keratin, and are bound together by tight junctions or desmosomes. A lipoprotein material is synthesized by the keratinocyte and when the keratinocytes are fully differentiated this fills the intercellular spaces.

As the keratinocytes differentiate they change in shape from cuboidal cells to flattened hexagonal plates and these become arranged in stacks above the cells that produce them. These stacks with the underlying cells that produce them have been called epidermal proliferative units (EPUs) [1]. Each such unit contains a dendritic cell or Langerhans cell. Although various origins and functions have been suggested for these cells, they are now known to originate from the bone marrow and have an important role in antigen presentation in skin immune responses.

This arrangement of cells in the epidermis can be seen by careful observation of paraffin sections but is most easily visualized by electron microscopy or by light microscopy on plastic sections of 1 µm stained with toluidine blue (Figure 1.2). It tends to be lost when the epidermis is in a highly proliferative state following injury or treatment with an irritant.

Although the epidermis is really a continuum, four main layers are recognized in the epidermis: the stratum germinativum (stratum basale or basal layer), the stratum spinosum (or spinous layer), the stratum granulosum (or granular layer) and the stratum corneum (or cornified layer). Strictly speaking, one should stick to one or other of these nomenclatures but they are frequently mixed, with the Latin version being used for all except the basal layer.

Basal layer

This consists of mainly cuboidal undifferentiated keratinocytes arranged as a single layer, being attached to each other by desmosomes and to the basement membrane by hemidesmosomes. This is the layer in which all the cell division of the epidermis takes place. In pigmented skin, melanocytes can be seen at the junction of the basal layer and the dermis. These have many processes that make contact with adjacent epidermal cells. Melanin granules produced by the melanocytes are extruded by these processes and taken up by the epidermal cells, which are consequently pigmented.

Stratum spinosum

Cells of the stratum spinosum range in shape from round to flattened, the cells appearing spinous due to the stretching out of the points of attachments or

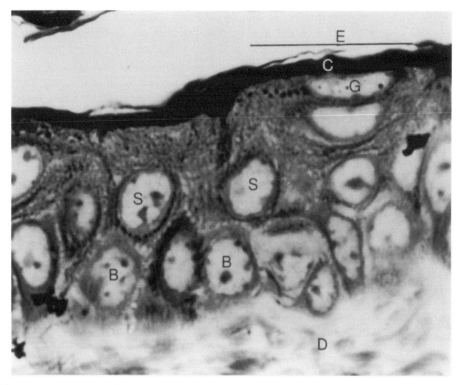

Figure 1.2   Mouse epidermis: 1 µm section plastic embedded stained with toluidine blue, showing (E) epidermal proliferative unit, keratinocytes of the (B) basal, (S) spinosum, and (G) granulosum layers, (C) stratum corneum, (D) dermis.

desmosomes. Tonofibrils can be seen stretching from the desmosomes into the cytoplasm and it is thought that these are important in maintaining the cohesion of the cells. It is in the stratum spinosum that keratinocytes synthesize keratin and no cell division takes place in this layer.

Stratum granulosum

The stratum granulosum is recognized by the presence of basophilic granules in the cytoplasm. These granules, together with the tonofibrils, polymerize to form the keratin of the stratum corneum. Under the electron microscope, membrane-coating granules can also be recognized and these are released into the intercellular space forming the lipid-rich intercellular cement. In the stratum granulosum the cells become much more flattened and evidence of stacking becomes apparent. The nucleus also degenerates so that by the time the cell reaches the stratum corneum the nucleus is no longer visible.

Stratum corneum

The stratum corneum consists of dead, flattened, squamous cells without nuclei that are arranged in stacks bound together by a lipid-rich cement. The cells contain a matrix of mature keratin which appears birefringent in the light microscope. In paraffin sections the stratum corneum tends to have a loose basket-weave appearance due to the leaching of the lipid-rich cement and the resultant artefactual separation of the squamous cells. Another layer, the stratum lucidum, is also described as lying between the stratum granulosum and the stratum corneum, however this is only seen in the thick plantar skin of the foot and is of uncertain significance.

1.2.2   Dermis (Corium)

The dermis is a connective tissue layer which underlies the epidermis. It is made up of two parts: a thin layer of loose connective tissue immediately underlying the epidermis, called the papillary layer, and the thicker, more dense, reticular layer.

The papillary layer contains a network of blood vessels, providing the epidermis with nutrients and lymphatic vessels which communicate with the local lymph node. Also present in this layer are nerve endings and nerve fibres. Elastic fibres pass vertically through it, connecting the basal lamina of the epidermis above with the reticular layer below.

The reticular layer consists mainly of bundles of collagen fibres with a fine network of elastic fibres and scattered fibroblasts, which synthesize both types of fibre. It is this layer that is mainly responsible for the strength and elasticity of the skin.

1.2.3   Hypodermis

Although the hypodermis is, strictly speaking, subcutaneous in terms of human anatomy, in most animal species it is regarded as part of the skin. As previously mentioned, it is composed of loose connective tissue and many fat cells (subcutaneous fat). It is bounded on the inside by the panniculus carnosus, a muscle layer loosely bound to the underlying musculature in most mammals by connective tissue. Cutaneous appendages such as hair follicles and sweat glands extend into the hypodermis. Unlike the epidermis, and the dermis and the panniculus carnosus, the thickness of the hypodermis can vary greatly with the physiological state of the animal. For instance, in animals with cyclical hair growth, the hypodermis can be five times thicker when hair growth is taking place. Also, in animals that store subcutaneous fat for use in the winter, the thickness of the hypodermis varies accordingly. It is important to recognize this in order not to mistake a normal physiological change for a pathological change.

1.2.4   Skin Appendages

All skin appendages (such as hair follicles, sebaceous glands, sweat glands, nails and scales) are of epidermal origin. The only ones with a dermal component are horns, where bone is included, and the centre of the shaft in bird feathers.

Hair

Hair follicles develop in the embryo from a downgrowth of the epidermis into the dermis. They are continuous with the epidermis and they give rise to the sebaceous glands as well as hairs.

The mature hair consists of a bulb and root contained in the follicle, and the shaft which protrudes from it. Within the shaft, three layers are recognizable: the outer cuticle which is made up of flattened overlapping scale-like cells, the cortex which is the main cornified layer of the hair, and the medulla which consists of shrunken cells and empty spaces in the centre of the hair. The hair is produced within the follicle as a result of cell division in a knot of cells at its base, called the matrix. This also gives rise to the internal root sheath, a transient layer between the follicle wall and the hair. The follicle wall, which is continuous with the surface epidermis, is also referred to as the external root sheath. Just above the matrix is a region where all these layers show keratohyalin granules, those of the internal root sheath being notable for being eosinophilic (trichohyalin). The internal root sheath breaks down before it is able to reach the sebaceous glands and the resulting space is filled with sebum from the sebaceous glands.

Hair growth within any particular follicle is cyclical [2], with a growth phase or anagen and a resting phase or telogen. Catagen is a short intermediate phase in which the growing follicle is converted to the resting follicle. In some animals, such as the mouse and the rabbit, hair growth is synchronized, starting in the ventral neck region and extending dorsally and then from the anterior to the posterior of the animal. Thus a section of the skin in such animals usually shows all hair follicles in the resting phase or all in the active phase, but sometimes a mixture is seen with some in the intermediate phase. In the resting phase the hair follicles and club hairs are largely contained within the dermis, whereas in the growth phase they are longer and extend well into the hypodermis. Towards the end of the growth phase, in animals with synchronized hair growth, the skin from the base of the panniculus carnosus to the skin surface is thicker than in the resting phase. This is largely due to an increase in thickness of the hypodermis, although some increase is seen in the thickness of the dermis. Also noticeable is an apparent increase in numbers of hair follicles and a reduction in interfollicular epidermis. Much of the increase in thickness in the dermis and the hypodermis is probably due to increased vascularization and fluid retention.

Although hair growth is a normal phenomenon, stimulation of entry into hair growth can be produced by hair plucking, skin damage and treatment with skin irritants.

Sebaceous glands

Sebaceous glands are composed of acini of large clear cells with a central nucleus and these open by a short duct into the upper part of the hair follicle. They are holocrine glands, that is, they produce a fatty material (sebum) within the cells, which then break down to release it. The sebum provides a waterproofing layer on the hair and skin surface. It is released continuously but secretion is stimulated by androgens (male sex hormones). They are better developed in some parts of the body than in others.

Sweat glands

Two types of sweat gland are recognized: apocrine, which release their secretion into the hair follicle and eccrine which release their secretion onto the skin surface.

Histologically, sweat glands are simple tubular glands consisting of a coiled secretory part, closely associated with blood capillaries and a thin duct. The main components of sweat are water, sodium chloride, urea, ammonia and uric acid.

Whereas eccrine sweat glands in man are present over the whole body, apocrine glands are present in restricted regions (e.g. axillae).

The cerumenous glands of the ear are modified sweat glands.

1.3 Biochemical and Cellular Mechanisms of Toxicity

When substances are tested for cutaneous effects, it is important to recognize that the lesions observed may not necessarily result from treatment, but may instead be due to a variety of other causes. To appreciate this, it is necessary to review these and the types of changes that they can produce before describing those induced by chemical agents.

1.3.1 Non-Chemical Agents

Physical damage

Before examining the effects of chemicals on the skin of animals, the hair must be removed with electric clippers. Even if no lesions are clearly visible, minor focal epidermal changes may be seen histologically within 2 to 3 days and it is important not to confuse these with an irritancy response. More severe physical damage can result in a typical wound healing response. It can also result in stimulation of hair growth and can act as a promoting stimulus in skin carcinogenicity studies [3].

Bacterial, viral and fungal infections

There are a number of skin lesions that can result from **bacterial**, **viral** or **fungal** infections. With **bacteria**, folliculitis is the most common lesion, but granulomatous lesions can also develop, whereas with **fungal** infections, localized inflammation and exfoliation is most common. The cause of these lesions can be recognized microscopically by the presence in the tissues of bacteria or fungal hyphae. Certain **viruses** can result in the development of papillomas (benign tumours).

Nutritional or vitamin deficiencies or excesses

Deficiencies of **vitamin A**, some of the **B vitamins** and **vitamin C** can all produce skin lesions, as can excess of **vitamin A**. With modern, balanced, laboratory animal diets however, skin lesions due to dietary deficiencies or excesses are rare in animal studies unless animals are deliberately put on altered diets or are given treatment which affects eating habits or digestion.

Inherited disorders

A number of inherited skin disorders are recognized in man ranging in severity from rare fatal disorders to minor localized disorders. Examples include xeroderma pigmentosum and psoriasis. In xeroderma pigmentosum there is a deficiency in the DNA repair mechanism with the result that exposure to **sunlight** is much more likely to give rise to dermatitis and skin cancer. In psoriasis there are localized patches of thickened flaking skin which are thought to result from an abnormality in keratinization. As many experimental rodents are genetically defined, inherited disorders are seldom encountered unless they are specifically bred for, e.g. hairless mice, nude mice and rats.

Radiation

Radiation, including **UV light**, is one of the most important causes of skin lesions in man. Acute effects of **UV light** include erythema following damage to the dermal blood vessels, blistering as a result of damage to the basal layer of the epidermis, and a more delayed desquamation of the epidermis. Long-term effects can include an increased risk of skin cancer or melanoma resulting from DNA damage in the epidermis or the melanocytes. Other forms of radiation that penetrate more deeply can result in hair loss (alopecia) owing to damage to dividing cells in the hair follicles.

1.3.2 Chemical Toxicity

Barrier properties, percutaneous absorption and toxicity

No matter how toxic a substance is, if it cannot penetrate the skin barrier it will not produce adverse effects. Hence it is important to consider what factors affect skin penetration and percutaneous absorption.

It has been demonstrated that the main barrier of the skin resides in the stratum corneum of the surface epidermis, since if this is removed by repeatedly stripping the skin with adhesive tape, the skin loses most of its barrier properties [4]. The barrier properties of the stratum corneum are due to alternating lipid and polar layers. The polar layers are the cornified squamous cells which are tightly joined end to end and the lipid layers are the intercellular lipid filling the spaces between the squamous cells. Lipid materials are prevented from entering by the polar layers, while aqueous materials are stopped by the lipid layers.

Substances penetrate the skin in three main ways: directly through the cells and the intercellular lipid of the stratum corneum, between the cells of the stratum corneum in the intercellular lipid, or via the hair follicles and other appendages (the involvement of sweat glands is questionable). Although it might be thought that penetration via the follicles would be easy, it should be remembered that the upper part of the follicle wall is continuous with the skin surface and therefore has similar barrier properties. Also the lower part of the follicle is either blocked by the inner root sheath of the growing hair or is filled with sebum around a club hair. Considering this, together with the fact that hair follicles account for only 0.1 to 0.2 per cent of the skin surface, it is not surprizing that most substances penetrate the skin mainly through the surface epidermis by one of the two routes mentioned. Despite this, absorption via the hair follicles can be important with substances that penetrate the stratum corneum poorly.

The skin barrier tends to be more effective against hydrophilic than lipophilic materials [5]. Substances which have both lipid and polar properties (e.g. **dimethylsulphoxide, detergents**) penetrate the most easily. The lipophilic or hydrophilic nature of the material affects which way the material penetrates the stratum corneum; if it is lipophilic it penetrates mainly between the cells, whereas if it is hydrophilic it penetrates through the cells. Thus, by taking the rather tortuous route around the squamous cells, lipophilic materials can avoid having to pass through an aqueous layer; whereas hydrophilic materials cannot avoid having to pass through a lipid barrier. This may explain why lipophilic materials penetrate more easily than hydrophilic materials. This barrier is also effective at preventing water loss.

Molecular size is also an important factor in skin absorption, the smaller the molecule, the more easily it penetrates; substances with a molecular weight of greater than 3000 tend to penetrate poorly. Electrolytes in aqueous solution generally penetrate the skin poorly, probably because of their polar nature and because water of ionization will increase their molecular size. As pH can affect the degree of ionization, it can have a marked effect on percutaneous absorption. An example of this is **benzoic acid**, which is much more rapidly absorbed at pH 2 (99.4 per cent undissociated) than at pH 6 (only 1.6 per cent undissociated) [4].

The effects of vehicles on the penetration of substances through the skin are complex. They can be best understood if it is borne in mind that it is the amount of substance dissolving in the stratum corneum cells or intercellular lipid per unit area that is important. Thus, if the solubility of the penetrant in the skin surface is greater than in the vehicle, skin absorption will be high. Hence a vehicle having a low affinity for the penetrant will maximize skin penetration. This is related to the partition coefficient of the substance between the stratum corneum and the vehicle. The viscosity of the vehicle also has some effect on skin absorption, with higher viscosity leading to a reduction in absorption. Some vehicles can increase the skin penetration by occluding the skin (e.g. **oils** and **greases**). This results in hydration of the stratum corneum and a physiological decrease in its barrier properties.

What we have discussed so far are vehicles that do not damage the barrier properties of the skin; however, many vehicles including most organic solvents do produce changes to the barrier. Such materials can greatly increase skin absorption, particularly if repeated application is involved. The changes produced in the skin by such vehicles may be limited to lipid removal from the stratum corneum (e.g. **acetone**), include mild epidermal damage and hyperplasia (e.g. **toluene**) or give rise to more severe skin damage (e.g. some **surfactants**).

It is important to realize that the rate of percutaneous absorption is different in different sites of the body [6] and in different species [7]. These differences are largely dependent on the thickness of the stratum corneum and the frequency of skin appendages. They are also dependent to some degree upon whether the penetrant used to assess the differences is lipophilic or hydrophilic. Thus in man, relative to forearm skin, absorption was found to be approximately equivalent for the palm of the hand, 2 times greater for the abdomen, 4 times for the scalp, 7 times for the axilla and 12 times for the scrotum. Comparing the skin absorption of different species with that in man, pig skin is approximately equivalent, rat skin is 2 to 3 times and rabbit skin is 3 to 4 times more absorbent.

Enzymatic activity of the skin

Although the main function of the epidermal keratinocytes is the production of keratin, they do have aryl hydrocarbon hydroxylase activity and cytochrome oxidase activity. Despite their much lower levels than in the liver (approximately 2 per cent of liver level), these are important in the activation of carcinogenic, polycyclic aromatic hydrocarbons to diol-epoxides, which bind to epidermal DNA (adduct formation). The presence of such adducts can give rise to mutations, some of which may result in initiation. Initiation is the first stage in cancer development.

The control of cell division is crucial to the homeostasis of normal skin, to regeneration following skin damage and to the development of cancer from initiated cells. This control is linked with protein kinase C, which lies in the cytoplasm of the cell just below the surface [8]. It is normally activated by diacylglycerols released by the cell membrane in response to an external stimulus. Activation of protein kinase C leads to a chain of events which results in the induction of ornithine decarboxylase and polyamine biosynthesis, which in turn leads to cell division. Certain substances which are able to promote the induction of cancer from initiated cells (e.g. **phorbol esters**), can directly activate protein kinase C and therefore markedly increase cell division.

Properties of chemicals in relation to their mechanism of action

A variety of toxicological changes in the skin can be produced by chemical agents. Depending on their main properties these may be categorized as follows:

1 Corrosive agents (acids, alkalis, etc.)
2 Skin irritants (acute or chronic)
3 Skin sensitizers
4 Systemically administered toxicants and allergens
5 Skin carcinogens

Corrosive agents (Table 1.1) These are materials which have a direct damaging effect on proteins and other cell constituents and examples include **strong acids**, **strong alkalis** and **phenol**. They are able to denature the barrier layer of the stratum

Table 1.1 Examples of primary irritants

Substance	Types of primary damage	Severity
Sulphuric acid	Denatures proteins	Corrosive
Sodium hydroxide	Denatures lipids and proteins	Corrosive
Phenol	Denatures lipids and proteins	Corrosive
Metallic salts of arsenic, mercury and cadmium	Can interact with skin proteins resulting in ulceration	Severe irritants
Surfactants e.g. sodium lauryl sulphate (10% aqueous)	Remove intercellular lipid and produce membrane damage in epidermis, SLS can denature dermal collagen	Mild to moderate irritant[a]
Formaldehyde (10% aqueous)	Reacts with proteins, damages epidermal barrier	Mild to moderate irritant[a]
Organic solvents, e.g. benzene, toluene	Remove intercellular lipids and damage epidermal cell membranes	Mildly irritant

[a] Depending on concentration and/or degree of occlusion.

corneum, penetrate through the epidermis and denature the dermal collagen. They are able to produce deep dermal damage which can extend into the hypodermis and result in the destruction of hair follicles. If exposure is sufficient this can produce permanent scarring.

Skin irritants (Table 1.1) There are a wide variety of skin irritants with differing physicochemical properties and the way in which they produce an irritant response varies accordingly. Whether or not a substance produces an irritant response depends upon its ability to pass through the skin barrier and damage epidermal cells and the dermal matrix. Also important is the rate of removal from the tissues by the blood stream and any tendency to accumulate within the tissues. Once a substance has penetrated the stratum corneum its migration through the epidermis and dermis and entry into blood vessels is likely to be affected by whether the substance is lipophilic or hydrophilic. As the epidermis contains more lipid than the dermis, lipophilic materials will tend to remain there longer. Such materials will also accumulate within hair follicles and sebaceous glands. In contrast, when hydrophilic materials have passed through the stratum corneum they would be expected to pass rapidly through the rest of the epidermis into the dermis and on to the general circulation. From this, it is not too surprising to find that with lipophilic irritants the primary changes are in the epidermis, whereas those which are more polar produce primary changes in the upper part of the dermis. The molecular size will also affect the rate at which a substance passes from the skin to the general circulation, as will the rate of blood flow and the permeability of blood vessel walls. Membrane damage of keratinocytes is a common finding with lipophilic organic solvents, and collagen denaturation in the dermis is a primary observation with some surfactants (e.g. **sodium lauryl sulphate**). Membrane damage to keratinocytes within the epidermis and to macrophages within the dermis stimulates them to release arachidonic acid and prostaglandins. These in turn stimulate the migration of inflammatory cells to the site of damage. Prominent among these inflammatory cells are polymorphonuclear cells, which phagocytose dead material and release lysosomal enzymes that can in certain circumstances increase tissue damage. At the same time vasodilation and an increase in the permeability of capillary walls takes place. This results in an increase in blood circulation to the skin and the leakage of fluid from the capillaries giving rise to oedema. How these changes and the subsequent regeneration relate to gross and microscopic observations will be discussed later.

Skin sensitizers (Table 1.2) These are chemicals which are capable of acting as haptens, that is they combine with proteins within tissues to produce an antigen. As mentioned previously, the Langerhans cells, which are histiocytic cells located in the epidermis, are involved in this interaction. The Langerhans cells then migrate to the draining lymph node and can set off a sensitization reaction. The morphological changes seen when a sensitizer is applied to sensitized skin are discussed later in this chapter.

Systemically administered toxicants and allergens Some toxicants and allergens given by other than dermal routes can produce changes in the skin. Thus dermatitis in man can be produced by non-dermal exposure to **arsenic**, **chromium**, **lead**, **silver**, **aniline** and **many drugs**. More insidious are substances which induce phototoxicity and photoallergic responses. These result in skin reactions when the individual is exposed to sunlight.

Table 1.2   Examples of sensitizers

Type or source of sensitizers	Examples of sensitizers
Aniline products	Azo dyes, trinitrotoluene (TNT)
Antibiotics	Neomycin, penicillin streptomycin
Dyes and dye-containing products	Paraphenylenediamine, paints, inks, lipstick and other cosmetic products
Metals and metal-containing compounds	Nickel, cobalt, chromates, arsenicals
Resins and polymers	Formaldehyde resins, epoxy resins, cellulose monomers, vinyl monomers, acrylic monomers
Rubber ingredients	Accelerators, antioxidants, vulcanizers
Perfume ingredients	Lavender oil, cinnamic acid
Plants, trees and derivatives	Ivy, primrose, chrysanthemum, bulbs of daffodil, tulip and hyacinth. Wood from pine, red cedar and mahogany. Creosote oil
Pharmaceutical products	Chlorothiazide, phenothiazines, procaines, tolbutamide

Skin carcinogens (Table 1.3)   It was in the skin that the concept of two-stage carcinogenesis was first proposed. The first stage of this process entails irreversible genetic change, called initiation, which can be produced by a single treatment with a carcinogenic substance (or initiating agent), and the second stage, called promotion, involves repeated application over a period of 6 to 12 months of a substance which produces sustained cell proliferation in the epidermis. Although the substance usually used as a promoter is **croton oil** or its most active principal, **12-*O*-tetradecanoyl phorbol-13-acetate (TPA)**, a variety of other irritant substances have been shown to have promoting activity (e.g. **Tween 60** and certain **other surfactants**, *n*-**dodecane** and other *n*-**paraffins, phenol** and to a lesser extent even irritant organic solvents such as **benzene** and **toluene**). In addition, carcinogenic substances such as **benzo(a)pyrene (BaP)** are capable of acting as promoters as well as initiators. Such carcinogens were called complete carcinogens, whereas those that produced few or no skin tumours in the absence of a promoter were called incomplete carcinogens or initiators. Recently, the mechanism of two-stage carcinogenesis has become better understood and how skin carcinogens and promoting agents interact will be described.

It is not too surprising to find that most of those carcinogens that do not require metabolism by living cells to become activated are able to produce skin cancer. These chemicals are termed proximate carcinogens and are usually activated by combining with water, for example *N*-**methylnitrosourea**, *N*-**methyl-*N*-nitro-*N*-nitrosoguanidine** and *β*-**propriolactone**. As mentioned previously, the epidermal cells of the skin do have cytochrome oxidase activity but skin cancer is not produced by all carcinogens. Of the carcinogens that require metabolic activation, the skin appears to be most sensitive to carcinogenic, **polycyclic aromatic hydrocarbons (PAHs)** such as **7,12-dimethylbenz(a)anthracene (DMBA)**, BaP, **3-methylcholanthrene** and **dibenz(ah)anthracene**. Although a few other carcinogens that require metabolism such as **4-nitroquinoline *n*-oxide** can also produce skin cancer,

Table 1.3   Examples of skin carcinogens and promoters

Substance	Number of aromatic rings	Carcinogenic activity in skin	Other comments
Polycyclic hydrocarbons			
Benzo(a)pyrene	5	+	
Benzo(e)pyrene	5	±	Initiator
Dibenz(a,h)anthracene	5	+	
Chrysene	4	±	Initiator
Benz(a)anthracene	4	±	Initiator
Pyrene	4	−	
Anthracene	3	−	
Proximate carcinogens			
N-Methylnitrosourea	NA	+	
N-Methyl-n-nitro-n-nitroso-guanidine	NA	+	
N-Ethyl-n-nitro-n-nitroso-guanidine	NA	+	
Melphalan	NA	+	
β-Propiolactone	NA	+	
Other compounds			
4-Nitroquinoline-n-oxide	NA	+	
Urethane	NA	±	Strong initiator
Tumour promoters			
Croton oil	NA	±[a]	
TPA (or PMA[b])	NA	±[a]	
Dihydroteleocidin B	NA	0	Strong promoters
Teleocidin	NA	0	
Benzoyl peroxide	NA	±[a]	
N-Dodecane	NA	−	
N-Tetradecane	NA	−	Moderate promoters
N-Hexadecane	NA	−	
Mezerein	NA	−	
Ethyl phenyl propiolate	NA	−	Weak promoters
Acetic acid	NA	−	

NA, not applicable. Carcinogenic activity: +, active; ±, weak or questionable; −, inactive; 0, no data.
[a] Any activity may be due to a non-genotoxic mechanism.
[b] Phorbol 12-myristate 13-acetate.

other carcinogens such as **2-naphthylamine** and **dimethylnitrosamine** do not. **PAHs** are metabolized to dihydrodiol epoxides which bind to the DNA of keratinocytes forming DNA adducts. Misrepair of such adducts can give rise to mutations within the basal layer of the epidermis. Some of these mutations may activate oncogenes of the *Harvey ras* (*H.ras*) type, which are now considered important in the initiation stage of skin cancer. A subsequent activation of *fos* oncogenes is thought to be important in the promotion and progression of cancer from initiated cells. Although prolonged treatment with carcinogens is effective in carrying out this second stage, some promoting agents such as **TPA** are also able to induce activation of *fos* oncogenes. In addition to this, the induction of epidermal hyperplasia is an important part of tumour promotion and progression and **TPA** is able to induce this by directly activating protein kinase C. However, it must be realized that initiated skin can be induced to develop skin cancer by a wide variety of irritant substances and even by repeated wounding of the skin.

1.4 Morphological Response to Injury

1.4.1 *Changes with Caustic Agents and Skin Irritants*

The morphological appearance of the various elements of the skin following treatment with caustic agents or skin irritants varies according to when the skin is observed. Because of the importance of maintaining the skin barrier, primary damage to the epidermis, dermis and skin appendages is rapidly followed by inflammatory and healing responses. As a consequence, primary damage, inflammation and healing responses are often seen together. The external signs of skin changes will be discussed first, followed by the histopathological changes.

Externally the clearest signs of skin irritation are reddening (erythema) and swelling (oedema). These changes are due to inflammation rather than to the primary damaging effect of a substance. Vesiculation is also sometimes seen in response to severe irritants. A sign of severe primary skin damage is an early whitening of the skin which is followed by marked erythema and oedema. Later a scab of necrotic tissue (eschar) becomes apparent, which is eventually lost from the surface of the skin. Other late signs of skin irritancy include pin scabbing (multiple small scabs), exfoliation (shedding of dead surface material) or desquamation (increased loss of surface squamous cells).

The pattern and severity of histological changes in the epidermis, dermis, hair follicles and other adnexa depend upon the nature of the substance and any vehicles employed, the degree of exposure in terms of concentration, time and frequency and the degree of occlusion, and other exposure conditions. The primary damage, the inflammatory responses and the healing (regenerative) responses in the various parts of the skin will each be described in turn, but it should be realized that, in irritant reactions, more than one of these findings will normally occur and that emphasis is given to the most severe finding observed. Where, however, the most severe finding is suspected to have been due to inadvertent physical injury, clearly it is important also to draw attention to the severest responses considered to result from exposure to the test substance. To illustrate the changes, examples of the reactions seen in rabbit [9] and mouse [10] skin will be shown.

Primary damage

Primary epidermal damage

Vacuolar degeneration (Figure 1.3a)   This is seen as a vacuolation of epidermal cells, mainly restricted to the cytoplasm but in more severe cases also affecting the nuclei. It can lead to hydropic degeneration (Figure 1.3b), necrosis and associated inflammatory changes. Vacuolar degeneration is seen with **organic solvents** and **detergents,** both of which can damage the cell membranes of keratinocytes. It is important to realize that tissue processing can result in an apparent vacuolation of epidermal cells and this should not be misinterpreted as vacuolar degeneration.

Spongiosis (Figure 1.3c)   This refers to an increase in intercellular space in the epidermis, making the spinous appearance of the keratinocytes in the stratum spinosum more apparent. Spongiosis is often produced by **organic solvents** and **detergents** which leach out the intercellular lipid.

Individual cell necrosis (Figure 1.3d)   Necrosis of individual cells within the epidermis can occur particularly in the basal layer where the dividing cells are more vulnerable than other cells. Increased eosinophilia of individual cells combined with nuclear changes such as karyorrhexis or karyolysis provide evidence for this. It may be seen with a variety of **irritants** but is particularly seen with **genotoxic agents**.

Epidermal necrosis (Figure 1.3e and 1.3f)   This can be recognized by an eosinophilia of the epidermal cells with condensation, pyknosis (shrinkage) or breakdown of the nuclei. It may occur immediately after a single treatment with **caustic agents** or **severe irritants** or after repeated treatments with **less severe irritants**.

Ulceration (Figure 1.3g)   This is the term used when skin damage is so severe that the epidermis is lost. It can be produced directly by certain **caustic agents** or can follow epidermal necrosis, particularly if this is followed by scratching.

Primary dermal damage

Dermal necrosis (Figure 1.4a and 1.4b)   This can recognized by an increase in eosinophilia of the dermal collagen accompanied by swelling and loss of its fibrous appearance. The fibroblasts are also necrotic. It can be produced directly by **caustic agents**, **severe irritants** and certain **surfactants**, or indirectly as a result of epidermal necrosis or ulceration.

Follicular damage

Degeneration and necrosis of the follicular wall   The upper part of the follicular wall can show signs of degeneration and necrosis which are similar to the surface epidermis. The sebaceous glands are also susceptible to damage, particularly by **lipophilic genotoxic agents** which may accumulate in them. This can result in a reduction in size or a depletion of sebaceous glands (sebaceous gland suppression).

Inflammatory changes

Inflammatory changes occur within the epidermis, the dermis and in association with hair follicles. Inflammatory changes in the dermis sometimes also extend into the hypodermis.

Epidermal oedema
Oedematous changes in the epidermis occur as a result of further development of vacuolar degeneration and spongiosis (e.g. Figure 1.3b). This includes intracellular and intercellular oedema, microvesicle formation and vesiculation (the formation of fluid-filled spaces within the epidermis).

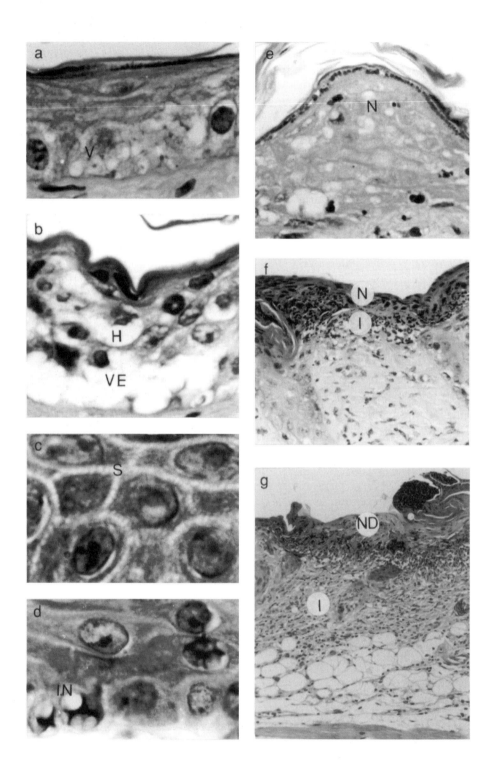

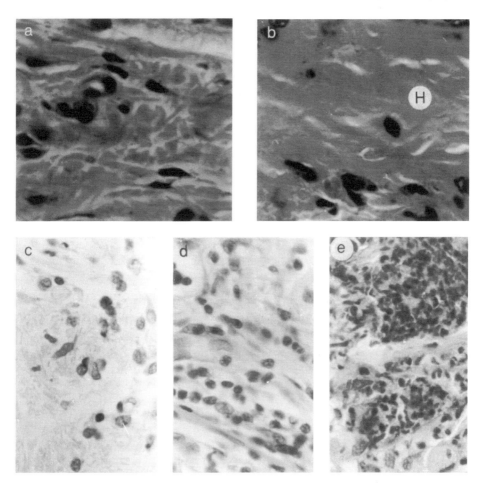

Figure 1.4 Dermal changes in rabbit skin, showing (a) normal collagen fibres in dermis and (b) loss of fibrous structure in necrotic dermis. (c) to (e) inflammatory cell infiltrate in dermis: (c) mild, (d) moderate and (e) marked. (H) indicates hyaline appearance of collagen. Changes produced by sodium lauryl sulphate.

Figure 1.4a to 1.4d were from a paper by Ingram and Grasso [9] and reproduced with permission from Blackwell Science Ltd.

Figure 1.3 Primary epidermal damage showing (a) vacuolar degeneration, (b) hydropic degeneration, (c) spongiosis, (d) individual cell necrosis, (e) and (f) epidermal necrosis and (g) ulceration. (V) indicates vacuolated basal cell, (H) keratinocyte with hydropic degeneration, (VE) hydropic cells breaking down to form vesicle, (S) increased space, (IN) individual necrotic cell, (N) necrotic epidermis showing no nuclear staining in (e) and pyknotic nuclei in (f), (ND) exposed necrotic dermis, (I) inflammatory cell infiltrate.

Figure 1.3c and 1.3d were from a paper by Ingram and Grasso [9] and reproduced with permission from Blackwell Science Ltd.

Figure 1.3a, 1.3b, 1.3f and 1.3g were from a paper by Ingram et al. [10] and reproduced with permission from John Wiley and Sons Ltd.

Epidermatitis
This is a term given to the presence of inflammatory cells within the epidermis, it is often seen in association with epidermal oedema. In irritation responses, poly-morphonuclear cells predominate, whereas in sensitization reactions lymphocytes are prominent; however a distinction between irritant and sensitization responses cannot be made on this basis.

Dermal oedema
This occurs as a result of blood vessel leakage as part of the inflammatory process. It can be recognized histologically by spaces adjacent to blood vessels and a general spacing of dermal elements. In some cases red cell leakage may occur. Unless associated with dermal necrosis or red cell leakage, it is often difficult to see histologically, as dehydration during tissue processing tends to reduce it.

Dermatitis (Figure 1.4c to 1.4e)
This follows oedema as part of the inflammatory process and is a migration of inflammatory cells into the dermis. It is strongly stimulated by dermal necrosis.

Folliculitis (Figure 1.5a)
This is recognized by the presence of inflammatory cells within follicles and in the surrounding dermis. It may be produced by skin irritants or bacterial infection. In severe cases it may be associated with necrosis or breakdown of the follicle wall. If this results in the leakage of sebum into the dermis, inflammation is greatly increased and a granulomatous response may develop.

Granulomatous response
This is characterized by an accumulation within the dermis or hypodermis of large numbers of macrophages with occasional multinucleate giant cells (formed by the fusion of macrophages), together with active fibroblasts. Other inflammatory cells are also usually present. The fibroblasts often produce a fibrous capsule around the lesion in order to isolate it.

Healing responses

Healing responses to skin irritants start very quickly in the epidermis (within 24 h), whereas resolution of dermal damage takes longer. Physical skin damage can produce similar responses.

Epidermal response to damage

Epidermal hyperplasia   Epidermal damage by an irritant results in a stimulation of the basal cells of the epidermis to divide. An increase in cell division starts after 24 h and the duration of increased cell division depends on the nature of the irritant and whether repeated treatments were involved. The increase in number of cells results in an increase in thickness of the epidermis, starting in the stratum spinosum, then in the stratum granulosum and finally in the stratum corneum.

Acanthosis (Figure 1.5b)
This is the term given to an increase in thickness of the stratum spinosum. Although it is usually due to an increase in cell division it can also result from a delay in differentiation.

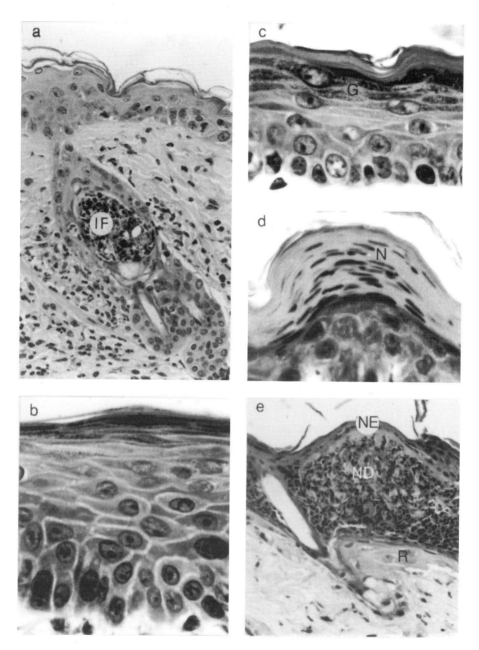

Figure 1.5 (a) Folliculitis in mouse skin, (b) to (e) healing responses. (a) shows inflammatory cells in follicle (IF), (b) marked acanthosis in rabbit skin, (c) early hyperkeratosis with stratum granulosum (G) three to four cells thick (normally one cell thick in rabbit back skin), (d) parakeratosis showing nuclei (N) in thickened stratum corneum, (e) undercutting of necrotic epidermal (NE) and necrotic dermal (ND) tissue by regenerated epidermis (R) in mouse skin.

Figure 1.5d is from a paper by Ingram and Grasso [9] and reproduced with permission from Blackwell Science Ltd.

Figure 1.5a is from a paper by Ingram *et al.* [10] and reproduced with permission from John Wiley and Sons Ltd.

Hyperkeratosis (Figure 1.5c)
This is indicated by an increase in the number of cell layers in the stratum granulosum and an increase in thickness of the stratum corneum. Whereas the former is easy to assess, the thickness of the stratum corneum is not, owing to the variable way the squamous cells separate in sections because of the leaching of lipids during tissue processing.

Parakeratosis (Figure 1.5d) This sometimes occurs following treatment with skin irritants and is characterized by the retention of nuclei in the stratum corneum and an absence of the stratum granulosum (absence of keratohyalin granules). In the stratum corneum of parakeratotic skin the keratin is abnormal and its barrier properties are reduced.

Repair of minor dermal damage
Minor dermal damage which results in inflamma-tory changes without dermal necrosis can be repaired by breakdown of damaged collagen by inflammatory cells and reformation by fibroblasts. Fibroblasts may be present in increased numbers during this repair process.

Repair of epidermal and dermal necrosis
Epidermal undercutting Where epidermal and underlying dermal necrosis have occurred, enzymes released by polymorphonuclear cells produce a separation of the necrotic tissue (containing dead inflammatory cells) from the living tissues. Cells from the adjacent living epidermis and the hair follicles migrate under the necrotic tissue until they form a complete epidermal layer. The cells then proliferate forming a new epidermis under the necrotic tissue, the latter becoming a surface scab (eschar) (see Figure 1.5e). Finally the surface eschar is lost and the lost dermal tissue is replaced by fibroblast proliferation and collagen synthesis. Where deep skin damage has occurred, an excess of collagen is formed, giving rise to scar tissue.

Repair processes in follicle
Being continuous with the skin surface, the wall of the hair follicle may exhibit hyperplasia but this is usually less marked than on the skin surface. Where folliculitis is present, this is usually resolved by the hair and attached inflammatory cells being lost, followed by hair regrowth (anagen). If hair follicles are totally destroyed, in a severe irritancy response, they do not regrow; however, if the bases of the follicles remain intact, they regenerate. Regenerating follicles appear as solid cords of cells and it is important that these are not mistaken for neoplastic infiltration.

1.4.2 *Responses to Skin Sensitizers (in Sensitized Subjects)*

In a response to a sensitizer, the first changes are inflammatory and these are followed by epidermal vesiculation or necrosis and dermal necrosis. Thus, although the sequence of development may be different to that following exposure to irritants, the end result appears similar histologically. The healing responses are similar to those seen with skin irritants. The differentiation between skin irritants and skin sensitizers is made more difficult by the fact that many sensitizers also have irritant properties and hence there may be a mixture of the two responses.

Contact urticaria

Contact urticaria is a transient appearance of elevated patches, often associated with itching, which occurs shortly after contact with an allergen. The change is produced by an alteration in vascular supply and if the site is washed thoroughly, this reaction will normally resolve without the development of true vesiculation.

1.4.3 Responses to Skin Carcinogens

Acute responses

Some skin carcinogens (i.e. proximate carcinogens) are highly reactive compounds and may act as severe irritants except at low concentrations. Even those which require metabolism (e.g. **DMBA**) may give rise to epidermal necrosis if applied repeatedly at high concentrations, particularly if treatment is repeated or is combined with a hyperplastic agent. At concentrations not producing severe irritation, the genotoxic effects of carcinogens may be shown by an enlargement of epidermal nuclei within 3 to 4 days of treatment [11]. This is followed by a period of epidermal hyperplasia in which the cells with enlarged nuclei appear to be lost from the skin surface [12].

Chronic responses

Before the chronic responses to carcinogens are discussed, it is important to consider the non-neoplastic lesions that occur in the skin of ageing animals and the spontaneous skin tumour incidence. Non-neoplastic lesions that may occur in chronic studies include histiocytosis, granulomas, various chronic irritancy and inflammatory responses, epidermoid and sebaceous cysts. The incidence of spontaneous skin tumours depends on the species involved. In mice and rats the incidence of spontaneous skin tumours is low and mainly confined to papillomas, squamous cell carcinomas and fibrosarcomas. Basal cell carcinomas, sebaceous adenomas, fibromas, schwannomas, lymphomas and mast cell tumours occur rarely. Mammary tumours may be seen, depending on where the skin is taken from; these are quite common in certain strains of mice and are known to have a viral aetiology. The incidence of spontaneous skin tumours (excluding mammary tumours) in a group of 50 untreated mice kept for 2 years is generally less than 4 per cent. A slight elevation of this spontaneous incidence can occur if chronic irritation is present (e.g. with solvent treatment). In dogs, histiocytomas and basal cell carcinomas are more common, but dogs are not used for studies of chronic skin carcinogenicity. If a skin carcinogen, e.g. **BaP** in acetone is applied to mouse skin twice or three times a week, tumours start to arise after 3 to 4 months. By 12 months, provided an optimum concentration is used, all animals would be expected to develop at least one skin tumour and many will develop multiple tumours.

The principal tumours that are induced in the skin by carcinogens are papillomas, keratoacanthomas, squamous cell carcinomas and, to a lesser extent, basal cell carcinomas. These tumours are all derived from the epidermis. Sarcomas derived from the dermis, hypodermis, or the underlying body wall are sometimes induced, however, it is often difficult to decide whether a low incidence of these is related to treatment, as the spontaneous incidence is higher than for epidermal tumours.

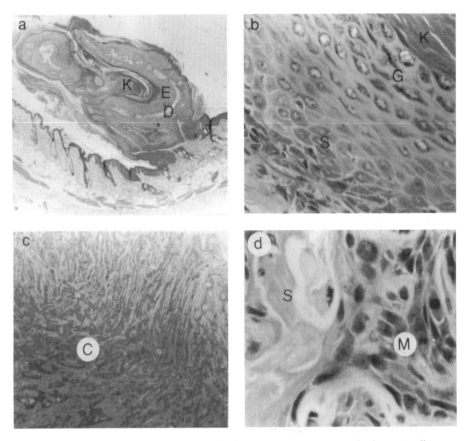

Figure 1.6 Tumours produced in mouse skin by a carcinogenic mineral oil. (a) Papilloma, showing its outward growth, the epidermal tissue (E) with the keratin (K) it produces and its supporting core of dermal (D) origin. (b) Detail of the same papilloma showing the retention of organised differentiation in the epidermal tissue with spinous (S), granular (G) and keratinized (K) layers. (c) Squamous cell carcinoma, showing cords (C) of tumour cells infiltrating dermal and underlying tissues. (d) Detail of the same carcinoma showing disorganized structure, cells showing squamous differentiation (S) and neighbouring cells in mitosis.

Papillomas (Figure 1.6a and 1.6b)

These are benign tumours arising as an outgrowth of the epidermis with a central core of connective tissue containing blood vessels. The surface of the outgrowth is usually folded, with keratin accumulating in the folds. Although the epidermal tissue is clearly acanthotic and the basal cells may appear abnormal, it still has an organization of squamous epithelium with recognizable layers. Papillomas may remain as they are, become constricted at their base and drop off (regress) or progress to malignant tumours (carcinomas). Progression to carcinoma is more likely if exposure to the carcinogen is continued or if a promoting agent is applied.

Keratoacanthomas

These are benign tumours believed by some to originate from hair follicles. They are typically flask shaped, with keratin in the centre and acanthotic epidermal tissue surrounding it. They are largely contained within the skin but may protrude to a variable extent above it. As with papillomas, the organization of the epidermal component into recognizable squamous epithelial layers is evident and the whole tumour is encapsulated by connective tissue. Keratoacanthomas can regress with loss of the central keratin to the outside, remain as they are, or progress to a carcinoma. Signs of a change to malignancy include infiltration of cells through the capsule and invasion of the panniculus carnosus.

Carcinomas (Figures 1.6c and 1.6d)

Skin carcinomas are malignant tumours characterized by a general disorganization of epidermal cells, with infiltration of cords or groups of cells into the dermis, hypodermis and panniculus carnosus. In some cases, migration (metastasis) of cells to the draining lymph nodes or to other organs takes place. Squamous cell carcinomas are much more commonly induced than basal cell carcinomas and are characterized by keratinizing cells in the centre of the cords, or nests of infiltrating cells. Basal cell carcinomas show little or no differentiation and the cells as a consequence show much more uniformity.

Sarcomas

In the skin these can arise from fibroblasts of the dermis and hypodermis (fibrosarcomas), from muscular tissue of the arrector pili muscle, the panniculus carnosus or the underlying body wall (rhabdomyosarcomas), or from the bone within the body wall (osteosarcomas). Of these, fibrosarcomas are most readily induced by carcinogens. Although the incidence of sarcomas produced by application of carcinogens to the skin surface is usually low, if they are injected subcutaneously a high incidence is obtained.

Melanotic tumours and melanomas

Melanotic tumours originating from the dermal melanocytes can be induced in hamsters, mice and guinea pigs by **DMBA** but not by other polycyclic hydrocarbons [13]. They normally only arise if a high level of **DMBA** treatment is given by a specific regimen in susceptible strains, and often combined with other treatments (e.g. **UV light**). They do not usually progress to malignant melanoma unless stimulated to do so (for example by **TPA**).

1.5 Testing for Toxicity

Although in many studies on skin toxicity, evaluations are limited to a gross examination of the skin surface, others require histological examination. In view of the difficulty in producing good skin sections, it is worthwhile drawing attention to various points that should be considered in section preparation.

1.5.1 Preparation of Skin for Histological Examination

Skin is a difficult tissue for four main reasons: it is elastic and tends to contract and curl up when removed; the surface is cornified and can harden with certain fixatives; it contains hard hairs that can disrupt the section during cutting; and hair follicles are angled in the skin and unless the skin is orientated carefully they will not be seen consistently in longitudinal section. Furthermore, skin sections need to be thin (around 3 µm) in order to examine the epidermis in any detail.

To prevent contraction and curling, skin should be placed on a piece of filing card with the inner side downwards before being placed in fixative. It is unnecessary to use any form of attachment as the skin will stick to the card. The skin should be placed flat on the card without excessive stretching. A good way of doing this is to cut the skin on three sides and peel it back, place a piece of card where the skin has been and then return the skin over the card to occupy nearly the same area as originally. The card with the skin attached may then be removed by cutting the fourth side and placed in the fixative, skin side downwards.

Avoidance of hardening fixatives is usually sufficient to prevent excessive hardening of the surface epidermis, and the disruptive effects of hair follicles can be minimized by cooling the block with ice and cutting the epidermal side first. The flattening of thin paraffin sections of skin can be a problem because of folding, but this can be circumvented by floating the sections on cold water on a slide before transferring to the hot bath.

Orientation of the skin section is most easily achieved by mounting the skin on a rectangular piece of card for fixation, the long axis coinciding with the direction of hair growth. For most purposes, sections parallel to the direction of hair growth are preferable, but in some circumstances, sections at right angles to this may be required.

Good skin sections should be obtained if these methods are used.

1.5.2 *Skin Irritancy Testing*

Although other species have been used for comparative irritancy studies, for example rats and minipigs, the skin of white rabbits is normally used in routine irritancy studies. This is because the pale pink colour of the shaved back skin allows skin reactions to be seen readily. The standard method of skin irritancy testing for many years has been the Draize test [141. As originally designed, the test involved the application of the test material on two, one inch-square (2.5 cm^2) patches to the shaved skin of six New Zealand White rabbits for 24 h under occlusive conditions. One of the two patches was applied to intact skin and the other to abraded skin. Each treated area of skin was examined after patch removal (24 h) and 48 h later (72 h) and assessed for erythema and oedema, each on a scale of 0 to 4. The erythema and oedema scores were totalled and the average score for intact and abraded skin at both times for the six rabbits was calculated, this being referred to as the irritation index.

The method used today is essentially the same as the original Draize test, except that the exposure period has been cut down to 4 h and a semi-occlusive patch is used. Abrasion of one of the skin areas has also been discontinued and the number of rabbits used has been reduced.

Much work has been carried out in recent years on *in vitro* methods for predicting skin and eye irritation. These have ranged from simply applying test chemicals to a variety of tissue culture cells, or even artificial gels, to more complex procedures such as measuring enzyme leakage from sheets of differentiating keratinocytes. Organ culture (isolated eyes) and chick embryos have also been used. These methods have had varying success, most being able to identify caustic substances and some being successful in ranking the irritancy of detergents. However, they are much less successful in correctly identifying mild and moderate irritants, particularly those that are lipid soluble. While some of these methods may be used to eliminate corrosive materials and prevent them from being tested on animals, they cannot yet be used for grading irritancy potential for the purpose of labelling products.

1.5.3 *Testing for Skin Sensitizers*

Although various tests have been proposed to detect skin sensitizers, the test described by Magnusson and Kligman utilizing guinea pigs has become the standard method [15]. This test involves an induction phase in which the test material is injected intradermally with and without Freund's adjuvant and also applied to the skin surface under occlusive conditions. To test for sensitization, the animals are challenged a fortnight later by dermal application of a non-irritating concentration of the test material in an appropriate solvent.

A new method still under evaluation is the local lymph node assay in the mouse [16]. In this, the test substance is applied in an appropriate vehicle to the mouse ear and cell proliferation in the draining lymph node is identified by injecting the animal with tritiated thymidine and measuring radioactivity in the node.

No *in vitro* methods are available for identifying skin sensitizers.

1.5.4 *Testing for Skin Carcinogens*

Although the first tests for skin carcinogenicity involved repeated applications to rabbit ears, these were soon replaced by studies in mice. A typical long-term skin-painting study in mice involves skin application of the test material 2 or 3 times a week to the shaved back skin for 2 years. Such studies will identify complete carcinogens. It is important that no more than slight skin irritation is produced in such studies, since substances producing severe irritation may produce skin tumours in mice by a non-genotoxic mechanism if treatment is continued long enough [17]. To ensure this, it is recommended that a pilot study is carried out in which the concentration of test material and its frequency of application is investigated. The irritancy of the vehicle and its effect on skin absorption must be borne in mind in deciding whether to use a vehicle and, if so, which one to use. Assuming that the background incidence of skin tumours in the strain of mice used is low and that the mice showed little signs of skin irritancy, the appearance of epidermal tumours in more than 2 out of 50 mice is generally regarded as necessary before a carcinogenic effect is claimed.

Initiating and promoting properties may also be tested for, but such studies should be interpreted with caution. To test for initiating properties, the test material is applied once or a few times over a week or two followed by treatment with a strong promoting substance (e.g. **TPA**) for several months. The appearance of skin tumours within this time is regarded as indicative of initiating activity. Promoting properties are examined by giving mice a single treatment of a carcinogen such as **DMBA** followed by repeated treatments with the test material. If a substance is shown to have clear initiating and promoting activity it is likely to be a skin carcinogen. However, if either or both responses are weak, results are difficult to interpret. This is particularly the case with initiation as prolonged treatment with **TPA** alone can produce a low incidence of skin cancer.

Because of the cost and time required for such studies, together with the desire to reduce animal testing, many attempts have been made to devise short-term biological assays for assessing likely skin carcinogenic potential. Examples of such assays include *in vivo* assays on mouse skin, such as the sebaceous gland suppression test [18] and the mouse skin nuclear enlargement test [19], and the *in vitro* modified Ames assay [20]. These tests have principally been developed to identify the skin carcinogenic potential of complex hydrocarbon mixtures such as oil products. Although all these assays have been used within the organizations which developed them, none have gained wide acceptance. The modified Ames assay has gained the widest support in the oil industry, but, although there is a reasonable correlation between activity in this test and the long-term carcinogenicity of many oil samples, there is evidence that the activity may not be due to the main carcinogenic components [21].

1.5.5 Subcutaneous Sarcoma

The induction of local sarcomas by repeated injection of test substances into the subcutaneous tissue of rats was, at one time, used widely as a test for carcinogenicity. The method involved injecting the test material, two or three times per week at the same site, into the connective tissue between the panniculus carnosus of the skin and the body musculature for up to a year or longer. The reliability of this method of testing for carcinogenicity was questioned by Grasso and co-workers [22, 23], who reported that a variety of substances which were able to produce tissue damage could produce subcutaneous sarcoma when administered in this way. In particular, they found that substances which were acidic, had surface active properties, were amphipathic (readily soluble in lipids and water) or were hypertonic, were likely to produce sarcomas. Such materials included **hydrochloric acid** and **sorbic acid** (acidic), **Tween 80** (a surface active agent), a variety of **food colours** (having one or more of the above properties) and **glucose** (hypertonic). Investigation of the earlier reactions produced by such substances, revealed that a granulomatous response with tissue damage resulted from repeated injections. This was followed by fibroblast proliferation and progression to tumour formation. Such responses were shown to be exacerbated by crystalline material, such as calcium salts, being deposited. Sarcomas can also result from test substances coming out of solution because of limited solubility and accumulating in the subcutaneous tissue as a result of repeated injections. Even inert solid materials have been shown to produce sarcomas when implanted under the skin, tumour formation depending on the physical form. For example, discs of film of a certain size induced tumours, whereas the same weight of powdered material did not.

Despite these arguments, potential carcinogenicity can be indicated by the appearance of sarcomas following subcutaneous injection. For instance, if a high incidence of tumours at the treatment site occurs within a few months of treatment, the substance is likely to have carcinogenic potential. This is particularly the case if a high incidence of tumours also occurs at other sites. The appearance of tumours following a single injection, or very few injections, is also suggestive of carcinogenic potential, but if the latent period is long, the possibility of crystal deposition being the cause should be considered.

From these considerations it is clear that any claim of carcinogenicity, based solely on the induction of subcutaneous sarcomas, should be regarded with suspicion and examined carefully on a case by case basis.

1.6 Conclusions

Prediction from animal studies of the likely skin effects in man, resulting from exposure to chemical substances and complex mixtures, is not always straight-forward. First, animals may be more or less sensitive than man to the chemical agents concerned and, second, the exposure conditions in animal tests may differ from those involved in human exposure.

With respect to skin irritancy, most animal species used for irritancy testing are more sensitive than man to most substances. Thus, the irritancy of a substance to man is liable to be overestimated by animal studies and this is particularly the case if occlusion is irrelevant to human exposure. Some attempt has been made to limit this overestimation by modifying the original Draize test protocol by reducing the length of the exposure period and the degree of occlusion. However, despite this, the irritancy of some products, such as detergents and cosmetic preparations, still tend to be overestimated. For this reason, open skin test methods and human skin testing have been used quite widely to assess such products. Although much work has been carried out into *in vitro* methods for predicting skin irritation, such studies are not sufficiently reliable to make predictions of irritation to man.

With respect to skin sensitization, animals are generally less sensitive than man and, as a result, weak sensitizers often give equivocal results. The greater sensitivity of guinea pigs to irritation increases the difficulty of identifying weak sensitizers that also have irritant properties (e.g. **formaldehyde**). There is therefore always a danger of not identifying mild sensitizers in animal studies and vigilance is required in reporting reacting individuals in human trials.

Long-term studies of skin painting in mice generally provide a good indication whether or not exposure to a substance is likely to give rise to skin cancer in man, but such studies will not indicate whether or not the material is capable of producing cancer in other organs. Although skin-painting studies have been used to test condensates of airborne pollutants with the aim of predicting their potential to induce lung cancer, such studies are hard to interpret and may give a misleading impression of the hazards to man. This is particularly the case if organic solvents are employed in skin-painting studies. Hence, the use of skin-painting studies is best restricted to materials where skin cancer is the main concern. Work is still going on towards developing an acceptable short-term assay for skin cancer and chemical analysis is widely used to reduce animal testing to a minimum.

Hence, in the assessment of irritant, sensitizing and carcinogenic hazards resulting from skin exposure to chemicals and complex mixtures there is, at present, no reliable substitute for animal or human studies. Although assessment of irritation, sensitization and to some extent skin carcinogenic potential rely mainly on surface observations, histopathological examination provides valuable further information into the nature of the response and is essential to the evaluation of long-term carcinogenicity studies.

References

1. ALLEN, T.D. and POTTEN, C.S. (1976) Significance of cell shape in tissue architecture, *Nature*, **264**, 545–547.
2. CHASE, H.B. (1954) Growth of the hair, *Physiology Review*, **34**, 113–126.
3. ARGYRIS, T.S. (1985) Promotion of epidermal carcinogenesis by repeated damage to mouse skin, *American Journal of Industrial Medicine*, **8**, 329–337.
4. MALKINSON, F.D. and GEHLMANN, L. (1977) Factors affecting percutaneous

absorption, in DRILL, V.A. and LAZAR, P. (Eds) *Cutaneous Toxicity*, pp. 63–81, New York: Academic Press.

5. COOPER, E.R. and BERNER, B. (1985) Skin permiability, in SKERROW, D. and SKERROW, C.J. (Eds) *Methods in Skin Research*, pp. 407–432, New York: John Wiley and Sons.

6. MAIBACH, H.I., FELDMANN, R.J., MILBY, T.H. and SERAT, W.F. (1971) Regional variation in percutaneous penetration in man, *Archives of Environmental Health*, **23**, 208–211.

7. WESTER, R.C. and MAIBACH, H.I. (1977) Percutaneous absorption in man and animal, in DRILL, V.A. and LAZAR, P. (Eds) *Cutaneous Toxicity*, pp. 111–126, New York: Academic Press.

8. RANDO, R.R. and KISHI, Y. (1992) Structural basis of protein kinase C activation by diacylglycerols and tumor promoters, *Biochemistry*, **31**, 2211–2218.

9. INGRAM, A.J. and GRASSO, P. (1975) Patch testing in the rabbit using a modified human patch test method. Application of histological and visual assessment, *British Journal of Dermatology*, **92**, 131–142.

10. INGRAM, A.J., KING, D.J., GRASSO, P. and SHARRATT, M. (1993) The early changes in mouse skin following topical application of a range of middle distillate oil products, *Journal of Applied Toxicology*, **13**, 247–257.

11. INGRAM, A.J. and GRASSO, P. (1985) Nuclear enlargement – an early change produced in mouse epidermis by carcinogenic chemicals applied topically in the presence of a promoter, *Journal of Applied Toxicology*, **5**, 53–60.

12. INGRAM, A.J. and GRASSO, P. (1977) Nuclear enlargement and DNA synthesis in mouse skin treated with carcinogen and promoter, *Experimental Pathology*, **14**, 233–242.

13. INGRAM, A.J. (1992) Review of chemical and UV-light induced melanomas in experimental animals in relation to human melanoma incidence, *Journal of Applied Toxicology*, **12**, 39–43.

14. DRAIZE, J.H., WOODWARD, G. and CALVERY, H.O. (1944) Methods for the study of irritation and toxicity of substances applied topically to the skin and mucous membranes, *Journal of Pharmacology and Experimental Therapeutics*, **82**, 377–390.

15. MAGNUSSON, B. and KLIGMAN, A.M. (1969) The identification of contact allergens by animal assay. The guinea pig maximization test, *Journal of Investigative Dermatology*, **52**, 268–276.

16. KIMBER, I. and DEARMAN, R.J. (1991) Investigation of lymph node cell proliferation as a possible immunological correlate of contact sensitizing potential, *Food and Chemical Toxicology*, **29**, 125–129.

17. INGRAM, A.J. and GRASSO, P. (1991) Evidence for and possible mechanisms of non-genotoxic carcinogenesis in mouse skin, *Mutation Research*, **248**, 333–340.

18. PERISTIANIS, G.C. (1989) Sebaceous gland suppression as a short-term test of the cutaneous carcinogenic activity of mineral oils, *Journal of Applied Toxicology*, **9**, 245–254.

19. INGRAM, A.J. and GRASSO, P. (1987) Nuclear enlargement produced in mouse skin by carcinogenic mineral oils, *Journal of Applied Toxicology*, **7**, 289–295.

20. BLACKBURN, G.R, DIETCH, R.A., SCHREINER, C.A. and MACKERER, C.R. (1986) Predicting carcinogenicity of petroleum distillation fractions using a modified *Salmonella* mutagenicity assay, *Cell Biology and Toxicology*, **2**, 63–84.

21. INGRAM, A.J., SCAMMELLS, D.V. and MAY, K. (1994) An investigation of the main mutagenic components of a carcinogenic oil by fraction and testing in the modified Ames Assay, *Journal of Applied Toxicology*, **14**, 173–179.

22. GRASSO, P. and GOLBERG, L. (1966) Subcutaneous sarcoma as an index of carcinogenic potency, *Food and Cosmetic Toxicology*, **4**, 297–320.

23. GRASSO, P., GANGOLLI, S.D., GOLBERG, L. and HOOSON, J. (1971) Physicochemical and other factors determining local sarcoma production by food additives, *Food and Cosmetic Toxicology*, **9**, 463–478.

2

The Digestive System I: The Gastrointestinal Tract and Exocrine Pancreas

GRAHAM R. BETTON

2.1 Introduction

The digestive system represents one of the largest organ systems in the body; it is involved in both the digestion and uptake of nutrients and it also plays a key role in intermediate metabolism, water and electrolyte homeostasis and the secretion of endogenous and exogenous waste products. It also represents the largest interface between the body and the environment, but unlike the skin, the digestive system is not readily assessed for local irritancy or other toxic effects. The physiological processes of the digestive system rank second only to the nervous system in terms of complexity. The autonomic nervous system, both sympathetic and parasympathetic, is intimately involved in the regulation of both gut motility and secretory activity. The diffuse neuroendocrine system is extensively represented in the gastrointestinal (GI) tract. This makes the gastrointestinal system the largest endocrine organ of the body, although its dispersed neuroendocrine cellular distribution makes it difficult to examine without special techniques which are generally outside the standard battery required in regulatory toxicology. The range of identified peptide hormones and neurotransmitters regulating gastrointestinal function increases yearly. A full understanding of both normal anatomy and physiology, as well as the responses to xenobiotics, is therefore essential in the study of the toxicology and safety evaluation of the GI tract.

A challenge for the toxicologist is also to understand the interdependencies between the digestive system and the other organ systems of the body following the administration of xenobiotics. The presence within the gut lumen of a complex and adaptable population of bacteria and other organisms, some symbiotic, others potential pathogens, provides biochemical pathways outside those found in mammalian cells which can significantly modify xenobiotics or their metabolites. The GI tract and its dependent glandular structures are also exceptionally diverse in terms of the microenvironment in the lumen, with large regional changes in pH, transit times, tonicity and other parameters which influence the ionic state of xenobiotics and hence their ability to cross the cell membrane of the lining epithelium. This review endeavours to provide the reader with information on both physiological and pathological processes in the GI tract resulting from exposure to xenobiotics.

2.2 Anatomy, Histology and Physiology

2.2.1 *Anatomy and Histology*

The rodent and the dog, representing the main species employed in toxicology testing, form the main subjects for a detailed discussion of anatomy and histology.

Oral cavity

The oral cavity of the dog is specialized for the hunting behaviour of the species and its carnivorous diet. Dentition thus combines highly developed canine teeth for combat and the capture of prey, with ridged premolar and molar teeth which are optimized for shearing. Grinding surfaces, as found in herbivores are barely developed. The permanent dentition of the upper jaw comprises 3 incisors, 1 canine, 4 premolars and 2 molars, with 3, 1, 4 and 3 teeth in the mandible, respectively. The deciduous dentition consisting of 3 incisors, 1 canine and 3 premolars in each jaw is normally completely replaced by the permanent dentition by 6 to 7 months of age. The fourth upper premolar and first lower molar are large carnassial teeth with apposing shearing faces. Tooth structure is composed of enamel, dentine and pulp cavity layers cemented into the jaw by cementum and collagen fibres and the dentition is orthodont, with the teeth ceasing to grow after eruption. The dental arcades divide the oral stratified squamous epithelium into the vestibule or labial mucosa and the oral mucosa proper [1].

The oral cavity of the rodent has evolved for a mainly herbivorous diet with specialized and powerful upper and lower pairs of incisors. The dentition is hypsodont, i.e. the teeth continue to grow throughout life. Enamel is present only on the labial surface of the incisors, resulting in a chisel-like wear pattern. The lips of rodents can close the wide diastema between the incisors and molars during gnawing activity [2]. The hamster possesses cheek pouches, lined by a stratified squamous epithelium, in which food can be stored prior to mastication. These pouches can be everted to carry out experimental studies on the topical activity of xenobiotics or carcinogenic processes.

In the dog and rodent the tongue functions for taste, mastication and grooming, and in the dog it also serves as an additional cooling surface when the core body temperature is elevated. Taste buds are specialized into filiform, fungiform, conical, foliate and circumvallate forms. In the rodent, serous and mucous lingual glands drain into the oral cavity along a line on the dorsum of the tongue. The oral cavity becomes the oropharynx at the caudal edge of the palate. The cavity passes towards the oesophagus with the larynx opening ventrally at the point of transition. The rat is an obligate nose breather with the epiglottis closing the oropharyngeal opening except during swallowing, whereas the dog can breathe through the mouth to increase the respiratory rate. The pharynx is also the site of the lymphoid tissue of the tonsil, which is rich in antigen-presenting cells for the induction of the immune response.

Salivary glands

In the dog, ducts of the serous parotid and mucous zygomatic salivary glands open into the dorsal vestibule whereas the mixed (seromucous) mandibular (submaxillary), and mucous sublingual salivary glands, open at the sublingual caruncle, rostral to the frenulum of the tongue.

Rodents have major and minor mucous sublingual salivary glands, mixed mandibular (submaxillary) glands, and serous parotid salivary glands. The intercalated duct cells of the salivary glands of the male mouse contain conspicuous granules of epidermal growth factor (EGF) which has actions on both GI secretion and growth [3]. Salivary secretion has a lubricative as well as a digestive function.

Oesophagus

The oesophagus in both the dog and rodent is lined by a stratified squamous epithelium. In the dog, submucosal mucous glands are present for lubricating the oesophagus during swallowing. The muscle wall of the oesophagus is composed of oblique coats of striated muscle in the dog and smooth muscle in the rodent, hence the ability of rodents to vomit. The oesophagus enters the stomach at the cardia and the reflux of food and gastric juice is prevented by the tone of the lower oesophageal sphincter which is regulated by cholinergic and serotonergic innervation.

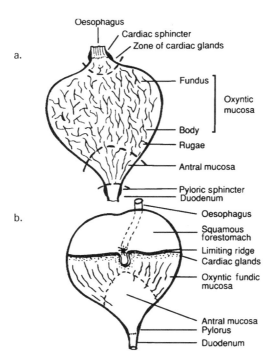

Figure 2.1 Anatomy of the dog and rodent stomach. The macroscopic appearance of the mucosal surface of the stomach after opening along the greater curvature is shown for the dog (a) and rat (b). The forestomach of the rodent is a non-glandular reservoir.

Stomach

The stomach of the dog (Figure 2.1a) is a simple distensible sac composed of a narrow band of mucous cardiac glands, the fundus and the body which are both lined by oxyntic mucosa, and the antrum which contains prominent lymphoid follicles and leads into the duodenum via the pyloric sphincter. In contrast, the rodent stomach (Figure 2.1b) is also sac-like in external shape but is divided into two parts by a prominent limiting ridge separating the stratified squamous epithelium-lined forestomach from the glandular stomach. The latter comprises a narrow band of mucous cardiac glands around the keyhole-shaped cardiac sphincter, an oxyntic fundus and body, and a smoother pale antrum leading into the pylorus.

   In the gastric fundus are the gastric glands. Above the glands, towards the lumen, are the gastric pits which open onto the surface epithelium. Mucus-secreting foveolar cells cover the luminal surface and line the gastric pits and provide a protective unstirred mucous layer on the surface of the lumen. In addition, active bicarbonate secretion by the foveolar cells creates a pH gradient across the mucous layer [4]. Cells of the oxyntic glands, chief cells and acid-secreting parietal cells, mucous neck cells, and neuroendocrine cells are illustrated in Figure 2.2. These cells have a long lifespan (100 days) compared with the 6 to 10-day lifespan of the foveolar cells of the gastric pits and the surface epithelium, and the cells of the antral mucosa [5]. The proliferative zone of the oxyntic mucosa is located at the base of the gastric pits (Figure 2.3a) and, therefore, relatively superficial erosions can impair the regenerative capacity of the mucosa. Differentiating cells from this zone migrate upwards into the gastric pits and down into the gastric glands. Less noticeable are the neuroendocrine cells of the gastric mucosa. These cells are are located as dispersed cells intercalated between the secretory cells, predominantly in the deepest third of the mucosa. The antral mucosa is much simpler histologically, with pits and short coiled glands, within which are located gastrin-secreting G cells and other neuroendocrine cell types (Figure 2.3b).

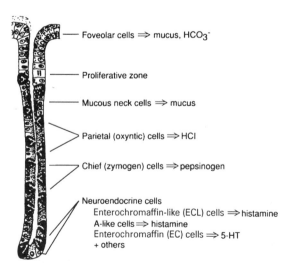

Figure 2.2 Gastric gland histology. Diagram of an oxyntic gland from the fundus of the stomach depicting the specialized cell types involved in secretion of acid, pepsinogen, mucus and bicarbonate. Note the superficial location of the proliferative zone.

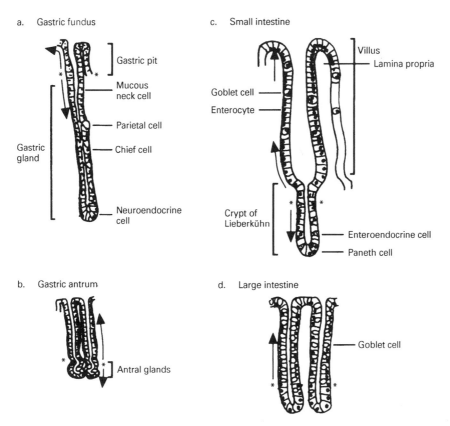

a. Gastric fundus
- Gastric pit
- Mucous neck cell
- Parietal cell
- Chief cell
- Neuroendocrine cell
- Gastric gland

b. Gastric antrum
- Antral glands

c. Small intestine
- Villus
- Lamina propria
- Goblet cell
- Enterocyte
- Crypt of Lieberkühn
- Enteroendocrine cell
- Paneth cell

d. Large intestine
- Goblet cell

Figure 2.3 Histological location of the proliferative zone and the migration of gastrointestinal cells. The location of the proliferative zone (∗) and the direction of cell migration (→) are shown for the gastric fundus oxyntic gland (a), the gastric antral gland (b), and the small intestine (c) and the large intestine (d). Note the superficial location of the proliferative zone of the gastric fundic glands compared with the deeper sites in the lower parts of the GI tract. In the small intestine, the proliferative zone is at the opening of the crypts of Lieberkühn.

A thin muscularis mucosae marks the boundary between the mucosa and the submucosa. Circular and longitudinal smooth muscle coats are locally developed into the oesophageal and pyloric sphincters.

Intestine

The small intestine of both the dog and rodent begins with the duodenum. This contains Brunner's glands in the submucosa in the first part of the duodenum distal to the pylorus [1, 2]. The bile duct and the dorsal and ventral pancreatic ducts open into the proximal duodenum via papillae. The duodenal–jejunal border is defined anatomically by the flexure at the end of the U-shaped course of the duodenum around the root of the supporting mesentery. Both the extensive jejunum and the ileum are suspended by mesentery. Within the mesenteric fan lie the prominent mesenteric lymph nodes which are situated along the branching cranial mesenteric artery. The gut associated lymphoid tissue (GALT) is represented by Peyer's patches which are present at increasing frequency in the ileal part of the small intestine in the rat but spread throughout the length of the small intestine in the dog.

The mucosal surface of the small intestine is maximized for secretory and absorptive functions by the presence of villi which are covered by columnar enterocytes, and these in turn have a microvillous brush border at their luminal surface (Figure 2.4). The enterocytes are interspersed with mucus-secreting goblet cells. The relative length of the small intestinal villi reduces progressively from the duodenum to the ileum. The proliferative zone of the small intestinal mucosa is at the opening of the crypts of Lieberkühn (Figure 2.3c). The crypt cells comprise stem cells, enteroendocrine (neuroendocrine) cells, columnar enterocytes, mucous goblet cells and granular Paneth cells (absent in the dog). The stem cell is pluripotential (Figure 2.5) with the greatest turnover taking place toward the villus tips by a process of cell migration up the villi.

The terminal ileum enters the colon via the ileocolic sphincter which has a

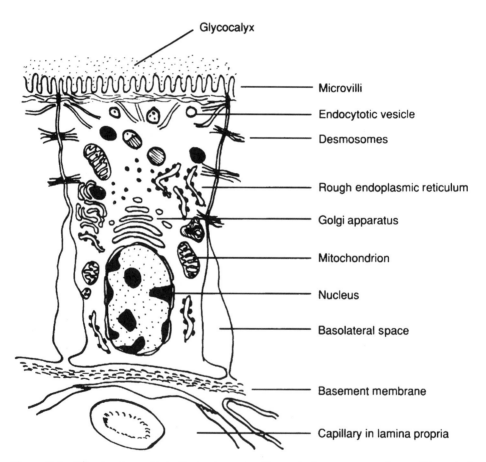

Figure 2.4 Ultrastructure of intestinal enterocyte. The typical appearance of a small intestinal enterocyte located on a villus. The microvillous border provides a large absorptive surface. Tight intercellular junctions and desmosomes prevent the entry of molecules between adjacent cells. Diffusion, transport, pinocytosis and endocytosis control the entry of molecules into the cell, and diffusion, transport and exocytosis across the basolateral membrane allow entry into the vessels of the lamina propria.

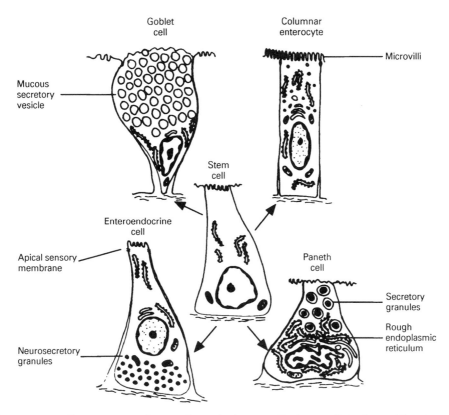

Figure 2.5 Differentiation pathways of intestinal crypt cells. Stem cells in the proliferative zone of the small intestinal crypt can differentiate into goblet cells and columnar enterocytes which migrate upwards to cover the villi. Enteroendocrine cells and Paneth cells are located in the base of the crypts (see Figure 2.3c). Loss of the stem cell compartment impairs the ability of the intestinal epithelium to regenerate after injury.

prominent ridge of lymphoid tissue in the dog. The caecocolic sphincter regulates entry of digested food into the blind-ended caecum. The large intestine is composed of the caecum, which is well developed in the rodent but minor in the dog, the colon, and the rectum, with its prominent lymphoid follicles, ending at the anus. In the dog, circumanal glands and a pair of anal sacs produce pheromones under androgen drive. There is no true appendix in the rodent and the dog, but the rabbit has a true appendix with a well-developed lymphoid structure. The large intestine lacks villi, although the surface area is increased by the presence of folds. The large intestinal mucosal glands are short and relatively simple with a predominance of mucus-secreting goblet cells (Figure 2.3d). The absorption and exchange of electrolytes in this region of the GI tract is of great physiological importance.

Pancreas

The exocrine pancreas is composed of loose lobular collections of acinar tissue located within the mesentery bounded by the duodenum; the blunt head of the pancreas is directed towards the stomach. The right pancreatic lobe lies in the mesoduodenum and the left lobe extends towards the spleen in the dorsal omentum.

The dorsal and ventral pancreatic ducts drain into the proximal duodenum adjacent to the bile duct. Embryologically, pancreatic tissue develops as a branching outgrowth of ducts from the primitive foregut. The pancreatic cells lining the intercalated ducts are responsible for elaborating the water and bicarbonate component of pancreatic secretion. The intercalated ducts lead to secretory acinar cells with apical eosinophilic zymogen granules which have trypsinogen, lipase and other enzymic activities. Following injury, regeneration of the acinar cells from ductular cells can be observed. Sometimes, the regenerating cells pass through a phase of hepatocytic differentiation. Insulin, secreted by endocrine pancreatic β-cells in the islets of Langerhans, stimulates the growth of the acinar cells of the exocrine pancreas. Acinar cell hypertrophy is sometimes observed around islets of Langerhans, the venous outflow from the islets supplies adjacent acinar cells. In addition to its actions on glucose metabolism, insulin also has important activities at growth factor receptors in the GI tract. Similarly, glucagon, secreted by the α-cells of the islets of Langerhans, and enteroglucagon secreted by A cells of the GI tract, both have metabolic, secretory and proliferative activities.

2.2.2 *Physiology*

Salivation

The types of secretion differ between the various salivary glands, that is, a mixed secretion from the mandibular (submaxillary) gland, a mucous secretion from the sublingual gland and a serous secretion from the parotid gland. Secretory products include water, electrolytes, enzymes (e.g. amylase), proteoglycans, immunoglobulin A, and EGF (especially in male mice). These secretions are regulated by β-adrenergic and cholinergic inputs, thyroxine and corticosteroids. A number of xenobiotics are actively transported into saliva, along with bicarbonate. The growth of salivary glands is promoted via β-adrenoreceptors [6].

Nausea and vomiting

Nausea and vomiting can be initiated by CNS effects (via the vestibular nucleus, the olfactory bulb or by the direct action of pharmacophores in the area postrema) or via topical effects on the upper GI tract or the stomach (e.g. irritants or corrosive substances). Salivation may precede vomiting, initiated via voluntary and autonomic neural pathways. Protracted salivation and vomiting may result in significant loss of potassium in these fluids.

Gastric secretion and mucosal protection factors

The stomach functions as both a storage compartment and as a site for the initial part of the digestive process. The secretions of the oxyntic mucosa lining the fundus and body of the stomach form the gastric juice. The non-glandular forestomach of the rodent provides additional storage capacity whereas the dog stomach is highly distensible, appropriate to its carnivorous diet. In the dog the regulation of gastric acid secretion is via food-stimulated cholinergic autonomic inputs and gastrin secretion [4], whereas the rodent is a basal acid secretor, again regulated via autonomic innervation and gastrin secretion from antral G cells of the neuroendocrine system. The level of circulating gastrin is determined by the luminal pH of the antral region of the stomach. Paracrine regulation of the gastrin-secreting G cells in the mucosa is mediated by a fall in somatostatin secretion by D cells which respond to a raised pH at their luminal surface (Figure 2.6). Gastrin exists in peptide forms of 34 and 17 amino acids and these are subject to further cleavage in the circulation [7] with the secretogogue N-terminal amino acids show close homology between species. The gastrin molecule is also closely homologous to cholecystokinin (CCK), which regulates bile and pancreatic acinar cell secretion [4], but secretagogue activity is confined to the stomach and, at high doses, the colon. Gastrin reaches the oxyntic mucosa via the circulation and acts on parietal cells via enterochromaffin-like cells (ECL cells) to effect acid secretion by the parietal cells (Figure 2.6). ECL cells are sited adjacent to parietal cells and the secretagogue action of gastrin is now considered to be mediated via the ECL cell. The ECL cell is stimulated to secrete histamine that in turn activates histamine H_2-receptors on the parietal cells, which are triggered to secrete acid via increased cyclic AMP and H^+, K^+-ATPase activation.

The gastric mucosa has developed mechanisms of protection against erosion by acidic gastric juice. A surface layer of unstirred mucus exists on the luminal surface

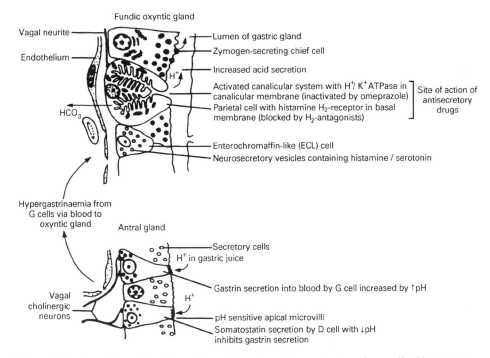

Figure 2.6 Regulation of gastric acid secretion via gastrin and enterochromaffin-like (ECL) cells. Regulation of gastric acid secretion from parietal cells is via vagal cholinergic and histamine signals from ECL cells (upper figure). Following the secretion of gastrin into the blood from the antral G cell (lower figure), ECL cells are stimulated to secrete histamine and serotonin as a result of gastrin binding to receptors on the basal surface of the cell. The secretion of gastrin is modulated by pH, autonomic innervation and paracrine somatostatin production. Acid secretion by the parietal cell is inhibited by histamine receptor antagonists or inhibitors of the H^+, K^+-ATPase acid secreting pump.

within which a pH gradient is created by active prostaglandin-stimulated bicarbonate secretion by foveolar cells (Figure 2.2). Throughout the GI tract, superficial epithelial cell populations show rapid turnover (lifespan about 6 days) and hence continual replacement from the proliferative zone is critical. Following superficial erosion, cells can spread out of gastric pits and reseal epithelial defects by forming new tight junctions. Interference with these mechanisms, e.g. a reduction in mucosal blood flow by the inhibition of prostaglandin $(PG)I_2$ (prostacyclin) synthesis, or hypotension, or mitotic inhibition by cytotoxic anti-cancer agents, will allow mucosal injury to develop. Trophic factors, which stimulate mucosal cell proliferation (e.g. PGE_2, EGF), therefore increase mucosal protection. Some strains of mice exhibit a spontaneous hyperplastic gastropathy, the severity of which can be modified by changes in diet [8].

Intestinal and pancreatic physiology

The entry of gastric juice into the duodenum requires peristaltic activity and the relaxation of the pyloric sphincter. The complex autonomic innervation of the intestinal tract is involved both in the control of gut motility and in secretory activity. Sympathetic stimulation promotes absorptive activity through the reduction of intracellular cyclic AMP, whereas cholinergic receptors initiate rises in intracellular calcium, and other second messengers, resulting in active secretion from the enterocyte into the gut lumen. Many other synergistic and antagonist mediators regulate the balance between absorptive and secretory activity. In addition, the GI tract has a rich and diverse neuroendocrine cell component with a wide variety of cell types (Table 2.1). Each cell type is regulated by specific agonist and antagonist

Table 2.1 Gastrointestinal neuroendocrine cell populations: distribution of cell types and peptide hormone secreted

Cell type	Location	Peptide hormone
ECL	Gastric fundus	None (histamine, 5-HT)
A	Gastric fundus, small intestine	Glucagon (250)
D	Gastric antrum, small and large intestine	Somatostatin (350)
D_1	Stomach, small and large intestine, pancreas	Vasoactive intestinal peptide (160)
G	Gastric antrum	Gastrin (300)
EC1	Small and large intestine	Substance P
EC2	Small and large intestine	Motilin
S	Small and large intestine	Secretin
I	Small intestine	Cholecystokinin
K	Small intestine	Gastric inhibitory peptide
L	Small and large intestine	Glicentin
N	Small and large intestine	Neurotensin
P	Stomach, small intestine	Bombesin (120)
PP	Pancreatic ducts	Pancreatic polypeptide, GHRH
A	Pancreatic islets, small intestine	Glucagon, CRH (250)
B	Pancreas	Insulin, TRH

GHRH, growth hormone releasing hormone; CRH, corticotrophin releasing hormone; TRH, thyrotrophin releasing hormone. ( ) indicates the size of the neurosecretory granule in nanometres.

molecular and neural signals which control secretion (Figure 2.7) or absorption (Figure 2.8). The specific peptide hormones which are secreted act locally (paracrine) or on distant sites (endocrine). The I cell, for example, regulates pancreatic acinar secretion and biliary secretion via CCK (pancreozymin) production in response to levels of lipid (in rodents) or signal peptide (in dog and man) present in the lower small intestine. Secretin, from intestinal S cells, stimulates bicarbonate secretion by pancreatic duct cells and the bile duct epithelium. Therefore, the scope for interference with these many and varied endocrine feedback loops is extensive.

The pH of the intestinal lumen changes from pH 2 in the stomach to pH 8 to 9 in the small intestine as a result of bicarbonate secretion by Brunner's glands, the bile duct epithelium in the liver, and pancreatic duct cells (Figure 2.9). The peptide hormone secretin is important in this response. The pH change is necessary for the saponification of fats which, in conjunctiton with the formation of fat micelles with bile acids produced by the liver, allows fat digestion to take place. Interference with this process results in steatorrhoea (undigested fat in the faeces). The intestinal

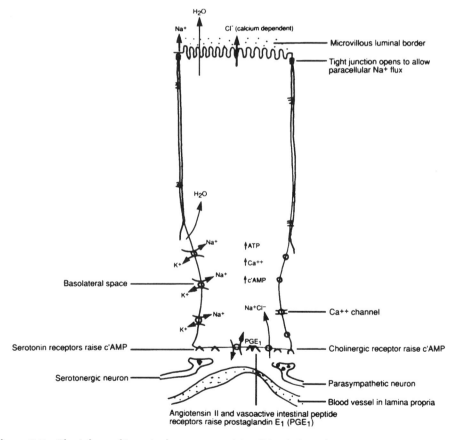

Figure 2.7 Physiology of intestinal secretory activity. Stimulation of entrocyte secretory activity is mediated via autonomic neuronal inputs (cholinergic and serotonergic), endocrine stimuli such as vasoactive intestinal peptide (VIP) and angiotensin II receptors. Receptors activate second messengers including prostaglandin (PG) E_1, cytosolic calcium and cyclic AMP. Na^+, K^+-ATPase pumps, and sodium, chloride and calcium channels are activated in turn.

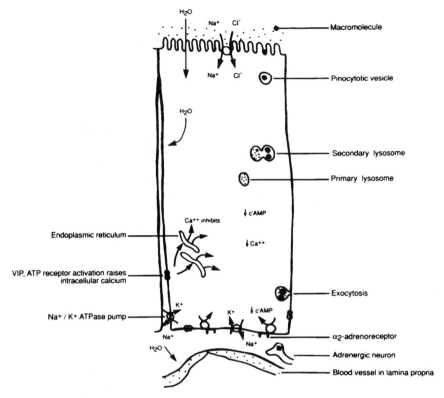

Figure 2.8 Physiology of intestinal absorption. Absorption of water and electrolytes via the apical microvillous border of the enterocyte is signalled by falls in cyclic AMP and free intracellular calcium after adrenoreceptor binding. ATP and vasoactive intestinal peptide (VIP) act at receptors on the basolateral membrane to raise cytosolic calcium and inhibit absorption.

epithelium is involved in a wide range of active and passive uptake processes, many of which are under strict endocrine and metabolic regulation. Regional pH differences in the intestine influence the ionization state of xenobiotics and thus target the site of absorption to those parts of the GI tract where non-ionized lipophilic molecules can readily cross cell membranes. Some molecules, such as cyano-cobalamin (vitamin B_{12}), require specific carriers (intrinsic factor) for receptor-mediated uptake and transport into the intestinal circulation. The intestine is also rich in a number of metabolizing enzyme systems. For example microperoxisomes are present in enterocytes, and cytochrome P-450s are abundant towards the enterocyte microvillous border at the villus tips [9]. The microvillous brush border of the enterocyte also possesses significant metabolic capability at the luminal surface, with the expression of enzymes such as maltase, sucrase, lactase and alkaline phosphatase. It should also be remembered that the gut microflora is capable of metabolizing many nutrients and xenobiotics. Furthermore, pH changes in the intestine can be employed to advantage, for example in the use of enteric-coated drug delivery systems. Endocrine status also significantly modifies digestion and absorption [10, 11], e.g. raised levels of growth hormone in pregnancy stimulates intestinal growth, with an increase in absorptive capability.

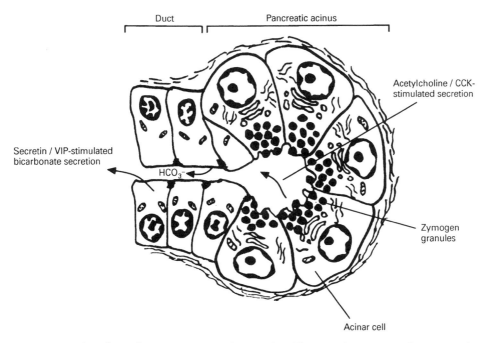

Duct | Pancreatic acinus

Acetylcholine / CCK-stimulated secretion

Secretin / VIP-stimulated bicarbonate secretion

HCO_3^-

Zymogen granules

Acinar cell

Figure 2.9 Physiology of exocrine pancreatic secretion. The exocrine pancreas is composed of duct cells and acinar cells. Duct cells secrete water and bicarbonate following secretin or vasoactive intestinal peptide (VIP) receptor activation, and acinar cells secrete zymogen granules into the lumen of the acinus following acetylcholine or cholecystokinin (CCK) receptor activation. Trypsinogen, lipase and other enzymes are secreted into the duodenum via the pancreatic duct as alkaline pancreatic juice.

The large intestine is mainly responsible for water resorption and maintaining electrolyte balance. Sodium/potassium exchange is regulated by angiotensin. The addition of non-absorbable or high-molecular-weight compounds to the diet can result in caecal distention, with bulky faeces or diarrhoea.

2.3 Biochemical and Cellular Mechanisms of Toxicity

2.3.1 *Mucosal Exposure to Xenobiotics*

The GI tract presents a very large total surface area to the environment due to its organization into villi, glands and cell surface microvillus structures. Within the lumen of the tract there is a wide range of pH from pH 2 in the stomach to pH 9 in the intestine. This range of pH can change the ionization state of nutrients and xenobiotics and provide opportunities for selective drug delivery. The low pH of the gastric mucosa provides a sink for basic xenobiotic molecules to be transported into the stomach lumen. Enzymic cleavage of prodrugs and toxin precursors may take place in the intestine. The absorptive surface of the gut is both large and highly active, with many transporters, some of which can allow macromolecules to enter the body. The entry of cytotoxins into the intestinal mucosa occurs via a variety of mechanisms including passive processes which are often dependent on the non-ionic form of the xenobiotic, uptake by carriers transporting a range of anions or cations or specific substrates, and by endocytosis or by entry into active transport pathways. Macromolecules can also be taken up through the specialized M cells overlying lymphoid mantle regions of the GALT (Figure 2.10) as part of the antigen uptake, processing and presentation sequence for the initiation of an immune response [12]. Conversely, overload with non-digestible or non-absorbable compounds can lead to diarrhoea or caecal enlargement [13]. The GI tract also serves as an excretory route for biliary excreted molecules and receives secretions from the salivary glands, liver and pancreas, as well as from GI glandular elements proper.

The epithelial barrier of the GI tract has a high rate of turnover and consequently the stem cells have a high mitotic index, rendering them sensitive to **cytotoxic drugs** [14, 15], **radiation** and some **DNA viruses**. Agents such as these typically affect the

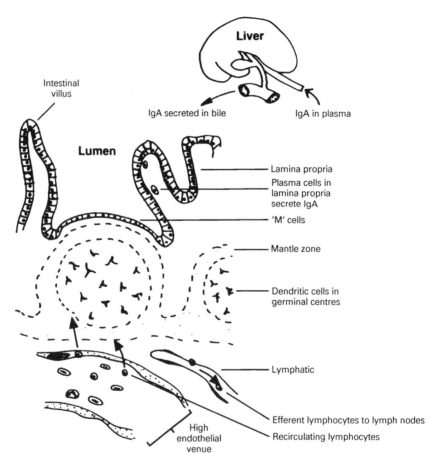

Figure 2.10 Gut-associated lymphoid tissue (GALT) and the mucosal immune response. Lymphocytes in the germinal centres and mantle zones of the Peyer's patch are presented with intestinal antigens taken up by specialized epithelial M cells. The antigens are presented to dendritic antigen-presenting cells in the germinal centres. B lymphocytes differentiate into immunoglobulin A (IgA)-secreting plasma cells after recirculation via the lymphatics and the blood. Some IgA is secreted in the bile and some is secreted into the lamina propria of the GI tract.

proliferative zone at crypt level leading to more severe injury and the impairment of regeneration. Systemic secondary toxic effects may result from **pathogenic bacterial invasion** or **toxin production**. Irritants (**plants, chemicals, heavy metals**) typically cause superficial injury to the mucosa, loss of villi, haemorrhage and inflammation. Factors which may affect GI toxicity therefore include the pH of dosing solutions (which are dependent on the pKa(s) of the xenobiotic molecule), the presence of excipients in the formulation, possible enterohepatic recirculation of parent drug or metabolites, dosing animals in a fed or fasted state, the status of the gut microflora and dietary composition.

2.3.2 *Mucosal Absorption Pathways*

As well as specialized transport pathways, the uptake of nutrients by intestinal enterocyte populations is affected by passive diffusion, ion pump channels, metal ion transporters, quaternary nitrogen transporters, amino acid transport and other structure-specific mechanisms (Figure 2.8). **Cholera toxin** and heat labile **bacterial endotoxins** induce adenyl cyclase activity which results in enterocytes switching into sustained secretory activity, with watery diarrhoea and electrolyte loss as an outcome. PGE_1 and PGE_2 produce similar changes with additional effects on gut motility.

Fats are taken up in the form of micelles with bile acids. Intracellular lipid is then assembled into chylomicrons and these enter the lymphatic system. High-molecular-weight molecules are taken up by pinocytosis by specialized M cells in Peyer's patches. Dendritic cells in the lymphoid follicles of the GALT present the processed antigens taken up by the M cells, and efferent lymphocytes undergo clonal expansion in the GALT and in the lymph nodes (primarily the mesenteric lymph nodes) to produce cell-mediated and humoral (IgA) responses (Figure 2.10). Macromolecules such as **high-molecular-weight paraffins** may enter macrophages in the lamina propia of the gut or in regional lymph nodes in a non-degradable form. Such macromolcules may accumulate within the lysosomal compartments of the phagocytic cell. In this way, therefore, a wide range of mechanisms exist for the entry of xenobiotics into the enterocyte, and subsequently into the extracellular fluid and the blood stream. Interference with secretory or absorptive pathways by receptor-mediated, or other actions can thus profoundly influence digestion through effects on motility and mucosal physiology. Impeding secretory and absorptive pathways may also cause secondary effects on water and electrolye balance and may influence other body systems, in particular the cardiovascular system.

2.3.3 *Mucosal Metabolism*

Enterocytes are rich in cytochrome P-450 mixed function oxidases, micro-peroxisomes, uridine diphosphate-glucuronyl transferases [9], *N*-acetyltransferases and other systems capable of xenobiotic metabolism. These may act to detoxify or activate compounds. Many of these metabolic activities are found at high concentrations in the enterocytes located at the villus tips in the upper small intestine. Treatment with P-450 enzyme inducers, either dietary (e.g. *Brassica spp.*), or xenobiotics (e.g. **methylcholanthrene, MCA**), increases expression in enterocytes. The stratified squamous epithelia of both the oesophagus and the rodent forestomach also contain P-450 mixed function oxidase isozymes capable of activating genotoxic carcinogens such as **MCA**.

2.3.4   Gut Microflora Metabolism

The normal gut microflora is composed of a balanced and diverse range of bacterial species with a wide variety of enzymic activities including many different hydrolases. Bacterial azo-reductases cleave the prodrug **sulphasalazine** to the active **5-aminosalicylic acid** in the colon. Bacterial glucuronidases deconjugate some xenobiotic or endogenous metabolites and conjugates (e.g. bile acids, thyroxine) secreted in the bile after phase 2 metabolism, aiding their enterohepatic recirculation. However, microfloral metabolism may generate toxic or carcinogenic agents from precursors, for example *Streptobacillus* glycosidase may produce **methylazoxy-methanol** from **cycasin**.

2.3.5   Motility Disorders

Regulation of GI contractility and secretion is highly complex, involving inputs from the CNS, autonomic nervous system, and many paracrine and endocrine hormones. The complex role of the sympathetic and parasympathetic nervous systems in swallowing, sphincter function and peristaltic activity, render the GI tract sensitive to a wide range of agents. **Organophosphorus**- or **acrylamide**-induced axonopathies can lead to megaloesophagus with the oesophagus becoming distended with food. *a*-**Adrenergic agonists** can increase peristaltic activity leading to the hyperactive conditions of intussusception or prolapse. Non-absorbable **sugar alcohols** (e.g. **xylitol**), **gums** and **fibre** can increase the bulk of the digesta leading to caecal distention [13] and diarrhoea.

2.3.6   Accumulation Enteropathies

The complex range of transport processes occurring in the gut may be overloaded or blocked by xenobiotics, e.g. by high doses of **quaternary ammonium compounds** [16]. Intestinal phospholipidosis may result from the inability of lysosomal enzymes to degrade **amphiphilic molecules**. Similarly, **high-molecular-weight molecules** may be transported into the lamina propria to accumulate as foamy macrophages or form macrophage aggregates in the regional (mesenteric) lymph nodes [17]. Inhibitors of protein synthesis, such as **puromycin** and **ethionine**, may lead to enterocyte lipid accumulation through lack of apoprotein synthesis [18]. Specialized M cells overlying Peyer's patch lymphoid tissue are able to endocytose macromolecules from the gut lumen and present processed antigens to the immune cells of the mantle zone (Figure 2.10). Macrophages of the lamina propria and the medulla of the mesenteric lymph nodes may also accumulate non-degradable macromolecules.

2.3.7 *Nutritional Factors*

High-fibre diets increase the bulk of the digesta and hence reduce transit time and this may reduce the availability of nutrients and xenobiotics. **Cholestyramine**, a bile acid sequestrant for the treatment of hypercholesterolaemia, can also bind fat soluble vitamins (A, E, K) leading to vitamin deficiencies. **Tetracycline antibiotics** can chelate divalent cations (Fe, Al, Mg, Ca, Cu etc.) leading to imbalances. Excess **dietary phosphates** can also compete with Ca^{++} uptake mechanisms which are under parathyroid hormone and 1,25-dihydroxycholecalciferol control.

2.4 Morphological Responses to Injury

2.4.1 *Oral Cavity*

The oral cavity is generally resistant to all except caustic substances. The cavity is only subjected to a transient exposure to toxicants in the diet, and there is a lack of exposure to test substances which are administered by gavage. An unusual feature of **calcium-channel blockers** [19], **valproic acid** and **cyclosporin A**, is gingival hyperplasia in dogs. The lesion has a characteristic gross appearance and results from fibroepithelial proliferation of the gingival margins. Similar changes have been reported in human patients receiving **antiepileptic compounds** (e.g. **phenytoin**) and **calcium-channel blockers**. Immunosuppressants, such as **corticosteroids**, may predispose to *Candida* infection in the oral cavity, with the white plaques of thrush present in the oral mucosa. **Tetracyclines** are incorporated into dentine during the period of tooth development and result in mottling after tooth eruption. Fluorosis also produces defects in enamel when **high fluorine diets** are administered chronically. Porphyrin may accumulate in enamel, either as a result of inborn errors of metabolism, or as a result of xenobiotics such as a **hexachlorobenzene, lead** or **griseofulvin** selectively inhibiting one or more of the enzymes involved in haem synthesis. Pink porphyrin deposits in enamel show a characteristic fluorescence in ultraviolet light. Cytotoxic anticancer agents such as **cyclophosphamide** cause malformation of the rapidly growing incisors and other teeth of rodents [20], which is related to the lifetime proliferation of the odontogenic epithelium in these species. Carbohydrates (e.g. **sucrose** and **xylitol**) administered in high amounts in the diet, induce dental caries formation, which is not a normal condition in rodent species [21].

2.4.2 *Salivary Glands*

Salivation is a classical feature of parasympathetic stimulation, and occurs, for example, in **organophosphorus** poisoning. Salivation may also be indicative of unpalatable test substances. Salivary acinar cell proliferation is stimulated via adrenergic receptors and chronic administration of agonists such as **isoprenaline** result in marked increases in salivary gland weight. Specific toxicities affecting the salivary gland are otherwise uncommon although the **sialodacryoadenitis virus** of rats can cause extensive pathology in disease outbreaks. In the dog, chronic administration of **sulphasalazine** and related molecules can induce an autoimmune keratoconjunctivitis sicca [22] which includes a mononuclear sialoadenitis component, resembling Sjögren's syndrome in man. Despite the extensive use of **sulphasalazine** in patients with ulcerative colitis, this effect remains species specific to the dog.

2.4.3   Oesophagus and Non-Glandular Forestomach

Because of the potential for delayed oesophageal transit times in the elderly, models have been developed for the study of the intra-oesophageal dissolution of tablet and capsule formulations of drugs [23]. Local corrosive effects, e.g. with β-**blockers**, have been described which have the potential for subsequent fibrous scar formation during repair, leading to oesophageal stricture and obstruction. Motility disorders of the autonomic nervous system of the oesophagus can be present as a congenital abnormality (megaloesophagus) or as a result of neuropathies following **acrylamide** or **organophosphorus** poisoning. Some **nitrosamines** are carcinogenic for the oesophageal squamous epithelium with the target site being correlated with the distribution of the cytochrome P-450 isozyme which is required for the metabolic activation of the (pro)carcinogen.

In the rodent, ulceration of the non-glandular forestomach may result from **non-steroidal anti-inflammatory drugs (NSAIDs)** and other treatments. High local exposure to gavage-administered compounds is a contributing factor. Lesions appear as pinhead, volcano-shaped, raised lesions with a central depressed ulcer surrounded by reactive hyperplasia of the stratified squamous epithelium. Similar lesions may be seen in aged rats with diminished food intake and here some generalized hyperkeratosis may also be seen.

Hyperplastic lesions of the rodent forestomach (Figure 2.11) have been reported with a wide range of compounds including the flavouring agent, **D-limonene** [24], the antioxidant, **butylated hydroxyanisole (BHA)** [25], **aristolochic acid** and a wide range of drugs and genotoxic carcinogens. In many cases, lifetime exposure progresses through stages of focal hyperplasia, papilloma and squamous cell carcinoma, where initiation by a genotoxic carcinogen and promotion by non-genotoxic agents such as **BHA** are involved [26]. The relevance of forestomach carcinogenesis in the rodent for human risk assessment of non-genotoxic compounds has been the subject of much debate, given the absence of a forestomach in man [25]. Cytochrome P-450 activity in the oesophageal and forestomach squamous epithelium has been correlated with the metabolic activation of genotoxic **nitrosamines** [27]. The histogenetic similarity of the oral and oesophageal mucosa in man to the rodent forestomach should be taken into account in any evaluation of safety. **Betel quid**, **tobacco** and **opium** are established carcinogens of these tissues in man.

2.4.4   Glandular Stomach

Lesions seen most commonly in this site are erosion or ulceration, and they are typically induced by **NSAIDs** [28] and **5-lipoxygenase inhibitors**. Interestingly, each of these two groups of drugs can protect against the ulcerogenic activity of the other. The role of prostacyclin (PGI_2) in maintaining the local mucosal blood flow

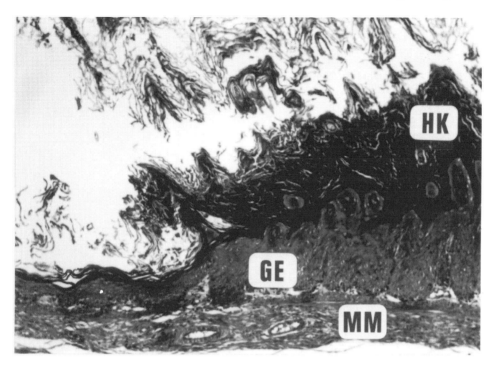

Figure 2.11 Hyperplasia and hyperkeratosis of the rat forestomach. Note focal area of hyperplasia with corrugation of the germinal epithelium (GE) above the muscularis mucosae (MM). Overlying keratinocytes are shed into the lumen from the area of hyperkeratosis (HK).

may be critical in the prevention of acute erosion of the gastric mucosa. **Angiotensin II antagonists**, and **acute blood loss**, can also lead to gastric ulceration (Figure 2.12). Erosion and ulceration can also result from the administration of a wide range of irritants (**ethanol, salt, acids, alkalis**), from 'stress', and from **ischaemia**. Reflux of bile into the gastric antrum may lead to ulceration by **bile acids**. Renal failure with associated uraemia has also been reported to lead to gastric mucosal erosion [29]. In addition, some agents may have a trophic (proliferative) action on the gastric glandular mucosa, e.g. **PGE$_2$** and **misoprostil** [30, 31]. These prostanoids may also confer cytoprotective properties, preventing ulceration.

The gross appearance of erosions or ulcerations will depend on the time between dosing and necropsy. Early lesions may result in haemorrhage which, on exposure to gastric acid, becomes a brown haematin deposit, typically along the raised folds of the stomach. If lesions involve full thickness damage, focal necrosis (Figure 2.12) is rapidly followed by ulcer formation. Since the proliferative zone of the gastric gland is relatively superficial (Figure 2.2), healing must take place from the ulcer border. **NSAIDs** will suppress the inflammatory reaction at the base of the mucosa.

Genotoxic gastric carcinogens include a large number of dietary [32] and xenobiotic **nitrosamines**, and other genotoxic chemicals. These may be proximate carcinogens or require metabolic activation, or nitrosation in the presence of nitrite in conjunction with low pH in the stomach, to produce adenocarcinoma of the exocrine epithelium. The antral (pyloric) region of the glandular stomach is a frequent site for tumour development. **N-(2-fluorenyl)acetamide, N-methyl-N'-nitro-N-nitrosoguanidine (MNNG), 1,2:5,6-dibenzanthracene** and **MCA** are

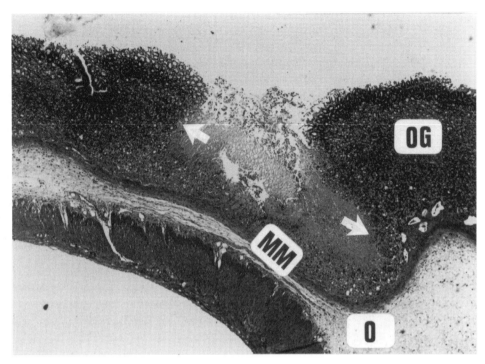

Figure 2.12   Acute ulceration of the rat gastric mucosa following angiotensin II antagonist treatment. Note pale well-demarcated lesion (↔) filled with necrotic glandular tissue following acute exposure to the drug. The oxyntic glands (OG) to either side are of normal appearance. There is no breach in the muscularis mucosae (MM). The submucosa shows inflammatory oedema (O).

typical genotoxic carcinogens, active in the stomach and other sites [33]. Many nitrosamines are forestomach and/or glandular stomach carcinogens in the rat, and the mode of administration in either the diet or drinking water determines the main target tissue, with either squamous cell carcinoma of the forestomach, or adenocarcinoma of the antral mucosa, as the outcome.

Some **secondary amines** can generate **nitrosamines** in the presence of nitrite. This conversion may involve bacterial metabolism. Certain drugs can also form *N*-nitro derivates under acidic conditions with nitrite (**piperazine, phenacetin, oxytetracycline, cimetidine, disulphiram, quinacrine, chlorpromazine**) but epidemiological evidence of human carcinogenicity involving these compounds is lacking. **Nitroso-cimetidine** has been shown to be non-carcinogenic in rats, probably as a result of rapid metabolism back to cimetidine.

Non-genotoxic gastric carcinogens include a new generation of potent, long-acting, antisecretory agents (**SK&F 93479, loxtidine, ICI 128,846** and **omeprazole**). These compounds were found to induce a novel oxyntic neuroendocrine hyperplasia and neoplasia in the stomach of the rat (Figure 2.13) and, in some cases, the mouse (Table 2.2). Induction of these 'carcinoid' tumours after 80 weeks of treatment was preceded by an early onset of hypergastrinaemia, and hyperplasia of oxyntic ECL cells which stain positively with Grimelius' method (argyrophilia), and for neuron-specific enolase, histidine decarboxylase and chromogranin A. The gastrin hypothesis (Figure 2.6) involves the pharmacological

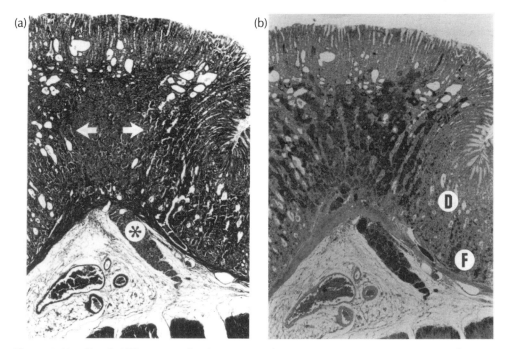

Figure 2.13 Gastric ECL neuroendocrine tumour after H$_2$-receptor antagonist treatment for 2 years in rats. (a) Haematoxylin and eosin section; intramucosal tumour (↔) showing a finger-like invasion of submucosa (∗). The surrounding oxyntic glands have dilated lumens. (b) Neuron-specific enolase (NSE) antibody staining showing NSE-positive cells filling the glands from the base within the tumour, and the submucosal area of invasion. Neighbouring oxyntic glands show diffuse (D) and focal (F) neuroendocrine cell hyperplasia.

Table 2.2 Enterochromaffin-like (ECL) cell tumour induction by antisecretory drugs

Lesion	Antisecretory drug					
	Cimetidine	Ranitidine	SK&F 93479	Loxtidine	BL6431	Omeprazole
Hypergastrinaemia	+	+	+++	+++	+++	+++++
Diffuse ECL cell hyperplasia	+	+	+++	+++	+++	++++
Focal ECL cell hyperplasia	−	+	+++	+++	+++	++++
ECL cell rat carcinoids (%M/%F)	−	ND/19	17/22	2/16	6/4	10/40
ECL cell mouse carcinoids	−	−	−	++	ND	−
Rat, no observed effect level (mg/kg per day)	950	c.2000	200	<50	55	<1

+ to +++++ indicates severity of lesion; ND, not determined.

blockade of acid secretion which leads to antral G cell hypersecretion of gastrin in response to elevated gastric pH. Hypergastrinaemia in turn causes ECL cell hyperplasia and neoplasia, and exocrine oxyntic glandular hypertrophy/hyperplasia (especially in the mouse) [34]. **Ciprofibrate** (a lipid-lowering drug) initially appeared to be an exception to the class specificity of ECL neuroendocrine tumour induction, until it too was shown to have antisecretory activity.

Some potent antisecretory agents (**omeprazole, SK&F 93479**) also produce increased eosinophilic granularity of chief cells (Figure 2.14). The mechanism for this has not been elucidated but it is also seen with unrelated agents such as **metabisulphite** [35]. Alternative hypotheses for ECL cell tumour induction include the proposal that gastrin may promote the action of exogenous or endogenous genotoxic nitrosamines [36]. However, genotoxic gastric carcinogens (e.g. **MNNG**), cause exocrine adenocarcinoma of the antrum, not fundic neuroendocrine tumours. The H_2-receptor antagonist **tiotidine** also produced adenomatous diverticulum and dysplasia/carcinoma of the antral mucosa by a mechanism probably related to a genotoxic mode of action. Less potent or shorter-acting compounds in this class of antisecretory agents were less prone to produce sufficient hypergastrinaemia to result in neoplasia in rodents, although lifetime administration of high doses did result in ECL neuroendocrine tumour development [37]. Surgical removal of most of the oxyntic mucosa by a 75 per cent fundectomy results in hypergastrinaemia, ECL cell proliferation and neoplasia. Conversely surgical removal of the antrum, the source of gastrin secretion, abolishes the ECL cell proliferation seen following **omeprazole** treatment. Therapeutic doses of these antisecretory drugs in man do not result in more than about a threefold peak rise in gastrin. This level is well below the gastrin

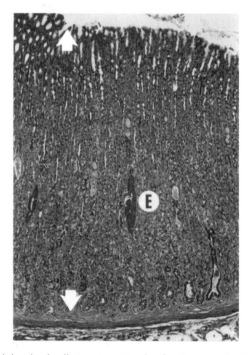

Figure 2.14   Eosinophilic chief cells in rat gastric glands. Mucosa of a 2-year-old rat treated with an H_2-receptor antagonist showing increased mucosal height (↔) and dark-staining clusters of eosinophilic chief cells (E) within the oxyntic glands.

levels associated with microcarcinoid development in patients who have chronic atrophic gastritis and a marked hypergastrinaemia sustained for many years [38].

2.4.5 Small and Large Intestine

The pyloric outflow enters the duodenum which possesses bicarbonate-secreting Brunner's glands. These glands show a vacuolated change in the dog following treatment with the β-blocker **atenolol** (Figure 2.15). No comparable changes have been observed in other animal species or in man. The epithelium of the GI tract is a site of rapid cell proliferation and, together with the bone marrow, is sensitive to **radiation** or **cytotoxic drugs** which target cells with rapid DNA or nucleotide synthesis. Given the short lifespan of intestinal enterocytes, these insults will result in rapid denudation of the villi, haemorrhage, ulceration and secondary gut microfloral invasion. The entry of bacteria or their toxins in this way can prove rapidly fatal, and the lipopolysaccharide cell wall component of Gram-negative bacteria (**endotoxin**) quickly induces congestion, hypotension, intravascular coagulation, shock and death. Gut sterilization with antibiotics can reduce or eliminate many of these effects. **Corrosive agents** typically produce only superficial and rapidly repaired lesions, whereas **cytotoxic drugs** can eliminate the proliferative stem-cell compartment which is required for repair. Lower-grade injury may result in villus stunting and clubbing, leading to a reduced absorptive area and subsequent

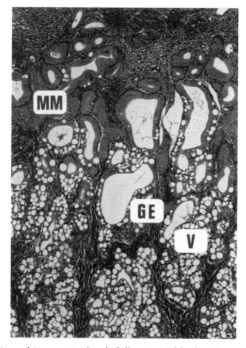

Figure 2.15 Vacuolation of Brunner's glands following β-blocker (atenolol) treatment in the dog. Brunner's glands extend through the muscularis mucosae (MM) into the submucosa. Following atenolol treatment, the epithelial cells (GE) of the glands develop cytoplasmic vacuolation (V).

malabsorption. Intestinal ulceration can occur in both the rodent and dog [39] following administration of a wide range of compounds including **NSAIDs**. Such lesions in the dog may be generalized or restricted to the mucosa overlying Peyer's patches. Deep ulcers carry a risk of necrosis and inflammation in the submucosa (Figure 2.16), muscularis externa and even the serosa, with possible subsequent perforation.

Accumulation enteropathies involving overload of the enterocyte cytoplasm with non-degraded xenobiotic [16] can lead to extensive vacuolar swelling of the cells (Figure 2.17) and cell death, resulting in the exposure and inflammation of the lamina propria. Chronic enteropathies are typically associated with chronic inflammatory conditions (hypersensitivity, ulcerative colitis), with the presence of lymphoid cells and macrophages in the lamina propria and submucosa. Also, in chronic inflammatory disease, there is often stunting of villi with a loss of absorptive area.

Malabsorption syndromes may also result from interference or overload of absorptive pathways, specific intestinal enzyme deficiencies, or loss of digestive enzyme secretion in the bile or pancreatic juice. Consequently, undigested or unabsorbed food often leads to bacterial fermentation and diarrhoea. In this condition, undigested fat or muscle fibres may be evident by faecal microscopy. Failure to absorb nutrients will be manifested in chronic loss of body weight.

Background infections may result from cross-infection or from xenobiotics causing the normal bacterial microflora to be replaced by pathogens. Tyzzer's

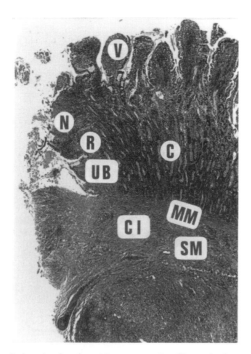

Figure 2.16   Duodenal ulcer in the dog. Note necrosis of intestinal mucosa (N) with loss of both villi (V) and crypts (C). Chronic inflammation and fibroplasia (CI) extend through muscularis mucosae (MM) into the submucosa (SM). There is a sharp demarcation of the ulcer border (UB) on the left with epithelial loss and regeneration (R).

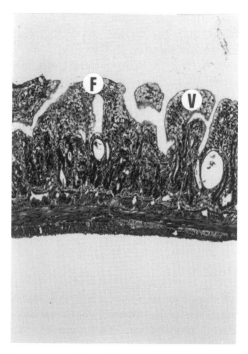

Figure 2.17 Accumulation enteropathy in the rat small intestine. Note vacuolated epithelium (V) and mucosal damage with both loss and fusion of villi (F), reducing the area for absorption.

disease (*Bacillus piliformis*) affects rabbits [40] and rodents and is manifest as colitis and hepatitis. *Helicobacter pylori* has been implicated in gastric ulcer disease in man [41] and *Campylobacter* spp. can cause diarrhoea in the dog and man. Transmissible ileal hyperplasia of hamsters is a proliferative response to *Citrobacter freundii* [42].

Gut microfloral modification is seen typically following chronic antibiotic administration. Animals maintained under gnotobiotic (germ free) conditions show a marked reduction in GALT and a generalized underdeveloped immune system, demonstrating the role of antigenic stimulation by the normal gut microflora. Modification of the microfloral spectrum by chronic, high-dose, antibiotic administration may have toxicological sequelae. Broad-spectrum antibiotics may lead to prolonged coagulation times through the elimination of **vitamin K**-forming bacteria. **Penicillin** and **erythromycin** cause a severe haemorrhagic colitis in guinea pigs and enterocolitis can be produced in hamsters and rabbits administered **lincomycin,** and related antibiotics, because of the overgrowth of pathogens. Pseudomembranous colitis in man is associated with **lincomycin** and **clindamycin** antibiotic administration. Abdominal pain, fever, leucocytosis, bloody diarrhoea and a fibrinous necrotizing colitis results from the growth in the gut of *Clostridium difficile*, which produces an exotoxin. **Clindamycin** may also interfere with colonic water transport pathways.

Intestinal carcinogenesis is uncommon and is typically confined to the colon where the turnover of epithelial cell populations is slower. This may perhaps allow time for the growth of transformed cells through a crypt dysplasia/adenoma/carcinoma sequence [43]. In man, the inherited disorder polyposis coli, and chronic ulcerative colitis, are important risk factors for development of colon carcinoma. Dietary **nitrate, low fibre, high fat intake,** and endogenous **bile acids** have been implicated in the development of these conditions [44].

Experimentally, **bracken fern, 3,2′-dimethyl-4-aminobiphenyl** and **dimethyl-hydrazine (DMH)** are potent colon carcinogens in the rat. **DMH** is metabolized by the gut microflora to **azomethane, azoxymethane** and finally to the proximate carcinogen **methylazoxymethanol (MAM). Cycasin** (from cycad plants) also liberates **MAM** through the action of glycosidases in the bacteria *Streptobacillus* and *Lactobacillus* spp.

Carrageenans are sulphated galactose polysaccharides which, if hydrolysed to low-molecular-weight fragments, can induce a chronic ulcerative colitis with macrophage infiltration in rodents. Chronic exposure to **carrageenans** results in mucous metaplasia, adenomatous polyp formation and, ultimately, colonic adenocarcinoma and squamous cell carcinoma [45].

2.4.6 *Exocrine Pancreas*

Target organ toxicity of the pancreas is uncommon. A number of **nitrosamines** at high doses can produce acute necrosis of both acinar and ductal elements. Regeneration is via ductal proliferation. The embryological origin of liver and exocrine pancreas, which develop as endodermal outgrowths of the gut, is shown by hepatocytic differentiation of regenerating exocrine tissue in some model systems in the hamster [46] and other rodents. **Copper deficient diets** facilitate the expression of this metaplastic change. The presence of **trypsinogen, lipase** and other potent digestive enzymes in the pancreas can result in the release of these enzymes into surrounding tissues following acute necrosis of pancreatic acinar tissue. The release of **lipase** results in fat necrosis, often followed by acute toxic shock.

Pancreatic hypertrophy and hyperplasia and the promotion of acinar neoplasia can be induced by feeding **high fat diets,** including **corn oil** when used as a vehicle, or by the use of **raw soya flour diets** [47, 48]. A heat-labile, **soya bean, trypsin inhibitor** prevents the digestion of a secreted marker peptide which is monitored by ileal I cells. Increased CCK secretion by these cells, in response to a perceived deficit in proteolysis, results in pancreatic hypersecretion, hypertrophy, focal hyperplasia and subsequent exocrine adenoma and adenocarcinoma development.

2.5 Testing for Toxicity

Evaluation of GI toxicity calls for the use of a wide range of routine and special investigational techniques. Vomiting is not uncommonly observed in dogs and it is important to determine whether it is due to CNS or a local GI effect. Local irritant effects usually result in vomiting immediately after dosing, whereas CNS effects typically appear after plasma levels of the compound rise, perhaps 1 to 2 hours after dosing. Administering the compound after feeding may ameliorate local GI effects. Irritants inducing gastric erosion or ulceration may be associated with symptoms of abdominal pain and if significant haemorrhage into the gut occurs, this will result in faeces which are black with the degradation products of haemoglobin. The use of test kits for occult blood (or more specifically haem) can be unreliable and a dog diet containing animal products may give false positive findings. Careful histological evaluation of accurately sampled tissue blocks is the method of choice in this situation. Because small punctate erosions can result in bleeding, with red cells interacting with gastric acid to produce brown haematin on the mucosal surface, the site of these lesions should be identified and separate blocks prepared from these, as the erosions may be less evident after fixation.

International regulatory guidelines specify the examination of the following levels of the GI tract: tongue, oesophagus, stomach (including forestomach in rodents), small intestine (duodenum, jejunum and ileum in a Swiss roll), large intestine (caecum, colon, rectum), liver and pancreas.

At necropsy, a macroscopic examination of the oral cavity is essential and in the rodent this is facilitated by removal of the lower jaw at necropsy. Any sites of ulceration, or reddening, or the development of a mass, should be taken for histology. Lesions of the teeth or gums require decalcified sections of the jaw or head to be taken. Standard rodent nasal cavity head sections should include sections of tooth roots which may be informative in the case of cytotoxic drugs causing tooth malformations. Porphyrin-related pink coloration of teeth shows a characteristic fluorescence in UV light. Collection of the tongue in rodents should include the band of lingual salivary glands behind the dorsum.

The oesophagus is normally sampled in the mid-thoracic region. After careful examination of the serosal surface of the abdominal viscera, the GI tract can be removed *in toto* by cutting along the mesenteric attachments. Given that most lesions will be present on the inner (mucosal) surface of the gut, careful opening of the length of the gut, except for short pieces taken for fixation (see below), is recommended. The stomach should be opened along the greater curvature, carefully examined and pinned out for fixation. The alternative procedure of inflating the stomach with fixative followed by opening and examination of the fixed tissue is less reliable for the detection of focal erosions. Although not required by guidelines, stomach weight can be a good measure of mucosal, and possibly muscularis, hypertrophy. If morphometric analysis of the mucosa is desired, pinning out to flatten the mucosa is essential and estimation of the total area of mucosa is indicated for the calculation of total mucosal volume.

The Swiss roll technique maximizes the area of small intestine examined but is only practicable in rodents. It is not widely used in regulatory toxicology, where a good macroscopic examination at necropsy, plus taking three segments of small intestine at the relevant levels, is generally considered adequate. Sections of intestine are best taken as segments (dog) or short unopened tubes (rodent) to permit rapid fixation, without eversion of the mucosa with contraction of the muscularis in fixative. The duodenum should be sampled close to the pylorus, to ensure inclusion of Brunner's glands, which are present only in the most proximal part. In the rodent, the duodenum can be left attached to the stomach and a longitudinal strip through the antrum, pylorus and proximal duodenum provides an optimal section. The position of Peyer's patches is usually evident on the serosal aspect and these should be included in the ileum block. Special staining techniques may require the use of frozen, Bouin's fixed or benzoquinone fixed tissue, to allow histochemical or immunocytochemical procedures to be applied, e.g. to demonstrate gastrin-secreting G cells (Figure 2.18).

A number of compounds can produce caecal enlargement due to osmotic, fermentational or neural effects and caecal weight can provide a reliable measure of an increase in size in the absence of pathological lesions.

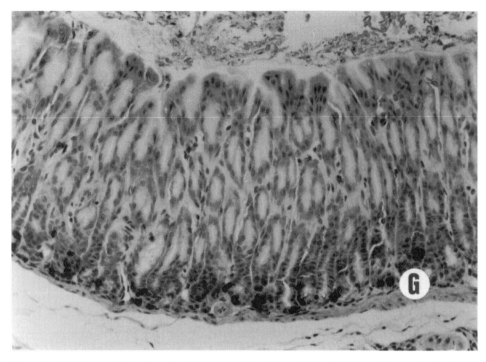

Figure 2.18 Immunohistochemical demonstration of antral G cells. Note dispersed, single, dark, gastrin-positive cells (G) located at the base of the antral glands.

Assessments of malabsorption and pancreatic insufficiency are well established for the dog as these are conditions presenting in clinical practice. They are not often applied to rodents or to regulatory toxicology studies. Microscopic examination of the faeces for evidence of undigested fat or muscle fibres is of limited value for animals fed laboratory chow. Intestinal alkaline phosphatase (ALP) can be specifically measured as an isozyme in the plasma but standard toxicological practice is to measure only total ALP activity. Pancreatic trypsinogen insufficiency tests use an orally administered BT-PABA substrate. Para-aminobenzoic acid (PABA) is cleaved by protease activity, absorbed and measured in plasma as a measure of pancreatic function. However, this test has generally been replaced by the measurement of trypsin-like immunoreactivity in plasma as a measure of pancreatic insufficiency [49]. However, the application of such techniques to rodents is wanting. One clinical pathology marker for GI erosion or ulceration is a regenerative anaemia. Lesser injury to the mucosa may result in the leakage of plasma proteins into the gut with a resultant hypoalbuminaemia. Malabsorption as a result of small intestinal pathology has been assessed using serum folate and vitamin B_{12} concentrations. Here, jejunal pathology is reflected in low folate, and ileal pathology in low B_{12} concentrations, respectively [50], these being the main sites of absorption of these vitamins. However, intestinal malabsorption must be differentiated from pancreatic insufficiency. It should also be noted that chronic GI disease may lead to protein deficiency, oedema and other complications. Clearly any digestive disturbance may result in impaired gain or maintenance of body weight.

GI peptides can be measured in the plasma. Collection of blood into tubes containing aprotinin (a protease inhibitor) is indicated to prevent protease degradation of the peptide prior to analysis. Given the minor sequence differences between species for these hormones, together with their presence as multiple forms in terms of chain length, sulphation and phosphorylation, careful validation of immunoassay conditions and antibody specificity is required.

A variety of investigational techniques are available for the study of GI toxicities. In dogs, gastroscopy using fibre optics can be used to serially monitor the appearance of the mucosa, and biopsy samples can be obtained for histopathology. Radiography, particularly fluoroscopy following the administration of barium meals, is a standard veterinary procedure and can be valuable in studying motility disorders. Endoscopy of the rat stomach is feasible using a human paediatric bronchoscope. Alternatively, the creation of a gastric fistula with a titanium port can allow chronic monitoring of gastric acid secretion [34], biopsy histology, and endoscopy. The action of cytotoxic drugs and carcinogens can be characterized by measurement of DNA synthesis and cell proliferation using tritiated thymidine or bromodeoxyuridine (BrDU) immunostaining. In the latter technique, BrDU, a thymidine analogue, is administered for a defined period either in the drinking water or by mini-pump. Tissues are then processed and BrDU incorporated into DNA is visualized by immunostaining with an anti-BrDU antibody. Proliferative events can thus be quantified to establish time, and dose–response relationships.

Scanning electron microscopy has provided an early marker for superficial injury to the GI epithelium, although the overlying mucous layer may obscure changes. Intestinal sampling using a biopsy capsule is feasible in the dog but this technique has not been applied to toxicology. Studies of changes in the large intestine are based primarily on pathology; rectal histology is important in establishing the potential irritancy of suppositories.

In vitro methodologies in GI toxicology range from isolated organ culture to cell culture techniques. Freshly isolated intestine, stripped of the muscularis externa, turned inside out and ligated to form a closed tube, can be used to study fluxes of water, electrolytes and organic molecules, including xenobiotics, across the gut epithelium. However, the viability of such systems in organ baths is generally short. Using enzymic digestion techniques applied from the serosal surface, mucosal epithelial cell suspensions can be prepared and purified by elutriation. Biochemical assays, and the *in vitro* study of secretion and the action of secretagogues and antagonists, has provided much detailed information on the pathophysiology of GI function. It should be remembered, however, that activity is an integral of several stimulatory and inhibitory pathways, including autonomic innervation, and hence cell systems are incomplete in these respects.

2.6 Conclusions

The GI tract represents one of the largest and most complex organs of the body and yet the level of toxicological knowledge on this system is low, compared with the extensive research base which exists for the liver and kidney. As a result, the sensitivity and predictiveness of GI findings in animals to human clinical experience is lower than for the better-researched target organs. Conversely, toxicological findings in the GI tract are less likely to be false positives. Considering that GI side-effects are frequent in clinical adverse event reporting, there is clearly scope for better evaluation of the system. NSAIDs have been widely studied in this regard, but species differences and idiosyncrasies in patient responses have complicated the search for a quantitative animal model. The dominant position of antisecretory drugs in global drug sales has attracted much debate about the relevance of rodent findings of ECL neoplasia for man: interestingly, work in animals has provoked a better appreciation of the biology of ECL cell microcarcinoids in man. The complexities of the autonomic nervous system, and the plethora of peptide mediators of secretion, motility and absorption in the GI tract, continue to be poorly understood and probably hold the secrets to irritable bowel syndrome and other unexplained clinical disorders. To the scientist interested in metabolism, the interaction of mammalian and bacterial metabolism, enterohepatic recirculation, changing pH and high local exposure, is a major challenge. Cancer of the GI tract remains a common and intractable cause of death in man and the role of the many natural and synthetic carcinogens in the daily diet continues to be a focus in cancer research. The GI tract therefore remains a major challenge to research and regulatory toxicologists alike.

References

1. EVANS, H.E. and CHRISTENSEN, G.C. (1979) *Miller's Anatomy of the Dog*, 2nd Edn, Philadelphia: W.B. Saunders.
2. HEBEL, R. and STROMBERG, M.N. (1976) *Anatomy of the Laboratory Rat*, Baltimore: Williams and Wilkins.
3. LI, A.K.C., SCHATTENKERK, M.E., HUFFMAN, R.G., ROSS, J.S. and MALT, R.A. (1983) Hypersecretion of submandibular saliva in male mice: trophic response in small intestine, *Gastroenterology*, **84**, 949–955.
4. JOHNSON, L.R. (1987) Regulation of gastrointestinal growth, in JOHNSON, L.R. (Ed.) *Physiology of the Gastrointesinal Tract*, 2nd Edn, pp. 301–333, New York: Raven.
5. HELANDER, H.F. (1981) The cells of the gastric mucosa, *International Review of Cytology*, **70**, 217–289.
6. SMITH, B. and BUTLER, M. (1978) The effects of long term propranolol on the salivary glands and intestinal serosa of the mouse, *Journal of Pathology*, **124**, 185–187.
7. DAUGHERTY, D. and YAMADA, T. (1989) Posttranslational processing of gastrin, *Physiological Reviews*, **69**, 482–502.
8. REHM, S., SOMMER, R. and DEERBERG, F. (1987) Spontaneous non-neoplastic gastric lesions in female Han:NMRI mice and influence of food restriction throughout life, *Veterinary Pathology*, **24**, 216–225.
9. KAMINSKY, L.S. and FASCO, M.J. (1992) Small intestinal cytochrome P450s, *CRC Critical Reviews in Toxicology*, **21**, 407–422.
10. LEVIN, R.J. (1969) The effect of hormones on the absorptive, metabolic and digestive functions of the small intestine, *Journal of Endocrinology*, **45**, 315–348.
11. HENNING, S.J. (1984) Hormonal and dietary regulation of intestinal enzyme development, in SCHILLER, C.M. (Ed.) *Intestinal Toxicology*, pp. 17–32, New York: Raven.
12. NAUKKARINEN, A. and SYRJANEN, K.J. (1986) Immunoresponse of the gastrointestinal tract, in ROZMAN, K. and HANNINEN, O. (Eds) *Gastrointestinal Toxicity*, pp. 213–245, Amsterdam: Elsevier.
13. LEEGWATER, D.C., DE GROOT, A.P. and VAN KALMTHOUT-KUYPER, M. (1974) The aetiology of caecal enlargement in the rat, *Food and Cosmetic Toxicology*, **24**, 687–697.
14. ALLAN, S.G. and SMYTH, J.F. (1986) Small intestinal mucosal toxicity of *cis*-platinum

– comparison of toxicity of platinum analogues and dexamethasone, *British Journal of Cancer*, **53**, 355–360.

15. BENNETT, R.E., HARRISON, M.W., BISHOP, C.J., SEARLE, J. and KERR, J.F.R. (1984) The role of apoptosis in the atrophy of small gut mucosa produced by repeated administration of cytosine arabinoside, *Journal of Pathology*, **142**, 259–263.

16. MURGATROYD, L.B. (1980) A morphological and histochemical study of a drug-induced enteropathy in the Alderley Park rat, *British Journal of Experimental Pathology*, **61**, 567–578.

17. GRAY, J.E., WEAVER, R.N., SINKULA, A.A., SCHURR, P.E. and MORAN, J. (1974) Drug-induced enteropathy characterised by lipid in macrophages, *Toxicology and Applied Pharmacology*, **27**, 147–157.

18. MAZUE, G., VIC, P., GOUY, D., REMANDET, B., LACHERETZ, F., BERTHIE, J., BARCHEWITZ, G. and GAGNOL, J.P. (1984) Recovery from amiodarone induced lipidosis in laboratory animals: a toxicological study, *Fundamental and Applied Toxicology*, **4**, 992–999.

19. HEIJL, L. and SUNDIN, Y. (1988) Nitrendipine induced gingival overgrowth in dogs, *Journal of Periodontology*, **60**, 104–112.

20. VAHLSING, H.L., FERINGA, E.R., BRITTEN, A.G. and KINNING, W.K. (1975) Dental abnormalities in rats after a single dose of cyclophosphamide, *Cancer Research*, **35**, 2199–2202.

21. GRENBY, T.H. and COLLEY, J. (1983) Dental effects of xylitol compared with other carbohydrates and polyols in the diet of laboratory rats, *Archives of Oral Biology*, **28**, 745–758.

22. KASWAN, R.L., MARTIN, C.L. and CHAPMAN, W.L. (1984) Keratoconjunctivitis sicca: histopathologic study of nictitating membrane and lacrimal glands from 28 dogs, *American Journal of Veterinary Research*, **45**, 112–118.

23. OLOVSON, S.-G., BJORKMAN, J.-A., EK, L. and HAVU, N. (1983) The ulcerogenic effect on the oesophagus of three β-adrenoceptor antagonists, investigated in a new porcine oesophagus test model, *Acta Pharmacologica et Toxicologica*, **53**, 385–391.

24. FIELD, W.E.H. and ROE, F.J.C. (1965) Tumour promotion in the forestomach epithelium of mice by oral administration of citrus oils, *Journal of the National Cancer Institute*, **35**, 771–787.

25. WESTER, P.W. and KROES, R. (1988) Forestomach carcinogens: pathology and relevance to man, *Toxicologic Pathology*, **16**, 165–171.

26. SHIRAI, T., FUKUSHIMA, S., OHSHIMA, M., MASUDA, A. and ITO, N. (1984) Effects of butylated hydroxyanisole, butylated hydroxytoluene and NaCl on gastric carcinogenesis initiated with *N*-methyl-*N'*-nitro-*N*-nitrosoguanidine in F344 rats, *Journal of the National Cancer Institute*, **72**, 1189–1198.

27. MIRVISH, S.S., WANG, M.-Y., SMITH, J.W., DESHPANDE, A.D., MAKARY, M.H. and ISSNBERG, P. (1985) β- to ω-Hydroxylation of the oesophageal carcinogen methyl-*n*-amylnitrosamine by the rat oesophagus and related tissues, *Cancer Research*, **45**, 577–583.

28. ELLIOTT, G.A., PURMALIS, A., VAN DER MEER, D.A. and DENLINGER, R.H. (1988) The proprionic acids, gastrointestinal toxicity in various species, *Toxicologic Pathology*, **16**, 245–250.

29. CHEVILLE, N.F. (1979) Uremic gastropathy in the dog, *Veterinary Pathology*, **16**, 292–309.

30. GANA, T.J., KOO, J. and MACPHERSON, B.R. (1992) Gross and histologic effects of topical misoprostol on canine gastric mucosa, *Experimental Toxicology and Pathology*, **44**, 40–46.

31. REINHART, W.H., MULLER, O. and HALTER, F. (1983) Influence of long term 16,16-dimethyl prostaglandin E_2 treatment on the rat gastrointestinal mucosa, *Gastroenterology*, **85**, 1003–1010.

32. SHEPHARD, S.E., SCHLATTER, C. and LUTZ, W.K. (1987) Assessment of the risk of formation of carcinogenic *N*-nitroso compounds from dietary precursors in the stomach, *Food and Cosmetic Toxicology*, **25**, 91–108.

33. THOMPSON, M.H. (1984) Aetiological factors in gastrointestinal carcinogenesis, *Scandinavian Journal of Gastroenterology*, **19** (Suppl 104), 80–97.

34. BETTON, G.R., DORMER, C.S., WELLS, T., PERT, P., PRICE, C.A. and BUCKLEY, P. (1988) Gastric ECL-cell hyperplasia and carcinoids in rodents following chronic administration of H_2-antagonists SK&F 93479 and oxmetidine and omeprazole, *Toxicologic Pathology*, **16**, 288–298.

35. BEEMS, R.B., SPIT, B.J., KOETER, H.B.W.M. and FERON, V.J. (1982) Nature and histogenesis of sulphite induced gastric lesions in rats, *Experimental and Molecular Pathology*, **36**, 316–325.

36. PENSTON, J. and WORMSLEY, K.G. (1987) Achlorhydria: hypergastrinaemia: carcinoids – a flawed hypothesis?, *Gut*, **28**, 488–505.

37. HAVU, N., MATTSON, H., EKMAN, L. and CARLSSON, E. (1990) Enterochromaffin-like cell carcinoids in the rat gastric mucosa following long term administration of ranitidine, *Digestion*, **45**, 189–195.

38. CREUTZFELDT, W. and LAMBERTS, R. (1991) Is hypergastrinaemia dangerous to man?, *Scandinavian Journal of Gastroenterology*, **26** (Suppl 180), 179–191.

39. STEWART, T.H.M., HETENYI, C., ROWSELL, H. and ORIZAGA, M. (1980) Ulcerative enterocolitis in dogs induced by drugs, *Journal of Pathology*, **131**, 363–378.

40. ALLEN, A.M., GANAWAY, J.R., MOORE, T.D. and KINARD, R.F. (1965) Taxers disease syndrome in laboratory rabbits, *American Journal of Pathology*, **46**, 859–881.

41. RATHBONE, B.J., WYATT, J.I. and HEATLEY, R.V. (1986) *Campylobacter pyloridis* – a new factor in peptic ulcer disease?, *Gut*, **27**, 635–641.

42. JACOBY, R.O. (1978) Transmissible ileal hyperplasia of hamsters, *American Journal of Pathology*, **91**, 433–450.

43. NAKAMURA, S. and KINO, I. (1985) Morphogenesis of experimental colonic neoplasms induced by dimethylhydrazine, in PFEIFFER, C.J. (Ed.) *Animal Models for Intestinal Disease*, pp. 99–122, Boca Raton: CRC Press.

44. WEISBURGER, J.H. and HORN, C.L. (1984) Human and laboratory studies on the causes and prevention of gastrointestinal cancer, *Scandinavian Journal of Gastroenterology*, **19** (Suppl 104), 15–26.

45. ISHIOKI, T., KUWABARA, N., OOHASHI, Y. and WAKABAYASHI, K. (1987) Induction of colorectal tumors in rats by sulphated polysaccharides, *CRC Critical Reviews in Toxicology*, **17**, 215–244.

46. MAKINO, T., USUDA, N., RAO, S., REDDY, J. and SCARPELLI, D.G. (1990) Transdifferentiation of ductular cells into hepatocytes in regenerating hamster pancreas, *Laboratory Investigation*, **62**, 552–561.

47. RAO, M.S. (1987) Animal models of exocrine pancreatic carcinogenesis, *Cancer and Metastasis Reviews*, **6**, 665–676.

48. EUSTIS, S.L. and BOORMAN, G.A. (1985) Proliferative lesions of the exocrine pancreas: relationship to corn oil gavage in the national toxicology program, *Journal of the National Cancer Institute*, **75**, 1067–1073.

49. WILLIAMS, D.A. (1985) The diagnosis of canine exocrine pancreatic insufficiency, *The Veterinary Annual*, **25**, 330–336.

50. BATT, R.M. and MORGAN, J.O. (1982) Role of serum folate and vitamin B_{12} concentrations in the differentiation of small intestinal abnormalities in the dog, *Research in Veterinary Science*, **32**, 17–22.

3

The Digestive System II:
The Hepatobiliary System

JOHN G. EVANS AND BRIAN G. LAKE

3.1 Introduction

Over 600 drugs and many man-made and natural chemicals have shown evidence of toxicity to the liver of man or laboratory animals. Furthermore, the liver has proved to be the predominant site of neoplastic development during bioassays for carcinogenicity in rats and mice. This has made the liver the most widely studied organ for the investigation of the mechanisms of toxicity and carcinogenicity. In addition, hepatocytes may be readily isolated from the liver and maintained in culture under controlled conditions for detailed examination of the cellular and biochemical events associated with toxicity.

3.2 Anatomy, Histology and Physiology

3.2.1 Anatomy

The liver is the body's largest visceral organ, accounting for between 2.5 and 5 per cent of the body weight, dependent on species. In man and laboratory animals the liver is a lobed structure and in all commonly used species other than the rat there is a gall bladder. In life the organ is found in the anterior abdominal cavity bounded cranially by the diaphragm and protected by the arc of the rib cage. Caudally, the liver is in contact with the right kidney, the stomach and other parts of the gastrointestinal tract. The normal liver is dark red in colour due to the large quantity of blood it contains.

The liver has a dual blood supply. Arterial blood enters the liver through the hepatic artery, a branch of the anterior mesenteric artery which comes directly off the abdominal aorta. There is also a venous supply that passes from the gut to the liver through the hepatic portal vein. The hepatic artery and the hepatic portal vein enter the liver at the hilus; both vessels branch as, or soon after, they enter the liver to supply the different lobes. Blood leaves the liver through the hepatic vein which joins the caudal vena cava. Also leaving the liver at the hilus is the common bile duct which carries bile from the liver to the duodenum. In species having a gall bladder, a short cystic duct joins the gall bladder to the common bile duct at the hilus.

3.2.2 *Histology*

The microscopic structure of the liver is determined by the vascular supply and associated connective tissue. Branches of the hepatic artery, portal vein and biliary system are found within connective tissue sheaths called portal tracts or triads. In addition to these three prominent structures there are nerves and lymphatics within these areas. With each division of the vessels and bile ducts the portal areas become smaller until they define the periphery of a classic hepatic lobule with a branch of the hepatic portal vein at the centre.

Branches of the portal vein form preterminal and then terminal vessels within the smallest portal tracts. The terminal vessels form venules which pass directly into the hepatic sinusoids. Blood entering the sinusoids drains across the lobule into a branch of the hepatic vein. In man this is a small terminal vein, whereas in the rat, veins as large as 200 µm may have sinusoids emptying directly into them.

The sinusoids are lined by endothelial cells and Kupffer cells. There are no tight junctions between endothelial cells within the sinusoids. In addition, there are many diaphragm-free fenestrations between the endothelial cells, allowing free access of plasma to the space of Disse and, therefore, to the plasma membrane of the hepatocytes.

Phagocytic Kupffer cells lie on the vascular side of the endothelium, although processes may pass through endothelial fenestrations into the space of Disse. Fat-storing (Ito) cells are found within the space of Disse, and occasional cells containing electron-dense granules (pit cells) may be seen. The latter are infrequently found and are thought to be natural killer cells.

Various morphological/physiological associations have been made to allow description of the microscopic anatomy of the liver (Figure 3.1). The first emphasizes the anatomical markers of the portal tract and central hepatic vein, and describes the flow of blood across the lobule from the portal area to the central vein. This is the 'classic' hepatic lobule and is conceived as being roughly hexagonal in

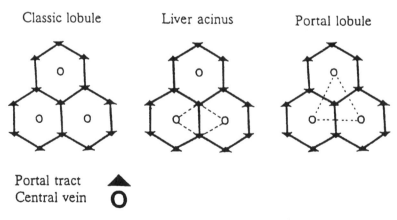

Classic lobule   Liver acinus   Portal lobule

Portal tract ▲
Central vein O

Figure 3.1   Primary hepatic units.

shape. This morphological form is rarely seen in practice, except in the pig, in which the periphery is outlined by a thin septum of connective tissue. None the less, histopathological descriptions of hepatic injury often make use of this concept of the hepatic lobule in order to describe the site of damage.

The second association, referred to as the portal lobule, considers the exocrine function of the liver, in which acini supplying a terminal bile duct are the primary hepatic unit. A third description of the primary hepatic unit was developed by Rappaport and his colleagues and was based on the observation that hepatic toxicity could not always be described in terms of the classic hepatic lobule. They proposed that the fundamental unit of the liver was the hepatic acinus [1]. This structure was an area of liver supplied by a terminal hepatic portal vein and artery. This also served as the primary metabolic unit of the liver, being dependent on the oxygen tension in its various parts; the further from the terminal vasculature, the lower the oxygen tension. In this regard three zones were defined: zones 1, 2 and 3, being equivalent to the periportal, mid-zonal and centrilobular areas of the classic hepatic lobule. The equivalence is not exact, however, as a single hepatic acinus will encompass parts from two or more classic lobules. Three or more simple acini form a complex acinus, while several complex acini form an acinar agglomerate. Thus, as in other glandular structures, there is a hierarchical structure to the liver based on a simple functional unit [1].

The hepatocyte is described as polyhedral in shape, although there may be some variation in different parts of the lobule. In man the average volume of the hepatocyte is approximately 11×10^3 μm^3. This is twice as large as that of the dog and rat, in which the average volume of hepatocytes is 4.8×10^3 μm^3. However, there is a size differential across the lobule, smaller hepatocytes being found in the periportal areas and larger hepatocytes in the vicinity of the central vein. This difference in size is also reflected in the mean density of hepatocytes from the different zones. This allows separation of the hepatocytes from the different zones by centrifugation on Ficoll density gradients.

The numerical proportion of cell types in human and rat liver are shown in Table 3.1. In man, 60 per cent of liver cells are hepatocytes, whereas in the rat this figure is 80 per cent. In both species, however, hepatocytes account for 80 per cent of hepatic volume [2].

The considerable metabolic activity of hepatocytes is reflected in the structure of the cells. The round, centrally placed, nucleus forms between 5 and 10 per cent of hepatocyte volume and has a prominent nucleolus with clumps of heterochromatin dispersed along the nuclear membrane and around the nucleolus. Ultrastructural

Table 3.1 Proportion (%) of cell types in normal human and rat liver

	Human	Rat
Hepatocyte	61	80
Sinusoidal	33	15
Bile duct	2.0	0.6
Connective tissue	2.2	0.2
Blood vessel	1.8	0.3

studies have shown that these clumps are in association with nuclear pores. The nucleolus is formed of two structural components: a granular and a fibrillar part. The nucleus has a double membrane, the outer part being continuous with the endoplasmic reticulum. The inner and outer parts are also fused at many points, forming pores through which macromolecules enter and exit the nucleus.

In newborn and fetal liver, the majority of hepatocytes are mononuclear and diploid. As the animal ages the ploidy of hepatocytes increases. This increase is species and sex dependent.

The plasma membrane has three surfaces: canalicular, sinusoidal and intercellular. The canalicular surface is a space between adjacent hepatocytes and accounts for approximately 13 per cent of the surface area of the hepatocyte cell membrane. The canaliculus is a tube-like structure that forms a network around hepatocytes and drains bile from the point of formation into bile ductules in the portal region. The canaliculus is sealed by a 'leaky' tight junction supported by desmosomes and microfilaments. The intercellular surfaces are held together by desmosomes, stud-like connections, and gap-junctions through which low-molecular-weight molecules may pass. The sinusoidal surface bears a considerable number of microvilli which increase the exposed surface of the hepatocyte to plasma in the space of Disse.

The endoplasmic reticulum (ER) accounts for approximately 15 per cent of cell volume. It is divided into rough (RER) and smooth (SER), depending on whether ribosomes are attached to the surface. In electron micrographs, the RER appears as membrane arrays studded with small particles, whereas the SER appears as vesicular profiles interspersed between other organelles. A number of Golgi complexes are also associated with the ER. In electron micrographs, the Golgi appears as a stack of plate-shaped cisternae with round vesicles appearing to separate at their periphery. There may be as many as 50 Golgi per hepatocyte and they are more numerous near the canalicular membrane.

Mitochondria appear as cylinders with a double membrane, the inner membrane being folded to form many cristae. This structure means there are two spaces within the mitochondria: the matrix space and intermembrane space. Mitochondria may also be identified at the light microscopic level by supravital staining with the redox dye, Janus green B. There are between 800 and 1000 mitochondria per cell.

Lysosomes and peroxisomes are membrane-bound structures. Lysosomes are rich in hydrolytic acid phosphatases showing optimal activity at a pH of around five. They are highly pleomorphic, showing either few internal structural features or containing dense pigment, myelin figures or partially digested organelles. A diagnostic feature is a membrane-bound structure which reacts positively for acid phosphatase. Both their size and number may increase in various disease states. Peroxisomes (microbodies) are similar structures bounded by a single membrane. They are approximately 0.2 to 0.4 µm in diameter and each hepatocyte contains approximately 200 to 250. Peroxisomes are involved in oxidative action involving molecular oxygen. As a result, hydrogen peroxide is produced which is destroyed by the activity of catalase. Catalase activity may be identified histochemically by the 3,3′-diaminobenzene (DAB) method. Mature peroxisomes of a number of species including the rat, but not man, contain a laminated nucleoid structure formed of uric oxidase. The half-life of peroxisomes is approximately 1.5 days and they may increase in number following treatment with a variety of agents including hypolipidaemic drugs and phthalate esters. Numbers may also be increased by dietary and hormonal factors and following partial hepatectomy.

As well as these well-defined organelles, the hepatocyte also contains a number of other elements. These include microtubules, intermediate filaments and micro-filaments. The role of microtubules in the liver is unclear but they may be involved in transport processes. Actin filaments are 6 nm in diameter, and are formed from a soluble pool of globular actin with which they are in dynamic equilibrium. Actin filaments form a structural skeleton throughout the hepatocyte but are particularly prominent in the pericanalicular and perisinusoidal regions. Accumulation of actin filaments has been found in the pericanalicular region during cholestasis. Myosin filaments are present in a ratio of 1 : 100 with actin and play an important regulatory role in cell motility. Intermediate filaments are 1 to 10 nm in diameter; they are present throughout the cytoplasm and form the support structure for the cell. They are particularly concentrated in the perinuclear region and along the border of the cell. They also form attachments to desmosomes and aggregate in certain forms of liver injury.

The compartmental structure of the hepatocyte is not a static one. Materials may be taken up by receptor-mediated endocytosis into clatharin-coated pits and vesicles. After fusion of the vesicles with lysosomes, the contents of the vesicles may be digested by lysosomal enzymes and the product used within the hepatocyte or secreted into bile.

As well as diversity based upon biochemical activity, hepatocytes in different regions show considerable structural diversity. The nuclei in hepatic acinar zone 1 are predominantly diploid, whereas increased ploidy is found in zone 3. Furthermore, rough endoplasmic reticulum is more numerous in the zone 1 region, whereas smooth endoplasmic reticulum predominates in zone 3. Mitochondria are larger and more numerous in zone 1, accounting for 20 per cent of cell volume, whereas in zone 3 they are smaller and less numerous, forming only 13 per cent of cell volume. These morphological differences are related to zonal differences in metabolic and catabolic patterns and undoubtedly play an important role in the differential toxicity that is frequently seen in the liver.

The mitotic index of hepatocytes in the normal rat liver is approximately 0.03 per cent and the average life of the cell is between 150 and 200 days.

3.2.3 *Physiology*

The physiology of the liver is complex but is based on its dual function of an endocrine and exocrine gland. Furthermore, Kupffer cells within the sinusoids serve to remove particulate material from the bloodstream and in so doing play an important role in the modulation of the immune mechanism and in the removal of damaged or dead cells from the circulation.

The liver, in its endocrine function, is the major site for the synthesis of most plasma proteins except immunoglobulins. These include albumin, almost all the blood clotting factors, acute phase proteins and the proteins involved in lipid transport. It is also the major site for the synthesis of cholesterol in the body and plays a pivotal role in intermediate metabolism. As a consequence of this extensive metabolic activity there is considerable heat production, which is important in maintaining body temperature [3].

The exocrine function of the liver is served by the production and excretion of bile into the intestine. Bile acids and salts function to emulsify fat prior to absorption from the gastrointestinal tract. Furthermore, bile forms an important vehicle for the excretion of lipid-soluble products of metabolism. These include certain products of xenobiotic metabolism and so the biliary system is an important conduit for certain detoxification mechanisms. The formation of bile is complex but involves both the active transport across the hepatocyte from the plasma to the canalicular membrane, followed by the passive transport of water via the tight junctions. Bile is probably later modified while in the lumen of the bile ducts [4].

The liver is the primary site of metabolic biotransformation [5]. It is not surprising, therefore, that the liver is also one of the major sites of toxicity, particularly from compounds that enter the body through the gastrointestinal tract. The major function of this metabolism is the conversion of lipophilic, water-insoluble, materials to water-soluble conjugates prior to excretion. This usually involves the generation of electrophilic species that may react with nucleophilic groups. During this process there is one- or two-step electron transfer from the substrate to the receiving group. The introduction, or unmasking of a functional group is described as phase I metabolism; the conjugation of phase I metabolites with a functional group, is described as phase II metabolism. The products of phase II metabolism generally show a considerable increase in water solubility and are, therefore, suitable for excretion via the kidney. Further metabolism of phase II products may occur in an additional third phase. If a functional group is already present on the molecule, phase II reactions may occur without the necessity of phase I reactions.

Oxidation, reduction and hydrolysis are the major phase I reactions and 90 per cent of phase I oxidation reactions are catalysed by the cytochrome P-450 mono-oxygenase system (microsomal enzymes; mixed function oxidases [MFO]), while flavin-containing mono-oxygenases and molybdenum hydroxylases (aldehyde oxidase, xanthine oxidase, etc.) together account for the remaining 10 per cent [6].

The subcellular localization of cytochrome P-450 has been accomplished by differential centrifugation of mechanically disrupted cells. The majority of the cytochrome P-450 is found in the microsomal fraction (consisting of disrupted particles of ER), although some activity is also found in the nuclear and mitochondrial fractions. Cytochrome P-450 forms a family of isoenzymes that show differing substrate specificities. Each has an iron protoporphyrin IX as the prosthetic group and the monomeric enzyme has a molecular weight of 45 000 to 55 000.

The enzyme complex is intermittently bound to the phospholipid membrane of the endoplasmic reticulum and the spatial conformation imposed by the membrane structure is a requirement for function.

Oxidative reactions may be summarized as follows:

$$RH + O_2 + NADPH + H^+ \rightarrow ROH + NADP^+ + H_2O$$

Substrate is bound to ferric iron of the enzyme complex which is then reduced to ferrous iron by reducing equivalents supplied by NADPH. Molecular oxygen then combines with the reduced complex and another electron and two hydrogens are added. Molecular rearrangement, the mechanism of which is not understood, then occurs resulting in regeneration of oxidized P-450, oxidized substrate and water.

P-450 haemoproteins are controlled by a superfamily of genes designated CYP. The proteins of members of any one family normally show greater than 40 per cent sequence homology and are defined by an Arabic numeral. Subfamilies are further identified by a letter followed by a number for the individual gene. Thirty gene families have so far been identified and it is estimated that there may be upwards of 200 P-450 genes in any one species. A more complete description is found in the review by Nelson *et al.* [7]

The activities of these enzymes show species, sex and age dependence. They may, as indicated, be induced and these factors may have a profound influence on the toxicity of chemicals that require metabolism before they express their toxicity.

In mammals the most important phase II reactions are glucuronidation, sulphation, acetylation, methylation and amino acid and glutathione conjugation. Because of the broad range of substrates, glucuronidation is the single most important reaction and these reactions are catalysed by uridine diphosphate (UDP)-glucuronosyltransferases and require UDP-glucuronic acid (UDPGA) to supply D-glucuronic acid. In the rat liver there are at least five UDP-glucuronosyltransferase isoenzymes showing different substrate specificities and some of these are inducible by phenobarbitone (PB) and other xenobiotics.

Glutathione *S*-transferases (GSH *S*-transferases) catalyse the initial step in the formation of mercapturic acid derivatives of xenobiotics through formation of a thioether bond between the tripeptide glutathione and the xenobiotic. GSH *S*-transferase activity is mainly cytoplasmic, although activity is also found in the nucleus, microsomes and mitochondria. As with other enzyme systems, the GSH *S*-transferases are inducible by a variety of compounds including PB and a number of antioxidants.

Cytosolic sulphotransferases conjugate inorganic sulphate to compounds with hydroxyl groups, forming sulphate esters or ethereal sulphates. N-acetyltransferases are cytosolic enzymes with acetyl-CoA as the cofactor. The activity of these enzymes shows polymorphism between species and between individual members of one species; individuals may be classified as fast or slow acetylators depending on their particular genetic make up. Expression of these alleles has considerable importance for both the toxicity and carcinogenicity of a number of xenobiotics.

Methylation and amino acid conjugation play a relatively minor role in xenobiotic phase II metabolism but are of primary importance in the metabolism of physiological substrates.

3.3 Biochemical and Cellular Mechanisms of Toxicity

In no case has a complete description for the biochemical or physiological mechanism of hepatotoxicity been given. None the less, there is compelling evidence which shows that many hepatotoxins require activation before toxicity is manifest and that two major mechanisms lead to cell injury: covalent binding of reactive metabolites and oxidative stress.

In this section, the action of hepatotoxins is illustrated using a number of examples. Those that require metabolic activation and lead to direct toxicity to either the hepatocyte or to the biliary epithelium have been described as intrinsic hepatotoxins. Others would appear to act through an indirect mechanism in which hepatic toxicity is not due to a direct action of the compound on the target cell but is mediated by cells of the immune system. Such mechanisms are often described as idiosyncratic as they are difficult to reproduce experimentally. However, these reactions may be important components of human clinical disease.

3.3.1 *Hepatocellular Toxicity*

Toxins requiring metabolic activation

CYP mediated

The most common forms of xenobiotic-induced hepatic injury follow a classic dose-related pattern. Whether injury is manifest depends on a number of variables: dose applied, metabolism and the state of the protective mechanisms. As previously indicated, the strategy of most of the systems involved in xenobiotic metabolism is aimed at increased water solubility prior to excretion. This is accomplished by the addition of polar groups to the molecule, either directly, if available, or following phase I metabolism. This process has the singular disadvantage that it may produce free radicals or reactive oxygen species.

Halohydrocarbons are amongst the most widely investigated hepatotoxins. These include **bromobenzene, carbon tetrachloride (CCl$_4$)** and **chloroform**. All these compounds show centrilobular toxicity in a variety of animal species and their toxicity is accepted as being dependent on the production of active species through metabolism.

Bromobenzene   This shows a complex metabolic pattern (Figure 3.2). The extent of the toxicity is dependent on covalent binding, which can be increased by enzyme inducers such as PB. Structural evidence of toxicity ensues when glutathione (GSH) levels fall to 20 per cent of control values, this reduction resulting from conjugation with **bromobenzene** metabolites. (The importance of GSH levels is shown by enhanced toxicity when GSH levels are reduced by pretreatment with diethyl maleate). Both the **3, 4'-** and **2, 3'-epoxides** are potential toxic species. It would seem, however, that it is the **3, 4'-epoxide** that is largely responsible for toxicity as strains of mice in which 2, 3'-epoxidation is the major pathway are relatively resistant to toxicity when compared with strains in which 3, 4'-epoxidation predominates. Pretreatment with 20-methylcholanthrene (20-MC) induces epoxide hydrolase resulting in the increased formation of the 3, 4'-dihydrodiol. Furthermore, 2, 3'-epoxidation, with the resultant formation of 2-bromophenol, is also increased. The induction of these two pathways by 20-MC results in decreased toxicity.

These data have shown that metabolism is an important feature of toxicity and that different pathways of metabolism may explain, in part at least, different individual susceptibility. Although **bromobenzene 3, 4'-epoxide** is reactive, it is still capable of leaving the site of initial formation and binding covalently at more distant sites. This balance between reactivity and relative stability may be important in determining the pattern of toxicity that results. The exact mechanism of toxicity of **bromobenzene** is unknown, although three potential mechanisms have been proposed: lipid peroxidation, arylation of low-molecular-weight compounds, and inhibition of enzyme activity through binding to SH groups.

Paracetamol   **Paracetamol (acetaminophen, *N*-acetyl-*p*-4-hydroxyacetanilide)** is a widely used antipyretic and analgesic agent. At toxic doses this compound also produces centrilobular hepatic necrosis with considerable species variation in susceptibility. Thus mice and hamsters are particularly sensitive while the rat is relatively resistant. Humans generally appear to be in the less sensitive category,

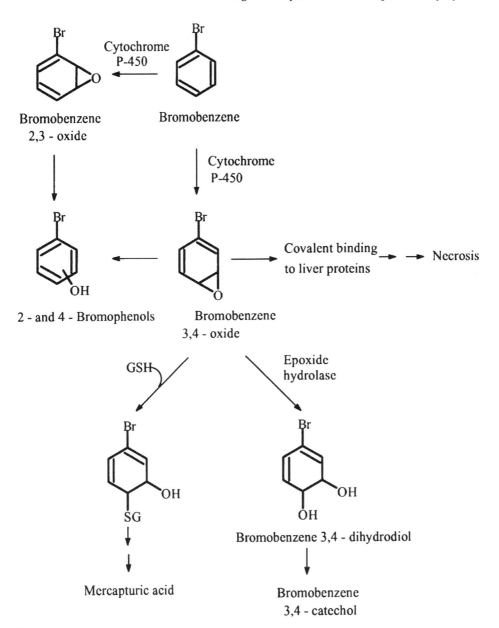

Figure 3.2 Metabolism of bromobenzene.

although approximately 5 per cent may behave in this respect more like the hamster and the mouse than the rat. In both man and rat, hepatic injury is the main manifestation of toxicity, although nephrotoxicity may also be observed. However, other than in the F-344 strain of rat, the renal tubular necrosis that is occasionally seen would appear to be secondary, in the majority of cases, to hepatic failure. As with other compounds, **paracetamol** requires activation by CYP enzymes before toxicity is observed (Figure 3.3).

Paracetamol metabolism seems relatively straightforward, although details of the

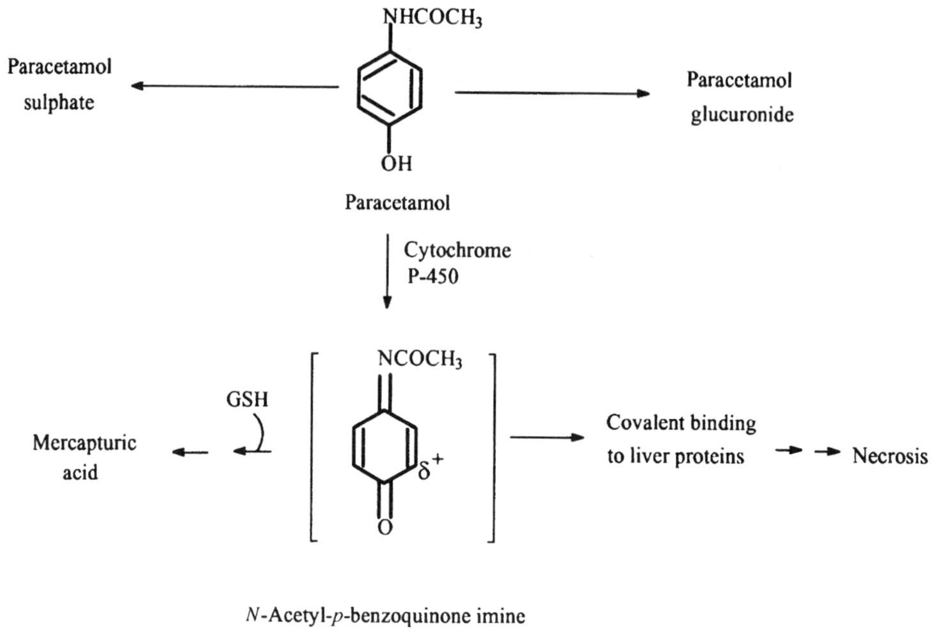

Figure 3.3 Metabolism of paracetamol.

mechanism are still controversial. The compound may undergo deacetylation to produce ***p*-aminophenol**, which may account for the nephrotoxicity seen in F-344 rats. Also, direct sulphation or glucuronidation through the phenolic hydroxyl group results in detoxification, whereas 2 electron oxidation leads to ***N*-acetyl-*p*-benzoquinoneimine** (**NAPQI**), the primary toxic product. Several proposed routes of **NAPQI** formation have been proposed: these include formation of an ***N*-hydroxyparacetamol** intermediate, a **3, 4-epoxide**, or through direct electron transfer via the formation of ferric cytochrome P-450 oxene complex. The latter route is presently the favoured mechanism of **NAPQI** formation. **NAPQI** has been shown to bind to GSH and sulphydryl groups of proteins, it is toxic to hepatocyte cultures and has been identified as a product in a reconstituted P-450 mixed function oxidase system [8].

That CYP activation is required is supported by the observation that piperonyl butoxide and cobaltous chloride inhibit the toxicity of **paracetamol** and that toxicity was enhanced by certain enzyme inducers. Specifically, **20-MC**-induced CYP1A1/2, and **ethanol**-induced CYP2B1 and CYP2E1, increase hepatotoxicity, whereas **PB**-induced CYP2B1/2 has a variable effect dependent on species. In the rat, there is little or no increase in toxicity following treatment with **PB**, while in the hamster, toxicity is considerably reduced due to the induction of glucuronyl transferase which results in an increase in the formation of the glucuronide.

Species and individual differences in the toxicity of **paracetamol** appear to be related to the amount of **NAPQI** formed. At non-toxic doses, approximately 70 per cent of the dose is excreted as the phenolic glucuronide and sulphate, 5 to 10 per cent as GSH-derived conjugates and about the same quantity as acetyl metabolites. In addition, in mice, a few cysteine and mercapturic acid derivatives of *p*-hydroquinone have been identified while *p*-aminophenol has been observed in the F-344 rat. As previously indicated, in susceptible species an increase in thioether metabolites has been described as a consequence of increased **NAPQI** formation. At toxic doses, irrespective of the species, there is considerable protein binding, 70 to 80 per cent of which is through 3-cysteinyl conjugation. This is accompanied by a marked reduction in the hepatic level of GSH. Immunocytochemical studies in a number of species have indicated that protein binding is not random and that binding to a 58 kDa protein may be a common feature.

It is apparent, however, that covalent binding is not sufficient for toxicity. Treatment of rats with positional isomers of **paracetamol** has shown equivalent total protein binding to that induced by toxic doses of **paracetamol** without equivalent toxicity. Furthermore, treatment with various sulphydryl groups, including *N*-acetyl-L-cysteine, up to 15 h after the administration of an otherwise toxic dose, prevents the expected toxicity. Such treatment does not affect protein-binding, as major binding will already have occurred, while the 3, 5-dimethyl derivative will produce toxicity in hepatocytes depleted of GSH without significant protein binding.

Experiments with certain antioxidants including **promethazine** and *a*-tocopherol have shown that hepatotoxicity, and to some degree the extent of lipid peroxidation, could be reduced. It has therefore been suggested that **paracetamol** induces toxicity by an oxidative mechanism. However, experiments in mice have shown that treatment with reduced iron could increase peroxidation by more than 20-fold without increased toxicity. Furthermore, chelation of endogenous iron markedly reduces peroxidation, while toxicity was unaffected. Studies in rats and cultured hepatocytes show a similar dissociation between toxicity and lipid peroxidation [8].

As with covalent binding, lipid peroxidation is not an absolute requirement for toxicity. It would seem probable, however, that a combination of the two events may play a role in the propagation of many toxicities, although neither seems essential. If there is a common association between covalent binding and oxidative damage it would seem to be related to the effect that each may have on the hepatic levels of GSH. It must be remembered that in the case of **paracetamol**, GSH levels are not reduced by oxidation but by covalent binding. However, toxicity can be prevented by treatment with the thiol reducing agent, **dithiotreitol**, or by the GSH precursor, *N*-acetyl-L-cysteine, and so the state of GSH in the hepatocyte would seem important in determining whether toxicity occurs or not [9].

Alcohol dehydrogenase mediated

Allyl alcohol The damage produced by the majority of hepatotoxins, at least initially, is in the centrilobular zone. This, as we have seen with **bromobenzene** and **paracetamol**, is due to the differential pattern of metabolism within the acinus. A number of compounds, however, produce the primary lesions at other sites. **Allyl alcohol** and its esters produce toxicity in the periportal region. Although metabolism may occur through the MFO system, the major metabolic pathway is the formation of the aldehyde, acrolein, by alcohol dehydrogenase. The alcohol dehydrogenases are cytosolic enzymes that are relatively evenly distributed throughout the hepatic lobule. They show substrate specificity, principally by metabolizing primary alcohols to their corresponding aldehyde. Acrolein is a highly reactive chemical that binds readily to macromolecules. This feature is thought in part responsible for the periportal site of injury, cells in the periportal areas being exposed first to the compound. However, there may be a degree of differential activity of alcohol dehydrogenase activity across the lobule, while concentrations of GSH at different sites may also be a contributing factor to the distribution of the toxicity [10].

Ethanol In humans, **alcohol** (**ethanol**) is undoubtedly the most important hepatic toxin [11]. Cirrhosis, the pathological consequence of chronic alcoholism, is the fourth commonest cause of death in middle-aged men. In man, alcohol-associated disease is complex but in the liver three clearly-defined conditions occur: (i) the accumulation of fat, (ii) alcoholic hepatitis, and (iii) cirrhosis. The consequences of these conditions in the body are considerable and include lactate acidosis, hypoglycaemia, reduced protein synthesis and derangement of steroid metabolism, in particular, oestrogens. As with other primary alcohols, **ethanol** is largely metabolized by alcohol dehydrogenase to acetaldehyde and then by acetaldehyde dehydrogenase to acetate. A small proportion, which may be increased in alcoholics, is metabolized by CYP enzymes.

Unlike **allyl alcohol**, the most marked effect of **ethanol** intoxication is on the centrilobular hepatocytes. The reason for this zonal distribution of alcohol-induced injury is unknown, although **ethanol** has the capacity to induce the CYP system, in particular CYP2E1. This would result in increased **ethanol** metabolism in the centrilobular area and so may result in toxicity. Furthermore, **ethanol** is not only a potential toxic agent but a rich energy source and the liver is the only significant site of its metabolism. There are no feedback mechanisms to control its metabolism and it is not stored or metabolized to any large extent in periportal tissues. As a result, in large doses, **ethanol** may replace almost all other substrates that are utilized in the liver for energy sources and so considerably disrupt normal physiological processes.

Acetaldehyde will form covalent bonds with a variety of macromolecules and will bind to circulating proteins including albumin. Free radicals (including the hydroxyl radical), lipid peroxidation, and reduced GSH levels are found following chronic **ethanol** intoxication. Antibodies against acetaldehyde protein adducts have been described in both humans and experimental animals and so immunological mechanisms may contribute to chronic injury.

3.3.2 *Biliary Toxicity*

Hepatocytes perform an exocrine function through the production and secretion of bile, and damage to this system leads to cholestasis (see later). If this is associated with obvious morphological evidence of hepatocellular damage then the condition has been described as hepatocanalicular cholestasis; if there is no obvious hepatocellular damage, the condition is described as bland cholestasis. The latter form has often been associated with the administration of **steroids** and so is referred to as steroid cholestasis. A third form of biliary injury is described as cholangiodestructive and is classically induced by such compounds as *a*-napthylisothiocyanate (ANIT), **paraquat** and **4,4'-diamino-diphenylmethane**. Contamination of flour by the last compound was the cause of Epping jaundice in England [12].

ANIT produces necrosis of the large interlobular bile ducts in the rat and mouse, whereas the dog and rabbit are resistant, with the hamster falling somewhere between the two. Pretreatment with **PB** increases the toxicity, while inhibitors of protein synthesis diminish the toxic response. α-Naphthylamine, carbon dioxide and sulphate are the only known metabolites of **ANIT** and the agent that induces cholestasis is unknown. Within 4 h of dosing, dilatation of the large interlobular bile duct is apparent. At 6 h, alterations are found to the tight junctions of hepatocytes. The morphological changes are associated with increased permeability of hepatocyte junctions, resulting in diffusion of osmotically active solutes from the bile into the plasma. The regurgitation of bile salts would seem to be the mechanism by which cholestasis is induced. Necrosis of the duct is evident at 24 h and there may be scattered foci of necrotic hepatocytes [13].

A number of drugs of which **phalloidin**, a tricyclic heptapeptide, is typical, produce cholestasis by interfering with the microfilament and microtubular cytoskeleton. **Phalloidin** is taken up into hepatocytes by transport mechanisms of bile acid and acts to stabilize microfilament structure. This would appear to decrease bile flow; unlike **ANIT** there is no regurgitation of bile [14].

A small and variable number of women exhibit cholestasis during pregnancy. In a number of countries, however, there is a high prevalence of cholestasis of pregnancy and studies have suggested that the predisposition is genetic. **Oral contraceptives** also induce intrahepatic cholestasis in these women. In contraceptives the active ingredient is **ethinyloestradiol**. Studies in rats have shown that a C_{18} steroid with a phenolic A ring is a requirement, whereas C_{19}, C_{21} and C_{24} steroids are inactive. Active compounds reduce bile flow by approximately 50 per cent, the reduction being largely associated with flow independent of bile acids. There is evidence suggesting that the mechanism of steroid-induced cholestasis is associated with decreased membrane fluidity and decreased N^+, K^+-ATPase activity. Cholestasis is thought to result from metabolism and formation of a D-ring glucuronide. It is hypothesized that such a glucuronide competes with bile acids for a carrier receptor [15].

Anabolic steroids have also been incriminated in cholestasis. A methyl group at C17 seems a requirement for this activity. Both bile acid dependent and independent flow are affected and it has been suggested that inhibition results from disruption of microfilaments and hence a decrease in canalicular motility.

The administration of **bile acids** will also induce canalicular damage. The bile acid **lithocholate** produces morphological changes in the canalicular membrane that are associated with a change in the cholesterol/phospholipid ratio in the membrane. This may alter membrane fluidity and permeability to ions and small non-ionic compounds. Cholestatic bile acids act as Ca^{2+} ionophores and increase cytosolic Ca^{2+}. This effect is dose-dependent and correlates with the potency of the bile acid as a cholestatic [16].

Jaundice induced by **chlorpromazine** shows an incidence in man of 1 to 2 per cent. The 7,8-dihydroxy metabolite of chlorpromazine and **chlorpromazine** itself can cause a reduction in the activity of Na^+, K^+-ATPase, and a decrease in membrane fluidity and cationic pumping.

3.3.3   *Immune-mediated Toxicity*

Immunological mechanisms play a pivotal role in hepatic injury induced by a variety of agents. By the nature of such injury, the pattern is not usually dose-related and is difficult to reproduce under experimental conditions.

In man, hepatic injury (allergic hepatitis) induced by drugs is characterized by the following features:

1 Follows repeated exposure
2 Dose-independent
3 Blood and tissue eosinophilia accompanied by fever
4 Specific sensitized T-lymphocytes or antibodies to:
   (a) drug or metabolite
   (b) normal liver tissue
   (c) modified liver tissue
5 Symptoms regress on cessation of treatment and promptly reappear on challenge

The presence of sensitized lymphocytes or of antibodies against tissue components need not indicate an immunological mechanism, as sensitization may also occur as a consequence of direct drug-induced injury.

Halothane

Halothane has been most widely studied and serves as a model of immunologically mediated hepatic injury. It also illustrates the difficulty of investigating immunological mechanisms of hepatic injury. The major proportion of inhaled anaesthetic is exhaled unchanged and only a small proportion undergoes metabolism, the major site being the liver. This involves oxidation by CYP enzymes to **trifluoroacetic acid**, although a small proportion may undergo reductive cleavage. Epidemiological data showed **halothane** was associated with hepatitis in a small proportion of patients who received multiple exposures to the anaesthetic. The time between exposure and the development of hepatitis decreased with successive exposures and antibodies against a number of tissue proteins could be detected in the sera of such patients. At first, 'halothane hepatitis' seemed to be restricted to obese middle-aged women, but subsequently similar affects were seen in males and children. Studies in animals failed to show a primary hepatotoxic effect, although toxicity may be demonstrated in rats made hyperoxic, or hypoxic after induction with **PB**. Because of the complexity of such models, their relevance to the human situation has been questioned [17].

Although the data from man and animals are complex and often conflicting, there is a general consensus that immune mechanisms play an important role in halothane hepatitis. Experimental evidence in animals has shown that a variety of antibodies to modified protein (mainly microsomal and plasma membrane) may be found under certain conditions and that the expression becomes greater following repeat exposure. However, antibodies against modified protein may be found in a number of instances in which the primary mechanism of damage is essentially cytotoxic. The role of hyper-sensitivity as the exciting mechanism of the tissue damage that is seen in conditions like halothane hepatitis is not as yet fully established, although, as in other forms of idiosyncratic injury, epidemiological evidence is strongly supportive of such a role.

3.4 Morphological Responses to Injury

3.4.1 Acute Injury

The morphological features of acute hepatic injury are usually characterized with respect to site, extent, and cytological changes, the last being expressed in terms of histological or ultrastructural features.

Site

The site of injury is described in terms of the major morphological landmarks, with periportal, mid-zonal or centrilobular describing the injury in relation to the portal tract and central vein (Figure 3.4). This terminology is convenient as it allows ready association with easily defined structural elements, although it may not be totally compatible with physiological and biochemical factors which may affect the pattern of distribution of the injury [1]. The site may also be species specific. **Aflatoxin B1** results in periportal injury in the rat and centrilobular injury in the mouse. Furthermore, pretreatment with enzyme inducers or other compounds may shift the site of injury. **Coumarin** produces centrilobular injury (Figure 3.5) in untreated rats but periportal damage in those previously exposed to **20-MC**.

Centrilobular   This is by far the most common site of hepatic damage, for two reasons: (i) the predominant distribution of the CYP enzymes at this site and (ii) relative anoxia.

Mid-zonal   This is a relatively rare site for injury and has been reported in the rat following treatment with the phytotoxin **ngaione** and after administration of **ferrous sulphate**.

Periportal   This was classically described following treatment with **elemental phosphorus**. Periportal injury is also found following treatment with **allyl alcohol** and its esters, the distribution of injury in this case being dependent on the activity of alcohol dehydrogenase and on the extreme reactivity of the reaction product, acrolein.

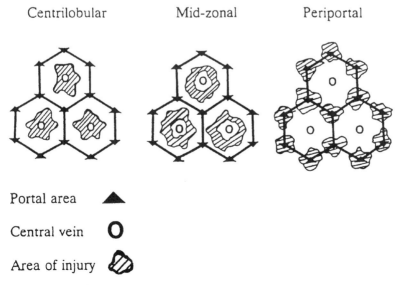

Figure caption text:

Centrilobular   Mid-zonal   Periportal

Portal area   ▲

Central vein   O

Area of injury   ⬭

Figure 3.4   Patterns of lobular injury.

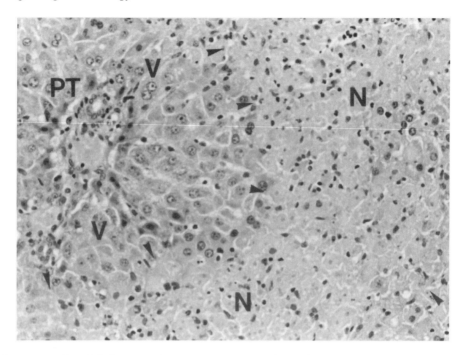

Figure 3.5 Centrilobular necrosis in a rat: note areas of coagulative necrosis (N) with viable tissue (V) surrounding a portal tract (PT). Arrowheads indicate the outer limit of viable hepatocytes. The area of necrosis extends in a bridging fashion between adjacent central veins (not seen in this photomicrograph).

Degree

The degree of injury is dependent on exposure, extent, and rate of metabolic activation. The extent of metabolism may be affected by a variety of factors including diet and previous exposure to enzyme inducers. If the degree of injury is dose dependent, then the site of injury at high doses may be less clear in respect to the anatomical landmarks. Injury may extend between adjacent lobules or indeed from the centrilobular to the periportal area. This pattern of injury emphasizes the metabolically equivalent areas within the liver as proposed by Rappaport [1], and in terms of the classic lobule is described as bridging.

If injury is marked and involves almost the whole of many lobules then the term pan-lobular or massive injury is used. Sometimes the different lobes may show considerable differences in the extent of injury. For example, **paracetamol** may produce massive necrosis in one lobe, and injury confined to the centrilobular area in another. This is particularly true in the case of susceptible species such as the hamster.

In the most severe injury, necrosis (cell death) is the most obvious manifestation. This, dependent on dose and compound, may be restricted to hepatocytes or also involve sinusoidal lining cells. Where hepatocytes and sinusoidal lining cells are involved not only will necrosis be apparent but there will be considerable haemorrhage and the lesion is described as haemorrhagic necrosis.

Cytology

Histological manifestation of injury can be described in terms of three major functional disturbances: (i) change in fluid balance, (ii) disturbance of lipid metabolism, and (iii) cell death.

Change in fluid balance Change in fluid balance occurs as a result of damage to membranes, resulting in failure of pumping mechanisms and as a consequence the perturbation in ionic balance. This results in accumulation of fluid within various cytoplasmic compartments. The overall effect is cell swelling. In its mildest form, the cytoplasm loses its normal texture in sections stained with haematoxylin and eosin and it becomes paler with a faintly granular appearance. This change is often described as cloudy swelling and is difficult to detect. In the most extreme case, clear vacuoles appear in the cell and this state is called hydropic change or hydropic degeneration.

Disturbance of lipid metabolism Accumulation of neutral lipid, lipidosis, is a common morphological manifestation of hepatic injury. This accumulation is generally caused by a failure of protein metabolism and hence a reduction in carrier molecules. In tissues processed for histology by conventional means, fat is removed by the solvents used, so that in sections stained with haematoxylin and eosin, all that remains is an empty vacuole within the cell. Fat can be demonstrated on sections that are cut from frozen tissue. The presence of lipid is then shown by stains which are soluble in the fat such as oil red 0 or osmium.

Lipid may be present in two major morphological forms, either as small vacuoles (microvesicular) or as large (macrovesicular), that may replace much of the normal cytoplasm and push the nucleus to one side.

It is generally held that the accumulation of fat within the cell is a more severe manifestation of cellular injury than that associated with the accumulation of water. Furthermore, cell death is more likely in situations in which extensive fatty change has occurred, although the two cannot be unequivocally be linked. Indeed, both the accumulation of water and of lipid within the cell may be completely reversible and have little effect on general cell function. The accumulation of lipid within the cell may also occur as a result of other non-toxic factors, such as the quantity and type of lipid present within the diet [18].

Cell death Cell death is the most extreme manifestation of toxic injury. Two major forms of cell death are recognized histologically: necrosis, in which a variable but large number of contiguous cells die, and apoptosis, in which individual or single cells are involved. Although in apoptosis the dying cells may be isolated, they may be widely scattered within the liver such that the total number may be quite high [19].

Necrotic cells may appear more eosinophilic than normal due to the cytoplasm becoming more acidic and the dissociation of ribosomes from the endoplasmic reticulum, while in other instances the cytoplasm may appear pale and swollen. The most characteristic feature of necrotic cells is the appearance of the nucleus. The nucleus may undergo karyolysis leaving only a faint outline in histological sections. It may become smaller and denser (pachychromatic) and eventually break into a number of small dense fragments (karyorrhexis). Build up of electrical charges on the nucleolemma are thought to cause the changes that lead to karyorrhexis. In the liver, the outline of dead cells may still be present although cytological detail is lost. In this form the necrosis is described as coagulative necrosis.

In contrast to necrosis, in which cell swelling and loss of cytological structure is the predominant feature, cell death by apoptosis is characterized by cell shrinkage. In addition, the nucleus takes on a characteristic appearance with condensation of chromatin as crescents along the nuclear membrane. As apoptosis proceeds, the cell breaks up into small pieces which include both nuclear and cytoplasmic material forming so-called apoptotic bodies. These may be taken up by surrounding epithelial cells or macrophages where they are degraded by lysosomal action.

Isolated dead cells having the morphological features of apoptosis may be seen in low numbers scattered throughout the normal liver. This may be consequent on the normal ageing process of cells and is associated with a low level of mitotic activity, presumably replacing the lost cells. Apoptotic bodies may also be found following treatment with a wide variety of agents such as **dimethylnitrosamine (DMN)**, which also produce frank necrosis. The apoptotic bodies may be seen prior to the development of necrosis or following the administration of low **DMN** doses. Apoptosis also plays an important role in the growth of altered foci within the liver, determining the rate of increase in size of the foci by balancing the gain in cell numbers as a result of mitotic activity, so limiting growth rate. It would appear, that in the rat at least, compounds such as **PB** reduce apoptosis, resulting in the rapid growth of foci. Apoptosis is also seen following the withdrawal of compounds that have caused hyperplasia and increased liver weight. In this case apoptosis is part of the normal homeostatic control, causing the liver to return to its pretreatment state.

Ultrastructure

Ultrastructural changes resulting from toxicity or any other form of cell injury are expressions of the changes previously described. Thus hydropic swelling and vacuolation appear as dilatation of the ultrastructural components, in particular the endoplasmic reticulum and mitochondria. A short description will be given of the major changes that are found [20, 21].

Contracted, electron-dense mitochondria with swollen cristae are associated with an uncoupling of oxidative phosphorylation and low ATP levels. Mitochondrial swelling in contrast, is associated with failure of the ATP-generated ion pumping mechanism, resulting in increased permeability of the membrane and the accumulation of fluid within the mitochondria. Massive or high amplitude swelling of mitochondria results from the intake of Ca^{2+} and activation of phospholipase A. There is an accumulation of degradation products of lipid metabolism in the inner membrane and increased permeability. Swelling of this type is generally considered irreversible and pathognomic of ensuing cell death. Enlargement of mitochondria can occur unrelated to osmotically determined swelling. A number of hepatotoxins produce a reversible enlargement of mitochondria. This seems to occur in part by fusion of one or more mitochondria, leading to giant or megamitochondria. Flocculant densities may be seen in mitochondria during injury caused by anoxia, toxicity, and as a result of other pathological mechanisms. Furthermore, other inclusions, often having a crystalline structure, are not infrequently seen. Their mechanism of formation is poorly understood.

The loss of cellular fluid balance is most apparent ultrastructurally by dilatation of the ER. In most extreme forms, the ER becomes vesicular and there is a loss of ribosomes from the RER. The ER and Golgi play an important role in lipid transport and lipoprotein synthesis. Cellular injury that blocks these processes may cause the accumulation of lipid within the membrane system. The SER is the structural home of the mixed function oxidase system and the induction of a number of these enzymes is accompanied by a massive proliferation of the SER. This ultrastructural change is apparent at the light microscope level by a ground glass eosinophilia of the cytoplasm of hypertrophic cells. With increased protein synthesis there is also an increase in Golgi and RER. Golgi appear greater in number and there is an increase in the number of tubular profiles and associated vesicles. Increase in RER is seen as a marked increase in the number of tubular profiles forming each stack of RER [22].

Sequestration of cytoplasmic materials may be seen in lysosomes forming autophagic vacuoles following cellular injury. Extensive degradation may result in the accumulation of large amounts of membrane material within lysosomes, the final product of which is extremely electron-dense residual material, seen in the light microscope as lipofuscin.

Extensive peroxisome proliferation in rats and mice may occur following exposure to a variety of agents including **hypolipidaemic drugs** and some **phthalate esters**. From less than 2 per cent of hepatic cytoplasmic volume, peroxisomes may increase to occupy upward of 20 per cent. This increase in volume is caused by both an increase in number of peroxisomes and an increase in the size of individual peroxisomes. These new peroxisomes lack the typical nucleoid core [23].

Ultrastructural changes to the plasma membrane are generally most apparent at the sinusoidal or canalicular surfaces. In the canaliculus, loss of microvilli and dilatation is a common morphological manifestation of injury. In addition there may be an increase in number and condensation of microfilaments in the immediate peri-canalicular region, while junctional complexes may become more pronounced. Desquamation of membrane within the canalicular space may also be observed, often appearing as myelin figures.

Obvious changes in the nucleus are associated with cell death. This is usually seen as clumping of the chromatin, particularly along the nuclear membrane. The nucleolus may also show extensive changes as a result of the inhibition of protein synthesis, with a reduction in nucleolar size and a change in the proportion of the fibrillar and granular components. In extreme instances there may be complete separation of the two parts with the formation of nucleolar caps and fragmentation of the nucleolus. In contrast, nucleolar enlargement is found when there is increased protein synthesis. This may be most obvious during cell division; in this instance, nucleolar size may be taken as a surrogate measure of synthetic activity within the nucleus in preparation for mitosis.

3.4.2 *Chronic Injury*

As in other tissues, the morphological manifestation of chronic injury in the liver is the result of two interlinked mechanisms: first, regeneration, with the replacement of lost cells and second, fibrosis, resulting in scarring. In the liver, the combination of these two events leads to the condition described as cirrhosis. In man this is an important disease as it is a common consequence of **alcohol (ethanol)** abuse, while a similar pathology may be induced in the rat by repeated exposure to CCl_4. Cirrhosis is characterized by diffuse fibrosis accompanied by focal hyperplasia, resulting in nodule formation (Figure 3.6). A further distinction based on the size of the nodules may also be made and the cirrhosis may be described as either micronodular or macronodular. Such distinction may not always be so clear, as cirrhosis may occur where nodules of a mixed size may be present. In cirrhosis, the normal architectural arrangement in the liver is disturbed, resulting in disruption of blood flow within the liver. Shunting of blood occurs between the portal supply and the vena cava, resulting in considerable physiological disturbance and eventually liver failure. In man, these physiological disturbances are of considerable importance, whereas in rodents such changes are rarely apparent [24].

Diffuse fibrosis without nodular hyperplasia should not be considered as cirrhosis. Repair by fibrosis alone may occur following a single treatment with a number of compounds, the best characterized of which are the **pyrrolizidone alkaloids**.

Focal granulomas may also be seen in the liver following treatment with a variety of compounds including **mineral oils**. The common feature of such compounds is that they are poorly digested by the lysosomal system and as a result accumulate within the cell.

The three conditions described: cirrhosis, fibrosis and granuloma formation are characterized by the production of collagen. While the exact mechanism in each case is unknown, it would seem that all involve the transformation of the cells of Ito to collagen-forming cells, possibly under the influence of factors derived from Kupffer cells or from damaged endothelial cells.

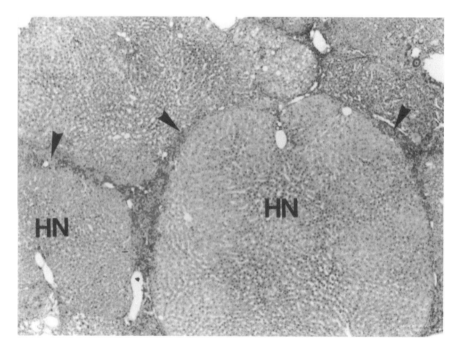

Figure 3.6 Cirrhosis in a rat: note hyperplastic nodules (HN) separated by delicate septa of connective tissue (arrowheads).

3.4.3 *Hypertrophy and Hyperplasia*

The conditions previously described are indicative of either acute or chronic injury to the liver. Adaptive changes may also seen, sometimes in association with obvious evidence of toxicity and sometimes without. Hypertrophy and hyperplasia are the primary examples of such conditions. The liver may may increase in size as a result of two fundamental processes. Hypertrophy results in an increase in size of individual cells without an increase in cell numbers (Figure 3.7). This is characterized biochemically by an increase in the total protein within the liver without an increase in total DNA. In contrast, hyperplasia is defined as an increase in liver size as result of an increase in cell numbers, with an associated increase in DNA. However, in reality the conditions are more complex. It is rare to find a purely hypertrophic or hyperplastic response in the liver and generally there is a mixture of both; when a pathologist makes a diagnosis of either from a histological slide, the inference is that the state described is predominant.

Hypertrophy is seen as an increase in size of individual cells. It is often focal and affects the cells of the centrilobular region. This is because the most common cause of cell hypertrophy is in association with induction of CYP enzymes and this effect is predominantly in the centrilobular region. However, there is often a transient mitotic effect that results in increased cell numbers. Furthermore, and particularly in mice, there may be a considerable increase in nuclear size. These two features mean that the total DNA content of the liver is increased, which is the characteristic biochemical feature of hyperplasia.

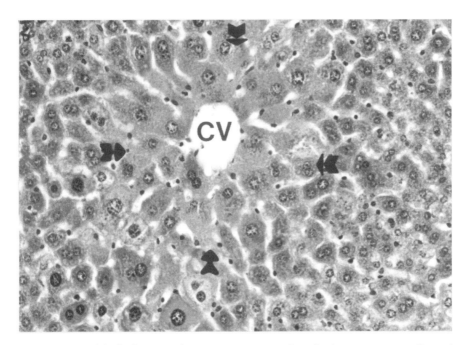

Figure 3.7 Centrilobular hypertrophy in a mouse given phenobarbitone: arrows indicate the limit of the hypertrophic cells around the central vein (CV).

Hyperplasia may be either diffuse, or focal. In some species, hyperplasia may result in plates of hepatocytes that are two cells thick, rather than the usual one cell thick. However, in rodents this is not commonly seen and hyperplasia is more often identified as an increase in cell and nuclear density. To confirm that hyperplasia has occurred, it is appropriate to conduct specific experiments using either tritiated thymidine or bromodeoxyuridine to show active DNA synthesis, although the cell cycle-associated antigen, proliferating-cell nuclear antigen (PCNA), may be used retrospectively as a marker of cell proliferation as the antigen is preserved during tissue processing. In the light of detailed biochemical studies and studies of ploidy within the liver, hyperplasia is now defined as an increase in the DNA content of liver whether due to increased nuclear size, and therefore DNA content, or to increased cell numbers, or indeed a mixture of the two.

3.4.4 *Carcinogenesis*

A list of primary hepatic neoplasms is shown in Table 3.2.

In most rat strains the lifetime incidence of primary hepatocellular tumours is less than 5 per cent. This contrasts with the mouse in which the lifetime incidence in CD-1 mice is 35 per cent for males and 5 per cent for females. In the B6C3F1 hybrid (the inbred mouse strain that is used in the USA National Toxicology Program) the incidence for males ranges between 25 and 40 per cent and between 4.6 and 9.7 per cent for females. In bioassays for carcinogenicity, the liver is the site that is most commonly affected. The induction of liver neoplasia has been the most thoroughly investigated carcinogenic process apart from experimentally induced skin cancer.

Cancer development in the liver is complex and is far from fully understood. Two major pathways have been described. One is through ductule (oval) cell proliferation leading to a lesion composed of an extensive connective tissue matrix investing a metaplastic ductal system. This has been called cholangiofibrosis or adenofibrosis, from which cholangiocarcinoma may, but does not inevitably, develop. The other is through altered hepatic foci, hepatic nodules and hepatocellular carcinoma. In both

Table 3.2 Primary hepatic neoplasms

Tissue of origin	Neoplasm
Hepatocellular	Adenoma (B) Adenocarcinoma (M)
Biliary	Cholangioma (B) Cholangiocarcinoma (M)
Vascular	Angioma (B) Angiosarcoma (M)
Connective tissue	Fibroma (B) Fibrosarcoma (M)
Mononuclear phagocytic system	Histiocytic neoplasms

B, benign; M, malignant.

systems there is the potential for the development of essentially benign lesions or indeed regression at certain stages [25, 26].

To an extent, the histopathogenesis of hepatic tumours may be model and species dependent and the study of hepatic tumour development has been confounded, particularly in the rat, by the cytotoxicity that often accompanied the administration of carcinogens. The discovery of carcinogenic compounds such as **nitrosamines** and **aflatoxin** that are relatively non-toxic at carcinogenic doses, together with the introduction of intermittent administration regimes, has largely overcome such problems, allowing an unhindered description of tumour development.

Development of hepatocellular neoplasia in rodents

It is now generally agreed that hepatocellular tumours develop from foci of altered hepatocytes. These foci are altered in respect of phenotypic expression as reflected in their histochemical appearance (Figure 3.8). They may show increased eosinophilia or basophilia or, because of the arrangement of RER, have a striped or tigroid appearance; they may appear vacuolated as a result of the presence of large quantities of starvation-resistant glycogen. In the rat many foci express foetal enzymes such as γ-glutamyl transferase (γ-GT) and the placental form of GSH S-transferase, or reductions in the activities of other enzymes such as Mg^{2+}-dependent ATPase and glucose-6-phosphatase. Functionally, foci may be resistant to loading with iron and they often show a relative deficiency of phase I enzymes, while phase II enzymes are increased. The reasons for these changes are not known. It has been proposed that many of the enzyme changes, and accumulation of starvation resistant glycogen, are

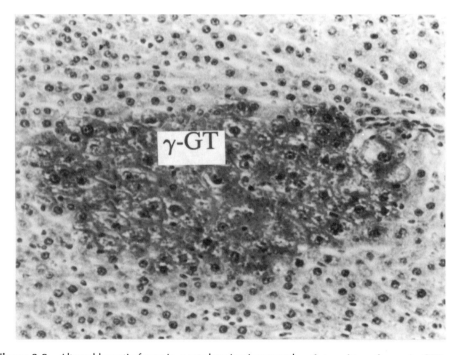

Figure 3.8   Altered hepatic focus in a rat showing increased γ-glutamyl transferase (γ-GT) activity.

evidence of a fundamental shift in carbohydrate metabolism to the pentose phosphate shunt, thus favouring the production of NADPH and anabolic rather than catabolic processes [27]. Furthermore, a reduction of phase I metabolism and an increase in phase II metabolism would act to protect the cells from a cytotoxic environment that might exist during continual administration of a carcinogenic agent, although it is difficult to see the advantage in such a shift in foci that arises spontaneously.

The changes are not seen in all foci. Indeed in foci that are found in the most widely used mouse model, in which neonatal animals are exposed to a single administration of a potent genotoxic carcinogen, or in those from control mice, induction of γ-GT and of the placental form of GSH S-transferase is not seen.

Whether all of the foci that have been described can develop into malignant tumours or indeed whether a proportion of the foci represent carcinoma *in situ* is not yet known. It may be that some foci represent carcinomas that require growth alone for them to exhibit their malignant potential; others may require the addition of further genetic alterations before they exhibit malignant behaviour: that is, the progressive acquisition of a malignant genotype and as a result, phenotype, which is implied in the term 'progression'. Another problem that has yet to be resolved is the origin of the altered foci. Many consider that they arise from mature hepatocytes as a result of genetic damage that occurs either spontaneously or from the application of genotoxic agents. Others have argued that they arise from a putative hepatic stem cell that resides at the junction of the biliary system and the hepatic plates within the canal of Herring. The pluripotential nature of such a stem cell would explain the often varied and sometimes mixed pattern of hepatic tumours that are seen [28].

Growth of foci leads to hepatic nodules. Nodules are distinguished from foci by

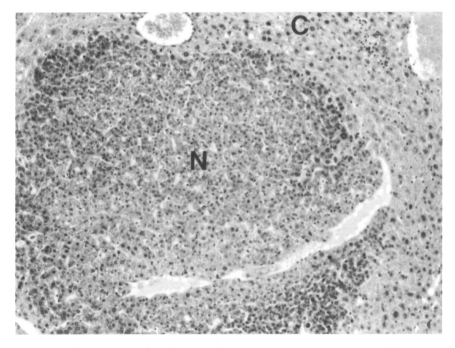

Figure 3.9 Simple hepatic nodule (N) in a mouse: the edge of the nodule is formed of small basophilic cells and there is some compression (C) of the surrounding tissue. Such nodules have been described as hyperplastic nodules or adenoma.

size, although they show tinctorial properties that are similar to foci (Figure 3.9). Nodules themselves may show progressive growth and acquire structural features that are associated with malignancy, although this is not inevitable. The uncertainty that is associated with potential behaviour has meant there has been extensive discussion as to the biological nature of nodules and their appropriate classification. There are experimental systems in which nodules induced by administration of a carcinogen will regress on removal of the exciting stimulus. The surgical production of a portacaval shunt will also result in the development of nodules within the liver, which regress on reconstitution of the normal blood flow. It is also clear that in some model systems, hepatic nodules will develop that do not progress to carcinoma but maintain themselves in an essentially benign form. These data suggest that hepatic nodules may exist in different biological forms: hyperplastic nodules that will regress, benign tumours or adenoma, and intermediate stages that will inevitably progress to malignacy. At present there are no histological features or reliable markers that will allow unequivocal identification of the potential of hepatic nodules.

Hepatocellular carcinoma may have a number of histological forms: glandular, trabecular (Figure 3.10), solid, and undifferentiated. On occasion, tumours will show a mixture of histological patterns. Such diagnostic exactitude probably has little relevance when assessing human risk. However, the distinction between benign and malignant may have to be made almost entirely on the histological character of the individual tumour, as the biological evidence of malignancy (that is metastasis) is often a late event in most rodent hepatocellular tumours, only being evident when the tumour is of a considerable size.

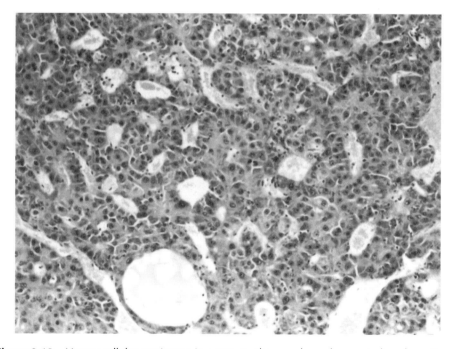

Figure 3.10 Hepatocellular carcinoma in a mouse: the neoplasm shows a trabecular pattern with marked thickening of the hepatic plates.

Other hepatic neoplasms

Other primary neoplasms of the liver are relatively uncommon. Vascular neoplasms are occasionally reported in the mouse, while in the rat they are extremely rare but may be induced by **vinyl chloride monomer**. Similarly, Kupffer cell sarcoma has been reported following exposure to **trypan blue**, certain **X-ray contrast media** and a number of **nitrosamines**.

3.4.5 Mechanisms of Neoplasia

As in other organ systems, the mechanism of tumour induction in the liver is conceived in the operational sense as a two-step process, that is, initiation followed by promotion. The initiation phase is thought to result from an irreversible effect involving direct interaction with DNA by so-called genotoxic agents, while promotion occurs as a result of the division of the initiated cells. Compounds that operate through the stage of promotion are often termed 'epigenetic or non-genotoxic carcinogens' [29]. Indeed, in both the rat and mouse there is no requirement for the animals to be exposed deliberately to a genotoxic carcinogen for neoplasia to develop, as all animals would appear to have within their livers a population of spontaneously initiated cells. As animals age, an increasing number of altered foci is seen. This is taken to imply spontaneous initiation, possibly as a result of low-level environmental exposure to genotoxic carcinogens or as a consequence of inherent metabolic processes leading to free radical formation, particularly various oxygen species [30].

Genotoxic carcinogens

Genotoxic agents generally require metabolic activation by the systems previously described, resulting in the formation of electrophilic species that will interact with nucleophilic sites on DNA (Figure 3.11). The formation of critical adducts then results in mutational changes in the genetic code, the primary event leading to cancer

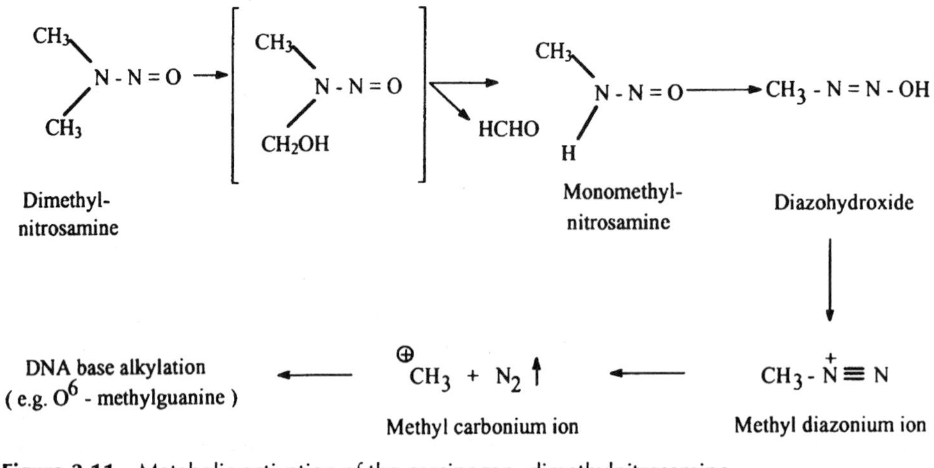

Figure 3.11   Metabolic activation of the carcinogen, dimethylnitrosamine.

formation. Other genetic or epigenetic mechanisms then result in clonal expansion of the transformed cell. For example, alkylating agents such as **diethylnitrosamine** (**DEN**) and **DMN** lead to alkylation of a number of sites on the DNA molecule. In particular, O^6-guanine and O^4-thymidine would appear to be critical sites in the initiation of carcinogenesis resulting in point mutations. In contrast, the premutagenic adduct of **aflatoxin** is the 8,9-epoxide, which may form a relatively bulky adduct leading to a considerable distortion of the DNA chain.

The initial biochemical lesions may be considered as premutagenic lesions. The function of the mutations that then ensue is poorly understood. However, tumours that develop in C3H and B6C3F1 hybrid strains of mice show a high incidence of mutation at codon 61 of the H-*ras* oncogene, although there is a question as to whether such mutations are a cause of transformation or a result.

Genetic analysis of recombinant inbred strains of mice derived from C57/BL and C3H/He mice has indicated that the difference in strain susceptibility to neoplastic development in mice may be controlled by two genetic loci, one of which plays a predominant (85 per cent) role. Further, this difference is not accounted for by metabolic differences, as base alkylation and repair are similar in the two strains. Indeed the difference appears to relate not to the initiating phase, but to the promotional stage, as a result of a much more rapid growth of altered foci in susceptible strains. The genes have been called hepatic cancer susceptibility (*hcs*) genes; they have yet to be fully characterized and their detailed biochemical mechanism of action is not known, but they may control mitotic activity within foci [31].

Non-genotoxic carcinogens

Two classes of chemicals have been widely investigated as liver carcinogens as they act in essentially different ways to that of genotoxic agents. As these are of considerable toxicological importance they will be considered in some detail. Both groups are non-genotoxic, at least in the conventional sense, in that they are negative in short-term tests for genotoxicity. The first group are those compounds that cause induction of the mixed function oxidase enzymes, the archetypal compound of which is **PB**. The second group is a heterogeneous group of compounds that have the common property of causing liver enlargement and proliferation of peroxisomes.

CYP inducers   When **PB** is given to rodents it produces liver enlargement as well as enzyme induction. The liver enlargement is caused initially by hyperplasia that is apparent during the first week of administration but is continued and increased by hypertrophy of cells in the centrilobular region. Hypertrophy results from proliferation of the SER, although there is also some increase in other organelles and nuclear enlargement. If **PB** is given to rats for periods in excess of 18 months, then there may be a small increase in the number of hepatic tumours in the treated animals. If treatment is preceded by a relatively short exposure to a potent genotoxic carcinogen such as **DEN**, then the administration of **PB** results in a considerable tumour burden.

The general consensus is that in such models, **PB** promotes initiated cells that become apparent as altered hepatic foci and then as frank neoplasms. Examination of foci has shown that their mitotic activity is up to 10 times greater than that in the rest of the liver. It might be expected, therefore, that foci would show rapid growth, but this is not the case, as there is a high rate of cell loss from foci due to apoptosis. One effect of **PB** administration on foci is similar to that which occurs in the rest of the liver, i.e. a transient hyperplastic response. The second effect, which is more profound in respect to the promoting activity of **PB**, is to reduce markedly the apoptotic activity within foci. In consequence the foci show rapid growth, and foci that previously would have been inapparent because of their small size can now be seen [30].

In mice, the effect of compounds such as **PB** is dependent on strain. In those strains that show a high spontaneous incidence of hepatic neoplasms, the effect of **PB** is to increase their number greatly with an apparent reduction in the latent period. In strains that show a low spontaneous incidence, **PB** only marginally increases the tumour incidence following prolonged administration. As in the rat, it has been argued that **PB** acts to promote spontaneously initiated cells. However, a number of features are inconsistent with this hypothesis. The first is that **PB** does not increase the incidence of malignant tumours and indeed it would appear to decrease it. Second, the foci and tumours that develop as a result of **PB** administration show a different phenotypic character to those that occur spontaneously. They are composed of large eosinophilic cells that contain large amounts of SER. This morphological feature is associated with considerable activity of the mixed function oxidase enzymes [32]. Furthermore, and in contrast to tumours that arise spontaneously, and following treatment of neonatal mice with **DEN**, they show activity of γ-GT, a very low frequency of H-*ras* activation, and cells isolated from them show poor growth in agar and on transplantation into nude mice [33].

Peroxisome proliferators Compounds that induce peroxisome proliferation form a chemically heterogeneous group. Those most intensely studied are the **phthalate esters**, the **hypolipidaemic agents** based on **clofibric acid**, and other unrelated chemicals such as **tibric acid** and **WY-14643**. The pleiotropic affect on the liver is to some extent species specific with both sensitive and insensitive species. Both rat and mouse are considered sensitive, the hamster is considerably less responsive, while the guinea pig and primates, including man, respond poorly. As with **PB**, liver enlargement is the most obvious feature of administration of peroxisome proliferators to sensitive species. This results from an essentially transient hyperplasia, followed by cellular hypertrophy, as a result of the massive expansion in size and number of peroxisomes, the volume proportion rising from somewhat less than 2 per cent in control animals to approximately 20 per cent in animals treated with the most potent agents. In addition to this massive increase in peroxisome volume there are also slight increases in mitochondria and SER. These morphological changes are associated with a 20 to 30-fold increase in fatty acid β-oxidation, whereas the activity of catalase is only increased two-fold [34].

Two major hypotheses have been proposed to explain the mechanism of peroxisome proliferation. The first is essentially a biochemical one, developed because of the diverse chemical nature of the compounds that induce peroxisome proliferation. This suggests that there is an inhibition of mitochondrial β-oxidation resulting in the accumulation of medium- and long-chain fatty acids. CYP4A1 and peroxisomes are then induced in an attempt to cope with the metabolic load [34]. The second hypothesis suggests that a cytoplasmic receptor is responsible for the induction. Several putative receptors belonging to the steroid hormone receptor superfamily, termed peroxisome proliferator-activated receptors (PPARs), have now been identified. In *in vitro* expression systems (e.g. COS 1 cells), PPARs have been shown to be activated by peroxisome proliferators and certain fatty acids. Activation, however, is complex and probably involves interaction between a number of activating and repressor factors, which may account for the known differences in tissue and species response [35, 36].

Chronic administration of agents that induce peroxisome proliferation results in accumulation of lipofuscin within the liver and the development of hepatocellular carcinoma in both rats and mice. Furthermore, examination of tumour development shows that they develop through a well-ordered sequence of events: basophilic foci give rise to regular basophilic nodules and then to well-differentiated trabecular carcinoma.

The foci and nodules that develop in the rat show a number of phenotypic differences from spontaneous neoplasms in this species. They are negative for γ-GT, and the placental form of GSH S-transferase, and they show low levels of metabolizing and detoxification enzymes and of epoxide hydrolase. At present there are two major factors that are thought to be important mechanistically in peroxisome-induced tumours. The first is the hyperplastic response and the second is oxidative stress. Neither of these factors seem sufficient alone to account for the carcinogenic effect of peroxisome proliferators, but a balance of the two may be critical in this respect. There is evidence in the case of certain of the more potent peroxisome proliferators that carcinogenesis might be associated with a chronic hyperplastic response and can only be demonstrated by the use of specialized techniques designed to detect a proliferative response over periods of a week or more, rather than hours or days. Chronic exposure to peroxisome proliferators does lead to prolonged oxidative stress and this may lead to DNA damage. Indeed, increased urinary levels of 8-hydroxydeoxyguanosine have been shown following chronic exposure to **ciprofibrate**. However, there is some uncertainty as to the source of this adduct and experiments in which the defence mechanisms against oxidative stress have been reduced have not resulted, as might be expected, in an increase in tumour development. In addition, the difference in enzyme induction between peroxisome proliferators that are relatively potent carcinogens, such as **WY-14643**, and those that are not, such as **di(2-ethylhexyl)phthalate (DEHP)**, would not seem sufficient to account for the different carcinogenic potency [34, 36].

Peroxisome proliferators increase both the number and size of foci, with the predominant effect appearing to be on growth. Thus peroxisome proliferators would appear to act as promoting agents. This view is supported by the observation that, as with **PB**, peroxisome proliferators have a much more profound effect in older rather than in younger animals, the presumption being that there are a greater number of spontaneously initiated foci in old animals.

3.5 Testing for Toxicity

In conventional toxicological procedures, the liver receives considerable attention as it is a common site of toxic injury. This assessment starts during the in-life phase of any study and is completed during necropsy and histopathological examination of the liver. Routine procedures that form a common assessment will be discussed first, followed by details of alternative methods that may be described as screens, and some techniques that may be used to investigate further the biochemical mechanisms of toxicity.

3.5.1 Clinical Chemistry

Blood samples for chemical analysis may be taken at various times during routine toxicological studies and may be processed as either plasma or serum depending on the examination that is required. For most purposes plasma is used, obtained by centrifugation of blood following collection into a suitable anticoagulant. The major biochemical tests reflect the major functions of the liver: protein synthesis and detoxification. Furthermore, enzymes may be released into the circulation during hepatic injury and a number of these may be more or less specific for hepatic injury, particularly when the pattern of their appearance in blood is considered.

Plasma proteins

The liver is the primary site of the synthesis of all the blood proteins other than immunoglobulins. Albumin is the major blood protein synthesized in the liver and it may be decreased during hepatic injury. The reduction, however, is not rapid because the half-life of this protein is several weeks. Furthermore, the plasma level may also be affected by dietary factors, kidney disease and hormonal balance. Indeed, as chronic nephrosis is a common finding in ageing rats, renal protein loss is the most common mechanism of reduced albumin levels in older rats.

Serum enzymes

Serum enzymes are probably the most widely used markers of hepatic injury both for the identification of the site of injury and in monitoring the progress of the injury. The enzymes fall into two broad classes: those that are used to monitor biliary injury and those used to detect parenchymal damage, although there is some overlap [37].

Biliary system　The most common enzyme markers of biliary injury are alkaline phosphatase (ALP), 5'-nucleotidase (5'-NT) and γ-GT. ALP is a family of enzymes with broad substrate specificity. It is present in high concentration in the biliary and canalicular membrane, and in cholestasis, serum levels may be considerably raised. It is probably of greater use in the dog rather than the rat as in the latter species the normal serum levels are relatively high with considerable fluctuation due to dietary factors. ALP may also be raised in other conditions unrelated to liver injury, in particular proliferative lesions of bone and in certain conditions affecting the GI tract. 5'-NT is found in the same sites as ALP and has been used to indicate and assess obstructive injury to the biliary system. γ-GT is a popular marker for biliary injury. In normal mature rat liver it can only be demonstrated in the biliary epithelium and not within the canalicular membrane nor within the hepatocyte cytoplasm. However, following treatment with a variety of hepatotoxins and with compounds that induce CYPs, the activity of this enzyme may be considerably increased at all three sites. As well as raised serum levels during cholestatic injury, there may be 10 to 20-fold increases in serum levels as a result of enzyme induction.

Furthermore, serum enzymes may also be raised, in certain instances, in animals that bear hepatocellular tumours.

Hepatocytes Several enzymes have been used to indicate or monitor the progression of parenchymal cell injury. A number of these are almost exclusively or mainly found in the liver and when serum levels are raised it is generally taken as indicative of hepatic injury. These include sorbitol dehydrogenase (SDH), ornithine carbamoyltransferase (OCT) and alanine transaminase (ALT). A number of other serum enzymes may also be raised during hepatic injury, such as aspartate transaminase (AST) and lactate dehydrogenase (LDH), although these enzymes may show marked increases following injury to other organs, particularly the kidney, skeletal muscle and heart. In routine monitoring, ALT and AST are the enzymes that are most commonly used, although SDH may be more specific and sensitive. The transaminases are preferred as SDH is very unstable and remains elevated for shorter periods. Once the specificity of liver injury has been established, then LDH may be a sensitive monitor of its progress. OCT is a mitochondrial enzyme that has proved a sensitive marker of hepatic injury. Furthermore, raised levels have correlated well with histological estimates of hepatic damage; however, the measurement is difficult to do and has not been widely used for routine purposes.

It must be remembered that changes in serum levels may not be comparable among different hepatotoxins or with the extent or degree of hepatic injury determined histologically. Thus **DMN** results in an extensive haemorrhagic necrosis whereas **CCl₄** results in necrosis that is not accompanied by haemorrhage. The former may therefore be considered as presenting injury of greater severity, although the latter shows a considerably greater elevation of serum enzymes. These differences may be accounted for by two aspects of the injury: first, by the dynamics of the injury, with the maintenance of damaged but viable cells that are able to release enzyme and, second, by haemodynamic factors associated with haemorrhage [38].

3.5.2 *Necropsy and Histopathological Examination*

In life, and immediately after death, the normal liver is a deep mahogany colour due to the large quantity of blood that it contains. During the course of liver injury there may be considerable changes in the colour of the liver, including pallor and exaggeration of the normal lobular pattern. Three main features are associated with change in the macroscopic appearance of the liver: alteration in blood distribution and haemorrhage, the pattern of necrosis and the accumulation of fat. Thus centrilobular necrosis with haemorrhage leads to pooling of blood in the centrilobular region that macroscopically appears as dark red spots less than 1 mm in diameter separated by paler parenchyma. In contrast, if there is extensive accumulation of lipid within the hepatocytes, the liver may appear swollen and pale tan in colour.

Liver weight forms an important criterion for detecting an effect on the liver. This may be expressed as absolute liver weight or, and often more usefully, as a percentage of body weight. An increase in liver weight is not an infrequent finding in toxicity studies. This is most often associated with enzyme induction, although an increase of upwards of 10 per cent may be associated with other factors such as increase in fluid content or the accumulation of fat.

Histological examination of the liver forms the single most important assessment of hepatic injury. The structural features of hepatic injury have been described previously and will not be discussed again. It is worth commenting, however, that evidence of injury may be extremely variable, within different areas of one liver lobe, and between different liver lobes. In order to make a proper assessment of the extent and severity of damage, sufficient samples are required. In the case of small rodents it is usual to prepare a section from each of the major lobes and it would not seem unreasonable to follow a similar procedure with larger animals. Histological examination may also be supported by electron microscopy (EM). As with light microscopy, care is required in EM of the liver both in terms of the site from which a sample is selected and in the number of samples as, and it cannot be emphasized enough, even examining relatively large numbers of samples at EM will represent only a very small area of the total liver volume. It is from this small area that the generality of an effect in the whole liver has to be drawn.

At both the light and EM level, estimates of effect may be made using simple arbitrary scoring systems either describing the changes as minimal, slight, moderate or severe or using some simple numeric scoring system. The problem with all these systems is the subjective nature of the estimate and the difficulty of making an overall assessment when different areas of the liver are affected to different degrees. To overcome these difficulties, more formal morphometric or stereological methods may be used. However, these are extremely time-consuming and may require perfusion fixation of the liver so that the in-life proportion of the sinusoid may be maintained and terminal anoxic affects within the hepatocytes are avoided. Furthermore, preliminary estimates of the extent of change may be needed so that an appropriate sampling schedule may be determined. None the less, such techniques may be extremely sensitive and are able to detect changes that may not be apparent to the naked eye. This is particularly true when an increase in the number or size of an organelle is suspected. For example, the volume of ER may increase upward of 90 per cent before this is detected by visual examination of electron micrographs and so stereological methods would be essential for detecting increases of this extent and less.

3.5.3 In vitro *Systems*

The techniques described above may be considered as standard methods and are commonly used in routine assessments of hepatic toxicity; however, the investigation of mechanisms has often relied on the techniques of organ and tissue culture, some of which are now used as screens for toxicity, especially when a class effect is suspected.

Isolated perfused livers have been used to investigate biochemical mechanisms of toxicity, particularly those associated with bile formation. The isolated liver is kept in a heated container and perfused via the hepatic portal vein with a physiological solution (with or without red blood cells) that supplies oxygen and other nutrients. The bile duct may be ligated and bile collected for chemical analysis. This technique has been used for metabolic investigations. However, the useful life of a liver kept under these conditions is limited to approximately 6 h as deterioration occurs rapidly. Furthermore, an isolation cabinet is required to maintain the liver and considerable surgical skill is needed for its isolation. For these reasons the technique has not been widely used [39].

Isolated hepatocytes have been used to investigate mechanisms of toxicity and have found limited use in some screening procedures. Cells are usually isolated from young animals by a two-step technique that results in a single cell preparation of hepatocytes showing up to 95 per cent viability. Cell suspensions may survive for up to 3 to 4 days, although metabolic studies are generally conducted within 6 h of isolation. As well as being used to investigate the metabolism and toxicity of a variety of compounds such as CCl_4, **bromobenzene** and **phthalate esters**, cultures of hepatocytes have been used to examine class effects and as preliminary screens to detect hepatotoxicity [40]. One of the main advantages of this system is that a number of identical cultures may be obtained from one liver and many replicate studies may be done. Cells may also be isolated from a number of species so that comparative studies may be performed. Furthermore, the amount of test material required is relatively low when compared with whole animal studies and this may be a considerable advantage when the quantity of test compound is small. The disadvantages of such a system are that the cells are isolated and so intercellular relationships are lost; also the process of enzyme digestion may itself damage the plasma membrane of the isolated cells and so affect the pumping mechanism of the cell. The problem of single isolated cells may be overcome in part by a technique that allows cellular couplets to form. Between each cellular couplet is a space that is equivalent to the canalicular space in the entire liver. Thus distinction is made in the culture system between the canalicular system and the rest of the plasma membrane and so, to a certain extent, transport mechanisms in the two surfaces may be studied. This, however, is limited as the canalicular space is little more than a sac with no movement of transported material from the site of production.

In order to overcome some of the problems associated with cell cultures, precision-cut liver slices have been introduced. Two primary factors are important in the successful application of this technique. The first is the introduction of techniques that minimize the mechanical damage inflicted during the preparation of the slice and the second is the maintenance of the slice in a viable condition. The former has been accomplished through the introduction of a mechanical tissue slicer in which a core of liver tissue of 1 cm diameter is cut in an oxygenated buffer. It is most common for the slices to be cut at 250 µm and a gentle current in the buffer carries the slice to a collecting basket. The success of the incubation system is based on the development of procedures that allow the section to be exposed sequentially to both the incubation media and the gaseous interface. In the most elegant system, the slices are held on a wire mesh that is maintained in a semicircular shape by stainless steel rings at each end. This structure is then placed inside a scintillation vial containing 1.5 to 2 ml of oxygenated media, sealed, and gently rotated on a heated roller. Hepatocytes may be maintained in a viable state for a sufficient period to allow investigative studies to be done. Furthermore, differential and site-specific toxicity as seen *in vivo* may be modelled in this system and studies on protein synthesis, ionic movement and xenobiotic metabolism have been undertaken [41].

3.6 Conclusions

Acute toxicity, chronic toxicity and carcinogenicity are frequently seen in the liver after the administration of xenobiotics. This is because of the relationship of the liver to one of the major portals of entry into the body and also because of its considerable metabolic capacity. Although there are species and strain differences in response, in many instances there are more cross-species similarities in response than there are differences. However, when differences between species do occur, usually they can be interpreted through a detailed examination of the mechanism of toxicity.

In experimental animals, the association between cause and effect may be made relatively easily. Experiments may be done under controlled conditions with a well-defined time course. This is not the case in clinical conditions, however, where the association between cause and effect may be difficult to make. Indeed the histological changes associated with xenobiotic-induced injury may be indistinguishable histologically from those induced by other causes, in particular those associated with viral hepatitis infection which may be a confounding concurrent disease process.

These comments notwithstanding, the area of greatest controversy has been evaluating the significance of the induction of neoplasia within the liver of rodents in respect to the assessment of human hazard and the evaluation of risk. In such assessments four major factors are considered: is the compound genotoxic as defined by conventional tests for genotoxicity; does the compound elicit an effect in one or more species; is there a clear dose response; are the neoplasms which are induced benign or malignant, or a mixture of the two?

In the worst case, in which a genotoxic compound produces malignant neoplasms after a relatively short latent period in both rat and mouse and possibly at multiple sites, then it would seem prudent to avoid human exposure if possible. However, man is exposed to a number of compounds that are potent hepatocarcinogens in rodents. Such exposure is usually inadvertent, the compounds being natural products (e.g. **aflatoxins**) or result from human activity that is difficult to avoid (e.g. **pyrolysis products** in cooked food). The analysis of experiments in animals in these situations is generally aimed at assessing the risk to man from low level exposure. In order to do this, extrapolation of the animal data is made using a mathematical model that describes a dose, and generally time, response. While most models show a good fit to experimental data in animals at high exposure levels, the estimates of low dose risk given by the different models is often widely divergent and as a result their utility has been questioned. Consequently, it has been argued that the most conservative of these models should be used when assessing risk to man, although the figures generated may have little scientific justification.

Non-genotoxic compounds that increase the incidence of neoplasia in rodent liver are considered to do so by promoting otherwise transformed cells. However, it is apparent that the mechanism of promotion will differ for different compounds as the neoplasms that develop may exhibit different biological properties. Thus a detailed investigation of each individual case may be required before a proper risk assessment can be made. It is now accepted that peroxisome proliferation does not occur in man to any significant extent and as this property would appear to be related to the carcinogenic effect in rodents it would seem unlikely that such a mechanism would account for any significant carcinogenic risk to man. In the case of **PB**, considerable epidemiological data have not shown any increased neoplastic risk to man from long-term exposure. Furthermore, even in rodents, a reasonably profound biological effect is required before a promoting effect is seen with peroxisome proliferators or **PB** and so a clear threshold level for neoplasia may be demonstrated.

References

1. RAPPAPORT, A.M. (1979) Physioanatomical basis of toxic liver injury, in FARBER, E. and FISHER, M.M. (Eds) *Toxic Injury of the Liver*, pp. 1–57, New York: Marcel Dekker.

2. MIYAI, K. (1991) Structural organization of the liver, in MEEKS, R.G., HARRISON, S.D. and BULL, R.J. (Eds) *Hepatotoxicology*, pp. 1–65, London: CRC Press.

3. JOHNSTON, D.G. and ALBERTI, K.G.M.M. (1985) The liver and endocrine function, in WRIGHT, R., MILLWARD-SADLER, G.H., ALBERTI, K.G.M.M. and KARRAN, S. (Eds) *Liver and Biliary Disease: Pathophysiology, Diagnosis and Management*, 2nd Edn, pp. 161–188, London: Baillière Tindall.

4. KLAASSEN, C.D. and WATKINS III, J.B. (1984) Mechanism of bile formation, hepatic uptake and biliary excretion, *Pharmacological Reviews*, **36**, 1–67.

5. CALDWELL, J. (1988) Biological implications of xenobiotic metabolism, in ARIAS, I.M., JAKOBY, W.H., POPPER, H., SCHACTER, D. and SHAFRITZ, D.A. (Eds) *The Liver: Biology and Pathobiology*, pp. 355–362, New York: Raven Press.

6. LINDAMOOD, C. (1991) Xenobiotic transformation, in MEEKS, R.G., HARRISON, S.D. and BULL, R.J. (Eds) *Hepatoxicology*, pp. 139–180, London: CRC Press.

7. NELSON, D.R., KAMATAKI, T., WAXMAN, D.J., GUENGERICH, F.P., ESTABROOK, R.W., FEYEREISEN, R., GONZALEZ, F.J., COON, M.J., GUNSALUS, I.C., GOTOH, O., OKUDA, K. and NEBERT, D.W. (1993) The P450 superfamily: update on new sequences, gene mapping, accession numbers, early trivial names of enzymes, and nomenclature, *DNA and Cell Biology*, **12**, 1–51.

8. BOOBIS, A.R., FAWTHORP, D.J. and DAVIES, D.S., (1992) Mechanism of cell injury, in: MCGEE, J.O'D., ISAACSON, P.G. and WRIGHT, N.A. (Eds) *Oxford Textbook of Pathology: Principles of Pathology*, Vol. 1, pp. 181–193, Oxford: Oxford University Press.

9. HORTON, A.A. and FAIRHURST, S. (1987) Lipid peroxidation and mechanisms of toxicity, *CRC Critical Reviews in Toxicology*, **18**, 27–79.

10. SWEENY, P.J. and DIASIO, R.B. (1991) The isolated hepatocyte and isolated perfused liver as models for studying drug and chemical-induced hepatotoxicity, in MEEKS, R.G., HARRISON, S.D. and BULL, R.J. (Eds) *Hepatotoxicology*, pp. 215–239, London: CRC Press.

11. LIEBER, C.S. (1988) The influence of alcohol on nutritional status, *Nutrition Reviews*, **46**, 241–254.

12. ZIMMERMAN, H.J. and LEWIS, J.H. (1987) Drug-induced cholestasis, *Medical Toxicology*, **2**, 112–160.

13. PLAA, G.L. and PRIESTLY, B.G. (1976) Intrahepatic cholestasis induced by drugs and chemicals, *Pharmacological Reviews*, **28**, 207–273.

14. PHILLIPS, M.J., POUCELL, S. and ODA, M. (1986) Biology of disease. Mechanisms of cholestasis, *Laboratory Investigation*, **54**, 593–608.

15. CHANGCHIT, A., DURHAM, S. and VORE, M. (1990) Characterization ^{3}H-estradiol-17β (β-D-glucuronide) binding sites in basolateral and canalicular liver plasma membranes, *Biochemical Pharmacology*, **40**, 1219–1225.

16. ANWER, M.S., ENGLEKING, L.R., NOLAN, K., SULLIVAN, D., ZIMNIAK, P. and LESTER, R. (1988) Hepatotoxic bile acids increase cystolic Ca^{++} activity of isolated rat hepatocytes, *Hepatotoxicology*, **8**, 887–891.

17. LIND, R.C., GANDOLFI, A.J., SIPES, I.G. and BROWN, B.R. (1985) Comparison of the requirements for hepatic injury with halothane and enflurane in rats, *Anaesthetics and Analgesia*, **64**, 955–963.

18. DIANZANI, M.U. (1991) Biochemical aspects of fatty liver, in MEEKS, R.G., HARRISON, S.D. and BULL, R.J. (Eds) *Hepatotoxicology*, pp. 327–399, London: CRC Press.

19. WYLLIE, A.H. and DUVALL, E. (1992) Cell injury and death, in McGEE, J.O'D., ISAACSON, P.G. and WRIGHT, N.A. (Eds) *Oxford Textbook of Pathology: Principles of Pathology*, Vol. 1, pp. 141–156, Oxford: Oxford University Press.

20. TRUMP, B.F., McDOWELL, E. M. and ARSTILA, A.U. (1980) Cellular reaction to injury, in LaVIA, M.F. and HILL, R.B. (Eds) *Principles of Pathobiology*, pp. 20–111, New York: Oxford University Press.

21. GHADIALLY, F.N. (1982) *Ultrastructural Pathology of the Cell and Matrix*, 2nd Edn, London: Butterworth.

22. DALLNER, G. and DE PIERRE, J. W. (1983) Membrane induction by drugs, *Methods in Enzymology*, **96**, 542–557.

23. COHEN, A.J. and GRASSO, P. (1981) Review of hepatic response to hypolipidaemic drugs in rodents and assessment of its toxicological significance to man, *Food and Cosmetic Toxicology*, **19**, 585–605.

24. TAMAYO, R.P. (1983) Is cirrhosis of the liver experimentally produced by CCl$_4$ an adequate model of human cirrhosis? *Hepatoroxicology*, **3**, 112–120.

25. FARBER, E. (1976) The pathology of experimental liver cancer, in CAMERON, H.M., LINSELL, D.A. and WARWICK, G.P. (Eds) *Liver Cell Cancer*, pp. 243–277, Amsterdam: Elsevier.

26. MOORE, M.A. and KITIGAWA, T. (1986) Hepatocarcinogenesis in the rat; effect of promoters and carcinogens *in vivo* and *in vitro*, *International Review in Cytology*, **101**, 125–173.

27. BANNASCH, P., ENZMANN, H., KLIMEK, F., WEBER, E. and ZERBAN, M. (1989) Significance of sequential cellular changes inside and outside foci of altered hepatocytes during hepatocarcinogenesis, *Toxicologic Pathology*, **4**, 617–628.

28. SELL, S. and DUNSFORD, M. (1989) Evidence for the stem cell origin of hepatocellular carcinoma and cholangiocarcinoma, *American Journal of Pathology*, **134**, 1347–1363.

29. WILLIAMS, G.M. (1981) Liver carcinogenesis: the role for some chemicals of an epigenetic mechanism of liver tumour promotion involving modifications of the cell membrane, *Food and Cosmetic Toxicology*, **19**, 577–583.

30. SCHULTE-HERMANN, R., TIMMERMANN-TROSIENER, I. and SCHUPPLER, J. (1983) Promotion of spontaneous pre-neoplastic cells in rat liver as a possible explanation of tumour production by non-mutagenic compounds, *Cancer Research*, **43**, 839–844.

31. DRINKWATER, N.R. and GINSLER, J.J. (1986) Genetic control of hepatocarcinogenesis in C57BL/6J and C3H/HeJ inbred mice, *Carcinogenesis*, **7**, 1701–1707.

32. EVANS, J.G., COLLINS, M.A., LAKE, B.G. and BUTLER, W.H. (1992) The histology and development of hepatic nodules in C3H/He and C57/BL mice following chronic phenobarbitone administration, *Toxicologic Pathology*, **20**, 585–594.

33. PEDRICK, M.S., RUMSBY, P.C., WRIGHT, V., PHILLIMORE, H.E., BUTLER, W.H. and EVANS, J.G. (1994) Growth characteristics and Ha-*ras* mutation of cell cultures isolated from chemically induced mouse liver tumours, *Carcinogenesis*, **15**, 1847–1852.

34. BENTLEY, P., CALDER, I., ELCOMBE, C., GRASSO, P., STRINGER, D. and WIEGAND, H.-J. (1993) Hepatic peroxisome proliferation in rodents and its significance for man, *Food and Chemical Toxicology*, **31**, 857–907.

35. ISSEMANN, I. and GREEN, S. (1990) Activation of a member of the steroid hormone receptor superfamily by peroxisome proliferators, *Nature*, **347**, 645–649.

36. LAKE, B.G. (1995) Mechanisms of hepatocarcinogenicity of peroxisome-proliferating drugs and chemicals, *Annual Review of Pharmacology and Toxicology*, **35**, 483–507.

37. CORNELIUS, C.E. (1991) Liver function tests in the differential diagnosis of hepatotoxicity, in MEEKS, R.G., HARRISON, S.D. and BULL, R.J. (Eds) *Hepatotoxicology*, pp. 181–239, London: CRC Press.

38. PRITCHARD, D.J., WRIGHT, M.G., SULSH, S. and BUTLER, W.H. (1987) The assessment of chemically induced liver injury in rats, *Journal of Applied Toxicology* **7**, 229–236.
39. WOLKOFF, A. W., JOHANSEN, K.L. and GOESER, T., 1987, The isolated perfused rat liver: preparation and application, *Analytical Biochemistry*, **167**, 1–14.
40. MCQUEEN, C.A. and WILLIAMS, G.M. (1987) Toxicological studies in cultured hepatocytes from various species, in RAUCHMAN, E.J. and PADILLA, G.H. (Eds) *The Isolated Hepatocyte: Use in Toxicology and Xenobiotic Biotransformation*, pp. 51–67, New York: Academic Press.
41. AZRI, S., GANDOLFI, A. J. and BRENDEL, K. (1990) Precision-cut liver slices: an *in vitro* system for profiling potential hepatotoxicants, *In Vitro Toxicology*, **3**, 309–320.

4

The Urinary System

PETER GREAVES

4.1 Introduction

A number of different factors make the kidney particularly susceptible to damage by a wide range of xenobiotics (Table 4.1). The kidney is exposed to high concentrations of circulating toxins because of its high blood flow. However, skeletal muscle, which is relatively resistant to toxins, also has a high blood flow. Hence, it is not high blood flow alone that makes the kidney sensitive to the effects of xenobiotics but also its unique functional organization.

For instance, circulating immune complexes are liable to be deposited in the kidneys because of the particularly large surface area of endothelial cells within the glomerular capillaries. The processes of glomerular filtration, tubular resorption and tubular secretion enhance the concentration of potentially toxic agents in the tubular cells. Changes in intratubular pH make certain compounds liable to precipitate within the tubular lumen giving rise to local tubular cell damage, inflammation and outflow obstruction. Renal tubular cells possess considerable metabolic and enzymatic activity making them susceptible to enzyme inhibitors and capable of generating toxic metabolites. The hypertonicity of the renal medulla can also enhance the concentration of drugs and metabolites within the interstitium. The dependency of the kidney on a high rate of oxygen consumption leads to the situation in which toxicity can be potentiated by the effects of anoxia.

Relatively few studies have correlated the adverse effects produced by xenobiotics in animals with those occurring in humans. The study by Fletcher [1] comparing toxic effects of drugs in animal studies with those subsequently occurring in humans, suggested that renal effects in animal studies occurred more frequently than subsequent renal effects developed in man.

4.2 Anatomy, Histology and Physiology

The complex structure of the kidney forms the basis for its diverse roles of excreting waste products, regulating body fluid balance and blood pressure as well as secretion

Table 4.1 Types of chemicals capable of producing renal toxicity

Type of principle change	Agent
Glomerulus – damage to filtration barrier	Protamine Penicillamine Puromycin
Glomerulonephritis	Immune complexes Mercury, gold salts Hydralazine Procainamide
Renal tubular necrosis	Mercury, cadmium Cisplatin Aminoglycoside antibiotics Cephalosporins Cyclosporin A Polymyxin B Amphotericin B Ethylene glycol Carbon tetrachloride Trichloroethylene κ immunoglobulin light chains
Renal tubular nuclear inclusions	Lead, bismuth
Renal tubular hyaline nephropathy (α_{2u}-globulin) in rats	Light petroleum hydrocarbons Levamisol BW540c BW58c
Crystal nephropathy	Ethylene glycol Methoxyfluorane Sulphonamides Adenine Acyclovir
Mineralization	Excessive milk and alkali intake Excessive vitamin D Acetazolamide
Interstitial nephritis	Sulphonamides Methicillin
Papillary necrosis	Non-steroidal analgesics Ethyleneimine 2-bromoethanamine
Urothelial damage	Physical agents Infections and infestations High urinary pH and sodium content Carbonic anhydrase inhibitors Bladder carcinogens (see Table 4.2)
Vascular alterations	Vasodilating antihypertensives Vasopressor agents Daunomycin

of hormones. A standardized nomenclature for the structures found in the kidney has been proposed by Kriz and colleagues [2] and renal histology has been reviewed in the detail needed by pathologists by Clapp [3]. In the laboratory rat, mouse, hamster, rabbit and dog, the kidney is composed of a single lobe, whereas in humans each kidney comprises between 10 and 14 lobes. Non-human primates possess kidneys similar to those in man, although they are unilobular in type.

4.2.1 Blood Supply

Each kidney is supplied by a main renal artery. In humans, this divides into segmental arteries which empty into interlobar arteries. These, in turn, give rise to arcuate arteries at the cortico-medullary junction. In unilobar kidneys, a similar pattern of segmental arteries also gives rise to arcuate arteries. The arcuate arteries traverse the renal parenchyma at the level of the cortico-medullary junction and give rise to interlobular (or cortical radial) arteries. Afferent arterioles originate from the interlobular arteries, each forming glomerular capillaries and efferent arteries. The medulla receives most of its blood supply through the efferent arteries that arise from glomeruli near the medulla and develop into arterial vasa recta (spuria). Arterial vasa recta turn back into venous vasa recta which empty into arcuate veins at the cortico-medullary junction. The efferent arteries arising from glomeruli near the cortex break up into a rich peritubular network of capillaries in the cortex. This network also eventually drains into arcuate veins.

4.2.2 Nephron

The main functional unit of the kidney is the nephron, composed of the glomerulus surrounded by the Bowman's space (renal corpuscle), the proximal tubule, thin limbs and the distal tubule which drains into the common collecting duct system (Figure 4.1). The renal tubular cells are representative of an important class of polarized cells involved in the transport of ions, water and macromolecules from one compartment to another. They perform this function by means of a surface membrane that is highly organized into distinct apical and basolateral domains containing different ion channels, transport proteins, enzymes and lipids [4]. For instance, the apical membrane which faces the urinary lumen contains sodium/ potassium antiporters and sodium-dependent glucose, amino acid and phosphate co-transporters which mediate the absorption of sodium from the glomerular filtrate into the cytoplasm. Sodium/potassium ATPase in the basolateral membrane then transports cytosolic sodium up an electrochemical gradient across the basolateral membrane into the extracellular fluid. Maintenance of cell polarity is dependent on the attachments between cells mediated by the calcium-dependent membrane glycoproteins called cellular adhesion molecules. Pathological insults such as produced by ischaemia have been shown to alter the membrane polarity of these molecules in the renal tubular cell [4].

Enzyme distribution along the nephron has been reviewed by Guder and Ross [5] and the biochemical asymmetry of surface membranes of epithelial cells by Fish and Molitoris [4].

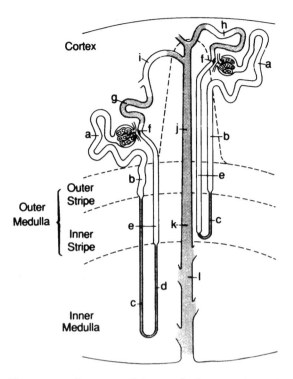

Figure 4.1 Illustration of the standard nomenclature for the nephron as defined by the Renal Commission of the International Union of Physiological Sciences [2]: (a) proximal convoluted tubule; (b) proximal straight tubule; (c) descending thin limb; (d) ascending thin limb; (e) distal straight tubule or thick ascending limb; (f) macular densa; (g) distal convoluted tubule; (h) connecting tubule; (i) connecting tubule of the juxtamedullary nephron; (j) cortical collecting duct; (k) outer medullary collecting duct; (l) inner medullary collecting duct.

4.2.3 *Glomerulus*

The glomerulus functions as a relatively selective macromolecular filter of the circulating blood. Structurally, the glomerulus represents a blind end of the proximal tubule invaginated by a tuft of capillaries. A thin fenestrated endothelium lines the lumen of the capillaries. The endothelial cytoplasm contains microfilaments and intermediate filaments and the endothelial cell surface carries a negative charge as a result of polyanionic glycoproteins. This negative charge contributes to the selectivity of the glomerular barrier. A mesangium, comprising mesangial cells and matrix, forms a central support for the capillary tuft. Ultrastructurally, mesangial cells are irregular with elongated cytoplasmic processes which are connected to the glomerular basement membrane directly or indirectly by microfibrils in the mesangial matrix. This suggests that they possess a contractile property, perhaps to counteract the distension caused by capillary and mesangial interstitial pressure [6]. The mesangial region is particularly exposed to circulating molecules because there is no basement membrane between the lumen of the glomerular capillary and the mesangial matrix. Mesangial cells have phagocytic properties and respond to a variety of factors such as interleukin I, platelet-derived growth factor and arachidonic acid metabolites.

The glomerular basement membrane can be demonstrated under light microscopy by periodic acid Schiff (PAS) and methenamine silver stains. Its major constituents are type IV collagen, proteoglycans rich in heparan sulphate, fibronectins and laminins. It is a size- and charge-selective barrier. Molecules smaller than 25 000 Da are usually able to cross the barrier and attain concentrations in glomerular filtrate of more than 50 per cent of their concentration in plasma.

The visceral epithelial cells, or podocytes, represent the largest cells in the glomerulus seen by light microscopy outside the basement membrane, where their prominent nuclei may bulge into the urinary space. Ultrastructural study has shown that podocytes have long cytoplasmic processes that surround the glomerular capillaries and divide into foot processes or pedicles which interdigitate with processes from other cells. Adjacent foot processes are separated by a filtration slit 25 to 60 nm wide which is bridged by a 4 to 6 nm filtration slit diaphragm, the precise function of which is unclear. Podocytes contain abundant rough endoplasmic reticulum, a well-developed Golgi apparatus, prominent lysosomes and numerous microtubules, microfilaments and intermediate filaments. Actin, myosin and α-actin have been located in the foot processes, whereas vimentin and tubulin appear to predominate in the cell body. The parietal layer of Bowman's capsule is usually lined by a single layer of flat squamous epithelium, but cuboidal epithelium has been described under certain circumstances in laboratory rodents and in man. In the mature male laboratory mouse or in female mice treated with male sex hormones, high cuboidal epithelium is commonly found. It is occasionally seen in laboratory rats and humans but rarely in other species.

4.2.4 *Proximal Tubule*

The proximal renal tubule has an important role in maintaining homeostasis of the organism, notably through the movement of water and sodium and chloride ions, but also by a great number of absorptive and secretory mechanisms of organic and inorganic substances. Morphologically, it is divided into an initial convoluted part and a straight portion. In some animals the proximal tubule has been subdivided into S1, S2 and S3 segments based on their ultrastructural features. The proximal convoluted tubules form the bulk of the cortical parenchyma. In histological sections, proximal tubular cells are cuboidal with a brush border, granular eosinophilic cytoplasm and round nuclei. The cell cytoplasm contains prominent lysosomes and numerous elongated mitochondria. Adjacent cells show complex basolateral interdigitations of their lateral borders. The proximal tubule is responsible for the reabsorption of about two-thirds of the glomerular infiltrate, which is coupled to the active transport of sodium mediated by the high sodium/potassium ATPase activity located in the basolateral membranes. The numerous mitochondria located close to the plasma membrane provide the energy required for active transport. The well-developed lysosomal apparatus provides the subcellular basis for the reabsorption and degradation of low-molecular-weight proteins such as albumin.

4.2.5 *Loop of Henle*

At the junction between the outer and inner stripe of the outer medulla, the proximal tubule abruptly becomes the descending thin limb of the loop of Henle. Juxtamedullary nephrons have long thin segments with the turn located near the papilla, whereas nephrons near the surface of the cortex have short thin segments. The thin limb of Henle's loop has an important role in the countercurrent multiplication component of urinary concentration. The thin descending limb is permeable to water but not to sodium ions so that passive absorption of water occurs. Conversely, the thin ascending limb is largely impermeable to water but has high permeability to sodium chloride. As a consequence, intratubular fluid entering the distal tubule is dilute and the surrounding interstitium hypertonic. Thus, the thin limb contributes to the maintenance of a hypertonic interstitium and delivery of a dilute fluid to the distal renal tubule.

4.2.6 Distal Tubule

The distal tubules, which comprise the thick ascending limb of the loop of Henle and the distal convoluted tubule, are somewhat similar to the proximal tubules, being eosinophilic with indistinct lateral borders because of basolateral membrane interdigitations and invaginations. They possess cytoplasmic basal striations due to the presence of elongated mitochondria but lack a brush border. Distal tubules are involved in the active reabsorption of sodium chloride and have high levels of sodium/potassium ATPase activity.

4.2.7 Collecting Duct System

The distal tubule is connected to the collecting duct system via a transitional connecting tubule. The collecting duct commences in the cortex and descends to the tip of the papilla. There is considerable heterogeneity along the collecting duct system but it is lined by two main cell types, the so-called principle cell and the intercalated or 'dark cell'. Although it is difficult to make the distinction on routine sections stained with haematoxylin and eosin, they can be visualized using toluidine blue, epon-embedded sections. The outer medullary collecting duct plays an important role in urine acidification. Cells possess sodium/potassium ATPase activity in their apical and basolateral membrane and high levels of carbonic anhydrase II. The inner medullary collecting duct represents the terminal part of the collecting duct and is believed to have an important role in urinary concentration; the reabsorption of urea and water in this segment causes the formation of concentrated urine.

4.2.8 Juxtaglomerular Apparatus

The juxtaglomerular apparatus is a functional unit important in tubuloglomerular feedback control of renal blood flow, glomerular filtration rate and possibly tubular control of renin secretion. The juxtaglomerular apparatus comprises afferent and efferent arterioles with granular renin-secreting cells, the macula densa, a specialized group of distal tubular cells and lacis cells, also called Goormaghtigh cells, polar cushion or extraglomerular mesangial cells. Immunocytochemical study has shown that much of the renin in the kidney is localized in the outer media of the afferent arterioles. The functional anatomy of the renin–angiotensin system has been summarized for pathologists by Lindop and Lever [7].

4.2.9 *Interstitium*

The interstitium is composed of an extracellular matrix containing sulphated and non-sulphated glycosaminoglycans and interstitial cells. Although it forms only a small proportion of renal mass, its relative volume increases from the cortex to the tip of the papilla and it may become altered in a variety of pathological states.

4.2.10 *Renal Pelvis*

The renal pelvis is a chamber with folds which extend into the medulla to form specialized fornices and ridges of the medullary outer zone, termed secondary pyramids. Transitional epithelium extends over the lining of the pelvis from the ureters to the insertion of the pelvis onto the renal parenchyma. From the point of insertion the thickness of the epithelium diminishes until a single layer of cells covered by microvilli remain over the true pyramid.

4.2.11 *Ureter and Bladder*

The ureters are designed to carry urine from the kidneys to the urinary bladder by peristalsis. The bladder is a large viscus that is able to distend to accommodate urine without changes in intraluminal pressure prior to the initiation of micturition. To achieve this, both the ureter and bladder have a similar structure, being lined by transitional epithelium or urothelium lying on a lamina propria surrounded by a layer of smooth muscle and adventitia. Transitional epithelium is stratified and the number of cell layers is variable between species. The number of urothelial cell layers seen in histological sections is somewhat dependent on the degree of stretching of the bladder or ureters prior to fixation. The basal layers are small polyhedral cells, whereas superficial cells are large polyhedral flattened cells which rest umbrella-like over smaller intermediate cells. Cell borders are highly interdigitated allowing increased epithelial area during stretching of the bladder or ureters. The luminal cell membrane is thicker than other cell surfaces and covered by a layer of extraneous, dense, filamentous material. This thickened membrane, termed an asymmetric unit membrane, is believed to serve as a selective barrier against loss of intracellular ions to the hyperosmotic urine. The superficial cells have tonofilaments, free ribosomes, some glycogen, a few mitochondria, a Golgi of medium size and flattened, discoid vesicles bounded by a trilaminar membrane which are incorporated into the surface membrane during stretching. For a detailed review of the structure of the ureters and bladder see Rhodin [8] and Reuter [9].

4.3 Biochemical and Cellular Mechanisms of Toxicity

4.3.1 *Glomerular Damage*

Although the glomerulus is exposed to circulating xenobiotics, it is a relatively uncommon site of toxic damage. However, circulating toxic chemicals may damage the glomerulus, leading to disturbance of the glomerular filtration barrier and proteinuria.

Agents such as **protamine** (a heparin antagonist) are believed to alter the polyanionic binding sites of the filtration barrier to produce proteinuria. **Penicillamine** causes structural alterations to basement membrane collagen. The deposition of excess endogenous substances such as immunoglobulin light chains or amyloid proteins produce structural defects in the glomerular basement membrane which lead to renal filtration deficiencies. The aminonucleoside, **puromycin**, damages epithelial cells (podocytes), which also leads to proteinuria.

Some chemicals disrupt endothelial or mesangial cells. Excessive quantities of circulating endogenous substances or injected macromolecules, such as **synthetic polymers**, **immunoglobulins** and **monoclonal antibodies**, which do not pass through the glomerular filtration membrane may be deposited at different locations within the glomerulus depending on their size, shape, viscosity and charge. Because of to the close proximity of mesangial cells to the circulation, these macromolecules easily enter the mesangium to be taken up within the mesangial cells.

The glomerulus may also be damaged through a number of different immunological processes. Immune complexes can be deposited in the glomerulus in several different ways. Circulating antibodies may either interact with antigens in plasma or with non-basement membrane, glomerular antibodies to become trapped *in situ*. Circulating immune complexes are usually deposited as granular deposits along the glomerular basement membrane. Although circulating immune complexes may penetrate the basement membrane into the subepithelial space, most seem to localize in the subendothelial region and the mesangium.

Antibodies to intrinsic components of the glomerular basement membrane may also develop. Spontaneously developing or induced antibodies reacting to the glomerular basement membrane are deposited as a smooth layer on the glomerular basement membrane with consequent filtration defects (antibasement-membrane disease or Masugi nephritis in the rat). Actual glomerular injury in glomerulonephritis appears dependent on activation of the complement system either through the classic or alternate pathway with activation of a variety of cytokines and the coagulation cascade.

Damage to the glomerular filtration mechanism allows protein to leak into the urine (proteinuria). If severe, this leads to such a massive loss of circulating albumin that oedema results (nephrotic syndrome). If, in addition, the capillary walls are disrupted, red blood cells also leak into the urine to produce haematuria (nephritic syndrome).

A number of drugs and chemicals including **mercury** and **gold salts**, **D-penicillamine**, **heroin**, **hydralazine**, and **procainamide** have been shown to produce different forms of glomerulonephritis in man through immunological mechanisms [10]. Although similar lesions have been reproduced in experimental animals and some mechanisms have been identified, findings are not entirely consistent between species. This is probably because these immune-related responses are genetically restricted. For example, it has been demonstrated that different rat strains vary in their susceptibility to the induction of glomerulonephritis by **mercury**. Brown Norway rats develop a severe antiglomerular basement membrane disease, whereas an immune complex nephritis associated with antinuclear antibodies occurs in the Wistar and the PVG/c strains. Other strains are resistant to mercury-induced glomerulonephritis [11, 12]. Hence, one chemical is capable of inducing variable immune responses among different strains of experimental animals and among humans which are accompanied by different morphological expressions of glomerular injury.

4.3.2 *Renal Tubular Injury*

The renal tubule is sensitive to toxic insults because of its ability to concentrate potentially toxic substances which enter the tubule either from the circulation, by filtration through the glomerulus, or from the blood stream, by active transport via the tubular cells into the tubular lumen. Hence, the renal tubule can be exposed to higher concentrations of potentially toxic substances than those present in the plasma. Although the renal tubule is well adapted to excrete toxic substances, its defence mechanisms can be overwhelmed, resulting in tubular cell damage. Moreover, because parts of the renal tubule are sensitive to anoxia, any associated circulatory disturbances can potentiate or complicate primary toxic tubular damage.

It has been suggested that renal tubular cells may be damaged by xenobiotics through several different mechanisms analogous to those believed to produce toxic reactions within the liver [13]. A chemical may interfere directly with essential metabolic or functional processes. A chemical may become metabolized within the renal cell to a highly reactive intermediate that binds covalently to protein or produces lipid peroxidation. Finally, a chemical may be metabolized by extrarenal enzymes to form a stable systemic metabolite, which then enters the kidney to produce renal toxicity by one of the above mechanisms.

A large number of xenobiotics can damage the renal tubule of man and laboratory animals, see Table 4.1 [14, 15]. Although sensitivity of the renal tubule to damage is variable between different species, these differences have not been well studied. However, only a few chemicals have shown complete species selectivity in renal toxicity.

Heavy metals such as **mercury** and **cadmium** are believed to produce tubular necrosis through a direct cytotoxic effect as they are potent inhibitors of a large number of cellular processes and as they are concentrated in the renal tubular cell. **Chromium** is excreted primarily via the kidneys, where it is also capable of producing tubular damage. **Lead** is also capable of producing damage to the renal tubular cell. Histologically, lead nephropathy is characterized by formation of dense, eosinophilic, acid-fast intranuclear inclusion bodies and disturbance to mitochondria which is associated with tubular dysfunction and characterized by amino aciduria, glycosuria, proteinuria and urinary casts. The inclusions are believed to be the result of the binding of lead with non-histone chromosomal protein. Excess ingestion of **bismuth** can also induce renal tubular damage associated with intranuclear and intracytoplasmic inclusions, believed to be composed of bismuth–protein complexes. These bodies are typically yellowish-brown, refractile and stain with PAS and Ziehl–Neelsen stains.

The platinum antineoplastic drug, **cisplatin**, produces tubular damage in both man and animals, although this may be the result of a metabolite of cisplatin rather than the parent drug. Tubular damage by heavy metals is potentiated by ischaemia secondary to associated vasoconstriction.

A wide variety of antibiotics have been shown to possess the potential to damage the renal tubule, although it is important to note that many of the reported nephrotoxic effects of antibiotics in humans are related to the circumstances under which they are used. The type of patient requiring an antibiotic is also likely to have pre-existing renal damage or an underlying disease process which is associated with electrolyte imbalance or alterations in renal blood flow [16].

Aminoglycoside antibiotics are well-known nephrotoxic drugs in both man and experimental animals. **Neomycin**, used mainly by the topical route is particularly nephrotoxic but **kanamycin**, **gentamicin** and **streptomycin** are examples of other aminoglycosides with nephrotoxic potential. These agents are excreted mainly by glomerular filtration whereupon some of the cationic drug binds to anionic phospholipids on the brush border of the tubular cells. This bound drug enters the lysosomes by endocytosis leading to an accumulation of drug in proximal tubular cells where it may persist for several days. This leads to the accumulation of characteristic, electron-dense lamellar lipid membranes within lysosomes (myeloid bodies) as well as overt tubular cell damage. Renal tubular damage is also produced by antibiotics of other classes, notably **polymyxin B**, **cephalosporins**, notably **cephaloridine**, and the polyene antifungal **amphotericin B**.

The immunosuppressive agent **cyclosporin A**, is a highly lipophilic drug which produces nephrotoxicity partly by altering renal haemodynamics, manifest by a decrease in glomerular filtration rate. The precise mechanism is unclear.

A number of volatile or halogenated hydrocarbons produce renal tubular necrosis. **Ethylene glycol**, a component of antifreeze, is one of the most nephrotoxic by virtue of a direct effect on tubular epithelial cells and rapid metabolism to oxalic acid, which forms masses of calcium oxalate in renal tubules. The result is a focal necrosis of tubular cells, dilatation of tubules proximal to the site of damage and obstruction and an inflammatory response within the interstitium. **Carbon tetrachloride**, a widely used industrial solvent, also has a direct toxic effect on the renal tubule. It produces damage to proximal tubules and its effects are potentiated by **ethanol** ingestion. **Trichloroethylene**, used as a cleaning agent, is another nephrotoxic hydrocarbon which produces proximal tubular damage and renal failure following excessive exposure.

In male but not female rats, light petroleum hydrocarbons have been shown to produce a renal tubular nephropathy characterized by accumulation of protein droplets in the renal tubular cells. Examples include unleaded gasoline and related products such as **decalin** (decahydronaphthalene), **JP5 jet fuel, Stoddard solvent 2,2,4-trimethylpentane, isophorone, 1,4-dichlorobenzene** and **d-limonene** (aromatic hydrocarbon) [17, 18]. The pharmacological agents, the pyrazoline **BW54OC**, the naphthoquinone **BW58C** and **levamisol** have also been shown to produce similar hyaline droplet accumulation [19].

It is believed that these agents or their metabolites bind to α_{2u}-globulin, a low-molecular-weight protein of 18 700 Da, which is synthesized in the liver of adult male rats and which passes into the glomerular filtrate. The chemical–protein complex is taken up by the proximal tubule through endocytosis where it accumulates in excess because it is resistant to degradation. The accumulation of excess droplets ultimately leads to disruption of tubular cells. As female rats and other species including humans neither synthesize this protein nor develop this disorder, it is believed that this particular type of nephropathy is specific to the male rat.

Although immunoglobulins are essential for health, their presence in excess within renal tubules can cause tubular damage in both man and animals. For example, the renal damage which develops in patients with myeloma is believed to be partly due to the direct tubular toxicity of monoclonal light chains (Bence-Jones proteins). An excess of certain types of monomeric or dimeric κ **light chains** (22 000 Da) enter the glomerular filtrate to be taken up by the renal tubules where they are capable of producing tubular dysfunction and overt tubular necrosis. Other macromolecules, such as circulating free **haemoglobin** in haemolytic states and **myoglobin** in rhabdomyolysis, also pass through the glomerular filter and enter the tubule where they may also produce tubular damage [20].

Localized tubular damage also occurs as a result of crystal formation of a wide variety of substances within the distal and collecting tubules. For instance, in humans with gout, endogenous **urates** may precipitate causing local destruction of the tubular wall and concomitant inflammation and a giant-cell reaction. Both **ethylene glycol** and **methoxyfluorane** produce precipitation of calcium oxalate crystals in the renal tubules.

Xenobiotics or their metabolites of low solubility may also precipitate in the renal tubule and when severe, urinary stasis, renal parenchymal inflammation and a foreign-body giant-cell response in the interstitial tissue results. For example, renal tubular crystal deposition has been reported with **sulphonamide** and **quinolone antibiotics, adenine,** the purine nucleoside antiviral analogue, **acyclovir** and a benzopyran−4-one, **PD119819** [21].

Disturbance of calcium balance may lead to the deposition of calcium salts in the kidneys. In humans, excessive intake of **vitamin D** is a well-known cause of nephrocalcinosis and this can be reproduced in experimental animals. Agents such as **acetazolamide** or excessive ingestion of **milk** and **alkali** for the treatment of peptic ulcers that produce disturbances in urinary acid−base balance may also induce nephrocalcinosis. The rat is particularly susceptible because manipulation of dietary mineral balance or administration of excess **calcium salts** readily induces nephrolithiasis.

4.3.3 *Interstitial Damage*

It may be difficult to determine histologically whether the interstitium is a primary site of toxic damage because the interstitium is almost invariably involved when there is severe tubular damage. However, primary interstitial nephritis, or perhaps more correctly described as 'tubulo-interstitial nephritis' appears to result from one of two principle mechanisms. Formation of antitubular basement membrane antibodies can give rise to tubulo-interstitial disease analogous to the manner in which antiglomerular antibasement membrane antibodies lead to glomerulonephritis. Examples of agents that are believed to produce interstitial damage by this mechanism are some **sulphonamides** and **penicillins,** notably **methicillin.**

Concentration of toxins or toxic metabolites in the interstitium may also lead to interstitial damage, examples being analgesic nephropathy. Despite extensive epidemiological and experimental investigation [22], the precise pathogenesis of the chronic interstitial nephritis, papillary necrosis and subsequent transitional cell tumours of urothelium, which is linked to the excessive ingestion of **analgesic agents** in humans, remains unclear. The epidemiology of papillary necrosis is complicated by the fact that a number of disease states, such as diabetes mellitus, urinary obstruction, sickle cell anaemia, jaundice and renal inflammation predispose to its development. Nevertheless, administration of **non-steroidal analgesics** and related experimental agents such as **ethyleneimine, 2-bromoethylamine hydrobromide** are capable of inducing papillary necrosis in laboratory animals, notably rats. Experimental studies have suggested the involvement of a number of mechanisms in the development of papillary necrosis, including direct toxicity of these agents or their metabolites, exacerbated by their concentration in the papilla, by dehydration, microvascular degeneration and medullary ischaemia, altered prostaglandin metabolism or disruption of the medullary matrix [22].

4.3.4 Urothelial Injury

The urothelium is normally only a slowly proliferating tissue, but it is capable of responding to injury by a marked proliferative response. As a consequence, hyperplasia represents one of the most common lesions of the urinary bladder and ureters. Proliferation of the urothelium is produced by a great variety of insults including **mechanical damage**, instillation of **water** or **saline, foreign bodies, freezing, ionizing radiation, chronic infection** and infestation with **parasites** such as *Trichosomoides crassicauda* in the rat. Most **genotoxic bladder carcinogens** (see below and Table 4.2) produce urothelial hyperplasia in common with a great number of non-carcinogens. It has also been shown that alterations in **urinary pH**, high **urinary sodium** and **bladder distension** are also capable of inducing urothelial hyperplasia. Drugs such as the **carbonic anhydrase inhibitors** that alter urinary pH and ion content have also been shown to produce mild urothelial damage acutely followed by hyperplasia [23, 24].

4.3.5 Disturbances in Blood Supply and Ischaemia

It should always be kept in mind that perturbations of the systemic circulation, either through spontaneous or induced disease, can adversely affect renal function or produce pathological renal alterations. Many systemic vascular disorders in humans such as atherosclerosis, hypertensive vascular disease and vasculitis can affect renal blood vessels and produce local ischaemia or infarction of renal tissue. Likewise, spontaneous arteritis in laboratory animals can develop within the renal vasculature. In rodent toxicity studies, vascular necrosis and inflammations, induced by administration of cardioactive drugs agents such as the **vasodilating antihypertensives** and **angiotensin**, as well as the anticancer anthracycline, **daunomycin**, and the mitomycin derivative, **BMY- 25282**, may also develop in the kidney [21].

Hypovolaemia or cardiovascular malfunction through a variety of causes may reduce renal perfusion to such an extent that renal function is compromised, sometimes so severely that renal failure occurs. This latter phenomenon is termed 'pre-renal failure' in contrast to 'post-renal failure' which occurs in response to severe urinary outflow obstruction. Administration of high doses of **digoxin** to dogs produces renal tubular dilatation and degeneration, possibly through lowered renal perfusion [21]. Moreover, because glomerular filtration rate may cease if the (negative) oncotic forces exceed the hydrolic forces (positive) in the glomerulus, renal failure can occur in hyperoncotic states in patients following the infusion of **high-molecular-weight dextran** to expand plasma volume [25].

4.3.6 Neoplasia

Primary renal tumours represent an important class of neoplasms in humans and they are found spontaneously in aged animals employed in carcinogenesis testing. The rat is the most frequently used laboratory animal in the study of renal carcinogenesis and a wide range of histological types of renal tumours have been induced in this species by treatment with over 100 different genotoxic chemicals (Table 4.2) [26, 27]. **Heterocyclic amines** and **amides** and **nitrosocompounds** have been the most commonly employed chemicals in the experimental investigation of renal carcinogenesis. Renal tumours have also been induced in rats by **ionizing radiation** and inoculation of neonates with **polyoma virus**.

In humans, the renal tumour most commonly linked to exposure to a xenobiotic is the transitional cell carcinoma of the renal pelvis which is associated with chronic

Table 4.2   Chemicals capable of inducing renal and
urinary bladder neoplasia in rats [26, 27, 29]

Renal cell adenoma and carcinoma
    Lead salts
    N-(4'-fluoro-4-biphenylyl)acetamide
    Formic acid
    Dimethylnitrosamine
    Diethylnitrosamine
    N-ethyl-N-hydroxyethylnitrosamine
    N-nitrosomorpholine
    Streptozotocin
    Cycasin
    Aflatoxin
    Daunomycin
    Nitrilotriacetate
    Tris(2,3-dibromopropyl)phosphate

Nephroblastoma
    Dimethylbenz[a]anthracene
    N-nitrosoethylurea

Renal mesenchymal tumour
    Dimethylnitrosamine
    N-nitrosomethylurea
    N-nitrosoethylurea
    Streptozotocin
    Cycasin
    Ethyl methane sulphonate
    1,2-dimethylhydrazine

Renal pelvic carcinoma
    N-[4-(5-nitro-2-furyl)-2-thiazolyl]formamide (FANFT)
    Di-isopropanolnitrosamine
    Bis-(2-oxopropyl)-nitrosamine
    Phenacetin

Urinary bladder carcinoma
    β-Naphthylamine
    N-butyl-N-(4-hydroxybutyl)-nitrosamine (BBN)
    N-[4-(5-nitro-2-furyl)-2-thiazolyl]formamide (FANFT)
    N-methyl-N-nitrosourea
    Cyclophosphamide
    Saccharin

analgesic abuse, particularly, **phenacetin**. **Phenacetin** is an aromatic amide with *N*-hydroxylated metabolites which appear to be potentially nephrotoxic.

A number of industrial chemicals have been incriminated in the induction of bladder cancer in humans, notably *β*-**naphthylamine**, **benzidine**, **4-amino-diphenyl** and **4-nitrodiphenyl**.

Whilst for many years *β*-**naphthylamine** was the only human bladder carcinogen known to induce tumours in experimental animals, a number of chemicals have now been shown capable of inducing neoplasms in the urinary bladder experimentally (Table 4.2) [28, 29]. Laboratory rodents and humans treated with the alkylating anticancer drug, **cyclophosphamide**, develop atypical and persistent hyperplasia and bladder neoplasia. Data obtained from biopsies and cytological preparations from human bladders and experimental studies have demonstrated a close relationship between cytological atypia and the development of bladder cancer.

Whereas these genotoxic agents appear to be clear examples of xenobiotics capable of inducing bladder neoplasia in both man and laboratory animals, in many instances where transitional cell tumours have been induced in laboratory animals by non-genotoxic agents, the relevance of the findings for man are less clear.

One of the main difficulties relates to the development of transitional cell neoplasms following the prolonged hyperplasia associated with the presence of treatment-induced bladder calculi or other extraneous materials in the bladder lumen. A close association between the presence of calculi and prolonged hyperplasia with development of bladder neoplasia has been established in a number of rodent models.

Weil and colleagues [30] showed that urothelial neoplasms which developed in rats treated with **diethylene glycol** were closely associated with bladder stones and that if the stones were removed, washed and reimplanted into the bladders of young rats, transitional tumours also resulted. Analogous effects have been shown in mice with bladders implanted with foreign bodies of various types, including **cholesterol** and **paraffin wax**. Although rats treated with **sulphonamides** develop bladder tumours, this has been shown to be linked to crystalluria and stone formation in an alkaline urine. Crystals, stones and the tumourigenic response disappear when the urine is acidified using ammonium chloride.

In view of the association between urinary tract lithiasis and the presence of foreign bodies with the development of urothelial neoplasia, a thorough examination for bladder calculi is essential in preclinical safety studies where bladder neoplasms are found.

4.4 Morphological Responses to Injury

4.4.1 Renal Weight Changes

Administration of xenobiotics may alter renal weight and as a consequence any renal weight changes in toxicity studies should be assessed with care. When increases in renal weight are manifestations of toxicity, they are frequently associated with macroscopic appearances of swelling and pallor of the kidney and evidence of significant damage on histological examination. When increases in renal weight occur in the absence of histopathological alterations, it is reasonable to assume that the changes are a manifestation of adaptive responses to increased physiological demands placed on the renal tissue in the elimination of the xenobiotic. Some xenobiotics, notably **angiotensin-converting enzyme (ACE) inhibitors**, have been associated with a reduction in renal weight without evidence of renal cellular damage, presumably as a result of reduced renal demand.

4.4.2 *Glomerular Hypertrophy*

Compensatory enlargement of the glomerular tuft is described following partial or unilateral nephrectomy, cyanotic heart disease, pulmonary hypertension and polycythaemia, possibly as a response to increased renal perfusion.

4.4.3 *Glomerular Atrophy*

The glomerulus can undergo atrophy as a result of ischaemic collapse in vascular disorders and vascular occlusion or as a result of compression by surrounding epithelial crescents (see below).

4.4.4 *Glomerulonephritis*

The term 'glomerulonephritis' implies an inflammatory process affecting the glomerular tuft, although clear evidence of inflammation within the glomerulus is frequently not present and diverse pathological reactions are included under this heading. The lack of overt inflammation may be partly due to the unique anatomy of the glomerulus, notably the lack of loose connective tissue which limits the range of expression of the inflammatory reaction.

Classification of glomerulonephritis occurring in humans is founded primarily on morphological and immunocytochemical criteria because of the lack of clear aetiological factors in many cases. To a certain extent, the morphological types found in man have been reproduced in laboratory animals by various immunological manipulations or administration of xenobiotics. However, the same agent may produce more than one type of change (Table 4.3). Unfortunately, the confusing terminology also confounds the exact correlation between human and animal glomerular diseases.

Virtually all species of animals can develop glomerulonephritis. Membranous or membrano-proliferative glomerulonephritis develops spontaneously in dogs although seldom in young laboratory-bred beagles. Some laboratory mouse strains, notably the New Zealand Black (NZB) develop glomerulonephritis that resembles that found in systemic lupus erythematosis (SLE) in man.

In the rat, the classical form of immune complex nephritis is serum sickness, which can be induced by the injection of a single large dose of foreign protein such as **bovine serum albumin**.

Heyman nephritis

This is a form of immune complex disease induced in the rat by injection of small quantities of **autologous renal tubular antigen** in Freund's adjuvant. This procedure probably induces production of autoantibodies which react with autologous antigens. Histologically, Heyman glomerulonephritis resembles human

Table 4.3 Glomerulonephritis produced by xenobiotics in man [10]

Morphological type	Typical morphology	Drugs implicated
Minimal change (lipoid nephrosis)	No light microscopic alterations, normal cellularity, fusion of foot processes seen at EM, epithelial cells sometimes vacuolated, no deposits	D-Penicillamine, probenicid, heroin, mercurial diuretics, gold salts
Membranous	Diffuse hyaline thickening of glomerular capillary walls, normal cellularity, silver stains show spiked basement membrane, granular patterns of immunoglobulin (IgG) along basement membrane, electron-dense subepithelial deposits	D-Penicillamine, gold salts, heroin, mercurial diuretics, trimethadione
Focal with systemic lupus-like syndrome	Variable lobular proliferation of mesangial cells, fibrinoid necrosis, red cells in glomerular space.	D-Penicillamine, procainamide, hydralazine, quinidine
Proliferative with crescents (Goodpasture's syndrome)	Proliferation of visceral and epithelial cells, crescents, typically linear antibasement-membrane immunoglobulin but granular patterns of immunoglobulin occur	D-Penicillamine
Mesangiocapillary (membranoproliferative)	Proliferative changes involving endothelial and mesangial cells, lobular pattern, doubling of basement membrane seen by silver stains, EM may show subendothelial deposits or dense deposits in lamina densa	Suphadiazine silver, heroin
Glomerulosclerosis	Focal or segmental glomerular sclerosis and hyalinization, collapse of basement membrane, disruption to epithelial cells	Heroin

114

membranous glomerulonephritis because of granular electron-dense deposits of IgG along the glomerulus basement membrane.

Antiglomerular basement membrane glomerulonephritis (Masugi nephritis in the rat)

This form of glomerulonephritis is produced by intravenous injection of **heterologous antibodies** against glomerular basement membrane. It is characterized by an infiltration of polymorphonuclear and mononuclear cells, variable swelling and extracapillary proliferation with formation of crescents. Immunocytochemical study reveals a linear binding of antibasement membrane antibody along the glomerular basement membrane.

Administration of agents such as **mercury** and **gold salts** and **D-penicillamine** to rats and mice has also been shown to be capable of inducing immune complex glomerulonephritis. However, its induction and expression is highly strain dependent (see above).

4.4.5 *Glomerular Vacuolation*

Vacuolation is seen in the glomerulus both as a spontaneous lesion or as a result of administration of drugs and chemicals. In some animals, particularly the beagle, foam cells containing lipid are considered a normal variation, although they may be more prevalent in older, obese animals. Variably sized, clear vacuoles have been described by light microscopic examination in the glomerular epithelial cells in laboratory rats treated with **anthracycline antibiotics** and other **anticancer drugs** (Figure 4.2). Their pathogenesis is uncertain although they may relate to drug-induced alterations in the plasma membrane of glomerular epithelial cells. **Puromycin**, an aminonucleoside cancer chemotherapeutic agent, also causes podocyte damage and proteinuria when administered to rats and this phenomenon has been used as an experimental model for the human 'minimal change' glomerulonephritis (Table 4.3).

4.4.6 *Glomerular Sclerosis (including chronic progressive nephropathy in rats)*

Glomerulosclerosis in man is a disease process characterized by sclerosis (excessive matrix) and presence of masses of proteinaceous material within capillary loops (hyalinization), particularly in juxtaglomerular glomeruli. It may be a focal (some glomeruli affected) or segmental (part of each glomerular tuft affected) process. Electron microscopy shows focal basement membrane collapse and disruption of epithelial cells and foot processes (Table 4.3). Its aetiology and pathogenesis is uncertain but glomerular sclerosis appears to be histogenetically related to 'minimal change' glomerulonephritis. Both types are believed to be due to a circulating molecule in patients that is probably not an immunoglobulin [31]. Injection of this circulating factor into rats has been shown to produce proteinuria. Glomerulosclerosis appears to be the most common form of glomerular damage in man which is associated with **heroin** abuse [10].

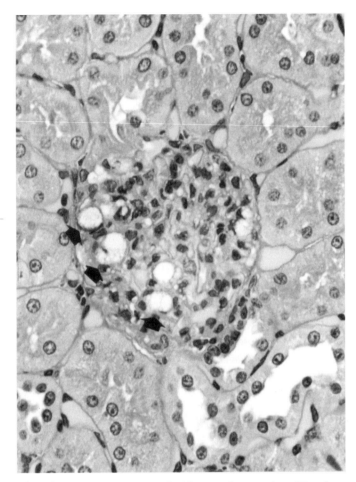

Figure 4.2   Kidney from a Wistar rat treated with an anticancer drug. The glomerulus shows vacuolation of the glomerular epithelial cells (arrows).

Although different to the human disease, glomerulosclerosis also represents a common spontaneous renal disease in the aged laboratory rat. It is an important condition because of the widespread use of rats in experimental toxicology and the fact that its development may be accelerated or retarded by treatment with a number of xenobiotics which modify renal function. Moreover, this form of glomerulosclerosis is associated with a number of histological features in common with the effects of tubular toxins so that it has the potential to confound the interpretation of toxicity studies performed in the rat. Its prevalence varies between rat strains but it is usually more common in males. Food or protein restriction retards its development and its onset can be accelerated by high calorie or high protein diet, salt loading or partial nephrectomy and the administration of xenobiotics that increase renal demand. For instance, its onset can be retarded by the administration of the inhibitor of prolactin secretion, **bromocriptine**. Drugs of quite different classes such as the antisecretory agent **omeprazole, dazoxiben**, a thromboxane synthetase inhibitor, **ibopamine**, and a dopamine analogue as well as **cyclosporin A** have been reported to exacerbate rat renal glomerulosclerosis in high-dose toxicology experiments.

The pathogenesis of the spontaneous rat condition remains uncertain but it seems to be primarily a basement membrane dysfunction as a result of changes in its amino acid composition and increased hydroxylation and glycosylation.

In its established form, the disease is characterized by enlargement, pallor and microcystic changes of the kidneys. Microscopic examination shows focal sclerosis of the glomerular tuft with little or no increase in cellularity, and periglomerular sclerosis and fibrosis. Thickening of the glomerular basement membrane is demonstrable by electron microscopy.

Renal tubules also show basement membrane thickening, sclerotic alteration and develop variable degrees of tubule cell degeneration, basophilia, atrophy, dilatation and cast formation. In advanced cases, tubular cells may show a variety of other alterations including accumulation of protein or pigment droplets, hypertrophy and hyperplasia. The interstitium may contain chronic inflammatory cells and show a fibroblastic reaction. Tubular changes in mild forms of disease may be found in quite young rats and may be difficult to distinguish from tubular damage induced by xenobiotics in short-term toxicity studies.

4.4.7 *Amyloidosis*

Amyloid accumulation develops in a number of chronic inflammatory conditions, following alterations in immune status and in diabetes mellitus in man. The rat remains relatively resistant to the development of amyloid, although it occurs spontaneously in untreated aged mice and hamsters. There are two major classes of amyloid fibrils, those composed of immunoglobulin light polypeptide chains and a similar group of proteins with an almost identical N-terminal amino acid sequence, designated A protein. Both are believed to originate from precursor proteins found within circulating plasma. It is the latter A type that is believed to form the major component of amyloid in experimental animals.

Man, mouse and hamster develop amyloid deposits in the glomeruli, and the tubules are also affected in severe cases. Pale aggregates of eosinophilic amyloid which stain red with Congo red are found within the glomeruli. Ultrastructural study shows amyloid fibrils within mesangial cells and around the capillary basement membrane. Extensive secondary changes develop in the renal tubules and the interstitium. The renal pelvis may eventually show infiltration by deposits of amyloid.

Experimental studies have shown that administration of agents that influence B- and T-cell function such as **thymic hormones** as well as **oestrogens** and **pituitary hormones** may alter the expression of amyloid [21]. Renal amyloid has been reported to develop in dogs treated with the antiarthritic organic gold drug, **auranofin** [32].

4.4.8 *Tubular Necrosis*

The histological features of tubular necrosis are generally fairly non-specific but vary with the time at which tissues are examined following the insult. The distribution of damage may also vary with the nature of the insult. At an early stage, affected tubules may contain degenerate tubular cells or cell debris. Subsequently, the tubules become dilated and lined by flattened regenerating cells characterized by basophilic cytoplasm, hyperchromatic irregular nuclei and occasional mitotic figures (Figure 4.3). Casts and

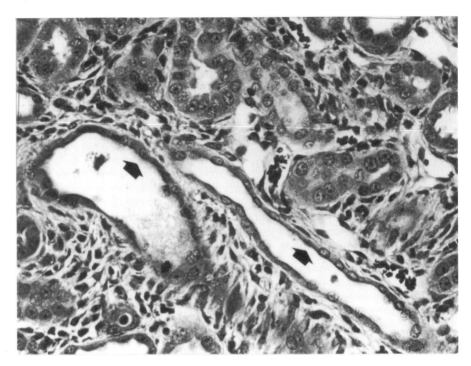

Figure 4.3 Section from the renal cortex of a Wistar rat treated with a novel drug that proved to produce excessive tubular necrosis. Damaged tubules are dilated and lined by flattened hyperchromatic cells (arrows). The interstitium shows infiltration by chronic inflammatory cells.

cell debris may be seen also in the distal tubules and collecting ducts. Oedema and inflammatory cells are found in the interstitial tissue.

4.4.9   Tubular Vacuolation

Vacuoles are seen in renal tubular cells under a variety of different circumstances both as spontaneous lesions and as a result of the effects of xenobiotics. As cytoplasmic vacuolation may result from cell damage and disruption of subcellular organelles and represent an early manifestation of tubular damage, it is important to assess the nature of any tubular cell vacuoles with care. Older terminologies for tubular vacuolation such as 'cloudy swelling' (Figure 4.4) are best avoided and more accurate descriptions based on an understanding of subcellular alterations should be used.

Tubular vacuoles can result from the presence of lipid droplets. Whilst these may be quite normal in certain species such as the dog, they may also be manifestations of mild tubular toxic damage. Lipid droplets are found in humans with diabetic nephropathy as well as the nephrotic syndrome (hence the term 'lipoid nephrosis', see Table 4.3 and Figure 4.4).

4.4.10   Hydropic Change

This is characterized histologically by pale-staining, swollen tubular cell cytoplasm containing fine and diffusely dispersed vacuoles (Figure 4.5). It represents a reversible

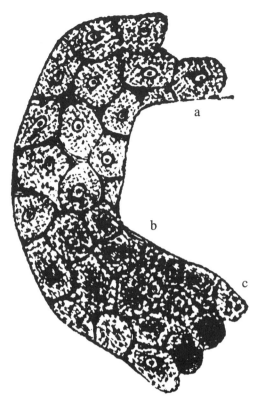

Figure 4.4 Woodcut from Virchow [35] accompanying an early description of cytological alterations within renal tubules. This represents a renal cortical tubule from a patient with 'Bright's disease' (glomerulonephritis) in which there is usually a nephrotic syndrome with excess protein in the renal tubule. It shows: (a) fairly normal epithelium; (b) cells showing 'cloudy swelling'; (c) early fatty change and degeneration.

alteration associated with a variety of pathological states in both humans and laboratory animals. Hydropic change occurs in man and laboratory animals following intravenous administration of **hypertonic sugar solutions** and **dextrans**, and in general disease states where there are severe electrolyte derangements. The vacuoles stain neither for glycogen nor lipid. Ultrastructural study has shown that the vacuoles developing after administration of **sugar solutions** and **dextrans** are lysosomal in nature, probably resulting from the pinocytosis of the infused carbohydrates.

Clear, PAS-positive staining vacuoles resulting from the accumulation of glycogen can be found in rats and humans with diabetes mellitus and their severity correlates with blood glucose levels.

4.4.11 Large Clear Vacuoles

These develop in proximal tubular cells and also occur in hypokalaemic states which result in impaired tubular concentrating mechanisms. Administration of **thiazide diuretics** is one of the main causes of potassium depletion in humans. Light microscopic examination shows the presence of large, clear vacuoles within the main

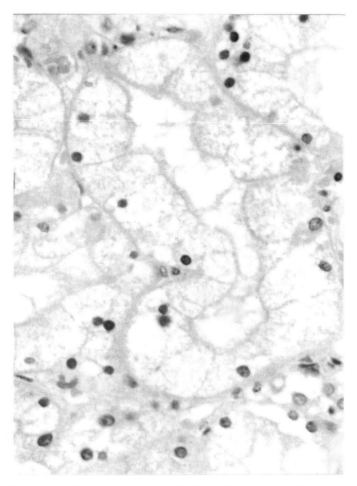

Figure 4.5 Renal cortex from a patient treated with an intravenous infusion of mannitol before death. Proximal tubular cells show typical swollen 'hydropic' appearances.

part of the tubular cell cytoplasm. Electron microscopic examination has shown that they partly result from distension of extracellular spaces with separation of the basal plasma membranes.

4.4.12 Tubular Hyaline Droplets

Dense, eosinophilic, rounded or angular droplets composed principally of proteinaceous material, usually within lysosomes of the proximal tubular cells are termed hyaline droplets (Figure 4.6). They can be well visualized using a toluidine blue stain. Electron microscopic examination shows their crystalloid nature, often accompanied by an ordered, electron-dense lattice structure of distinct periodicity, features consistent with crystalline protein or a similar macromolecule (Figure 4.7). These bodies are usually intimately associated with lysosomes and have high lysosomal enzyme activity. They occur under a variety of circumstances in both man and laboratory animals but they become particularly large or prominent when there is

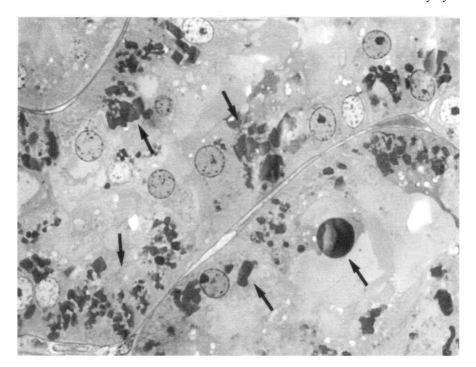

Figure 4.6 Section of kidney from a male Wistar rat treated with a xenobiotic that induced the accumulation of hyaline droplets in the cells of proximal renal tubule. Typical angular and rounded droplets (arrows) are visible in this plastic-embedded section stained with toluidine blue.

enhanced protein accumulation within the proximal tubule. This may be the result of increased protein catabolism, administration of proteins by the parenteral route or disturbance of the protein catabolic activity of the proximal tubular cell.

Administration of **volatile hydrocarbons** and some drugs (see above) to male rats has also been shown to produce hyaline droplets composed principally of the normal male rat urinary protein α_{2u}-globulin. Tubular cell overload by these droplets and crystals leads to chronic tubular cell damage. As this globulin is not present in humans, this form of xenobiotic-induced alteration is believed to be rat specific.

4.4.13 *Tubular Crystal Deposition*

Xenobiotics or endogenous compounds of low solubility have a tendency to precipitate in the distal nephron where the urine reaches its greatest concentration (Figures 4.8 and 4.9). Crystal deposition has been reported for a number of drugs when administered in high doses either to laboratory animals or to humans. Examples include **sulphonamides** and the antiviral drug, **acyclovir**. Crystals are seen predominantly in the collecting ducts where they may be accompanied by an inflammatory reaction, foreign-body giant cells, tubular dilatation and tubular epithelial hyperplasia. Some particularly insoluble agents may be precipitated in the proximal parts of the nephron. Unlike protein crystalloids, drug crystals often dissolve from the tissues during histological processing, leaving empty clefts within the tissue sections.

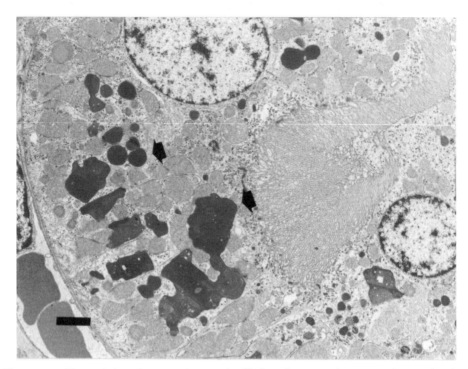

Figure 4.7 Transmission electron micrograph of kidney from a male Wistar rat treated with a xenobiotic (levamisol) that produced hyaline droplets in the proximal tubules. Typical, moderately electron-dense, rounded and angular deposits can be seen in the proximal tubular cell cytoplasm (arrows). Bar = 2 μm. Illustration from *Histopathology of Preclinical Toxicity Studies* by courtesy of Elsevier Science Publishers and Dr N.G. Read.

4.4.14 *Pigmentation of Tubular Cells*

Lipofuscin, characterized as small yellowish-brown droplets in the cytoplasm of the proximal renal tubular cell, may be seen in laboratory animals with advancing age. Certain classes of drug such as the **benzodiazepines** potentiate the development of lipofuscin droplets in renal tubules. Bile pigment can be seen when there is bilirubinaemia.

Haemoglobin may be found in the renal tubules in haemolytic states but a more common expression of haemolysis is the presence of iron in renal tubular cells or in the urine. Free haemoglobin enters the renal tubules where it is catabolized and the haem iron is incorporated into storage protein (ferritin and haemosiderin). It can be demonstrated histochemically by Perls' (Prussian blue) stain for iron. Perls' positive iron droplets may also be seen when there are other causes of high iron turnover in the kidney.

4.4.15 *Tubular Nuclear Inclusions*

Two metals are known to produce intranuclear inclusions, **lead** and **bismuth**. Ingestion of excess **lead** is capable of producing renal tubular damage characterized

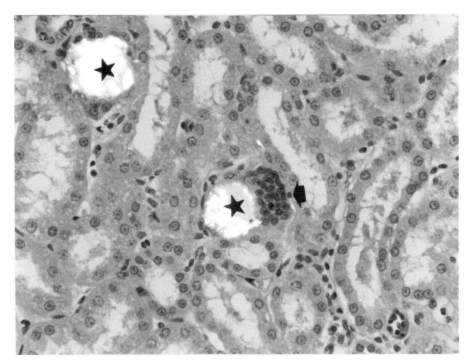

Figure 4.8 Section of a kidney from a cynomolgus monkey showing the presence of birefringent oxalate crystals (stars) within proximal tubular cells, accompanied by foreign-body giant cells (arrow). Polarized light.

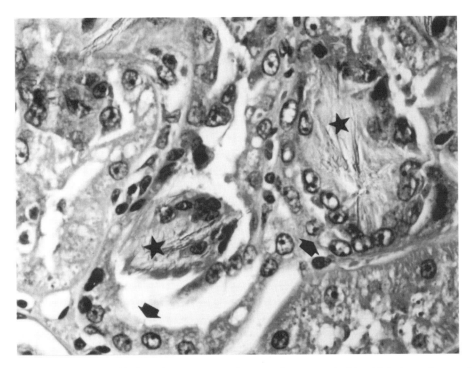

Figure 4.9 Section of kidney from a cynomolgus monkey treated with a high dose of a novel drug which formed crystals within the renal tubules. In this field, foreign-body giant cells have formed around elongated drug crystals (stars) which have caused tubular damage (arrows).

123

histologically by the presence of typical dense, eosinophilic, acid-fast inclusion bodies, usually with a halo, predominantly in the proximal tubular cell nuclei but also occasionally in the cytoplasm. Electron microscopic examination shows electron-dense bodies with a dense central core surrounded by a cortex of matted and radiating filaments [33]. **Bismuth** also produces large spherical intranuclear acid-fast inclusions, with occasional cytoplasmic forms, typically yellowish brown and refractile. Ultrastructurally, these are typically round with a sharp margin, unlike lead-induced inclusions.

4.4.16 *Tubular Hypertrophy*

Hypertrophy of the renal tubules or collecting ducts is found in response to increased renal demand that occurs following **partial nephrectomy, diets high in protein** or **sodium chloride** or following administration of certain diuretic drugs such as **furosemide** and **indacrinone**. Studies in animals following **partial nephrectomy** or given **high protein diets** have shown that the proximal tubule develops the greatest hypertrophic response, whereas following **sodium chloride** or **diuretic** treatment the distal convoluted tubule shows greater hypertrophy. Moreover, it has been shown that following **partial nephrectomy** or administration of **high protein diets** there is a close link between hypertrophy of the proximal tubular cell and elevation of glomerular filtration rate, although the precise relationship between the ultrafiltration dynamics and hypertrophy is uncertain.

Minor degrees of hypertrophy are difficult to characterize in histological sections and accurate morphological characterization of hypertrophy requires morphometric analysis. Morphometric analysis has shown that although increased tubular cell proliferation (hyperplasia) also occurs in response to increased tubular demand, this is usually limited to younger animals.

4.4.17 *Tubular Hyperplasia*

Chronic renal tubular damage may lead to hyperplasia of the renal tubular epithelium. This may occur in response to spontaneous disease such as in the aged rat afflicted with chronic glomerular sclerosis or following the administration of xenobiotics which produce chronic renal injury. For instance, administration of the antineoplastic drug, **cisplatin**, has been shown to produce tubular necrosis followed by the development of tubular cystic lesions or tubular hyperplasia in man and in the rat. Other xenobiotics have been shown to produce analogous alterations which in some instances appear to be the prelude to the development of renal tubular neoplasia (see below).

4.4.18 *Interstitial Nephritis*

Although interstitial inflammation accompanies a variety of renal conditions such as glomerulonephritis and pyelonephritis, the term 'interstitial nephritis' is reserved for primary inflammatory disease of the interstitium. In man, it is a well-recognized complication of **methicillin** therapy but it is also reported following **interferon** administration. It appears to be immunologically mediated with formation of antitubular basement membrane antibody. Immunologically-induced interstitial nephritis occurs spontaneously in mice and can be induced in brown Norway rats and some strains of mice using similar methods to those used for producing glomerulonephritis.

It is characterized histologically by an infiltration of varying numbers of polymorphonuclear cells, lymphocytes, and plasma cells with oedema and eventually fibrosis within the interstitial tissue. Tubular loss is variable but does subsequently occur.

4.4.19 Vascular Changes and Infarction

The blood vessels of the kidney are affected by pathological changes found in other parts of the cardiovascular system. In laboratory animals, the various forms of spontaneous arteritis can occur in the renal vasculature. In man, the kidney is the site of atherosclerosis and hypertensive alterations. Whilst the renal vascular bed is not particularly predisposed to develop alterations in response to the administration of xenobiotics compared with mesenteric or coronary arteries, renal arteritis is reported in rats given high doses of **vasopressors**, vasoconstrictor or vasodilating **antihypertensive agents**. Some **anticancer** and **immunomodulatory** agents have also been shown to produce arteritis in the rat kidney (see above).

Histologically, arteritis is characterized by varying degrees of endothelial damage and proliferation, medial necrosis, infiltration by neutrophils and/or chronic inflammatory cells, thrombosis, perivascular oedema and haemorrhage. When vascular damage is severe, occlusion by thrombosis may result. This may lead to a typical wedge-shaped infarction, characterized by a zone of necrotic parenchyma surrounded by a rim of inflammatory tissue. Older lesions show varying degrees of repair and scarring, with collapse of renal tubules and thickening of tubular basement membrane.

Administration of **cardioactive drugs** and **pressor agents** may also give rise to medial hypertrophy and arterial sclerosis in the kidney vasculature similar to that found in other vascular beds.

4.4.20 Hypertrophy and Hyperplasia of the Juxtaglomerular Apparatus

Hypertrophy, hyperplasia, and increased granularity associated with an extension of immunostaining for renin along the vasculature have been demonstrated in the kidneys of laboratory animals in which there is chronic stimulation of the renin–angiotensin system and an increased demand for renin (Figure 4.10). The granules can be visualized using special techniques such as the Bowie and Hartcroft stain, immunostaining for renin or plastic-embedded sections stained with toluidine blue. These changes have been observed in experimental animals following adrenalectomy, sodium depletion, experimental renal ischaemia, hypertension and following the administration of **ACE inhibitors**. Similar changes have been observed in humans.

4.4.21 Papillary Necrosis

The fully developed typical lesion is characterized by confluent necrosis of the tip of the renal papilla which may be shed into the renal pelvis. Mild lesions may just

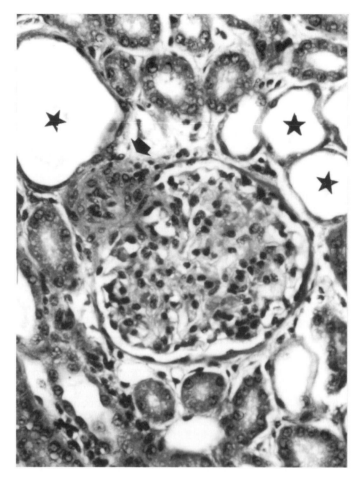

Figure 4.10 Kidney from a Wistar rat treated with a high dose of an ACE inhibitor. There is evidence of renal tubular damage with dilation of some tubules which are lined by abnormal flattened epithelium (stars) and hyperplasia of the juxtaglomerular apparatus adjacent to the glomerular tuft (arrow).

involve the apex or tip of the papilla but when severe, the necrosis can extend to the inner medulla (Figure 4.11). An inflammatory reaction may develop at the border between the necrotic and unaffected tissue, although this is not usually a prominent feature. Haemorrhage, casts, cell debris and mineral may also be present in the remaining viable medullary tissue, and ulceration and reactive alterations may be visible in the transitional epithelium lining the pelvis.

Papillary necrosis occurs in both man and laboratory animals, where its development has been primarily associated with the chronic administration of **non-steroidal anti-inflammatory** drugs.

4.4.22 *Mineralization*

Mineralization can be divided into two main types, dystrophic and metastatic. Dystrophic mineralization is usually closely associated with local tissue damage,

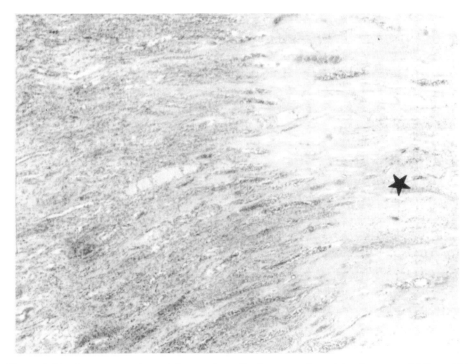

Figure 4.11 Low power view of the renal papilla from a patient dying from renal failure. This section shows the typical appearance of advanced renal papillary necrosis in which the apex of the papilla is almost completely necrotic (star) and surrounded by a zone of haemorrhagic tissue.

whereas metastatic mineralization is the result of mineral imbalance, frequently related to an altered renal tubular process.

Different forms of metastatic mineralization have been observed in the kidneys of man and animals, some spontaneous in nature or related to diet and others induced by a wide range of xenobiotics. Deposits of mineral may form in the renal tubule (intratubular lithiasis) or in or adjacent to the renal pelvis. They are characterized as aggregates of amorphous material usually staining intensely blue with haematoxylin (Figure 4.12).

Renal calcium deposition has been reported following administration of substances that alter the calcium balance in the nephron such as **calcium** itself, **vitamin D, oxalates, phosphates, parathyroid hormone**, and **carbonic anhydrase inhibitors** such as **acetazolamide, modified starches, sugar alcohols** and **lactose**.

4.4.23 Hydronephrosis

Hydronephrosis is characterized by a pathological dilation of the renal pelvis, associated with evidence of renal parenchymal damage. It usually results from the urinary outflow obstruction that can be produced by the precipitation by xenobiotics of crystals and calculi in the renal outflow tract, but may be congenital in origin.

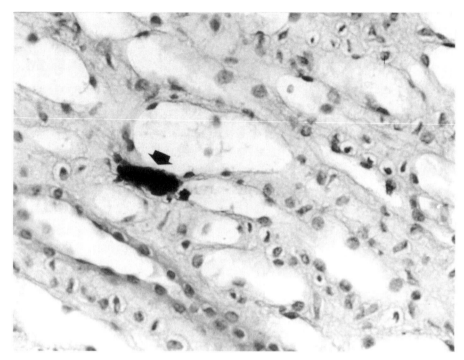

Figure 4.12 Section of renal medulla of an untreated beagle dog, showing mild lithiasis characterized by the presence of small, intensely staining fragments of mineralized material in the tubules (arrow).

4.4.24 *Pyelonephritis*

This condition is characterized by the presence of a primary inflammatory process in the renal pelvis. It usually results from an ascending urinary tract infection, frequently potentiated by some underlying urinary tract condition that favours infection through urinary stasis and outflow obstruction. It can occur following the administration of xenobiotics that produce renal stasis, crystal deposition and outflow obstruction.

4.4.25 *Renal Neoplasia*

The histological appearances, biological behaviour and age relationship of renal tumours found in laboratory animals are usually similar to those occurring in humans showing epithelial, mesenchymal or embryonic differentiation. Consequently, they are classified histologically into tumours of epithelial, mesenchymal, embryonal and mixed cell types.

Adenoma and adenocarcinoma

These form the largest histological group. They are composed of tubule-like cells with a wide range of histological and cytological appearances ranging from eosinophilic (oncocytic), basophilic, or clear cells arranged in solid, tubular or papillary growth patterns. They are believed to develop from cortical epithelial cells.

In rodents, the distinction between focal hyperplasia, adenoma and adenocarcinoma remains somewhat arbitrary. Focal hyperplasia is usually considered to be a localized proliferation of tubular epithelial cells remaining within the confines of a single renal tubule. Extension of the proliferation beyond the confines of a single tubule is considered to be evidence of autonomous growth and therefore defined as an adenoma. Adenomas remain well demarcated with little or no cellular pleomorphism and mitotic activity. Typical adenocarcinomas are large and characterized by cellular pleomorphism, mitotic activity, vascularisation, haemorrhage and necrosis with infiltration of the surrounding parenchyma by tumour cells. Ultimately, renal carcinomas tend to seed metastatic deposits via the blood stream.

Nephroblastoma

This is a tumour that affects younger animals or human infants, characterized histologically by varying proportions of proliferating blastematous, primitive epithelial and stromal cells as well as primitive glomeruli of variable maturation (Figure 4.13).

Mesenchymal tumour

The so-called mesenchymal tumour of the rat kidney is a highly characteristic neoplasm which develops commonly following administration of **dimethylnitrosamine** and other

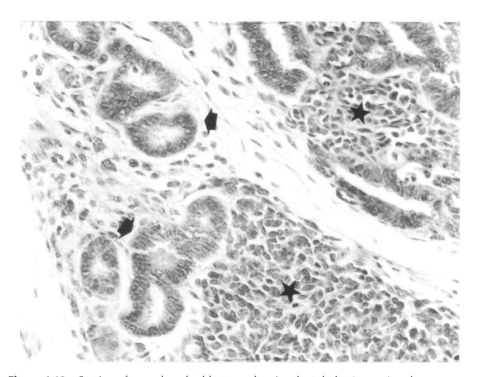

Figure 4.13 Section of a renal nephroblastoma showing the tubular (arrows) and undifferentiated patterns (stars).

129

nitroso compounds. It is composed of a heterologous mixture of fibroblast-like spindle or stellate cells, elements of skeletal muscle, vascular, cartilaginous or osteoid differentiation. It has been suggested that they develop from primitive stem cells of connective tissue or vasculature within the renal interstitium [26].

Benign mesenchymal tumours develop spontaneously in laboratory animals. These are usually composed of mature fat and smooth muscle cells, lipoblasts, prominent blood vessels and immature spindle cells. Although these tumours may show mitotic activity and haemorrhage, they are generally considered to be benign.

Oestrogen-induced renal tumour of the hamster

A unique nephroblastoma-like tumour of uncertain histogenesis can be induced in the kidney of Syrian hamsters treated with **oestrogens** for periods upwards of 200 days. These tumours develop as solid nodules within the renal parenchyma. Histologically, they are composed of nests or sheets or blocks of solid blastemic cells, zones showing trabecular, tubular, papillary and cystic appearances. Ultrastructural examination shows that these different patterns are closely intermingled and show both glandular and undifferentiated cells. This tumour may be of epithelial type or dysembryonic in nature, although immunohistochemical study has suggested that it possesses characteristics of renal interstitial cells.

Transitional cell or urothelial tumour

Neoplasms falling under this heading are histologically similar to those occurring in the bladder. They develop in the renal pelvis (see below). In humans, these tumours have been associated with papillary necrosis and the chronic ingestion of large amounts of **phenacetin**-containing analgesics.

4.4.26   *Inflammation of the Urinary Bladder, Cystitis*

Inflammation of the bladder is an uncommon spontaneous finding amongst most laboratory animal populations but it is seen in some colonies of aged rats, mice and hamsters in association with urinary tract pathology, such as urolithiasis, pyelonephritis, prostatitis, and urethral stasis or in the rat, infestations such as *Trichosomoides crassicauda*.

Some xenobiotics or their urinary metabolites are associated with erosion, haemorrhage and inflammation of the bladder mucosa. A notable example is the anticancer drug, **cyclophosphamide**, which is activated by hepatic microsomal enzymes to potent alkylating cytotoxic metabolites. Administration of this agent is associated with the development of haemorrhagic cystitis characterized by epithelial loss, inflammation and oedema in the bladder mucosa of patients with cancer, and this effect can be reproduced in laboratory animals (Figure 4.14).

The crystalluria produced by administration of high doses of poorly insoluble xenobiotics in toxicity studies can induce haematuria, with haemorrhage, ulceration and inflammation of the urothelium. There is evidence that drug crystals can be nephrotoxic in human patients if they are formed *in vivo*.

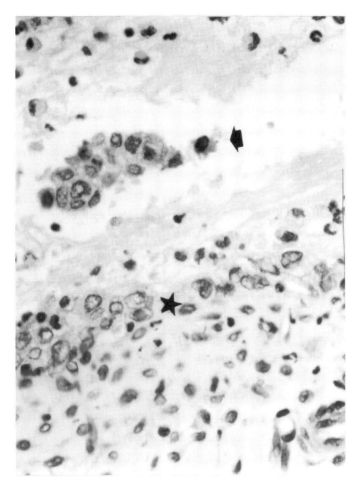

Figure 4.14 Bladder mucosa from a Wistar rat treated for 2 days with cyclophosphamide. There is almost complete loss of the transitional epithelium with cell debris evident in the bladder lumen (arrow) and degenerate cells still attached to the bladder wall (star), where there is also a mild inflammatory infiltrate.

4.4.27 *Bladder Mineralization, Calcification, Calculi, Stones*

Mineralization in the bladder can take the form of a single large calculus or multiple and often facetted bladder stones. They are found sporadically in most colonies of rats, mice and hamsters, but only very occasionally in laboratory beagles and non-human primates. The cause of the spontaneous development of bladder calculi is unclear, although diet and hormone balance are important. Bladder surface glycosaminoglycans may be important antiadherence factors which prevent calcium, which is often supersaturated in the urine, from depositing on the bladder surface and forming a nidus for stone formation. Other factors which influence the development of urolithiasis include urinary tract infections, presence of foreign bodies, drug crystals and anatomical abnormalities of the urinary outflow tract.

Composition of urinary tract calculi is variable, but in the rat they are usually mixed, comprising proteins, calcium carbonates, calcium or ammonium magnesium phosphates.

The presence of bladder stones or calculi is typically associated with transitional cell hyperplasia. This may be marked and accompanied by submucosal inflammation and fibrosis (see below).

4.4.28   Urothelial Hyperplasia

Hyperplasia of transitional bladder epithelium occurs in response to a variety of adverse stimuli including chronic inflammation, urinary stasis, presence of calculi, crystals, parasites or other foreign bodies as well as following administration of xenobiotics.

Simple focal or diffuse hyperplasia is characterized by an increase in the number of epithelial cell layers compared with normal control animals. In making comparisons of epithelial thickness between control and treated groups, it is important to employ a uniform sampling and fixation procedure. This is ideally performed after inflation of the bladder with fixative. Fixation of the collapsed bladder may increase the apparent thickness of the mucosa in histological sections.

Marked hyperplasia is associated with the development of infolding, cystic downgrowth of the epithelium into the bladder wall or the formation of small papillary mucosal structures (Figure 4.15). Studies of the rat urinary bladder

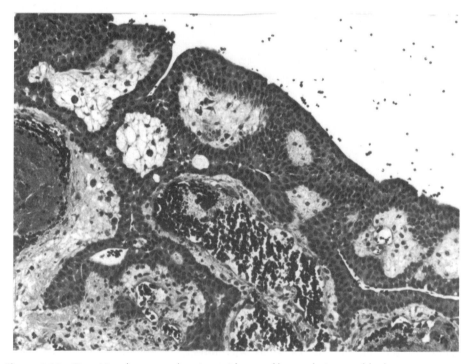

Figure 4.15   Transitional mucosa showing evidence of hyperplasia, notably the pseudopapillomatous appearance and the increased number of cell layers within the epithelium.

following single episodes of **surgical trauma, freezing** damage or intravesicular instillation of **formalin** have shown that florid changes of this type are fully reversible within 3 or 4 weeks and lead to no long-term hyperplastic or neoplastic sequelae.

A nodular form of hyperplasia is also recognized in the rat. This is represented by a nodular downgrowth of well-circumscribed, well-differentiated transitional cells, extending beneath the normal epithelial limits [28].

Scanning electron microscopy has been shown to be a very sensitive technique for the detection of mucosal bladder lesions and characteristic surface changes have also been described in urothelial hyperplasia (Figures 4.16 and 4.17). In the normal rat bladder, the large superficial polygonal cells exfoliate to reveal underlying round intermediate cells with uniform short microvilli. As these intermediate cells mature, their microvilli merge and develop into so-called 'ropy microridges'. Thus, the rate of exfoliation and replacement of urothelium can be estimated from the extent of the surface with ropy microridges and uniform microvilli. In rats, in reactive hyperplasias of the urinary bladder produced by **local trauma, formalin** instillation or following dosing with **saccharin**, increased numbers of zones showing ropy microridges and uniform short microvilli are found. Epithelial cells in marked or prolonged reactive hyperplastic states also develop pleomorphic surface microvilli, which have been associated with early lesions of experimental bladder cancer.

Whereas reactive hyperplasia is usually observed in association with some clear evidence of bladder pathology, uncomplicated reactive hyperplasia can occur

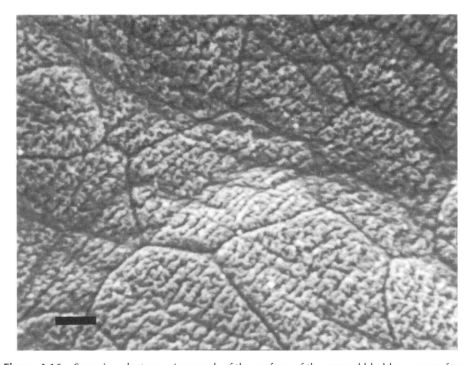

Figure 4.16 Scanning electron micrograph of the surface of the normal bladder mucosa from a Wistar rat showing an intact pavement of scalloped cells. Bar = 12 μm. Illustration from *Histopathology of Preclinical Toxicity Studies* by courtesy of Elsevier Science Publishers and Dr N.G. Read.

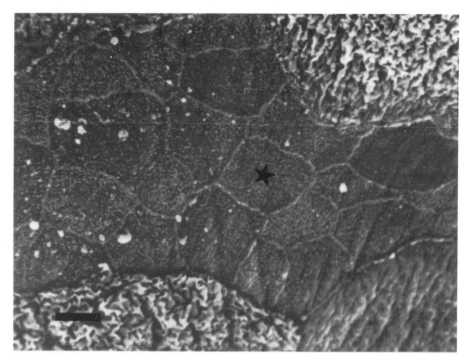

Figure 4.17 Similar micrograph to Figure 4.16 but after treatment with a drug which caused mild damage to the urothelium. There has been a shedding of superficial cells to reveal intermediate cells (star) with short stubby microvilli. The remaining superficial epithelial cells show prominent superficial ridges. Bar = 5 μm. Illustration from *Histopathology of Preclinical Toxicity Studies* by courtesy of Elsevier Science Publishers and Dr N.G. Read.

following the administration of xenobiotics without evidence of lithiasis or crystal formation.

An important part of the evaluation of bladder hyperplasia in toxicity studies is the characterization of any atypical or dysplastic cytological features; such features have traditionally been associated with the progression of urothelial hyperplasia to bladder neoplasia in a number of experimental rodent models and in man. Atypia of bladder epithelium is characterized by a disturbance of the normal regular cell polarity and maturation, nuclear hyperchromasia and pleomorphism, giant cells, prominent nucleoli, chromatin clumping and the presence of mitoses, particularly in upper parts of the epithelium.

4.4.29 Neoplasia of the Urinary Bladder

Tumours of the urinary bladder are uncommon in most untreated laboratory rodents, dogs and primates, although they can be induced by treatment with a number of carcinogens. Histologically, experimental bladder neoplasms resemble those found in man and a similar classification is applicable. However, although the same principles are used for the classification of human and experimental transitional cell neoplasms, it is important to be aware of the differences in emphasis given to their histopathological diagnoses. One difficulty is the separation of transitional cell papilloma from a highly differentiated transitional papillary cell carcinoma. In line with the diagnosis of other tumour types in rodent carcinogenicity studies, non-invasive papillary tumours with only slight cellular atypia are generally classified as papillomas, whereas in humans such lesions are generally considered to behave as low-grade carcinomas. Moreover, in common with other organs, a range of transitional cell hyperplasias are also recognized in the assessment of proliferative bladder lesions in carcinogenicity studies, whereas such lesions are not frequently recognized in the human bladder [28, 29].

Most bladder tumours are of epithelial nature, although the bladder wall is occasionally also the site of development of mesenchymal tumours.

Transitional cell papilloma

Transitional cell papillomas are single or multiple, pedunculated growths composed of arborescent, delicate branching villi with a fibromuscular stroma. They are covered by transitional epithelium which possesses the uniform appearance of normal bladder epithelium, devoid of significant cellular atypia or anaplasia. These tumours can ulcerate or develop squamous metaplasia. The stroma may be oedematous and contain inflammatory cells. Invasion of the stalk is not seen.

Transitional cell carcinoma

These take the form of papillomatous or sessile growths, distinguished from the papilloma by a greater degree of epithelial atypia including hyperchromasia, nuclear pleomorphism and mitotic activity as well as the variable presence of spindle-shaped, rounded or columnar cells and evidence of stromal invasion. Squamous metaplasia may be seen, although metastatic deposits are infrequent in most series reported in laboratory animals.

Other tumour types

Other tumour types reported in smaller numbers include squamous cell carcinoma, adenocarcinoma, undifferentiated carcinoma, carcinomas showing mixed patterns of differentiation and mesenchymal tumours showing fibrohistiocytic, smooth muscle or vascular differentiation [29].

4.5   Testing for Toxicity

Histopathological assessment is the cornerstone of assessment of renal toxicity, although a number of other techniques and methods are important, particularly in the elucidation of mechanisms of toxicity or monitoring renal function during life. However, it has been suggested that whilst histopathology in toxicity studies produces good information about the nature of the toxic effects, it may be less sensitive as a screening tool than quantitative urinanalysis [34].

Although renal weight changes are a useful guide to renal toxicity, it is essential that assessment of renal toxicity includes careful visual inspection of the renal parenchyma at necropsy for appearances of toxicity such as swelling, pallor, congestion and haemorrhage and this should be followed by careful histopathological examination.

Inspection of the contents of the renal pelvis and bladder for crystals and mineral and cellular debris is also important at necropsy because these substances may be lost in subsequent tissue handling and processing.

Conventional fixation and processing followed by haematoxylin and eosin staining supplemented by PAS is usually appropriate for most conventional toxicity studies. It is important that all parts of the nephron are examined microscopically, so histological sections should comprise both cortex and medulla and include the tip of the papilla.

A number of special techniques are available for more detailed study of xenobiotic-induced alterations in the nephron. Electron microscopy has a time-honoured place in the study of pathological alterations in both the glomerulus and renal tubule, although perfusion fixation may be needed for good preservation of tubular cells for ultrastructural study. Light microscopy of plastic-embedded sections 1 to 3 μm thick is a useful compromise which provides excellent resolution of renal structures.

Histochemical demonstrations of enzyme activities are useful as markers for components of the nephron and for correlation between structural alteration and functional changes. For instance, lysosomal enzyme activity is highest in the proximal tubule, reflecting the role of this segment in degradation of reabsorbed macromolecules. Therefore, enzyme cytochemical demonstration of acid phosphatase or other lysosomal enzymes may help in the assessment of alterations in the proximal tubule. Demonstration of acid phosphatase at electron microscopic level can be used in the characterisation of induced alterations in proximal tubular lysosomes. Important cytochemical markers are brush border enzymes, alkaline phosphatase, 5'-nucleotidase and γ-glutamyl transpeptidase, which are useful in the study of chemically-induced tubular damage.

Immunocytochemistry can also be used to demonstrate the presence of brush border enzymes such as γ-glutamyl transpeptidase. Tamm–Horsfall proteins, localized at the surface membrane of the thick ascending loop of Henle, and renin in the juxtaglomerular apparatus, can also be demonstrated by immunocytochemistry.

Histological study of the bladder mucosa requires special care at fixation. The best orientation of the epithelium is obtained following inflation of the bladder with fixative at autopsy as this removes folds which can give a misleading impression of the thickness of the epithelium. Scanning electron microscopy is a useful special technique for the examination of the superficial transitional epithelium damaged by xenobiotics.

The disadvantage of histopathology is that it requires tissue samples either obtained at necropsy or by biopsy. Hence, analyses of blood and urine provide non-invasive methods of assessment of renal function and are methods that can be used both in animal toxicity studies and in humans. Common urinary measurements include urine volume, osmolarity, pH, electrolytes, glucose, protein and urinary sediment, particularly red and white blood cells and casts. Careful characterization of urinary protein may give more specific information about glomerular or tubular function. Fent and colleagues [34] have suggested that repeated quantitative urinalysis in small numbers of rats may be a sensitive screening tool for nephrotoxicity. However, for effective urinalysis it is important that urine is collected without contamination with faeces, food and other extraneous materials.

Measurement of enzyme activity in the urine is also a useful complementary, non-invasive technique for the assessment of tubular toxicity in man and laboratory animals because cellular enzymes such as *N*-acetyl-β-D-glucosaminidase from damaged tubular cells spill into the urine in increased amounts. High resolution ¹H NMR has also been used in the detection of biochemical alterations to urine in toxicity studies [15], although experience in this laboratory suggests that results are not always consistent in the study of different xenobiotics.

Measurement of blood electrolytes, urea and creatinine are also helpful in the study of renal alteration. In special instances it may be necessary to make detailed functional measurements. Use of a marker such as inulin (molecular weight approximately 5200) which enters the glomerular filtrate but is not reabsorbed, can provide an assessment of glomerular filtration. Measurement of *p*-aminohippuric acid, which is completely cleared from the plasma by the kidney as it is both filtered and secreted by the tubules, is a good assessment of renal plasma flow. The endogenous substances, creatinine and urea, normally depend largely on glomerular filtration for their excretion into the urine so that measurement of their clearances provide a more convenient measure of glomerular filtration.

4.6 Conclusions

The kidney represents an organ frequently affected by xenobiotics because of its unique functional and structural organization and its pivotal role in the control of body homeostasis and the elimination of xenobiotics. Although the correlation of renal effects of xenobiotics in laboratory animals and man appear to be reasonable, the relevance of renal findings in experimental studies to humans unfortunately frequently remains uncertain. As a consequence, assessment of pathological alterations in the kidney in animals following exposure to chemicals needs to take place in the context of a good understanding of normal renal physiology and structure of the species being studied, information about the systemic effects and the disposition, metabolism and elimination of the xenobiotic under investigation.

References

1. FLETCHER, A.P. (1978) Drug safety tests and subsequent clinical experience, *Journal of the Royal Society of Medicine*, **71**, 693–696.
2. KRIZ, W., BANKIR, L., BULGER, R.E., BURG, M.B., GONCHAREVSKAYA, O.A., IMAI, M., KAISSLING, B., MAUNSBACH, A.B., MOFFAT, D.B., MOREL, F., MORGAN, T.O., NATOCHIN, Y.V., TISCHER, C.C., VENKATACHALAM, M.A., WHITTEMBURY, G. and WRIGHT, F.S. (1988) A standard nomenclature for structures of the kidney, *Kidney International*, **16**, 290–300.
3. CLAPP, W.L. (1992) Adult kidney, in STERNBERG S.S. (Ed.) *Histology for Pathologists*, Ch. 36, pp. 677–707, New York: Raven Press.
4. FISH, E.M. and MOLITORIS, B.A. (1994) Mechanisms of disease: Alterations in epithelial polarity and the pathogenesis of disease states, *New England Journal of Medicine*, **330**, 1580–1588.
5. GUDER, W.G. and ROSS, B.B. (1984) Enzyme distribution along the nephron, *Kidney International*, **26**, 101–111.
6. KRIZ, W., ELGAR, M., LEMLEY, K. and SAKAI, T. (1990) Structure of the glomerular mesangium: a biomechanical interpretation, *Kidney International*, **38** (Suppl. 30), S2–S9.
7. LINDOP, G.M.B. and LEVER, A.F. (1986) Anatomy of the renin–angiotensin system in the normal and pathological kidney, *Histopathology*, **10**, 335–362.

8. RHODIN, J.A.G. (1974) The urinary system, in *Histology, a Text and Atlas*, Ch. 32, pp. 647–674, New York: Oxford University Press.

9. REUTER, V.E. (1992) Urinary bladder and ureter, in STERNBERG, S.S. (Ed.) *Histology for Pathologists*, Ch. 37, pp. 709–720, New York: Raven Press.

10. JAO, W. (1982) The kidney and urinary tract, in RIDDELL, R.H. (Ed.) *Pathology of Drug-Induced and Toxic Diseases*, Ch. 11, pp. 229–278, New York: Churchill Livingstone.

11. DRUET, E., SAPIN, C., FOURNIE, G., MANDET, C., GÜNTER, E. and DRUET, P. (1982) Genetic control of susceptibility to mercury-induced immune nephritis in various strains of rat, *Clinical Immunology and Immunopathology*, **25**, 203–212.

12. HOEDEMAEKER, P.J., FLEUREN, G.J. and WEENING, J.J., (1986) Immune mechanisms in injury to glomeruli and tubulo-interstitial tissue, in JONES, T.C., MOHR U. and HUNT, R.D. (Eds) *Monographs on Pathology of Laboratory Animals, Urinary System*, pp. 151–174, Berlin: Springer-Verlag.

13. RUSH, G.F., SMITH, J.H., NEWTON, J.F. and HOOK, J.B. (1984) Chemically induced nephrotoxicity: role of metabolic activation, *CRC Critical Reviews in Toxicology*, **13**, 99–160.

14. ALDEN, C.L. and FRITH, C.H. (1991) Urinary system, in HASCHEK, W.M. and ROUSSEAUX, C.G. (Eds) *Handbook of Toxicologic Pathology*, Ch. 15, pp. 316–387, San Diego: Academic Press.

15. LOCK, E.A. (1993) Responses of the kidney to toxic compounds, in BALLANTYNE, B., MARRS, T. and TURNER, P. (Eds) *General and Applied Toxicology*, Vol. 1, Ch. 25, pp. 507–536, Basingstoke: Macmillan Press.

16. APPEL, G.B. and NEU, H.C. (1977) The nephrotoxicity of antimicrobial agents, *New England Journal of Medicine*, **296**, 663–670.

17. ALDEN, C.L. (1986) A review of unique male rat hydrocarbon nephropathy, *Toxicologic Pathology*, **14**, 109–111.

18. SWENBERG, J.A., SHORT, B., BORGHOFF, S., STRASSER, J. and CHARBONNEAU, M. (1989) The comparative pathobiology of α_{2u}-globulin nephropathy, *Toxicology and Applied Pharmacology*, **97**, 35–46.

19. READ, N.G., ASTBURY, P.A., MORGAN, R.J.I., PARSONS, D.N. and PORT, C.P. (1988) Induction and exacerbation of hyaline droplet formation in the proximal tubular cells of the kidneys from male rats receiving a variety of pharmacological agents, *Toxicology*, **52**, 81–101.

20. SANDERS, P.W., HERRERA, G.A. and GALLA, J.H. (1987) Human Bence-Jones protein toxicity in rat proximal tubule epithelium *in vivo*, *Kidney International*, **32**, 851–861.

21. GREAVES, P. (1990) Urinary tract, in *Histopathology of Preclinical Toxicity Studies. Interpretation and Relevance in Drug Safety Evaluation*, Ch. 9, pp. 497–583, Amsterdam: Elsevier.

22. BACH, P.H. and BRIDGES, J.W. (1985) Chemically induced renal papillary necrosis and upper urothelial carcinoma. Part 1 and 2, *CRC Critical Reviews in Toxicology*, **15**, 217–439.

23. DURAND-CAVAGNA, R., OWEN R.A., GORDON, L.R., PETER, C.P. and BOUSSUQUET-LEROUX, C. (1992) Urothelial hyperplasia induced by carbonic anhydrase inhibitors (CAIs) in animals and its relationship to urinary Na and pH, *Fundamental and Applied Toxicology*, **18**, 137–143.

24. SHIOYA, S., NAGAMI-OGUIHARA, R., OGUIHARA, S., KIMURA, T., IMAIDA, K. and FUKUSHIMA, S. (1994) Roles of bladder distension, urinary pH and urinary sodium ion concentration in cell proliferation of urinary bladder epithelium in rats ingesting sodium salts, *Food and Chemical Toxicology*, **32**, 165–171.

25. MORAN, M. and KAPSNER, C. (1987) Acute renal failure associated with elevated oncotic pressure, *New England Journal of Medicine*, **317**, 150–153.

26. HARD, G.C. (1986) Experimental models for the sequential analysis of chemically-induced renal carcinogenesis, *Toxicologic Pathology*, **14**, 112–122.
27. HARD, G.C. (1990) Tumours of the kidney, renal pelvis and ureter, in TURUSOV, V.S. and MOHR, U. (Eds), *Pathology of Laboratory Animals, Tumours of the Rat*, Vol. 1, 2nd Edn, pp. 301–344, Lyon: International Agency for Research on Cancer.
28. SQUIRE, R.A. (1986) Classification and differential diagnosis of neoplasms, urinary bladder, rat, in JONES, T.C., MOHR, U. and HUNT, R.D. (Eds) *Monographs on Pathology of Laboratory Animals, Urinary System*, pp. 311–317, Berlin: Springer-Verlag.
29. KUNZE, E. and CHOWANIEC, J. (1990) Tumours of the urinary bladder, in TURUSOV, V.S. and MOHR, U. (Eds), *Pathology of Laboratory Animals, Tumours of the Rat*, Vol. 1, 2nd Edn, pp. 345–397, Lyon: International Agency for Research on Cancer.
30. WEIL, C.S., CARPENTER, C.P. and SMYTH, H.F. (1965) Urinary bladder response to diethylene glycol. Calculi and tumours following repeated feeding and implants, *Archives of Environmental Health*, **11**, 569–581.
31. RITZ, E. (1994) Pathogenesis of 'idiopathic' nephrotic syndrome, *New England Journal of Medicine*, **330**, 61–62.
32. BLOOM, J.C., THIEM, P.A. and MORGAN, D.G. (1987) The role of conventional pathology and toxicology in the evaluation of the immunotoxic potential of xenobiotics, *Toxicologic Pathology*, **15**, 283–293.
33. GHADIALLY, F.N. (1982) Intranuclear lead and bismuth inclusions, in *Ultrastructural Pathology of the Cell and Matrix*, Ch. 1, pp. 96–102, London: Butterworths.
34. FENT, K., MAYER, E. and ZBINDEN, G. (1988) Nephrotoxicity screening in rats: a validation study, *Archives of Toxicology*, **61**, 349–358.
35. VIRCHOW, R. (1862) *Die Cellularpathologie*, Ch. 14, p. 275, Berlin: Hirchwald.

The Cardiovascular System

KEVIN R. ISAACS

5.1 Introduction

Widespread cardiovascular disease in the Western world has led to the development of a large number of cardioactive compounds with the potential to induce unwanted effects in addition to their therapeutic actions. A wide range of compounds in daily use in industry and domestic life also presents a potential hazard to the cardiovascular system as a result of accidental exposure. Changes that are detected in animal toxicity studies must be translated into a protocol for the investigation of their effects in man, and care must be taken to ensure that toxicology testing will provide relevant, and meaningful results.

The majority of animal studies are conducted in rodents and beagle dogs which may show a range of pharmacological, metabolic, pharmacokinetic and pathological effects that differ in important respects from responses in man. The use of other species to complement or replace studies with dogs and rats (e.g. non-human primates, guinea pigs, hamsters) may not provide a complete answer and the results of toxicity studies must always be subject to critical appraisal.

Cardiovascular disease is often treated with compounds that exert their effects on the vasculature, as well as the heart, and although the potential for toxicity is great, the incidence of vascular toxicity is comparatively low.

This chapter is divided into two sections: (Section A) The Heart and (Section B) The Vascular System, with a general conclusion.

Section A: The Heart

5.2 Anatomy, Histology and Physiology

5.2.1 Gross Anatomy

In simplistic terms, the heart consists of two pairs of two-chambered pumps equipped with 'non-return' valves. During fetal development the heart is converted from a simple muscular tube by a process of convolution and remodelling that results in separation of the right and left circulatory channels. Disturbance of this process may be seen as a range of developmental abnormalities (e.g. persistent ductus arteriosus, septal defects, situs inversus, etc.).

Blood from the systemic circulation enters the right atrium from the vena cava, at low pressure, and is forced into the right ventricle via the right atrioventricular valve (tricuspid valve) and then to the lungs, through the pulmonary valve and pulmonary arteries, by contraction of the right ventricle. Oxygenated blood, again at low pressure, enters the left atrium from the pulmonary veins and is ejected through the left atrioventricular valve (mitral valve) into the left ventricle which contracts to send blood to the tissues through the aortic valve and aorta.

The right side of the heart, supplying the lungs, operates at lower pressures than the left, which provides the systemic circulation, and the relative pressures encountered in each chamber are reflected in the thickness of walls.

The heart is situated in the mediastinum and is enveloped by a fibroserous sac, the pericardium. The visceral layer of the pericardium is known as the epicardium and overlies the muscular layers of the heart, the myocardium. The internal lining of the heart, the endocardium, consists of an inner endothelial layer with a subendocardium that contains connective tissue, blood vessels, nerves and conducting fibres (Purkinje fibres) in the ventricles.

The left and right coronary arteries arise from the base of the aorta and encircle the heart in the coronary groove with radiating, penetrating vessels that enter the myocardium and subsequently divide to form a rich capillary bed. Venous drainage tends to parallel the arterial supply and terminates in the left atrium via the coronary sinus. The pattern of the coronary vasculature varies between, and to a lesser degree within, species. Lymphatics, which are concentrated in the epicardium, converge into larger vessels alongside veins and arteries and eventually drain into the tracheobronchial lymph nodes.

The cardiac conduction system consists of the sinoatrial (SA) node, located at the junction of the anterior vena cava and right ventricle; the atrioventricular (AV) node and common bundle situated beneath the septal leaflet of the right atrioventricular valve; and the left and right bundle branches that run through the interventricular septum before dispersing over the ventricle as Purkinje fibres.

Innervation is mediated by the sympathetic (cardiac plexus) and parasympathetic divisions (vagus nerve) of the autonomic nervous system.

5.2.2 *Histology*

Myocardium

The myocardium is principally composed of contractile cells, the myocytes, with a rich supply of blood vessels in a fine matrix of connective tissue, nerves and lymphatics.

Myocytes

Ventricular myocytes are branching, roughly cylindrical cells, joined by intercalated discs that couple the cells to form a functional electrical and mechanical syncytium. Each cell has one or two centrally located nuclei which are associated with a small zone containing other subcellular organelles (Golgi complex, mitochondria, lysosomes, glycogen etc.).

Contractile elements comprise 50 per cent of the cell volume and are separated into fibrils by mitochondria (35 per cent of cell volume), sarcoplasmic reticulum, T-tubules, glycogen particles and other organelles. The arrangement of the contractile elements results in the formation of obvious bands divided into three zones (A-band, I-band and Z-band). Mitochondria, which provide the energy for contraction, are numerous. The sarcoplasmic reticulum and T-system are a network of fine intracellular tubules responsible for the uptake and release of calcium ions during the contraction–relaxation cycle.

Atrial myocytes are essentially similar to ventricular myocytes but differ in some ultrastructural features, most notably the presence of granules containing various atrial natriuretic peptides.

Conducting fibres

The nodal tissues and the bundle of His generally consist of small spindle cells with few myofibrils, although there are variations in fine structure in each site. Purkinje fibres, which appear in the bundle branches and predominate in the ventricles, contain myofibrils at the periphery and lack T-tubules. Smaller transitional cells establish contact with ordinary myocytes.

Interstitial tissues

Collagen fibres form a diffuse structural network for the co-ordinated contraction of myocytes, with cartilage (and bone in some species) providing rigidity at the heart base. Cellular components of the interstitium include fibroblasts, myofibroblasts (especially in valves), undifferentiated mesenchymal cells, Anitschkow cells (which may be activated fibroblasts), macrophages and mast cells. Elastic fibres are infrequent and small. Blood vessels and unmyelinated nerves accompany each other throughout the myocardium.

Pericardium

The parietal pericardium (the outer layer of the pericardial sac) is composed of fibrous connective tissue with an inner layer of mesothelial cells, and the visceral pericardium (or epicardium) consists of a layer of mesothelial cells with an underlying submesothelial layer. The submesothelial layer is well-developed in the atria with abundant collagen and elastin fibres, but is almost unnoticeable in the ventricles.

Endocardium

The inner lining of the heart is thicker in the atria than in the ventricles and is more prominent in the right than the left side of the heart. There are five layers: endothelium, inner connective tissue layer, elastic layer, smooth muscle layer and outer connective tissue layer.

Cardiac valves

Valve leaflets are fibrous flaps that originate in circular collagenous structures at the heart base and extend into the lumen of the chambers to prevent backflow of blood as the chambers contract. Atrioventricular valves extend into the lumen and are connected to papillary muscles on the opposite wall of the ventricle by fibrous cords (chordae tendineae). The pulmonary and aortic valves form discrete semilunar cusps and have three perceptible layers: the fibrosa, the spongiosa and the ventricularis. The right-side valves are thinner than left-side valves, reflecting the differences in pressure between the systemic and pulmonary circulation.

5.2.3 *Physiology*

Cardiac impulse

The electrical impulse usually originates in the SA node and travels rapidly through the atria to the AV node, where transmission is slowed before the bundles of His and Purkinje fibres conduct the impulse rapidly from the AV node, through the Purkinje cells to the ventricular myocardium. The co-ordinated spread of the impulse and the anatomic arrangement of myocyte and conducting bundles ensures the efficient operation of the heart as a pump under normal conditions.

Electrical activity is mediated by the flow of sodium, potassium, calcium and chloride ions in individual myocytes and conducting fibres. Depolarization of the cell membrane is initiated by a variety of electrical currents and chemical mediators to a threshold value that triggers an action potential with either a slow or fast response.

Fast response cells depolarize from a resting potential of −90 mV to −70 mV and the fast sodium channels open (phase 0) to elicit the action potential with a resultant internal potential of +30 mV. Repolarization (phase 1) commences with the influx of chloride ions and the efflux of potassium ions. During the plateau (phase 2), calcium and sodium ions enter the cell to initiate contraction of the myocytes. Phase 3 is accompanied by an increased permeability to potassium ions with the slow sodium and calcium channels diminishing. Completion of repolarization (phase 4) is the final result.

Slow response fibres, found in the SA and AV nodes, have a resting potential of −60 mV with the slow sodium and calcium channels being activated at a threshold of −40 mV. Phase 4 of slow fibres shows a continuous decline in potential as sodium enters the cell to trigger another action potential, thus providing a rhythmic pacemaking activity. The SA node, with the most rapid pacemaker rhythm, usually overrides other slow fibres to elicit a spreading action potential.

Excitation–contraction coupling

Myocyte contraction is achieved by the sliding of myosin filaments past actin filaments in each fibril from a fixed point in the intercalated disc. The process is mediated by changes in intracellular calcium ion concentration, and myosin ATPase, in the presence of magnesium ions, acts as the energy source. The force and rate of contraction is determined by the concentration of calcium which is released from the sarcoplasmic reticulum by the action potential, whilst reuptake of calcium into the sarcoplasmic reticulum results in reversal of the myosin–actin interaction to relax the myocyte.

Myocardial metabolism

Myocytes have a high metabolic rate which is sustained by the production of high-energy phosphates (ATP or creatine phosphate) in mitochondria from energy sources like lactate, glucose, fatty acids and triglycerides. Protective metabolic systems (e.g. catalase, glutathione peroxidase) for the removal of potentially damaging reactive radicals are relatively limited, rendering the myocardium vulnerable to oxidative membrane damage.

Nervous control of the heart

Vagal parasympathetic fibres principally innervate the atria, SA and AV nodes. Release of their neurotransmitter, acetylcholine, results in a reduction of contraction velocity in the AV node, a decreased force of contraction in atria and ventricles and a decrease in heart rate by slowing depolarization in the SA node. Noradrenaline from the sympathetic nerve fibres increases influx through slow calcium channels of the conducting fibres, thus accelerating the rate of depolarization of slow fibres leading to an increase in heart rate (positive chronotropy). An increase in the force of contraction of myofibrils (positive inotropy), mediated by cAMP, is another action of sympathetic nerve stimulation. Systemic release of catecholamines (adrenaline) by the adrenal glands has a similar effect to sympathetic stimulation of the heart.

5.3. Biochemical and Cellular Mechanisms of Toxicity

The heart is unavoidably exposed to high concentrations of all absorbed test compounds, and their metabolites, for prolonged periods irrespective of the route of administration. Although the heart has a large physiological reserve, toxic reactions in the heart have serious implications because of the lack of regenerative capacity of myocytes in the case of sublethal effects.

5.3.1 *Developmental Abnormalities*

Incomplete remodelling of the primitive heart during organogenesis can lead to a number of sublethal defects, some of which are seen as spontaneous, congenital defects. Ventricular and atrial septal defects (usually fistulae) have been seen following prenatal treatment with **thalidomide** in man, with **phenobarbital** and **caffeine** in rats and **acetylsalicylic acid** in dogs. Perinatal dosing of rats with **opiates** or **ethanol** leads to a persistent lack of responsiveness to sympathetic stimulation, and exposure of neonatal rats to **lead** is associated with an increased propensity to noradrenaline-induced arrhythmia [1].

5.3.2 *Physiological Mechanisms*

Effects on ion movement

A wide range of compounds exert effects upon ion transport with potentially catastrophic effects on impulse conduction and excitation–contraction coupling. Disturbances in ion transport may be systemic in origin (diuretic-induced potassium deficiency, hypercalcaemia) or local effects on specific membrane sites (**tetrodotoxin, cardiac glycosides, anthracyclines**). Alterations in the cardiac impulse are seen as arrhythmia, ectopic beats, heart block, tachycardia, bradycardia, etc., whereas changes in excitation–contraction coupling may lead to positive or negative inotropy [2].

5.3.3 *Biochemical Mechanisms*

The metabolic rate of the myocardium is high, and may predispose the heart to the toxic effects of certain compounds as well as hypoxia. Mitochondrial enzyme inhibitors (**cyanide**), uncoupling agents (**dinitrophenol, cobalt, lead**) or other agents affecting mitochondria (**monensin, acriflavin**) can precipitate generalized myocyte degeneration or necrosis [3].

If myocytic metabolic transformation of **allylamine**, an industrial intermediate, to **acrolein** exceeds the capacity of glutathione conjugation to neutralize it, myocardial necrosis is the result [4]. Metabolism of **anthracyclines** (e.g. **doxorubicin**) within myocytes leads to the generation of toxic oxygen radicals that may exceed the capacity of endogenous catalases to neutralize their damaging effects on intracellular membranes [5, 6].

Hypothyroidism, diabetes mellitus and prolonged fasting cause alterations in lipid metabolism that may result in neutral lipid droplets appearing in myocytes.

5.3.4 *Pharmacological Mechanisms*

Drugs with known pharmacological effects on the heart are specifically developed as therapeutic entities. The administration of potent, active therapeutic agents at massive doses may be associated with exaggerated pharmacology irrespective of any associated abnormal metabolic and pharmacokinetic patterns. The interpretation and extrapolation of toxic reactions at the highest limits of dosing requires care and experience and must be made in the context of the pharmacology, metabolism, distribution and excretion for test species and the target population (humans).

Exaggerated pharmacological alterations in the heart of dogs dosed with cardiovascular therapeutic compounds are well documented [7, 8]. Peripheral vasodilatation in dogs results in a reflex tachycardia with an increase in myocardial oxygen demand. As a result of this high demand and poor capillary perfusion in the subendocardium of the left ventricular papillary muscles, focal myocardial necrosis is a common reaction. Increased contractility, induced by positive inotropic agents, is associated with turbulent blood flow within the heart chambers of dogs and mechanical disruption is responsible for the endocardial haemorrhage and fibroplasia (so-called 'jet lesions').

As the intended target population (heart failure patients) has a reduced cardiac output, these compounds are intended to bring contractility and heart rate into the normal range and the reactions seen at high dosages are not considered to be predictive of potential toxic effects in patients.

5.3.5 *Immunologically Mediated Toxicity*

Systemic anaphylaxis with the release of vasoactive substances, like histamine, has different implications for different species. In man, coronary vasoconstriction can lead to arrhythmia or heart block, whereas dogs exhibit peripheral vasodilation with potentially fatal hypotension. Although **penicillin**-induced anaphylaxis and immune-complex-mediated myocarditis (**methyldopa**) occur in man, similar hypersensitivity reactions in animal tests are rare and extrapolation to man is fraught with difficulty.

5.4 Morphological Responses to Injury

5.4.1 *Non-neoplastic Changes*

No morphological change

No morphological change may be detected with a variety of cardiotoxic compounds, especially if the effects are peracute and involve disturbances of impulse conduction or excitation–contraction coupling. Heart block and arrhythmias often lead to death with no detectable histopathological change.

Scar formation

As myocytes lose the ability to regenerate at an early stage of neonatal development, degenerative lesions heal with interstitial fibrosis (scar formation, Figure 5.1). There is compensatory myocyte hypertrophy in response to the increased haemodynamic load rather than the regenerative hyperplasia that is seen in epithelial tissues.

Hypertrophy

An increase in myofibril mass, in the absence of degenerative change, is seen as a response of cardiac muscle to an increased haemodynamic load (as in trained athletes). A change is initially encountered as an increase in weight and may be discovered in hearts with congenital defects, valvular pathology, hypertension, hyperthyroidism and with some drugs (**potassium channel agonists, noradrenaline, vasodilating agents, calcium channel blockers, *α*- and *β*-blockers**). Unless the change is relatively marked it may be difficult to detect a morphological alteration in myocytes and special techniques may be required to confirm an effect of treatment (and, more importantly, a no-effect level). In the absence of other pathological changes, this process may be regarded as an adaptive response to treatment.

Atrophy

Drug-induced decreases in heart weight as a result of reduced haemodynamic load have been reported with **angiotensin-converting-enzyme inhibitors** and **atriopeptin III**. Ageing and cachectic animals may also undergo atrophic changes in the heart, as well as in other tissues.

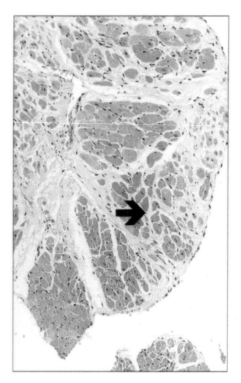

Figure 5.1 Heart from a marmoset showing marked interstitial fibrosis. The arrow indicates the separation of cardiac myocytes by mature collagen fibres, with very few fibrocyte nuclei.

Necrosis

Increased cytoplasmic eosinophilia with nuclear pyknosis or karyorrhexis are the cardinal features of myocyte necrosis. Depending on the circumstances, there may be associated infiltration by inflammatory cells (polymorphs, lymphocytes and macrophages), and finally fibrosis. Various morphological subtypes of myocardial necrosis have been described (e.g. coagulative, contraction band), but are not usually recorded in routine toxicity studies. Infiltration of necrotic areas by macrophages occurs within 24 to 48 h (Figure 5.2) and is usually accompanied by a few polymorphs. As the sarcoplasmic debris is removed there is progressive deposition of collagen by fibroblasts, and capillary formation. Small lesions tend to heal quite rapidly until the affected area is replaced by collagen and a few fibroblasts (scar tissue). In larger lesions the process may take 6 to 8 weeks.

The distribution of necrosis may be a characteristic feature of the exciting agent. Multifocal necrosis in the left ventricular subendocardial zone and papillary muscles, with subsequent invasion by macrophages and replacement fibrosis, is typical of lesions induced by vasoactive amines (**noradrenaline, adrenaline, isoprenaline, salbutamol, allylamine**). An exaggerated pharmacological response to these compounds leads to an increased myocardial oxygen demand, coronary arterial constriction and tachycardia with lesions principally affecting the subendocardium and papillary muscles [9]. Myocardial necrosis, in the papillary muscles of dogs treated with positive inotropic or vasodilating agents, is also thought to be essentially

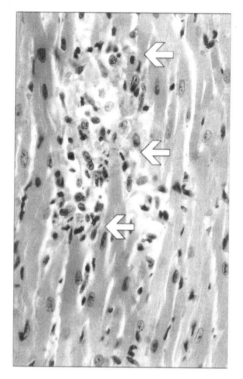

Figure 5.2 A small focus of myocyte loss in a rat with mononuclear cell infiltration (delineated by arrows). This change represents the healing process following a localized area of necrosis and, in some instances, necrotic remnants may still be seen. This appearance is typical of the minor lesions that are commonly encountered as a spontaneous change in animals from toxicology studies.

ischaemic in origin, as a result of poor collateral blood circulation and increased oxygen demand at this site.

Infarction

Infarction specifically refers to necrosis resulting from vascular occlusion, and should only be used to describe changes that can be unequivocally linked to vascular obstruction. This condition is extremely rare in the species commonly used for toxicity testing.

Mineralization

Dystrophic mineralization (predominantly calcification), as a sequel to myocardial damage, is rapid in onset and may be widespread in cases of necrosis induced by **monensin** toxicity or **selenium/vitamin E deficiency**. Metastatic mineralization is associated with a generalized disturbance of calcium/phosphate metabolism (e.g. in renal failure), and is seen as a multifocal change in a wide range of tissues, including the myocardium.

Vacuolar degeneration

Widespread degeneration of myocytes and Purkinje cells with vacuolation, myofibrillar loss, necrosis and ventricular dilatation has been induced in a wide range of species treated with the anthracyclines (**doxorubicin, daunorubicin**), **cyclophosphamide** and other anticancer drugs. The effect is attributed to the formation of free oxygen radicals with subsequent intracellular membrane damage. The lesion may be difficult to detect at light microscopy in short-term tests and ultrastructural methods may be required.

Myocytolysis

Loss of myofibrils, seen as cytoplasmic pallor and loss of cross-striations at light microscopy, has been reported with **furazolidone** in birds [10], **potassium deficiency** and **plasmocid** toxicity in rats [11]. This change may be more easily appreciated with electron microscopy.

The resultant loss of contractility and resilience of the myocardium may lead to dilatation of the ventricles and heart failure.

Fatty change

Accumulation of neutral lipids in the cytoplasm of myocytes is demonstrable as small, clear vacuoles in sections stained with H and E and as red or black droplets by specific staining procedures in frozen sections (oil red O, Sudan III respectively). This change is considered to be degenerative and, therefore, reversible and may be seen as a non-specific change as a result of a number of conditions (e.g. anaemia, fasting) or as an effect of treatment on lipid metabolism (e.g. **oxfenicine, erucic acid, glucocorticoids**).

Lipofuscin pigment

Lipofuscin pigment, the end-product of endogenous membrane and organelle breakdown by lysosomes, is seen as residual bodies in electron micrographs, and can be demonstrated by specific staining procedures for light microscopy (periodic acid Schiff [PAS], Schmorl's, autofluorescence with H and E). This condition occurs spontaneously, with an increase in severity with age. Cachectic conditions (e.g. severe renal disease, leukaemias) can accelerate the process, and similar changes have been seen as a toxic response in rats treated with **Brown FK, anthracyclines** and **chloroquine**.

Endocardial and epicardial changes

Haemorrhage, haemosiderin deposition, inflammation and fibrosis affecting the atrioventricular valves of dogs are seen following the administration of positive inotropic/vasodilating agents. The changes are a consequence of the mechanical stresses associated with turbulent blood flow induced by an exaggerated, pharmacological inotropic effect.

Atrial lesions

Atrial lesions characterized by haemorrhage, fibrosis, focal myocyte necrosis and arterial degeneration were originally reported in dogs and pigs treated with **minoxidil** [7], but have since arisen in studies with other vasodilating agents (**hydralazine, theobromine, nicorandil**). Although their pathogenesis has not been fully elucidated, there has been no evidence of similar effects in man following post-mortem studies conducted in patients treated with **minoxidil**.

Thrombi

Atrial thrombi may be observed with cardiotoxic drugs as a sequel to underlying myocardial damage, and are commonly encountered as a secondary effect in uraemic animals (renal failure). Ventricular or valvular thrombi are rarely seen, except in the presence of inflammatory conditions (e.g. indwelling cardiac catheters, bacterial endocarditis).

5.4.2 Tumours

Cardiac tumours are relatively rare, especially as a consequence of treatment.

Spindle cell tumours

Endocardial spindle cell tumours (Figure 5.3), generally diagnosed as Schwann cell tumours [12], occur spontaneously and have also been induced by treatment in studies conducted in rats with a range of compounds including **urethan, ethylnitrosourea (ENU), methylnitrosourea (MNU), 1-aryl-3,3 dialkyltriazenes, 1,2-diethylhydrazine** and **2-acetylaminofluorene (2-AAF) derivatives**.

Other tumours

Atriocaval and pericardial mesotheliomas are rare tumours of the cardiac serosa, which may be induced by the intrathoracic installation of durable fibrous material.

The heart may be the site for deposition of malignant cells in multicentric tumours (e.g. leukaemias, malignant lymphoma), especially as a result of local infiltration from the thymus.

Metastasis of tumours from other sites is uncommon, but there may be deposits in the endocardium, epicardium or myocardium (e.g. malignant pulmonary tumours in mice).

5.4.3 Spontaneous Pathology

The occurrence of spontaneous lesions is a complicating factor in all toxicity studies. It may be difficult, if not impossible, to separate spontaneous and induced lesions on morphological grounds, especially if the effects are minor.

Spontaneous foci of necrosis in the myocardium are commonplace, and rats are afflicted with myocardial necrosis and fibrosis (sometimes referred to as a spontaneous cardiomyopathy) that increases in incidence and severity with age [13], although the cause is unknown. The interpretation of treatment-related disturbances in such conditions (often diminishing in rats showing restricted growth) must be

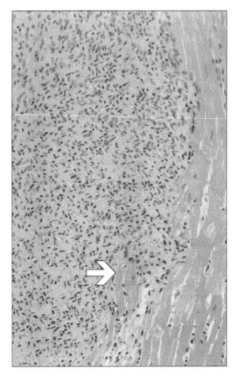

Figure 5.3 To the left of the section is a mass of neoplastic Schwann cells, in a rat heart, with their characteristic spindle cell appearance. The arrow indicates the border with normal cardiac myocytes.

made with due regard to all possible contributing factors (diet, stress, age, contemporaneous control data, etc.).

5.5 Testing for Toxicity

5.5.1 *Physiological Methods*

Myocardial contractile function and electrical activity can be monitored in a number of *in vivo* and *in vitro* models. In routine toxicity testing, measurements of ECG, heart rate and blood pressure are the most common procedures. Specific effects of treatment require the formulation of a more detailed testing schedule to uncover their cause.

5.5.2 *Plasma and Serum Enzymes*

In theory, myocardial damage may be associated with the leakage of intracellular enzymes into the bloodstream, which could be detectable as an elevation above normal levels by biochemical analysis. In practice, the measurement of creatine kinase, lactic dehydrogenase, aspartate transaminase or alkaline phosphatase enzyme levels rarely provides useful information with regard to cardiotoxicity.

As the release of enzymes in acute injury may be sudden, and transient, elevated enzyme levels may only be apparent for a very short period after treatment. With low-level chronic changes, enzyme levels are unlikely to differ significantly from control values.

5.5.3 *Morphological Methods*

The heart is not a homogeneous structure, and effects of treatment may be relatively site specific, so care must be taken to ensure that a thorough examination of the heart is undertaken as a matter of routine.

Necropsy

The objectives of a routine necropsy in toxicology studies are to examine, remove and preserve the tissues specified in the protocol and to ensure that any potentially treatment-related changes are adequately documented and sampled. The necropsy procedure also ensures that sufficient material and information is provided for the histotechnologist to embed the correct site(s) for the pathologist to evaluate by light microscopy.

In small laboratory rodents, the macroscopic examination of the heart of offers limited scope for the identification of lesions as only the epicardial surface is available for scrutiny. In larger species (dog, non-human primate), the heart should be opened prior to fixation in order to permit the examination of all internal surfaces. This enables the identification of lesions for subsequent processing and facilitates subsequent fixation.

The heart is usually weighed and fixed by immersion in 10 per cent neutral buffered formalin (NBF). In special circumstances, the heart may be fixed by perfusion methods or components of the heart may be dissected free and weighed separately, but this is not a standard requirement.

Tissue sampling

Only a small proportion of the heart is processed for histological examination, so it is important that the selection of sites to be examined microscopically is conducted in a systematic manner. The following structures should be considered for any routine examination:

- Both atria
- Both atrioventricular valves
- Pulmonary valve
- Aortic valve
- Left papillary muscles
- Interventricular septum
- Coronary circumflex arteries
- Coronary ventricular and atrial branch arteries
- Elements of the conducting system
- Gross abnormalities

This regime can be achieved with 9 or 10 sections, in larger species (Figures 5.4a to 5.4d), and provides a good basic survey. In laboratory rodents, sections through both ventricles and the apex and base of the heart are normally examined (Figures 5.5a and 5.5b). It is important that identical sites are examined for every animal on test to allow direct comparisons to be made.

Staining

H and E is adequate as the routine stain for most studies but additional special stains may be helpful for the identification of specific changes:

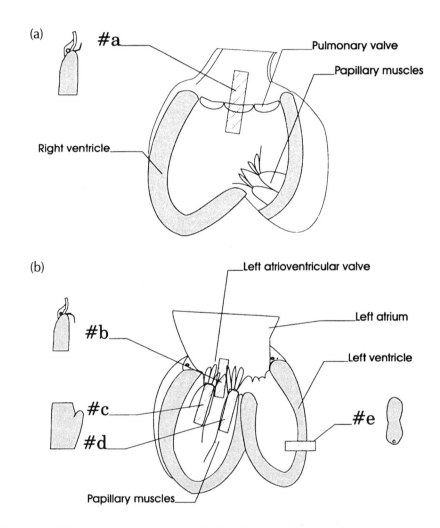

Figure 5.4 Dissection of canine heart following fixation. For a thorough survey of the canine heart, the following samples may be taken at histological processing. The heart should have been opened at necropsy, as described in the text. For routine studies, fewer samples may be required (e.g. #a, #b, #c, #f).

(c)

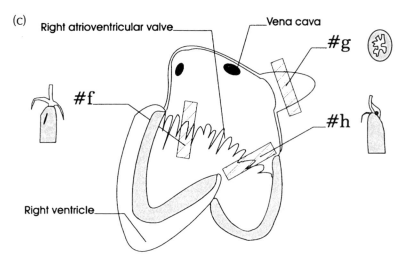

(d)

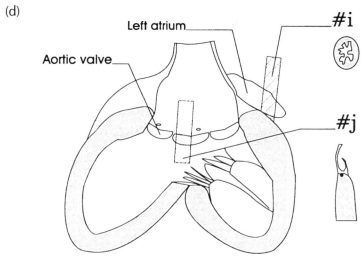

Key to Figure 5.4a to 5.4d.

Block	Structures sampled
#a	Right ventricle, pulmonary artery, right circumflex artery, pulmonary valve
#b	Left ventricle, left atrium, left circumflex artery, left ventricular artery, left atrioventricular valve
#c and d	Left papillary muscles
#e	Interventricular septum, left interventricular artery
#f	Interventricular septum, left septal artery, left atrioventricular valve, right atrioventricular valve, atrioventricular node
#g	Right atrium, right atrial artery
#h	Right ventricle, right atrium, right circumflex artery, right ventricular artery, right atrioventricular valve
#i	Left atrium, left atrial artery
#j	Left ventricle, aortic valve, left circumflex artery

Figure 5.4 *Continued*

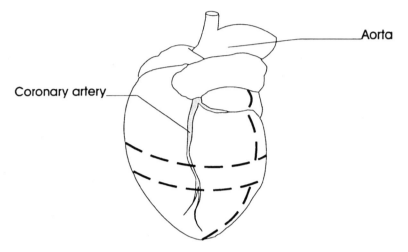

Figure 5.5a Planes of section for rodent heart, at histological processing. The central area and one half of each longitudinal section are embedded.

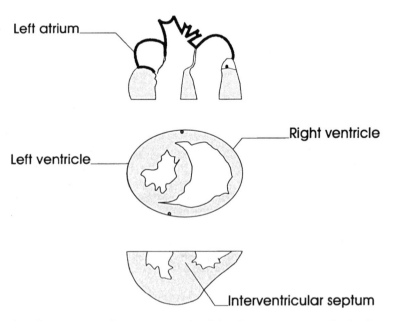

Figure 5.5b The sections as they appear on the slide. This arrangement is both effective and economical.

- Oil red O or Sudan IV (neutral lipids)
- Perls' Prussian blue (haemosiderin)
- Elastic van Gieson (fibrosis, elastic fibres)
- Trichrome stains (fibrosis, degeneration)
- Phosphotungstic acid haematoxylin (PTAH) (cross-striations, fibrin)
- Von Kossa or Alizarin red (mineralization)

Histopathology

The principal aim of the histopathological evaluation is to assess and record any pertinent histological changes and provide a valid comparison between control and treated animals. Additional considerations include the provision of data for comparison with contemporaneous studies, and to elucidate the pathogenesis of any lesions encountered.

The terms used in the diagnosis of lesions are often a reflection of the experience and expertise of the pathologist performing the evaluation. Complete consensus between pathologists is rare and the formulation and application of an internationally recognized lexicon of diagnostic terms may eventually facilitate the standardization of results presented to regulatory authorities.

Irrespective of any diagnostic terms that are used, any findings that are recorded should adequately and concisely reflect the qualitative nature of any change and attempt to quantify the changes with regard to severity and extent.

5.5.4 *Special Techniques*

It may be justifiable to perform a number of special procedures to characterize further, or investigate, the pathogenesis of previously detected lesions. It should be emphasized that such techniques are usually restricted to specific investigative studies rather than included in routine toxicology studies.

Electron microscopy

The value of ultrastructural techniques lies in the detection of early, transient, reversible or minor changes that are not readily detected by light microscopy. As the sample size for electron microscopy is small, the sites to be examined must be selected very carefully. For the same reason, the use of electron microscopy (EM) as a 'screening' procedure is not recommended. The use of perfusion techniques for tissue preservation is expensive and less sophisticated methods (mincing of selected tissue sites under fixative solution) may be adequate. Both scanning electron microscopy (SEM) and transmission electron microscopy (TEM) techniques are used in the investigation of cardiovascular disease and the pathologist is advised to work in conjunction with an experienced ultrastructural pathologist in the preparation and execution of investigative studies.

Other techniques

A variety of other special techniques can be utilized to expand an investigative programme further.

Vascular permeability can be assessed with tracers (horseradish peroxidase) and enzyme biochemistry can be investigated using phosphatases, esterases or dehydrogenases as markers in frozen sections.

The incorporation of H^3-leucine can be measured by autoradiography to investigate the distribution of newly synthesized proteins in hypertrophic cardiac myocytes.

The demonstration of glycosaminoglycans in vessel walls or valve leaflets by histochemical methods may be a useful indicator of an early increase in haemodynamic stress.

In investigative studies where extensive, acute myocardial necrosis is expected, it may be advisable to use the 'breadloaf' system of opening the heart before incubating the slices in nitro-blue tetrazolium (NBT) in Sörenson's buffer. Normal myocardium reduces the NBT to a dark blue colour, but necrotic cells lose their enzymes and stain faintly to allow the identification of gross areas of myocardial necrosis at each level.

Investigations into the effects of treatment on valve morphology have included the dissection and weighing of the valve leaflets, and the dissection and weighing of individual heart chambers may be of use in the investigation of cardiac hypertrophy.

Section B: The Vascular System

5.2 Anatomy, Histology and Physiology

The circulatory system is a system of closed channels that can contract and expand to regulate the flow, and pressure, of blood to the tissues as a result of neural, humoral and local metabolic changes. The capacity of the system greatly exceeds its normal volume and vascular tone is altered to modulate the supply to individual tissues. The passage of blood, sometimes at high pressures and flow rates, is governed by physical laws (affecting laminar flow, turbulence, viscosity, etc.) that have a dramatic effect on the conformation of the vessel walls.

5.2.1 Anatomy

The anatomical distribution of blood and lymphatic vessels follows a similar pattern in mammals with a few major variations between species and some minor differences between individuals. Standard anatomy texts should be consulted to gain familiarity with the species commonly used for toxicology testing.

5.2.2 Histology

Most vessels are essentially similar in design with three layers:

1 Tunica intima: an endothelium overlying a basal lamina.

2 Tunica media: bundles of smooth muscles in longitudinal and circumferential arrays.

3   Tunica adventitia: a circumferential band of collagen, elastic fibres and nerves with small, nutrient blood vessels (vasa vasorum) in large arteries.

Arteries are subdivided into functional groups:

Elastic (conducting) arteries

The major component is a wide tunica media consisting of layers of elastin fibres and smooth muscle encircled by an internal and external elastic lamina. The tunica adventitia is collagenous with prominent vasa vasorum, and the tunica intima has a distinct basal lamina. A typical example is the aorta.

Muscular (distributing) arteries

The tunica intima consists of an endothelial layer overlying the internal elastic lamina. There is a muscular tunica media and a collagenous adventitia.

Arterioles

These channels are less than 100 µm in diameter, have only two or three layers of smooth muscle in the tunica media and a thin tunica adventitia. Variations in muscular tone of these vessels exert the greatest effect on systemic blood flow and pressure.

Capillaries

These are small vessels, only 5 to 10 µm in diameter, consisting of an endothelium, basal lamina and a layer of supporting cells (pericytes). The endothelium shows functional variations and may be continuous (the majority of tissues), fenestrated (endocrine tissues) or discontinuous (renal glomeruli). They are the site of blood–tissue exchange and operate at low transmural pressures. There is a net outflow of fluid into the extracellular space at the arteriolar end and a net influx at the venular end of capillary beds.

Veins

The venous system has a massive reserve volume (four to five times that of arteries) and veins have thin walls in relation to a large lumen with a prominent tunica adventitia (limb veins also have relatively thick tunica media) and valves to prevent the retrograde flow of blood. The proximal portion of pulmonary veins in rodents is surrounded by myocardial muscle, and valves are absent in all species.

Lymphatic vessels and capillaries

These lack the basal lamina seen in capillaries, whilst larger lymphatic vessels are equipped with valves and are almost indistinguishable from veins.

Anatomical and physiological variations

There are some minor species-specific variations in the histological structure of blood vessels where a more detailed knowledge may be required when investigating specific changes. For example, the pulmonary arteries in the rat show regional variations in medial thickness which may be misinterpreted as hypertrophy. Similarly, the arteries of the canine papillary muscles show adaptations to the normal physiological stresses placed upon them, as duplication of the internal elastic lamina and medial thickening, which should not be regarded as pathological changes.

Specialized structures

Vascular beds in a range of sites show distinct anatomical and physiological variations which are related to functional adaptations (Table 5.1).

Endothelium

The endothelium is not just an inert, semipermeable, barrier but an active, secretory tissue with an important role in the maintenance of vascular tone and repair of injury (e.g. secretion of factor VIII, plasminogen activator and inhibitor, serotonin, bradykinin, collagen, fibronectin, glycosaminoglycans [GAGs], elastin, passage of inflammatory cells). Endothelial cell junctions are a means of transendothelial transport and vary in their permeability depending on their site.

Some vasoactive substances (e.g. bradykinin, acetylcholine, ATP) depend upon an intact endothelium to exert their vasodilatory effects and removal of the endothelium may abolish or reverse their usual effects.

Vascular smooth muscle

The contractile elements in smooth muscle (actin and myosin filaments) are similar to cardiac and skeletal muscle but lack the alignment of fibres to give a striated

Table 5.1 Vascular beds with anatomical and physiological variations

Tissue	Structure	Function
Aorta	Aortic Body	Chemoreceptor
Carotid artery	Carotid body Carotid sinus	Chemoreceptor Baroreceptor
Kidney	Juxtaglomerular apparatus Glomerulus Medullary vessels	Blood pressure regulation Plasma ultrafiltration Countercurrent ion exchange
Testes	Pampiniform plexus	Heat exchange
Liver	Hepatic portal vein	Metabolic regulation
Hypothalamus	Hypothalamic portal system	Pituitary hormone regulation
Penis	Corpora cavernosa	Erection

appearance. In addition to determining vascular tone, smooth muscle cells are capable of proliferating and migrating into the tunica intima, secreting collagen, elastin, GAGs and showing phagocytic activity.

The action potential and contractile function of vascular smooth muscles is principally mediated by calcium ions. Calcium channel antagonists (e.g. **verapamil, nifedipine**), used in the treatment of hypertension, act upon resistance vessels which depend upon calcium influx for contraction of their smooth muscle walls.

Connective tissues

Supporting tissues are most prominent in the tunica adventitia, but are present as a 'skeleton' throughout the vessel wall. Fibrocytes and collagen provide tensile strength and elastic fibres contribute to the resilience of the wall to expansile forces. Extracellular spaces contain small quantities of GAGs (possibly acting as a shock-absorbing gel), and an increase is often seen as a response to increased transmural stress.

Blood

Blood is a medium for the provision of essential nutrients, gases, hormones, electrolytes, fluid and components of the immune system in addition to the transport of waste materials to excretory organs and temperature regulation. The principal exchange of fluids, proteins and metabolites within the extracellular spaces of tissues occurs across the capillary endothelium (e.g. gas exchange in the lung, glomerular filtrate in the kidneys).

The physical properties of blood are important in determining the response of blood vessels to physiological and pharmacological changes. Viscosity, which is determined by plasma protein concentrations and cellular density, affects flow characteristics according to physical laws. Plasma protein and electrolyte levels determine the plasma osmotic potential (oncotic pressure), thus influencing fluid exchange across capillary walls. The net transfer of fluids depends upon hydrostatic pressure within capillaries, plasma oncotic pressure, the permeability of the endothelium and drainage of extracellular spaces by lymphatics. An imbalance in favour of efflux (e.g. hypertension, lymphatic blockage, hypoproteinaemia, capillary damage) is often apparent at necropsy and microscopy as simple (i.e. non-inflammatory) oedema of affected tissues.

5.2.3 *Physiology*

Nervous and humoral control of vessels

Nervous control of vessel diameter is mainly exerted by sympathetic adrenergic fibres to arteries, arterioles and veins, although other neurotransmitters may be involved (acetylcholine, serotonin, nitric oxide). Humoral factors (e.g. prostacyclin and other prostaglandins, angiotensin II, CO_2, H^+, PO_2) are also of central importance in the systemic and local control of blood supply and the fine regulation of blood flow is a complex interaction of many factors.

Blood vessels show regional variations in their response to exogenous vasoactive compounds. **Noradrenaline** exerts a widespread vasoconstrictor activity, **ergot alkaloids** act preferentially on veins and **hydralazine** is a potent dilator of arterioles.

5.3 Biochemical and Cellular Mechanisms of Toxicity

As with the heart, the vasculature is exposed to most absorbed, or injected, xenobiotics for prolonged periods, although plasma binding and enzymatic removal of some substances (e.g. acetylcholine) may restrict any toxic potential. The toxic effects of treatment may involve an exaggerated pharmacological response, like sustained vasoconstriction, or a direct interaction with the components of the vascular wall (e.g. **allylamine**).

5.3.1 *Developmental Abnormalities*

Although alterations in the pattern of vascular supply may be induced by prenatal treatment, they are unlikely to be discovered by routine methods, unless the changes have a marked effect on the development of a particular tissue.

5.3.2 *Biochemical Mechanisms*

As in the myocardium, the metabolism of **allylamine** to **acrolein** leads to nuclear damage of smooth muscles and subsequent intimal proliferation. The normal metabolism of the endothelium may be compromised by hypertonic solutions (**urea, NaCl, mannitol**) and subsequent disruption of tight junctions can lead to cerebral oedema.

5.3.3 *Physiological Mechanisms*

Injection of biologically inert substances such as **methylcellulose** or **complex polysaccharides** may stimulate a non-specific, physiological inflammatory response to the introduction of foreign material. The principal findings are granulomatous lesions affecting a large number of vessels, principally the pulmonary vessels, renal glomeruli and spleen.

Hypoxia in rats causes an increase in pulmonary arterial pressure with an increase in the medial thickness and extent of muscular arteries. Hyperoxia also leads to medial thickening of muscular pulmonary arteries as well as right ventricular hypertrophy, but the mechanism is unclear.

Hypertonic solutions of **NaCl** can lead to shrinkage of endothelial cells with separation of tight junctions and cerebral oedema. An excessive intravenous infusion of physiological fluids can lead to hypervolaemia with subsequent pulmonary oedema, and hyperbaric oxygen induces hypertrophic changes in pulmonary capillaries.

5.3.4 *Pharmacological Mechanisms*

Excessive doses of vasoactive agents are associated with a range of clinical and pathological findings that may not be reflected in morphological alterations to the vessels themselves. Systemic vasodilatation, with hypovolaemia as a consequence, leads to a sustained reflex tachycardia that induces cardiac damage in dogs with no evidence of damage to systemic blood vessels. **Ergot alkaloids**, when administered to rats, lead to prolonged vasoconstriction and subsequent ischaemic necrosis of the tail (dry gangrene).

Treatment with **fenoldopam mesylate** (a dopamine agonist) by intravenous infusion in rats resulted in focal necrosis of the tunica media, with haemorrhage, in medium-sized arteries of the gastrointestinal tract and kidneys [14]. It is thought that the effect is a non-specific response to excessive vasodilatation. Similar lesions have been reported [15] with phosphodiesterase III inhibitors (**ICI 153,110**) and **LY 195115** and medial necrosis at the same sites is also seen with vasoconstrictors e.g. **angiotensin** [16]. It would appear, therefore, that excessive transmural forces (dilatory or constrictive) are capable of inducing vascular smooth muscle damage.

The specific effect of angiotensin-converting enzyme (ACE) inhibitors on the renin-producing cells of the glomerular afferent arterioles results in marked hypertrophy of this zone as part of a homeostatic mechanism and is merely an adaptive response to treatment (Figure 5.6).

The repair and maintenance of blood vessels depends on an interaction between clotting factors in the blood (platelets, clotting factors) and components of the vessel wall. Although haemorrhagic diseases can be a result of vascular damage, the administration of agents that interfere with platelet function or the clotting cascade (**coumarins, fibrinolytics, heparin**) may exert no direct effect on the vessels themselves but will induce perivascular haemorrhages (especially in the bladder and stomach) that may be confused with vascular lesions.

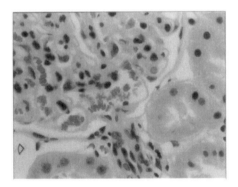 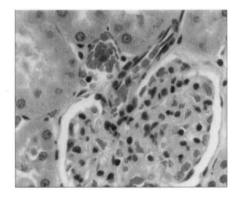

Figure 5.6 The photograph on the left illustrates a glomerulus, with its afferent arteriole (centre to top right), from a control rat. The vessel wall is thin and inconspicuous and is difficult to see in routine sections. The photograph on the right shows slight hypertrophy of the afferent arteriole (centre to bottom right) as a result of blockade of the renin–angiotensin system. The enlargement of the arteriole in this site is associated with proliferation of renin-producing smooth muscle cells as part of a homeostatic, hormonal mechanism. This lesion illustrates the potential for changes attributable to the specialized nature of blood vessels in certain sites, rather than alterations in haemodynamics.

5.3.5 *Immunologically Mediated Toxicity*

With the advent of biosynthetic proteins and peptides as therapeutic entities, animal tests may be complicated by immune reactions, with manifestations of vascular disease, as an expected but undesirable effect of treatment.

Many immune-mediated diseases are characterized by changes in vessels of the skin, kidneys and joints and will not be considered specifically in this chapter. For instance, systemic sensitization to proteins, or compounds acting as haptens, can lead to hypersensitivity type III angiitis of small vessels, an important complication of treatment with **penicillin, methyldopa** and **sulphonamides** in man. Immune responses are not dose or time dependent and are usually easily differentiated from direct drug-mediated effects.

Lymphokines and other mediators of immune or inflammatory responses are currently synthesized as therapeutic agents and administration to animals may result in dramatic vascular changes, e.g. lymphocytic infiltration of pulmonary arterioles and venules in mice and rats treated with **interleukin 2** [17].

5.4 Morphological Responses to Injury

Because of the apparent simplicity of vessel structure, it is relatively easy to detect structural changes in routine H and E sections. In most cases, diagnoses of vascular disease are collated with the organ affected, and may represent specific disease entities rather than a generalized process specifically affecting blood vessels. Vascular ectasia, the expansion of sinusoids in endocrine tissue, is commonly seen in ageing rodents and is probably associated with focal loss of parenchymal cells. It would be misleading to include such conditions as examples of generalized vascular disease.

5.4.1 *Non-neoplastic Changes*

The response of vessels to treatment is relatively limited and many changes are non-specific with few clues to their pathogenesis. In addition, the functional effects of any lesions may not be related to the magnitude of the change in affected vessels, and relatively florid lesions (e.g. intimal proliferation) may have no functional consequences whilst vasoconstriction, with no morphological change, may result in ischaemic necrosis. Widespread capillary damage or clotting defects may lead to fatal haemorrhage with only minor vascular changes (e.g. **coumarins**), whereas intimal proliferation in canine coronary arteries does not appear to have any functional consequences.

Haemodynamic changes

Physical forces acting on the vessel walls are important factors in the production of vascular disease. Excessive dilatation or shearing forces can cause endothelial disruption, rupture of the internal elastic lamina, smooth muscle hypertrophy or necrosis with healing lesions characterized by intimal proliferation. It is possible that physical forces acting on vessel walls form part of a 'common final pathway' for many types of vascular toxic change.

164

Atherosclerosis

Atherosclerosis, an extremely rare lesion of dogs and rodents is not commonly encountered in toxicity testing and is more likely to be seen in rabbits, non-human primates or pigs as a result of intentional dietary or genetic manipulations. Lesions encountered in toxicity studies are likely to be early manifestations of disease with focal intimal aggregations of foamy cells (probably derived from smooth muscles) rather than advanced changes with fibrosis and thrombus formation that are seen in man.

Intimal proliferation

Intimal proliferation is commonly seen in hypertension and arteritis but has also been reported in a range of vessels following administration of **allylamine** to rats, and in the coronary arteries of dogs treated with **phosphodiesterase (PDE) III inhibitors** (Figure 5.7). The intima is expanded by the influx and proliferation of smooth muscle cells with prominent GAGs production and slight endothelial hypertrophy.

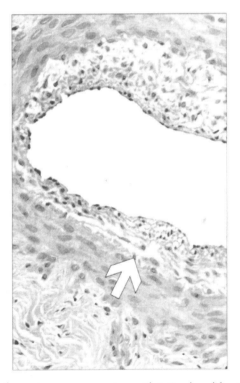

Figure 5.7 A section of a canine coronary artery with intimal proliferation. The arrow indicates the location of the internal elastic lamina. The thickened tunica intima consists, principally, of smooth muscle proliferation with glycosaminoglycan production (clear spaces towards top of photograph). There is minor hypertrophy and hyperplasia of the overlying endothelium. This change is characteristic of the coronary arteriopathy seen in dogs treated with phosphodiesterase III inhibitors.

Spontaneous intimal proliferation is seen at branching points of arteries and in areas of arterial motility (e.g. papillary and atrial branches of coronary arteries) and can be regarded as a physiological adaptation to transmural stress. An increase in motility, as expected, leads to an exacerbation of spontaneous changes. Areas of chronic inflammation may also result in intimal thickening of associated vessels (e.g. gastric ulcers).

Coronary vascular lesions induced with vasodilating and inotropic agents in dogs may resemble spontaneous lesions, and an effect of treatment may only be seen as intimal or adventitial changes in branches of the coronary arteries that are not usually affected by spontaneous changes [8].

Medial necrosis

Medial necrosis, with accompanying haemorrhage, has been reported in muscular arteries following treatment with vasoactive agents (e.g. **fenoldopam mesylate, minoxidil, SK&F 94654, hydralazine, angiotensin**) in rats, non-human primates, pigs and dogs (Figure 5.8). The splanchnic beds are more prone to change in rats with the coronary vessels often at risk in larger species. The lesion usually undergoes repair with intimal proliferation, adventitial fibrosis and occasionally, formation of small, intramural blood vessels which give a 'Swiss cheese' appearance to the vessel wall.

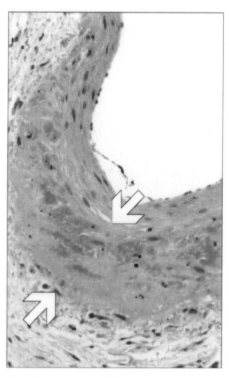

Figure 5.8 Canine artery showing necrosis of the outer half of the tunica media (between the arrows). There are remnants of pyknotic nuclei and small (dark) areas of haemorrhage. The separation of the endothelium from the internal elastic lamina, overlying the lesion, is artefactual.

Medial hypertrophy

Medial hypertrophy and hyperplasia is seen as thickening of the tunica media and is commonly associated with hypertension, **ergot** poisoning and **hyperbaric oxygen** (the latter affecting the pulmonary arteries). Normal anatomical variations in wall thickness must be taken into account when considering a diagnosis of medial hypertrophy.

Adventitial oedema, haemorrhage and fibrosis

Separation of the adventitial collagen fibres by GAGs (adventitial oedema) is seen in the coronary arteries of dogs treated with some **vasodilating agents** and may be a response to increased transmural stress. An increase in adventitial collagen, sometimes associated with haemorrhage and formation of new blood vessels (neovascularization), is seen as a more severe, or as a chronic manifestation, of the same change (Figure 5.9)

Fibrinoid necrosis

Fibrinoid necrosis is a term used to describe necrosis of the vessel wall with serum proteins and fibrin accumulation to produce uniform, eosinophilic, amorphous areas.

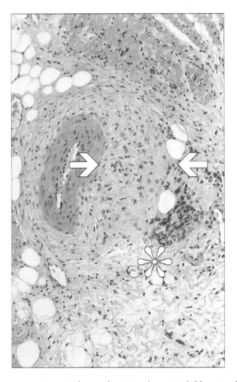

Figure 5.9 Canine coronary artery with moderate adventitial fibrosis (between the arrows). As this lesion is relatively recent there are numerous fibroblasts, but long-standing lesions tend to consist of mature collagen deposits with few cells. Just above and to the right of the asterisk is indicated the site of a small focus of mononuclear cells with haemosiderin-laden macrophages which is a sequel to a previous perivascular haemorrhage.

Endothelial loss with thrombi may be seen. **Organic mercurial compounds** and **lead** toxicity may produce this change in cerebral vessels. Fibrinoid necrosis is characteristic of necrotizing vasculitis (seen in dogs as 'beagle pain syndrome' [see below]) where there is also a florid adventitial polymorphonuclear leucocyte infiltration.

Arteritis/periarteritis

Arteritis/periarteritis refers to inflammatory changes affecting all elements of the vessel wall, often with haemorrhage, inflammatory cell infiltration and fibroplasia (see spontaneous changes below). Areas adjacent to frank inflammatory lesions may only show intimal proliferation and adventitial fibrosis. Degeneration may be seen in all three tunics in severe lesions resulting in weakening of the vessel wall and subsequent aneurysmal dilatation with thrombus formation.

Capillary damage

Damage to capillaries, leading to intratesticular haemorrhage, is seen with **cadmium** toxicity in rats, although capillary pathology is rarely reported.

Spontaneous expansion of capillary channels and sinusoids, with associated parenchymal degeneration, is commonly seen in ageing rodents as vascular ectasia (syn. angiectasis, telangiectasis) of endocrine organs and the liver.

Hypersensitivity angiitis

Hypersensitivity angiitis is seen in small arterioles, capillaries and venules as vascular and perivascular aggregations of lymphocytes, macrophages and occasional eosinophils. As with most immune-mediated diseases, the reaction is not dose or time dependent. Immune-mediated vascular disease is often relatively site specific (e.g. glomerulonephritis, lupus erythematosus in the kidneys).

Mineralization

Mineralization usually affects elastic fibres and is seen in a wide range of sites in metastatic calcification following renal failure or **hypervitaminosis D** (e.g. aorta, mesenteric, renal, gastric, testicular and coronary arteries).

Amyloidosis

Amyloidosis is a common and debilitating disease of mice and hamsters (very rare in rats) with deposits of amorphous, eosinophilic material in a large number of vessels (especially renal glomeruli and renal, pulmonary, testicular and mesenteric arteries) with the potential for thrombosis and subsequent ischaemic damage to the tissues supplied. A protein-losing nephropathy with severe hypoproteinaemia may result in widespread subcutaneous and interstitial oedema with ascites and hydrothorax.

Thrombi

Thrombi are formed in response to endothelial discontinuity and can affect vessels of all sizes. Early thrombi, consisting of platelets and fibrin, are gradually infiltrated by macrophages, fibroblasts and new capillaries (organization) with the proliferation of endothelial cells that re-establish single or multiple patent channels (recanalization). Venous thrombi are commonly encountered in veins in intravascular studies but arterial thrombi are rare. Detachment of thrombi into the circulation is called embolization, and colonization of thrombi by pathogenic bacteria results in septic thrombi (and emboli). Emboli formed by skin and hairshaft fragments are not uncommon in the lungs of animals from intravenous infusion or injection studies.

In studies using in-dwelling catheters thromboembolism, and septic thrombi, are not uncommon and bacterial colonization, with inflammation of the valvular endocardium (bacterial endocarditis), may ensue.

5.4.2 *Tumours*

Because of the ubiquitous nature of blood and lymph vessels, tumours of the vascular system may affect any organ or tissue, although the spleen, liver and subcutaneous tissues are the most usual sites for spontaneous lesions.

Haemangioma

Haemangioma is a benign, non-invasive, proliferation of blood-filled spaces lined by well-differentiated endothelial cells within a prominent fibrous matrix. In some instances, especially in young animals, such structures are regarded as developmental abnormalities rather than neoplasms and are termed 'vascular hamartoma'.

In old animals there may be a non-neoplastic proliferation of widely dilated vascular spaces with associated haemorrhage and fibrosis. The mesenteric lymph nodes of some rat strains, and the uterus and ovaries of mice, are commonly affected and the lesions are often recorded as angiectasis or vascular ectasia. Differential diagnosis of angiectasis from haemangioma or haemangiosarcoma can be very difficult.

Haemangiosarcoma

Haemangiosarcoma (Figure 5.10) is the malignant counterpart of haemangioma and is characterized by the proliferation of large, hyperchromatic endothelial cells sometimes with bizarre nuclei. The tumour may be relatively fibrous or extremely vascular with haemorrhages, thrombosis and local invasion of surrounding tissues. Metastasis is relatively uncommon, but may be seen in the lungs, spleen and liver depending on the primary site.

Induced tumours have been recorded in a variety of sites with a range of xenobiotics and procedures. There may be a predilection for a specific tissue (e.g. liver with **vinyl chloride**) and the process may be considered to be a manifestation of specific-organ toxicity. An alternative view regards vascular tumours as multicentric (i.e. not site specific) in origin and requires the inclusion of vascular neoplasia from all sites in any analysis of effects of treatment (as for haematopoietic tumours.)

Other tumours

Other components of the vascular wall (smooth muscle, fibroblasts or nervous tissue) can become neoplastic but it is unlikely that many tumours (especially large

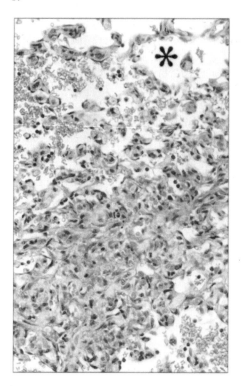

Figure 5.10 A section showing the typical appearance of a haemangiosarcoma in the mouse. There are many irregular vascular channels, of varying size (the asterisk denotes a large channel), with a more solid area at the bottom of the picture. The endothelial cells making up the neoplasm are larger than normal, with considerable variation in size and an increase in nuclear : cytoplasmic ratio.

ones) would be considered to have arisen from blood vessels rather than the tissues they supply. In some cases tumours with vascular and fibrous components may be considered to have arisen from vascular pericytes (haemangiopericytomas), but are rarely a significant diagnostic problem.

Specialized vascular structures (e.g. carotid and aortic bodies) may become neoplastic, but have not been reported as specific target tissues for potential carcinogens.

Tumours of lymphatic vessels pose a diagnostic problem to the pathologist as they are not easily distinguished from haemangiocellular tumours. Fortunately they are very rare and have not been identified as a primary site for carcinogens.

5.4.3 Spontaneous Pathology

Three diseases of laboratory animals have led to serious difficulties in the assessment of vascular toxicity.

Beagle pain syndrome

Idiopathic necrotizing arteritis or 'beagle pain syndrome' manifests itself as fibrinoid necrosis, or as a more quiescent, healing arteritis/periarteritis, predom-inantly in the coronary, vertebral, gastric, vesical, mediastinal and thymic vessels [18]. The condition may be severe and lead to the euthanasia of the animal, or may be seen as recurrent attacks of fever, malaise, altered gait and stiffness of the neck. As a non-specific effect, possibly allied to the stress of treatment, the condition may be consistently seen only in animals from treated groups (e.g. some **benzi-midazoles**) but without a clear dose-response. The cause of the condition is unknown and, although immune mechanisms have been postulated, there is some evidence to suggest that there may be a viral origin [19]. Although there has been no evidence to suggest that this condition is predictive of toxic effects in man, the occurrence of this disease in toxicity studies has delayed the development of several compounds.

Extramural coronary arteritis

Idiopathic extramural coronary arteritis is seen in a small percentage of control dogs (up to 7 per cent in some laboratories) and may present changes that are difficult to distinguish from the coronary arterial lesions induced by **vasodilating/inotropic agents** [20]. The predilection of the spontaneous lesion for the circumflex coronary vessels, rather than the extramural and intramural branches, and the consistent inflammatory nature of the condition may be helpful in the differential diagnosis, although a careful examination of the coronary vasculature is required to eliminate the possibility of an effect of treatment.

Arteritis/periarteritis

Arteritis/periarteritis affecting vessels in a wide variety of sites, but with a predilection for mesenteric arteries, is a common spontaneous finding in ageing rats. As the condition may be influenced by level of nutrition as well as of treatment e.g. **caffeine** [21] and **PDE III inhibitors** [15], any changes in the incidence or severity of this lesion must be interpreted with caution.

5.5 Testing for Toxicity

5.5.1 *Physiological Methods*

Blood pressure and flow measurements

Simple measurements of systemic pressure are feasible in most species for routine toxicology testing, although the information derived may be relatively non-specific. The assessment of blood flow in particular tissues is restricted to investigative studies.

Sophisticated techniques have been employed to monitor pressure and flow in a variety of specific tissues by the surgical implantation of miniature transducers and the administration of intravascular tracers.

5.5.2 *Morphological Methods*

Necropsy

Because blood vessels are ubiquitous, most routine sections contain a wide range of vessels. At necropsy it is unlikely that many lesions will be attributed to particular blood vessels and most changes (e.g. haemorrhage, oedema, vasculitis) will usually be ascribed to specific tissues or organs.

Apart from the aorta in large animals, blood vessels are rarely opened and the adventitial surface is usually the only site open to scrutiny at necropsy. Most large or medium-sized vessels are easily located in non-rodent species, but the most easily visible vascular beds in rodents (apart from the retina) can be found in the limbs, mesentery and pampiniform plexus of the testis.

Intravascular studies

A proportion of routine toxicology studies involve the administration of compounds by the intravenous route using a needle or catheter into the limb veins of larger species, and the tail vein of rats. Repeated administration over a period of weeks results in a number of puncture wounds at each site, and affected areas show different stages in the development of any effects of treatment, whether it is a simple healing process or a reaction to local irritancy.

Tissue sampling

With compounds exerting obvious systemic vascular effects, it is advisable to examine and preserve a greater range of vessels than normal. There is no problem in locating major vessels in larger species, but the selection of sites may be more difficult in rodents and the thoracic and abdominal aorta, limb and mesenteric vessels may be sampled consistently.

Intravascular studies require special attention to the examination and sampling of the injection sites. In rodents, the tail is usually sampled in its entirety and three (or more) sites selected for transverse sections, following careful decalcification. In larger species, the injection sites (usually the limb veins), are dissected free, with the underlying subcutis, and attached to card before fixation and processing.

Staining

In the majority of instances, H and E staining is sufficient for the detection of most changes.

Special stains that are commonly used to assist in diagnosis include:

- Alcian blue (GAGs)
- Perls' Prussian blue (haemosiderin)
- Elastic van Gieson (elastic fibres)
- Masson's trichrome or van Gieson (connective tissue)
- PTAH (fibrin)
- Von Kossa or Alizarin red (mineralization)

Histopathology

As with the heart, the same general principles apply to the diagnosis and recording of findings. The recording of findings should be more detailed for intravascular studies, where the grading of lesions to detect a 'no-effect-level' is of great importance.

Where there are vascular lesions, as a result of treatment, special stains may assume greater importance in the detection of minor or subtle effects (e.g. GAGs in vessel walls, damage to the internal elastic lamina).

5.5.3   Special Techniques

Investigative techniques with blood vessels encompass the borderline between physiology, pharmacology and pathology. Multidisciplinary investigations are often required to elucidate the pathogenesis of a drug-induced change and a variety of techniques are available.

Electron microscopy

TEM and SEM are useful adjuncts in the investigation of induced lesions, but should be used with caution (if at all) in routine toxicity studies. Preparation of vascular tissues usually involves perfusion fixation techniques to attempt to preserve the vessels under normal physiological conditions.

Swelling, degeneration and desquamation of endothelial cells can be dramatically demonstrated by SEM, whilst changes to the basement membrane and vessel walls are more readily appreciated using TEM.

Tracers

Monastral blue, Evan's blue or horseradish peroxidase, administered intravenously before necropsy, can be employed to detect functional changes in vascular permeability. A loss of vascular integrity can be detected by the leakage of these markers at the macroscopic and microscopic level.

Isolated vascular beds in vivo and ex vivo

The effects of novel compounds can be investigated by the isolation of vascular beds in living animals (e.g. mesenteric vessels, superficial vessels in the skin) or as isolated preparations in nutritive media.

Isolated vascular muscle strips

Isolated, human, vascular muscle strips have been useful in providing comparative information when extrapolating the results of animal studies to man.

Tissue culture

Vascular smooth muscles and endothelial cells can be sustained in tissue culture and their reaction to various stimuli (physical, pharmacological or toxic) assessed.

5.6   Conclusions

The assessment of the potential toxic effects of xenobiotics on the cardiovascular system involves a structured, multidisciplinary approach that extends from early, routine studies to sophisticated investigations of specific problems. Routine, regulatory studies are designed to detect relatively major changes in structure and function, and provide the starting point for any further work. It is, however, prudent to extend the range of investigations conducted in routine studies when using agents with known cardiovascular pharmacological activity.

The heart is affected by a wide range of compounds which may exert physical, metabolic, pharmacological or morphological effects. The outcome of exposure to these agents may be functional, structural or both. Depending on the severity and extent of these effects, the well-being and viability of the animal may be compromised. Some morphological changes, like lipofuscin deposition, may have no functional implications, whereas hypokalaemia may prove fatal with no morphological alteration.

The range of reactions to treatment in blood vessels is limited, and the pathogenesis of any lesions may be difficult to determine in morphological studies. As with the heart, functional changes, like prolonged vasoconstriction, may result in ischaemia and necrosis of tissues with no obvious morphological change in vessels. In contrast, pronounced thickening of the wall of coronary arteries in the dog usually results in no functional alteration in the myocardium.

In common with most toxicological investigations, the animals used in routine studies may not be ideal models for the extrapolation of results to man. Decisions regarding the safety of any compounds tested must take into account all relevant information derived from a range of investigations. Differences in anatomy, physiology, metabolism, pharmacokinetics, pharmacology and pathology between laboratory animals and man all have a bearing on the potential risk to man. There are no simple formulae that can be applied, and experience, judgement and attention to detail are essential in the planning and execution of toxicology studies.

References

1. JACKSON, B.A. (1981) Developmental cardiotoxic effects of chemicals, in *Cardiac Toxicology*, Vol. III, pp. 163–176, Boca Raton, Florida: CRC Press.
2. SPERELAKIS, N. (1981) Effects of cardiotoxic agents on the electrical properties of myocardial cells, in *Cardiac Toxicology*, Vol. I, pp. 39–108, Boca Raton, Florida: CRC Press.
3. CONFER, A.W., REAVIS, D.U. and PANCIERA, R.J. (1983) Light and electron microscopic changes in cardiac and skeletal muscle of sheep with experimental monensin toxicosis, *Veterinary Pathology*, **20**, 590–602.
4. BOOR, P.J. (1983) Allylamine cardiotoxicity: metabolism and mechanism, in *Myocardial Injury*, pp. 533–543, New York: Plenum.
5. DOROSHOW, J.H., LOCKER, G.Y. and MYERS, C.E. (1980) Enzymatic defenses of the mouse heart against reactive oxygen metabolites: alterations produced by doxorubicin, *Journal of Clinical Investigation*, **65**, 128–135.
6. HERMAN, E.H. (1981) Cardiotoxicity of antineoplastic agents, in *Cardiac Toxicology*, Vol. II, pp. 165–187, Boca Raton, Florida: CRC Press.
7. DOGTEROM, P. and ZBINDEN, G. (1992) Cardiotoxicity of vasodilators and positive inotropic/vasodilating drugs in dogs: an overview, *Critical Reviews in Toxicology*, **22**, 203–241.
8. ISAACS, K.R., JOSEPH, E.C. and BETTON, G.R. (1989) Coronary vascular lesions in dogs treated with phosphodiesterase III inhibitors, *Toxicologic Pathology*, **17**, 153–163.
9. LEHR, D. (1981) Studies on the cardiotoxicity of α- and β-adrenergic amines, in *Cardiac Toxicology*, Vol. II, pp. 75–112, Boca Raton, Florida: CRC Press.

10. CZARNECKI, C.M. (1980) Furazolidone-induced cardiomyopathy – Biomedical model for the study of cardiac hypertrophy and congestive heart failure, *Avian Diseases*, **24**, 120–138.

11. D'AGOSTINO, A.N. (1963) An electron microscopic study of skeletal and cardiac muscle of the rat poisoned by plasmocid, *Laboratory Investigation*, **12**, 1060–1071.

12. BERMAN, J.J., RICE, J.M. and REDDICK, R. (1980) Endocardial schwannomas in rats, *Archives of Pathology and Laboratory Medicine*, **104**, 187–191.

13. GREAVES, P. and FACCINI, J.M. (1992) *Rat Histopathology, a Glossary for Use in Toxicity and Carcinogenicity Studies*, 2nd Edn, Amsterdam: Elsevier Science Publishers.

14. YUHAS, E.M., MORGAN, D.G., ARENA, E., KUPP, R.P., SAUNDERS, L.Z. and LEWIS, H.B. (1985) Arterial medial necrosis and hemorrhage induced in rats by intravenous infusion of fenoldopam mesylate, a dopaminergic vasodilator, *American Journal of Pathology*, **119**, 83–91.

15. WESTWOOD, F.R., ISWARAN, T.J. and GREAVES, P. (1989) Pathologic changes in blood vessels following administration of an inotropic vasodilator (ICI 153,011) to the rat, *Fundamental and Applied Toxicology*, **14**, 797–809.

16. THORBALL, N. and OLSEN, F. (1974) Ultrastructural pathological changes in intestinal submucosal arteries in angiotensin induced acute hypertension in rats. *Acta Pathologica, Microbiologica et Immunologica Scandinavica* (A), **82**, 703–713.

17. ANDERSON, T.D. and HAYES, T.J. (1989) Toxicity of human recombinant interleukin-2 in rats. Pathologic changes are characterized by marked lymphocytic and eosinophilic proliferation and multisystem involvement, *Laboratory Investigation*, **60**, 331–346.

18. HAYES, T.J., ROBERTS, G.K.S. and HALLIWELL, W.H. (1989) An idiopathic febrile necrotizing arteritis syndrome in the dog: beagle pain syndrome, *Toxicologic Pathology*, **17**, 138–144.

19. FELSBURG, P.J., HOGENESCH, H., SOMBERG, R.L., SNYDER, P.W. and GLICKMAN, L.T. (1992) Immunologic abnormalities in canine juvenile polyarteritis syndrome: a naturally occurring animal model of Kawasaki disease, *Clinical Immunology and Immunopathology*, **65**, 110–118.

20. HARTMAN, H.A. (1989) Spontaneous extramural coronary arteritis in dogs. *Toxicologic Pathology*, **17**, 138–144.

21. JOHANSSON, S. (1981) Cardiovascular lesions in Sprague–Dawley rats induced by long-term treatment with caffeine, *Acta Pathologica, Microbiologica et Immunologica Scandinavica* (A), **89**, 185–191.

Additional Reading

BALAZS, T. (Ed.) (1981) *Cardiac Toxicology*, Vols I, II, III, Boca Raton, Florida: CRC Press.

BENIRSCHKE, K., GARNER, F.M. and JONES, T.C. (1978) *Pathology of Laboratory Animals*, Vol. 1, New York: Springer-Verlag.

BOORMAN, G.A., EUSTIS, S.L., ELWELL, M.R., MONTGOMERY, Jr. C.A. and MACKENZIE, W.F. (Eds) (1990) *Pathology of the Fischer Rat, Reference and Atlas*, London: Academic Press.

EVANS, H.E. and CHRISTENSEN, G.C. (1979) The Heart and Arteries, in *Miller's Anatomy of the Dog*, 2nd Edn, pp. 632–651, Philadelphia: W.B. Saunders Company.

GOPINATH, C., PRENTICE, D.E. and LEWIS, D.J. (1987) *Current Histopathology – Atlas of Experimental Toxicological Pathology*, Vol. 13, Lancaster: MTP Press Limited.

GREAVES, P. (1990) *Histopathology of Preclinical Toxicity Studies, Interpretation and Relevance in Drug Safety Evaluation*, Amsterdam: Elsevier Science Publishers.

HASCHEK, W.M. and ROUSSEAUX, C.G., (Eds) (1991) *Handbook of Toxicologic Pathology*, London: Academic Press.

JONES, T.C., MOHR, U. and HUNT, R.D. (Eds) (1991) *Monographs on Pathology of Laboratory Animals, Cardiovascular and Musculoskeletal Systems*, New York: Springer-Verlag.

JUBB, K.V.F., KENNEDY, P.C. and PALMER, N. (Eds) (1985) *Pathology of Domestic Animals*, 3rd Edn, London: Academic Press.

MOHR, U., DUNGWORTH, D.L. and CAPEN, C.C. (Eds) (1992) *Pathobiology of the Aging Rat*, Vol. 1, Washington, D.C.: ILSI Press.

ROBBINS, S.L., COTRAN, R.S. and KUMAR, V. (Eds) (1984) *Pathologic Basis of Disease*, Philadelphia: W.B. Saunders Company.

SCHNEIDER, P. (1990) Hemodynamically induced heart lesions in the dog after the administration of cardio-active substances, *Experimental Pathology*, **40**, 155–168.

TURUSOV, V.S. (Ed.) (1979) *Pathology of Tumours in Laboratory Animals, Tumours of the Mouse*, Vol. II, Lyon: IARC Scientific Publications.

TURUSOV, V.S. and MOHR, U. (Eds) (1990) *Pathology of Tumours in Laboratory Animals, Tumours of the Rat*, Vol. I, 2nd Edn, Lyon: IARC Scientific Publications.

VAN VLEET, J.F. and FERRANS, V.J. (1986) Myocardial diseases of animals, *American Journal of Pathology*, **24**, 98–178

6

The Haematopoietic System

C. MICHAEL ANDREWS

6.1 Introduction

The importance of blood examination in toxicity studies is a direct consequence of the intimate exposure of experimental compounds to the cellular and humoral components of the blood (Table 6.1) Blood is a rapidly dividing tissue and blood-forming capacity has a high potential for expansion. In man, under normal conditions, the turnover of blood cells is considerable, of the order of 2 to 3×10^{11} cells per day, but in times of increased demand, the enlargement of haematopoietic tissue can be up to eight times the normal value. Therefore, the consequences of toxicity to circulating blood cells, or their precursors, may be very serious and ultimately result in profound anaemia, haemorrhage or overwhelming infection. In one survey of drug-related blood dyscrasias, whilst this form of adverse reaction constituted only 10 per cent of all those reported, 40 per cent had a fatal outcome [1]. In the development of novel pharmaceutical entities, the occurrence of transient and reversible suppression of bone marrow production is not uncommonly encountered at high dosages. However, only if the proposed therapy is for life-threatening disease may haematotoxic side-effects be allowable in clinical practice, and in such cases the toxicity will limit the therapeutic dose. Nevertheless, it is not possible using conventional toxicity study design to predict the *idiosyncratic* failure of the bone marrow which is seen occasionally in man in response to treatment with certain drugs (e.g. **chloramphenicol, phenylbutazone**). In these albeit rare reactions, marrow failure may be total (aplastic anaemia) and without successful therapy, such as bone marrow transplantation, lead to death. Because of the limitations of conventional screening for haematotoxicity, methods such as *in vitro* marrow culture and marrow transplantation into sublethally irradiated mice are becoming increasingly commonplace. These techniques can throw light on damage to the earliest haematopoietic precursors, the pluripotent stem cells, whose alteration might ultimately lead to marrow failure or neoplastic change. Meanwhile, the ease with which biopsies of blood may be taken has always allowed for sequential monitoring of toxic changes to blood and bone marrow, and blood examination has, therefore, always been a standard component of toxicity screening. Indeed, as

Table 6.1 Examples of haematotoxic effects on a range of targets, showing toxic agent, action and mechanism

Toxic agent	Action	Mechanism
Bone marrow		
Aminopterin	Bone marrow suppression (predictable)	Unknown
Chloramphenicol	Bone marrow suppression (idiosyncratic)	Stem cell damage
Benzene	Leukaemia	Stem cell damage
Erythrocytes		
Oestrogen	Anaemia (bone marrow suppression)	Erythropoietin $\downarrow$
Butoxyethanol	Anaemia (haemolytic)	Membrane damage
α-Methyldopa	Anaemia (haemolytic)	Immune-mediated
Aniline	Anaemia (haemolytic, methaemoglobinaemia)	Oxidative haemolysis
Pb, Hg, Al	Anaemia (microcytic)	Haem synthesis $\downarrow$
Isoniazid	Anaemia (sideroblastic)	Pyridoxine metabolism
Phenytoin, AZT	Anaemia (megaloblastic)	Folate metabolism
Neutrophils		
Corticosteroids	Neutrophilia	Decreased neutrophil half-life
Adrenaline	Neutrophilia	Neutrophil demargination
Pb, Hg	Neutrophilia	Tissue damage
β-Lactam antibiotics	Neutropenia	Immune-mediated
Ethinyl estradiol	Neutropenia	Marrow suppression
Lymphocytes		
Corticosteroids	Lymphocytopenia	T lymphocyte destruction
Busulphan	Lymphocytopenia	B lymphocyte depression
Platelets		
AZT, BHT	Thrombocytosis	Unknown
Chlorothiazide	Thrombocytopenia	Marrow suppression
Quinidine	Thrombocytopenia	Immune-mediated
Aspirin	Decreased platelet aggregation	Thromboxane metabolism
Heparin	Decreased platelet aggregation	Thrombin generation $\downarrow$
Penicillin	Platelet aggregation $\downarrow$ and adhesion $\downarrow$	? Platelet binding
Coagulation cascade		
Antibiotics, warfarin	Coagulation factor synthesis $\downarrow$	Vitamin K metabolism
Chlorpromazine	Decreased coagulation activity	Immune-mediated

$\downarrow$, decreased; AZT, azidothymidine; BHT, butylated hydroxytoluene.

techniques improve, it will be possible to apply more and increasingly sensitive measurements to the very small blood samples available from some laboratory species.

6.2 Anatomy, Histology and Physiology

6.2.1 *Anatomy*

Bone marrow

This tissue produces blood cells in the adult life of higher mammals and is found in the central cavities of the long bones (e.g. femur, tibia). When performing marrow biopsies in adult dogs, it is usually necessary to take samples from the sternum or a rib, as the femoral marrow cavity may be almost entirely replaced by fat. In the rat and mouse, however, the relatively high turnover of cells and their shorter lifespan means that the bone marrow cavity is fully populated throughout life; indeed, haematopoiesis also persists in extramedullary sites, principally the spleen, and it is this organ that provides the primary erythropoietic response. All lineages of blood cells are derived from common precursors, the pluripotent stem cells, which are found in greater numbers with increasing radial distance from the long bone axis [2]. The haematopoietic tissue is based around structural reticuloendothelial cells which form the inner surfaces of venous sinuses. Associated with the reticuloendothelial cells are fat cells and fibroblasts. It is the interaction of these various cell types, through the mediation of adhesion molecules and the soluble cytokines which the cells secrete, which control the proliferation, lineage-evolution and maturation of haematopoiesis.

Spleen and lymphoreticular tissue

Since this tissue is dealt with at length elsewhere (Chapter 7), it will not be discussed in greater detail here, other than to point out the major features as they impinge on general haematological function. Essentially, the spleen and lymph nodes are organizations of lymphocytes and macrophages constructed to detect foreign antigens as the blood supply perfuses through them. The interaction of macrophages and subpopulations of lymphocytes brings about the presentation and recognition of antigens, cell-mediated killing and antibody production, through the stimulation and proliferation of specific clones of lymphocytes.

The spleen is an important site of extramedullary haematopoiesis, especially in rodents [3]. In addition, a proportion of blood bathing the spleen passes directly from the arterial to the venous circulation by way of splenic sinuses, entering the sinuses by interendothelial slits. These slits effectively 'sieve' the blood, trapping large intraerythroid inclusions such as Heinz bodies and Howell–Jolly bodies (see Section 6.4). This important function of the spleen is therefore lost when the organ is removed following surgery, and increased numbers of such red cell inclusions are seen in the stained blood film.

As well as extramedullary haematopoiesis and sieving, the spleen sequesters a pool of erythrocytes, leucocytes and platelets whose numbers in peripheral blood increase after splenectomy, or by sympathetic stimulation which causes contraction of the muscular capsule of the organ. Splenic contraction shows considerable species variation, being maximal in the horse and some dog breeds, where haematocrit (the proportion of blood occupied by erythrocytes) may be increased by 50 per cent. Contraction of the spleen may be stress-induced, and may be reversed by the effects of anaesthetics.

Blood

Blood consists of the cellular elements, leucocytes (white cells), erythrocytes (red cells) and platelets, circulating in a complex fluid matrix, the plasma. The circulation provides a transport system for those elements contained within it, and as such it should be borne in mind that a blood sample can only provide a snapshot of a dynamic system. With the exception of erythrocytes, the other cell types are on their way to a location where their function is required. All the cell types are constantly leaving the circulation and being replaced at differing rates.

There is considerable homeostasis with regard to plasma volume, pH and constituents. However, water movement into and from plasma (e.g. as a result of excessive hydration from fluid intake, or dehydration from vomiting or diarrhoea) may lead to haemodilution or haemoconcentration.

Plasma proteins are generally viewed as being in the domain of clinical biochemistry, but the examination of coagulation factors, which constitute a major component of plasma, are considered below as part of haematology. After clotting, with the depletion of fibrinogen and many coagulation factors from the plasma, the resultant fluid is serum.

Erythrocyte development

The generation of anucleate, biconcave, discoid, haemoglobin-containing cells is achieved normally in four cell divisions from the first recognizable erythroid precursor, the pronormoblast (Figure 6.1), under the the stimulatory influence of erythropoietin. With the extrusion of the nucleus, the resulting immature erythrocyte is termed a reticulocyte, owing to the appearance of clumps of residual cytoplasmic RNA when stained. The reticulocyte persists for about 2 days after release into the circulation. An important factor limiting cell division is the attainment of an intracellular haemoglobin concentration (mean cell haemoglobin concentration, MCHC) of 33 per cent. The transient circulation of the reticulocyte and the

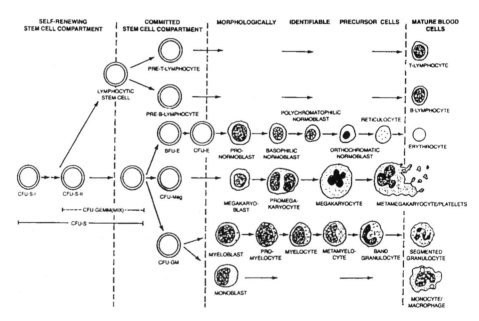

Figure 6.1 Differentiation and maturation of blood cells. CFU-S, CFU-E, CFU-Meg, CFU-GM, CFU-GEMM(MIX); colony-forming unit – spleen, erythroid, megakaryocyte, granulocyte–macrophage, granulocyte–erythroid–macrophage–megakaryocyte (mixed), respectively; BFU-E, burst-forming unit – erythroid. CFU-S-II are distinguished from CFU-S-I by their increased proliferative capacity and decreased capability for self-renewal. Note that monocytes and lymphocytes retain the ability to proliferate once they have left the circulation. Stem cells are depicted as open circles as they possess no distinctive morphological features. Reproduced, with permission, from [4].

attainment of a MCHC of 33 per cent are consistent features of all mammalian species, whereas erythrocyte volume (mean cell volume, MCV) and erythrocyte count vary considerably [5].

Leucocyte development

Granulocytes (neutrophils, eosinophils and basophils) and monocytes are derived from a common precursor, the granulocyte–macrophage colony-forming unit (CFU-GM) under the influence of the cytokine, granulocyte–macrophage colony stimulating factor (GM-CSF), and interleukin 3 (IL-3) and lineage-specific cytokines (Figure 6.1). At the final granulocyte stage capable of cell division, the myelocyte, secondary lineage-specific granules (neutrophilic, eosinophilic or basophilic) begin to appear. From the metamyelocyte stage onwards, the nucleus of the granulocyte indents and lobulation starts, producing the characteristic polymorphonuclear appearance. The number of nuclear lobes in circulating neutrophils (and other granulocytes) therefore reflects cell maturity.

Monocytes of all mammalian species have a kidney-shaped nucleus with lacy chromatin, palely basophilic 'ground glass' cytoplasm with frequent vacuolation and occasional azurophil granules.

Most mature lymphocytes are small cells with scanty, pale blue cytoplasm, but in a variable proportion there is more abundant cytoplasm, and the overall size approaches that of granulocytes and monocytes. Lymphocytes are derived from divergent lineages, and have quite separate functions. It is not possible using routine staining to distinguish the subtypes, this can only be achieved by cytochemical or immunocytochemical staining. The lymphocyte is the predominant leucocyte type in the peripheral blood of the rat and mouse, whereas in dogs and primates, neutrophils often exceed lymphocytes, as is normally seen in man.

Platelet formation

The mature megakaryocyte is a polyploid cell (up to 64 n in the rat) with cytoplasm that becomes increasingly granular with maturity. The mechanism by which platelets (which are aggregates of megakaryocyte granular cytoplasm) are released from their parent cell is unclear, but appears to be by fragmentation of the cytoplasm. This process may take place in an extramedullary location, possibly the lung. The cytokine, thrombopoietin, stimulates megakaryocyte proliferation, platelet production, and differentiation from the common stem cell, the CFU-GEMM (MIX) (Figure 6.1). As with erythrocytes, the lifespan of platelets varies from species to species: in man it is 10 days, in the dog 8 days, in the rat 4.5 days and in the mouse 4 days. Similarly, mean platelet volume is lower (and platelet count greater) in rodents than in man; in dogs and cats platelet volume is higher than in man.

6.2.2 *Histology*

Blood and bone marrow smears (Figures 6.2, 6.3 and 6.4) are usually stained with a Romanowsky stain (e.g. May–Grünwald, Giemsa, Wright, Leishman, etc.) which stain basic components orange-red (eosinophilia) and acidic components blue (basophilia). Nuclei appear purple, cytoplasm varying shades of blue, and

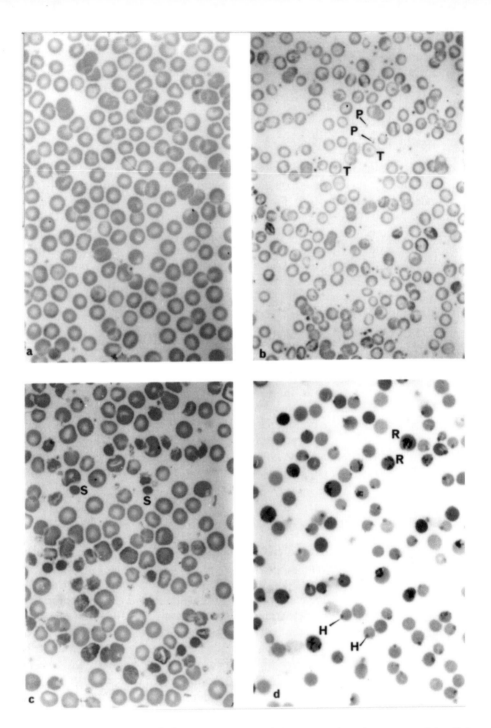

Figure 6.2 Erythrocyte morphology. (a) Rat: normal (i.e. normochromic, normocytic) cells in an untreated animal (May–Grünwald–Giemsa). (b) Rat: hypochromia and microcytosis following gastrointestinal bleeding with resultant iron deficiency. Target cells (T) and increased platelet (P) numbers (thrombocytosis) are present (May–Grünwald–Giemsa). (c) Rat: spherocytosis (S) and polychromasia resulting from oxidant haemolysis following the administration of the azo dye red 2G (May–Grünwald–Giemsa). (d) Marmoset: reticulocytes (R) and Heinz bodies (H) in an animal with wasting marmoset syndrome (new methylene blue). Reproduced, with permission, from [6].

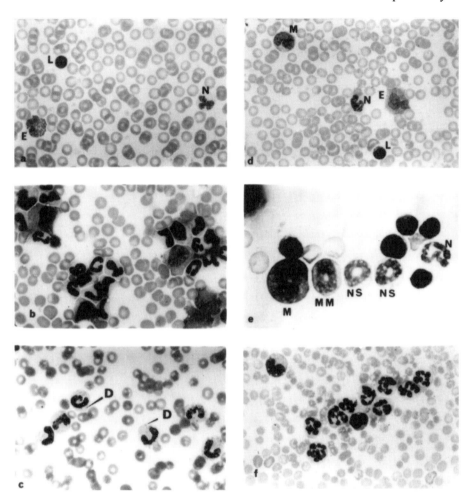

Figure 6.3 Leucocyte morphology. (a) Dog, peripheral blood: normal eosinophil (E), lymphocyte (L) and neutrophil (N). Variations in neutrophil granulation are peculiar to some species. In the dog, secondary granulation is very pale, reflecting the absence of stainable alkaline phosphatase (May–Grünwald–Giemsa). (b) Dog, bone marrow: normal neutrophil maturation; recovery from agranulocytosis following the administration of the oestrogen ethinyl estradiol (May–Grünwald–Giemsa). (c) Dog, peripheral blood: left shifted neutrophils containing Döhle bodies (D) in a chronic infection (May–Grünwald–Giemsa). (d) Rat, peripheral blood: normal monocyte (M), neutrophil (N), eosinophil (E) and lymphocyte (L). In rodent species, metamyelocytes are 'doughnut' shaped, and the resultant neutrophil possesses nuclear lobes linked in a ring (May–Grünwald–Giemsa). (e) Rat, bone marrow: normal neutrophil maturation. Here, the sequence of five cells illustrates the progression from myelocyte (M) to mature neutrophil (N). MM, metamyelocyte; NS, non-segmented neutrophil ('stab cell') (May–Grünwald–Giemsa). (f) Rat, peripheral blood: neutrophilia with right shift (nuclear hypersegmentation); inflammation of the eye (May–Grünwald–Giemsa). Reproduced with permission from [6].

cytoplasmic granules are differentiated according to lineage. Marrow sections (Figure 6.4) may for convenience be stained with haematoxylin and eosin (H and E). Whilst the examination of a smear preparation is necessary for either the recognition of individual stages of maturation or the performance of a myelogram or myeloid–erythroid ratio (see Section 6.5.3), the cellularity of the marrow can only accurately

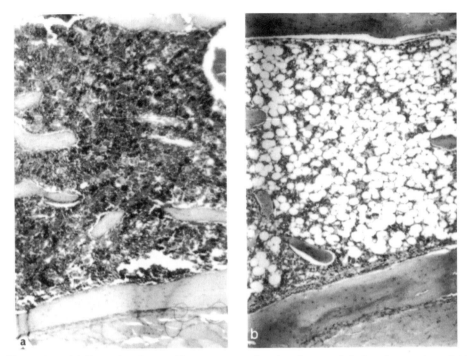

Figure 6.4 (a) Control rat femoral bone marrow showing dense cellularity of normal myeloid and erythroid haematopoiesis. (b) Marrow hypoplasia induced by the administration of azathioprine; hypocellularity and many large fat spaces are evident. Reproduced with permission from [6].

be assessed from a marrow section. In addition to cytochemical methods (see Section 6.5.3) it is possible to establish the lineage and maturity of blood cells by identifying antigens expressed on the cell membrane using antibody–enzyme complexes and the staining of cells in smears or sections *in situ*. Alternatively, cell suspensions may be characterized by flow cytometry

6.2.3 *Physiology*

Erythrocyte biology

Erythrocyte function The function of the red blood cell (RBC) is to transport oxygen to the tissues. The principal promoter of red cell production is erythropoietin, which is secreted in response to variation in circulating oxygen tension by renal cortical interstitial cells. The net effect of decreased haemoglobin concentration, where the bone marrow is functional, is therefore: (i) lowered tissue oxygen delivery, (ii) increased erythropoietin secretion from the kidney and (iii) stimulation of erythrocyte production, which is seen as reticulocytosis (Figure 6.2d). Conversely, in situations where plasma volume is decreased, typically following dehydration or lowered water intake (a possible concomitant of decreased food consumption in rodents), haemoconcentration occurs. This causes erythropoietin levels and reticulocyte counts to fall.

Haem synthesis Haem synthesis is effected via a pathway starting with the condensation of succinyl CoA and glycine into δ-aminolevulinic acid, the generation of a succession of porphyrin rings and the eventual incorporation of a single atom of iron. The final step is effected in the mitochondria of the intermediate (polychromatophilic) normoblasts of the bone marrow under the influence of the enzyme ferrochelatase.

Iron Iron is first absorbed by the gut from dietary sources and transported as a complex with transferrin to the marrow, from where it is transferred to erythroid precursors by endocytosis. Iron stores may be assessed by staining marrow with Perls' Prussian blue method or by measurement of plasma ferritin.

Folic acid and vitamin B_{12} Vitamin B_{12} and folic acid are required in the synthesis of nucleic acids and their deficiency (dietary, malabsorption, lack of binding proteins, increased utilization in neoplasia) is soon reflected in abnormal haematopoiesis (megaloblastosis), and peripheral cytopenias.

Energy requirements Energy is required by the erythrocyte (although not for oxygen take-up or delivery) especially in the maintenance of a reduction potential to prevent the oxidation of haemoglobin. In the mature red cell, the glycolytic pathway and the pentose-phosphate shunt are the only sources of high-energy phosphate and reduced glutathione. Energy is also needed to maintain the biconcave shape of the erythrocyte membrane.

Red cell lifespan After the extrusion and loss of the nucleus, the lifespan of the erythocyte is limited, in man, to 120 days. In most other mammalian species, red cell lifespan is shorter: in the dog, 110 days; in the rat, 60 days; and in the mouse, 40 days. It is possible to predict red cell lifespan in different species from adult body weight using the following approximation [7]:

$$\bar{\tau} = 68.9 M^{0.132}$$

where $\bar{\tau}$ = mean RBC lifespan (days); M = body weight (kg)

To maintain circulating red cell numbers, marrow turnover must reflect the rate of removal of cells from the circulation. Consequently, the number of immature erythrocytes (reticulocytes) is inversely proportional to red cell lifespan.

Erythrocyte senescence and haemoglobin breakdown Senescent red cells are removed from the circulation by macrophages of the reticuloendothelial system, in the spleen, liver and marrow. Haemoglobin is catabolized to globin, the amino acids of which re-enter the protein synthesis pool. Haem is degraded via biliverdin to urobilinogen and bilirubin and excreted in the urine and bile, respectively.

Leucocyte biology

Neutrophils The functions of neutrophil granulocytes are twofold. They are a major component of the inflammatory response and they also have an important role in bacterial killing. With an increased demand for neutrophils in either function, marrow production is upregulated by growth factors. Unlike erythropoiesis, where the demand for red cell upregulation is detected by tissue hypoxia, the sensor for granulopoiesis is unknown. Circulating neutrophils have a half-life of only a few hours (man, 6.5 h; dog, 5.5 h) and their numbers are balanced by a 'marginating' pool of mature cells which are loosely bound to capillary endothelial cells. Physiological factors which cause demargination of neutrophils, and a resulting neutrophilia, include exercise and stress. This response is transient and reversible but a sustained neutrophilia, mediated by corticosteroids, is seen with the chronic action of these stimuli.

Chronic myeloid leukaemia (i.e. a leukaemia involving granulocytes) is rare in rodents, reflecting the relative predominance of lymphoid cells in these species. However, some rat strains do show a low spontaneous incidence of this leukaemia.

Eosinophils Eosinophils are involved in allergic responses and are found particularly in the lung and gut. Approximately 1 per cent are found in the circulation; the half-life in man is similar to the neutrophil (6.5 h), but in the dog, eosinophils only circulate for approximately 30 min.

Basophils Basophils contain large quantities of histamine. They are also involved in the allergic response and are related to tissue mast cells. Large numbers of mast cells are sometimes seen in rat bone marrow. Increased circulating numbers of basophils are seen in association with allergy or inflammation.

Monocytes Monocytes are amoeboid phagocytes, ultimately bound for sites such as the liver, spleen, alveoli, and peritoneum. In these tissues they become fixed macrophages and may subsequently proliferate. As fixed macrophages they perform a diverse range of functions, principally scavenging (e.g. removal of senescent erythrocytes), but in combination with lymphocytes they are involved in antigenic recognition. They are sensitive to, and also secrete, a range of cytokines, as well as modulating the inflammatory response and secreting lysozyme.

Lymphocytes Lymphocytes, although appearing relatively homogeneous in their morphology, belong to one of two lineages: B and T lymphocytes. Both are derived from a common precursor, and mature in bone marrow and thymus respectively. The function of B cells is primarily that of antibody production and the final stage of B-cell development is the marrow plasma cell. In addition to this morphologically distinct cell type, circulating B lymphocytes may be in a resting state as memory cells. Memory cells may circulate for many years, and may express activation markers on their membranes as a result of stimulation and interaction with T-helper cells and monocytes.

T lymphocytes may be recognized by their differential expression of surface antigens and are sudivided into helper/effector and suppressor/cytotoxic lineages. Characteristic cell surface antigens are classified in groupings with the same specificity, 'clusters of differentiation'. These are assigned CD numbers. All T lymphocytes express CD3, whilst CD4 and CD8 expression denote T-helper/effector and T-suppressor/cytotoxic subtypes, respectively. In addition to the activation of B lymphocytes, and the modification of cytotoxic responses, T lymphocytes secrete cytokines, most importantly the interleukins, IL-1 and IL-6. These have wide-ranging stimulatory effects, for example, on primitive haematopoietic cells, B lymphocyte proliferation and differentiation, and the production of acute phase proteins from hepatocytes.

Platelet biology

Platelet function The primary role of the platelet is front-line defence in haemostasis. Initially, in haemostasis, platelets adhere to the endothelium of damaged blood vessels.

Then, as the platelet undergoes a shape change, a series of granule-bound proteins are secreted, promoting the aggregation of more platelets to those already adhering, and stimulating the coagulation pathway. Platelets are intimately involved in many subsequent steps of the haemostatic mechanism. They provide a surface for the assembly of several enzyme complexes that form during the coagulation sequence, they provide up to 20 per cent of coagulation factor V, they participate in the activation of Factor X and the activation of the surface contact phase of coagulation, and they also promote the retraction of the fibrin clot. Adhesion takes place between the platelet membrane and subendothelial components such as collagen and fibronectin, under the influence of von Willebrand factor and membrane glycoprotein receptors. Collagen, as well as inducing platelet adhesion, also stimulates platelet aggregation. ADP and thromboxane A_2 are secreted by adherent platelets. ADP is also released from damaged tissue and erythrocytes, and ADP therefore may be involved in the initiation of platelet involvement in haemostasis. Fibrinogen, as well as taking part in the coagulation cascade, is also involved as a cofactor in platelet aggregation.

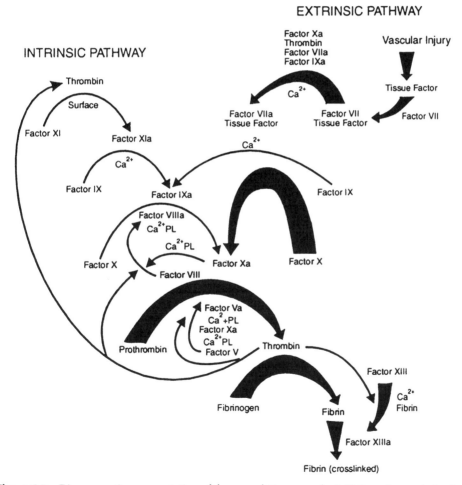

Figure 6.5 Diagrammatic representation of the coagulation cascade. Initiation of coagulation by tissue factor activation via the extrinsic pathway is shown in heavy arrows. Activated coagulation factors are denoted by 'a'; PL refers to phospholipid. Reproduced with permission from [8].

Haemostasis

The coagulation cascade   Haemostasis is achieved by a delicate balance of the continual activation of coagulation and the removal of the end product, the fibrin clot (fibrinolysis). In the principal (extrinsic) pathway of coagulation (Figure 6.5), the initiating stimulus is the release into the blood of tissue factor from damaged tissue. There then follows a series of steps culminating in the production of stable fibrin polymer. Coagulation is also initiated by the contact of coagulation factors with the exposed surface of endothelial cells, and the stimulation of this intrinsic pathway is promoted by the generation of thrombin. In many of the steps of the coagulation 'cascade', calcium is a requirement. Phospholipid is also required and is supplied by platelets.

Synthesis of coagulation factors   The majority of coagulation factors are produced by the liver, but non-hepatic endothelial cells, monocytes and megakaryocytes are also responsible. Some factors (II, VII, IX and X) are derived from vitamin K, which is synthesized by gut bacteria. Fibrinogen is generated by the liver in large quantities (roughly 2 g/l of plasma, with a half-life of about 3 days).

Fibrinolysis   Breakdown of the fibrin clot (fibrinolysis) is achieved by activating plasminogen to plasmin, which in turn degrades fibrin. Activators of plasminogen include streptokinase, urokinase and tissue plasminogen activator, all of which have been isolated and synthesized for therapy in the aftermath of thrombosis.

6.3   Biochemical and Cellular Mechanisms of Toxicity

6.3.1   *Metabolism*

It is important to consider whether toxicity of any kind is caused by a parent compound or its metabolites. Many *in vitro* systems may only reflect direct toxicity, such as the inactivation of coagulation factors, direct lysis of erythrocytes, or the inhibition of growth in haematopoietic culture systems. In such cases, results may only be extrapolated to the *in vivo* situation where the compound under test is not modified by host metabolic processes. Thus, although the myelosuppressive activity of **chloramphenicol** is usually ascribed to the parent compound, the nitroso form shows a far greater inhibitory effect in mouse haematopoietic culture assays, and there is considerable variation in the susceptibility of cells from different mouse strains. In man, **nitrosochloramphenicol** has not been identified as a metabolite of chloramphenicol, further hampering any extrapolation from *in vitro* toxicity studies to the therapeutic situation. **2-butoxyethanol**, a cleaning agent, is inactive in the *in vitro* haemolysis screen in rats, whilst oral administration in this species produces a haemolytic anaemia. The major metabolite of **2-butoxyethanol, butoxyacetic acid**, however, produces marked swelling and lysis of erythrocytes *in vitro*. Furthermore, as with **chloramphenicol**, there is considerable variation in the susceptibility of red cells from different species to this lytic effect. Much of the metabolism of **1,2-diethyl-3-hydroxypyridin-4-one (CP94),** a synthetic iron chelator, is via the the glucuronic acid pathway in the guinea pig. As such it shows little systemic toxicity, but also clears no iron from the liver. In contrast, only 14 per cent of **CP94** is glucuronated by the rat. However, in this species, **CP94** is an efficient chelator, but at the expense of considerable toxicity, causing myelosuppression.

6.3.2 Myelosuppression

The downregulation of marrow haematopoiesis is an extremely important aspect of toxicity, as was mentioned in Section 6.1. Any or all of the cell types produced in bone marrow may be affected, that is, granulocytopenia, thrombocytopenia or anaemia may occur. These effects are frequently encountered during acute toxicity studies, while dose ranging studies are being carried out, and the changes are usually dose-related and reversible on withdrawal of the test compound. Frequently, the initial treatment of a repeat-dose regimen will cause temporary myelosuppression. This may only be detectable by a residual effect at the first scheduled bleed (say, 2 weeks later), when depressed cell counts are seen. When subsequent samples are taken, resolution of the effect may be complete. Alternatively, evidence of a 'rebound' effect may be present [9] (see Section 6.3.3). The mechanisms involved in such dose-dependent myelosuppressive effects are predictable and relate to inhibitory effects on primitive cells in the marrow, such as BFU-E and CFU-GM (Figure 6.1). The inhibition of these primitive cells would be manifested as erythroid hypoplasia and granulocytopenia, respectively, and may be due to direct cytotoxicity, inhibition, or blocking of specific growth factors, or a result of interference with some fundamental process such as DNA replication. For example, erythropoietin production has been reported to be suppressed by **oestrogens**. Other known bone marrow depressants, whose action is dose-dependent and reversible, include **aminopterin**, a folic acid antagonist, and **benzene**.

More seriously, a very small number of susceptible individuals may unexpectedly succumb to *irreversible* myelosuppression in a *dose-independent* manner, perhaps after a course of therapy has been discontinued. In these cases, it is postulated that the effects are at the primitive cell level, and some kind of genotoxic damage has been inflicted on an already sensitized cell line. A wide range of compounds in a variety of classes have been implicated in inducing these effects and drugs often associated with marrow hypoplasia include **chloramphenicol, phenytoin** (an anticonvulsant) and **gold compounds** (used in the therapy of rheumatoid arthritis). A similar series of events has been proposed for the induction of leukaemia, but instead of the cell line possessing a reduced ability to proliferate, a leukaemic clone, endowed with a growth advantage, evolves. It would appear, therefore, that bone marrow aplasia and leukaemia may belong to a spectrum of evolutionary events. Myelodysplastic syndrome (MDS) in man is a clonal and potentially preleukaemic syndrome, with leukaemia supervening on a long-standing refractory anaemia. Chromosome damage is frequently apparent in MDS, and an aplastic presentation is commonly seen.

6.3.3 Hyperplasia of Haematopoietic Elements

Neutrophilia

A raised neutrophil count (neutrophilia) is seen in cases of bacterial infection and a wide range of inflammatory conditions. In addition, a variety of chemicals such as

lead, mercury, phenacetin and **pyridine** may induce neutrophilia as a result of tissue damage or hypersensitivity. Also, neutrophilia is often seen in laboratory animals as a secondary event in neoplastic conditions or following haemorrhage. **Corticosteroids**, the physiological mediators of neutrophilia, when administered therapeutically, exert their effects by delaying the release of cells from the blood into the tissues. Neutrophil half-life is thereby increased.

Eosinophilia

Eosinophilia is seen in dermatitis, occasionally in allergic reactions to drugs such as **salicylates**, and especially in parasitic infections. This last situation may be seen in toxicological studies, when wild-caught primates are used. Increased eosinophil numbers may be seen in the wall of the rat gut and peripheral blood following the use of dietary expanders such as **modified starches** and **sugars** (e.g. **sorbitol, mannitol, lactose, polyethylene glycol**).

Basophilia

Increased circulating numbers of basophils are seen in association with allergies or inflammation but also in some endocrine disorders, iron deficiency, and in chronic myeloid leukaemia. Basophil or mast cell leukaemia is a rare disorder sometimes seen in rodents and other laboratory species.

Monocytosis

Monocytosis is commonly seen together with neutrophilia in laboratory species; it is sometimes seen acutely after trauma (e.g. accidental lung-dosing of rodents by gavage needle) where the increase in cell number may be quite marked and characterized by the presence of early monocyte forms. Monocytosis has been described resulting from the administration of the antipsychotic drug **chlorpromazine**. Pure monocytic leukaemia does not occur in laboratory animals, although a proportion of rodent chronic myeloid leukaemias show partial monocytic differentiation. However, the histiocytic variant of lymphoma is commonly seen in both rats and mice. In such cases, proliferation of lymphoid and monocytic cell types coexists.

Lymphocytosis

Increased lymphocyte numbers may be seen in viral infections. Occasional circulating plasma cells may also be seen in viral disease; increased numbers may be present peripherally following immunization or in myeloma. Large numbers of plasma cells are sometimes seen in marrow smears of mice with myeloid hyperplasia.

Reticulocytosis

All haematopoiesis is suppressed by single large doses of some cytotoxic drugs (e.g. antineoplastic agents such as **busulphan** or **cyclophosphamide**), but following a short period of hypoplasia, marrow activity is generally spontaneously restored, often resulting in a hyperplastic rebound or 'overshoot'. Thus, reticulocyte counts may be increased above the normal range for a time. Similarly, leucocyte 'overshoot'

8 days after cyclophosphamide administration is utilized in the harvesting of peripheral blood stem cells for transplantation. Erythroid hyperplasia of the bone marrow (and spleen, in rodents) is the expected concomitant of increased erythrocyte loss (i.e. haemorrhage) or destruction (i.e. haemolysis).

Increased numbers of erythrocytes are seen in peripheral blood following decreased food intake and in haemoconcentration due to fluid loss (e.g. in diarrhoea or vomiting). The increased erythrocyte counts in these situations may therefore only reflect the change in overall blood volume, rather than alterations in the production or fate of cells.

Thrombocytosis

Hyperplasia of platelets may be seen following a variety of events. For example, after acute blood loss, where the humoral mediator, thrombopoietin is involved, or following trauma, such as bone fracture or surgical procedures. The cytotoxic drug **5-fluorouracil** causes an immediate fall and then a sustained increase in platelet numbers. Other compounds causing thrombocytosis are the drug **azidothymidine (AZT)** and **butylated hydroxytoluene (BHT)**, a food additive. The mechanisms involved in drug-related thrombocytosis are unclear, although cytokines including stem cell factor and interleukin 6 (IL-6) have been implicated. Thrombocytosis is often synchronous with reticulocytosis, supporting the hypothesis that erythropoietin has a stimulatory effect on megakaryocytes.

All the above proliferative events are essentially adaptive, and reversion to a normal condition would be expected on, or a short time after, withdrawal of the stimulus. However, hyperplasia may warn of preneoplastic change, for example in MDS an excess of blast cells may be seen in the bone marrow. Similarly, *in vitro* colony formation of mouse myeloid precursors is actually stimulated at micromolar concentrations of **hydroquinone** (a benzene metabolite) and the cytotoxic agents **busulphan** and **cyclophosphamide** whereas at lower concentrations, colony formation is inhibited. It is of interest to note that these three compounds induce leukaemia in mice.

Myeloproliferative disorders in man (for example polycythaemia vera, principally a proliferation of the erythroid lineage) show a tendency to culminate in malignancy, usually myeloblastic leukaemia. These disorders have not been identified readily in laboratory animals, but it is still important to distinguish between benign hyperplasias and leukaemias. Morphological characteristics are of value in these cases, and it is generally true that hyperplasia gives rise to a range of mature cell types, whereas neo-plasia (leukaemia) is characterized by less mature forms. Where uncertainty remains, cytochemical, and membrane markers can be of use. For example, chronic myeloid leukaemia may be distinguised from myeloid hyperplasia by the lower levels of intra-cellular alkaline phosphatase in the leukaemic condition. Also, positivity for the antigens TdT and Ki-67 indicates 'high-grade' malignancy in lymphoproliferative conditions.

6.3.4 Leukaemogenesis

The development of leukaemia, in that it is not a highly predictable, dose-related phenomenon in man, would appear to require at least two events that cause genetic damage to haematopoietic precursor cells. Aetiological stimuli in leukaemogenesis include viruses (such as feline leukaemia virus and Friend murine leukaemia virus) and possibly other infectious agents which may account for the clustering of human leukaemias; radiation (notably in man, following the atomic explosions in Japan), and exposure to chemical clastogens (e.g. **benzene** or its metabolites). A primary insult by any of these agents results in genetic damage, which will be met by cellular DNA repair mechanisms. In many cases, the damage is reversible. For example, the folic acid antagonist **methotrexate** causes transient *in vitro* DNA damage, whereas therapeutic use of the drug is not associated with the development of malignancy. A secondary insult may overcome natural DNA repair capability resulting in permanent chromosome damage and disinhibition of the proliferation of an abnormal clone. Chromosomal abnormalities are detectable in over two-thirds of human leukaemias; several types of abnormality have been associated with specific leukaemia subgroups and provide important prognostic information.

Leukaemia in man and animals is divided into two types, acute and chronic, according to the rapidity of its progress. Acute and chronic forms are closely mirrored by the types of cell which predominate and this allows the classification into myeloid and lymphoid forms. In acute leukaemia, a homogeneous picture of primitive and blast-like types are encountered in the blood and marrow, whereas in chronic leukaemia, more mature cells from a wider spectrum of developmental stages are seen. Myeloid leukaemia may be induced in rats with very small quantities of **dimethylbenzanthracene (DMBA)** or with **ionizing radiation** and its morphological characteristics have been described as resembling the acute form of the disease, which is not seen spontaneously in the rat. The chronic form may be seen (rarely) in some rat strains, but not in mice. Again, the leukaemia type induced in mice by the carcinogen **1,3-butadiene** is thymic lymphoma, the spontaneous incidence of which is negligible. Similarly, mice given **DMBA** develop lymphoid lymphomas/leukaemias, and not myeloid leukaemia, whereas rats given the organophosphate **dimethyl morpholinophosphoramidate** develop lymphoid leukaemia, but mice are not susceptible.

6.3.5 *Inhibition of Haem Synthesis*

Metals with an inhibitory effect on enzymes of this pathway include **mercury** and **aluminium**. As with iron deficiency, the net result is a reduced rate of haemoglobin synthesis. Erythrocyte maturation requires adequate levels of haemoglobin before cell division ceases. Additional divisions of erythrocyte precursors result in smaller mature cells (i.e. MCV is decreased); if the level of haemoglobin synthesis is still inadequate, the resultant cells will also have lower MCHC values. A slight reduction in MCV is not infrequently encountered in toxicity studies when there is a also a drop in the haemoglobin level, suggesting that many compounds may possess the ability to inhibit haem synthesis as well as affect the maturation of early erythroid cells. In these cases, the erythrocyte count is not always depressed to the same degree as haemoglobin and haematocrit values, and indeed the RBC count may even show a slight increase, reflecting the extra marrow division.

Failure to incorporate iron into haem results in sideroblastic anaemia, with the presence of iron-containing granules in erythrocytes. This condition is seen with **lead** toxicity, where inhibition of several of the enzymes of the haem synthesis pathway occurs. Sideroblastic anaemia may also develop as a secondary condition following treatment with the antituberculous drug **isoniazid**, or with **chloramphenicol**. With excessive **alcohol** intake, sideroblastic anaemia results from altered pyridoxine metabolism.

6.3.6 *Interference with B$_{12}$ and Folate Metabolism*

Malabsorption is a common cause of interference with folate metabolism. However, certain agents cause a similar effect with the resulting development of megaloblastic erythrocytes. Such agents include **alcohol**, dihydrofolate reductase inhibitors such as **methotrexate**, and antimetabolites such as the pyrimidine analogue **AZT**, the last drug also causing myelosuppression. Anticonvulsants (e.g. **phenytoin**) and the anaesthetic gas **nitrous oxide** also cause megaloblastosis.

6.3.7 *Immune-mediated Cytopenias*

Blood cells may be depleted as a result of immune activation. Such autoimmune states can cause haemolytic anaemia, selective granulocytopenia or thrombo-cytopenia. In some granulocytopenias and thrombocytopenias, it is sometimes possible to detect antibodies with specificity for therapeutic agents (e.g. **phenyl-butazone**), in others (e.g. **β-lactam antibiotic**-induced granulocytopenia), drug–hapten complexes may form on the membrane of the cells. In immune red cell destruction (autoimmune haemolytic anaemia), antibodies to drugs (e.g. **α-methyldopa**) may coincidentally possess the same specificity as red cell membrane proteins. In the case of immune complex formation, complement may be bound to the erythrocyte, leading to intravascular destruction of the cell. Alternatively, the biconcave shape of the erythrocyte may be lost, and it becomes spherical (spherocyte formation, Figure 6.2c). Again, as occurs with **penicillin**, the drug may bind to the erythrocyte membrane, and drug–antibody complexes may subsequently form. In these examples involving the erythrocyte, antibody can be demonstrated on the cells by the direct antiglobulin (or direct Coombs') test. **Cephalosporins** may also give a positive Coombs' test. Usually **cephalosporins** cause configurational changes to the erythrocyte membrane components and non-specific binding of plasma proteins (including immunoglobulins) occurs, resulting in an artefactual false-positive Coombs' reaction. In such cases, erythrocyte survival is generally unaffected, but haptenic or immune-complex haemolytic anaemia may sometimes be seen following cephalosporin therapy.

    Corticosteroids cause immunosuppression, with an associated lymphocytopenia and eosinopenia; similar effects may be seen in stressed animals.

6.3.8 *Oxidative Haemolysis*

Inhibition of erythrocyte enzymes, particularly those of the pentose-phosphate pathway, may cause haemolysis. Haemoglobin may be oxidized to methaemoglobin in the presence of oxidant compounds, to which the red cell is unduly sensitive. Denatured globin chains may then form intracellular inclusions (Heinz bodies,

Figure 6.2d), which attach to the inner leaflet of the cell membrane. Many oxidant compounds (e.g. **aniline**, and **azo compounds**), when given at sufficient levels either *in vivo* or *in vitro* will overcome the reducing potential of the erythrocyte. In human patients with glucose-6-phosphate dehydrogenase deficiency, the abnormal sensitivity to the oxidant properties of, for example, **primaquine** or the **pollen of the bean *Vicia fava***, may cause haemolytic crises which are life threatening.

6.3.9 Coagulation

Coumarin-like compounds such as **warfarin** inhibit the γ-carboxylation of coagulation factors II, VII, IX and X and thus prolong clotting times. **Cephalosporins** are also responsible for the prolongation of clotting times due to a similar mode of action. Other antibiotics which cause the eradication of gut flora, and thereby lower levels of available vitamin K, produce a similar effect and prolong clotting. Any toxic compound causing liver damage (e.g. **paracetamol**) will also lower the output and concentration of coagulation factors.

Pregnancy and **oral contraceptives** cause an increase in the concentration of a number of coagulation factors with a corresponding shortening of coagulation times (prothrombin time and activated partial thromboplastin time, see Section 6.5.4). Fibrinogen is an acute phase reactant, and levels increase many fold during inflammation. Fibrinogen measurement is therefore a useful screen for inflammatory changes.

6.3.10 Platelet Function

When platelet numbers or function are drastically reduced, bleeding will take place even with an otherwise intact coagulation system. Platelet aggregation in response to a number of stimuli (e.g. thrombin, ADP, collagen or adrenaline) is increased in **tobacco** smokers and oral **contraceptives** cause an increase in ADP-induced platelet aggregation. However, many compounds cause a decrease in platelet aggregability, especially in response to ADP. Such compounds include **ethanol**, **penicillin** and **phenylbutazone**. In normal platelet metabolism, thromboxane A_2 is generated from prostaglandin H_2, which in turn is derived from arachidonic acid. These synthetic steps may be blocked by the inhibition of either thromboxane synthase (e.g. by **dazoxiben**) or cyclo-oxygenase (e.g. by **aspirin**). This type of blocking activity forms the basic action of several antiplatelet compounds used therapeutically in the control of thrombosis. Other experimental compounds have been developed specifically to block platelet binding sites, for instance, to inhibit the binding of fibrinogen.

6.4 Morphological Responses to Injury

6.4.1 Bone Marrow Hypoplasia

In hypoplastic conditions where a single cell line is involved, the bone marrow smear will show a lack of the affected cell type. However occasionally 'maturation arrest' may be seen, where a specific lineage is represented, but only as far as a particular developmental stage. Alternatively, there may be no specific morphological features associated with a hypoplasia. In severe cases of hypoplasia no recognizable cells from myeloid (granulocytic) or erythroid lineages will be identified, but only lymphocytes, plasma cells and reticuloendothelial macrophages will be evident. In marrow hypoplasia, myeloid–erythroid ratios should be interpreted with caution, and only taken into account with all other available haematological findings (see Section 6.5.3). The histological marrow section is particularly useful in confiming hypoplasia or aplasia since spatial relationships are preserved in these sections, and overall cellularity can be assessed (Figure 6.4).

6.4.2 *Erythrocyte Abnormalities*

At present, microscopic examination of the stained blood film is still the definitive screen for cellular abnormality. However, automated blood analysers are now capable of performing many measurements which may give an indication of morphological change, for example, red cell (volume) distribution width, RDW. Nevertheless, microscopy can uncover specific morphological abnormalities which point to underlying pathological mechanisms. RDW is a measure of *anisocytosis* (variability of cell size) which may be due to a mixture of normal-sized erythrocytes (normocytes) (Figure 6.2a), small cells (microcytes) (Figure 6.2b) or large cells (macrocytes). Variation in shape from the discoid norm is termed *poikilocytosis*, which may not be detectable by automated analysis. Within these broad desciptions of abnormality, specific morphological changes are listed below.

Microcytosis

Microcytes are small erythrocytes, i.e. cells with a low MCV. Microcyte formation (Figure 6.2b) is associated with the inhibition of haem and/or globin synthesis, and it may also be seen in the presence of sphered or fragmented cells. It should be noted that reticulocytes are larger than mature erythrocytes and therefore a lowered MCV in a group of treated animals may indicate reticulocytopenia rather than microcytosis.

Hypochromia

The erythrocytes of all mammals when fully loaded with haemoglobin appear to possess a pale central region, roughly one-third of the total cell area. When this proportion is exceeded, cells are judged to be hypochromic (Figure 6.2b). The response is associated with an inhibition of haem or globin synthesis. Affected cells have low MCHC. The single most common cause of depleted iron stores in laboratory animals, where dietary deficiency is unlikely, is chronic haemorrhage and this will be manifested with the production of microcytic, hypochromic erythrocytes. Hypochromia may be seen in **lead**-induced sideroblastic anaemia.

Polychromasia

This term indicates the differential staining of reticulocytes and red cells. Reticulocytes have a slightly blue-grey appearance due to residual RNA with Romanowsky stains and they possess a characteristic reticular (net-like) pattern with supravital stains (Figure 6.2d). Increased polychromasia is seen in regenerative anaemias, i.e. where a reticulocytosis is present.

Macrocytosis

Macrocytes are large erythrocytes. Polychromatic cells (reticulocytes) are also larger than mature red cells (Figure 6.2c). However, increased size of mature erythrocytes (macrocytosis) is often the first indicator of megaloblastic change and in this case the cells will have a raised MCV. In megaloblastosis, the blood film may show neutrophils with hypersegmented nuclei (Figure 6.3f), and the bone marrow may also show a range of developmental changes, for example, very large erythroid precursors with relatively immature nuclear development, and giant metamyelocytes. Megaloblastosis may be caused by anticonvulsants, e.g. **phenytoin**, or by antimetabolites such as **methotrexate**, or **nitrous oxide**. Macrocytosis may also be seen following therapy with cytotoxic drugs such as **cyclophosphamide**, and in liver disease, or with excessive **alcohol** intake.

Spherocytosis

In spherocytes (Figure 6.2c), the area of central pallor of the erythrocyte is lost and the cells often appear to take on a coppery hue. Spherocytes are often seen in cases of immune haemolytic anaemia, for example due to **penicillin, cephalosporins**, or *α*-**methyldopa**. The MCHC is raised in spherocytosis.

Heinz bodies

These erythrocyte inclusions (see Section 6.3.8) do not take up Romanowsky stains, but may be apparent as pale bulges at the periphery of the red cell. However, with supravital stains such as new methylene blue and brilliant cresyl blue, the inclusions appear turquoise (Figure 6.2d). Heinz body formation may be seen in conditions of oxidative haemolysis due to **pyridine, aniline, phenylhydrazine** or with other **azo compounds.** Heinz bodies are removed from the erythrocytes in the spleen, and in this situation a specific type of poikilocyte, sometimes called a 'bite' cell, may be seen in the peripheral blood. Free (i.e. extraerythrocytic) Heinz bodies may be seen in blood films of rodents in cases of oxidative haemolysis. Heinz body anaemia may be encountered in marmosets, often in association with 'wasting marmoset syndrome'. The primary defect in the marmoset erythrocyte may, however, lie in the lipid composition of the cell membrane, rather than enzyme (e.g. glucose-6-phosphate) deficiency.

Howell–Jolly bodies

These are nuclear remnants and are the micronuclei of the eponymous test for mutagenicity. Howell–Jolly bodies are seen in increased numbers in certain dyserythropoietic anaemias, and in splenic dysfunction. They are a normal feature of the blood of mice and marmosets.

Basophilic stippling

In conditions inducing reticulocytosis, basophilic stippling may be seen in mature erythrocytes and is due to the presence of aggregates of rough endoplasmic reticulum. This condition may also be seen in the erythrocyte in *β*-thalassaemia and here it is due to free globin α-chains. In **lead** poisoning, inhibition of pyrimidine 5'-nucleotidase in the erythrocyte causes basophilic stippling due to the failure of RNA degradation.

Siderotic (iron-containing) granules (Pappenheimer bodies) in the erythrocyte give an appearance similar to basophilic stippling, but here there are usually small numbers of granules in a cluster near the edge of the cell. Siderotic granules may be seen after **isoniazid** therapy or in splenic malfunction.

Stomatocytes

Stomatocytes are seen where there is imbalance in circulating lipid levels, notably the cholesterol/lecithin ratio. Equilibration between the plasma and constituents of the erythrocyte membrane lipid leads to a shape change in the erythrocyte when the outer leaflet of the membrane becomes disproportionately large. This condition is seen with excessive **alcohol** intake and in the presence of cationic lipid soluble drugs such as **phenothiazines**.

Target cells

Lipid imbalances similar to those which cause stomatocyte formation may also lead to the formation of target cells (Figure 6.2b). These are often seen in liver disease, and also where there is hypochromia due to iron deficiency.

Schistocytes

This term refers to cellular fragmentation which may be seen in disseminated intravascular coagulation or following mechanical haemolysis (e.g. after heart valve replacement, or extracorporeal circulation).

6.4.3 Leucocyte Abnormalities

Neutrophil maturity may be assessed by the development of nuclear lobes. Neutrophil immaturity is denoted by a shift from the normal nuclear lobe number (three to five in the dog and man) to the non-lobed metamyelocyte stage ('left shift'). In rodents, immaturity is characterized by the presence of 'doughnut'-shaped nuclei (Figure 6.3d). Immaturity of the neutrophil is seen where there is an increased demand for neutrophils (e.g. in inflammation or bacterial infection) which outstrips the production of cells in the marrow, and consequently immature cells are released prematurely into the circulation (Figure 6.3c).

Right shift

This neutrophil change (nuclear hypersegmentation) is often seen in conjunction with megaloblastic development (see Section 6.4.2.), but also in cases where the removal of mature neutrophils from the circulation is delayed, as in **corticosteroid** administration.

Granulation variation

Differences in the appearance of neutrophil granulation are helpful in establishing pathological mechanisms. In man, most primates and the rat, the secondary granules of neutrophils appear pink with Romanowsky stains. In the dog, this pink coloration of the granules is almost absent, making the assessment of hypogranulation almost impossible. Hypogranulation is also a feature of myeloid leukaemic change, and represents maturation arrest of the cytoplasm at the promyelocyte stage.

'Toxic' granulation

This form of neutrophil granulation is seen in acute infections. In man the granules may be punctate and purplish, representing a persistence of primary granules in neutrophils prematurely released from the bone marrow. However, in the dog and rat, the most prominent neutrophil alteration evident in acute infections is basophilia of the cytoplasm, rather than any change in the appearance of the granulation.

Döhle bodies

Döhle bodies (Figure 6.3c) are large bluish cytoplasmic inclusions in the neutrophil resulting from the aggregation of rough endoplasmic reticulum. They are seen in neutrophils in similar circumstances to 'toxic' granulation changes, but have also been reported following **cyclophosphamide** administration.

Lymphocytes

Slight variations may exist in lymphocyte morphology (Figure 6.3a and d). Larger types may be seen with more abundant cytoplasm and occasionally nucleoli are visible in these cells. In viral infections, many lymphocytes may show deep cytoplasmic basophilia and nuclear immaturity (i.e. the presence of nucleoli and a lack of nuclear condensation). These cells are referred to variously as 'atypical' or 'reactive' lymphocytes. Such lymphocytes are seen typically in man in large numbers in infectious mononucleosis, but a moderate proportion of lymphocytes may exhibit such features in young animals of other species, especially the dog.

Vacuolation of lymphocytes may be seen where phospholipidosis has been caused by amphiphilic compounds such as **chlorphentermine**. Electron microscopy of the bodies which correspond to the vacuoles reveals a multilamellar structure.

A few large lymphocytes in healthy animals may possess azurophil (red) granules. These so-called large granular lymphocytes are antigenically distinct from T and B cells, and possess natural killer activity. They are able to kill tumour cells without prior stimulation.

6.5 Testing for Toxicity

6.5.1 *Regulatory Requirements: the Full Blood Count*

The standard core of haematology measurements stipulated for clinical pathology investigations in toxicity studies is that required by the Food and Drug Administration's Red Book guidelines. This consists of an assessment of erythrocyte count, haemoglobin and haematocrit, total and differential leucocyte count, and some indication of 'clotting potential' [10]. If the minimum requirements are followed, erythrocyte indices (that is, MCV, MCH (mean cell haemoglobin), MCHC) need not be measured, which may lead to difficulties in the interpretation of an underlying pathology when changes do occur in the values of the 'standard core' measurements. However, most modern blood analysers are capable of generating erythrocyte indices as part of the full blood count, and are able to do this using the small volumes of blood available at rodent interim bleeds.

A similar range of tests is required by European Community regulations, for example in the Notification Scheme on New Substances, but again, 'clotting potential' may be interpreted here simply as a platelet count. However, the European Community regulations stipulate that in chronic and carcinogenicity studies, a differential leucocyte count may be performed in the absence of a total leucocyte count. Analysis of such leucocyte data (i.e. percentages only) may be extremely problematic [11] as there can be no way of knowing what the *overall* concentration (i.e. the absolute count) of any cell type is. Where a differential leucocyte count is performed on a blood film by eye, examination of erythrocyte morphology should also be performed. Some automated blood analysers are now able to measure and report such parameters as RDW or grade the degree of micro- and macrocytosis (see Section 6.4.2).

The performance of a platelet count is often taken to be sufficient for the assessment of 'clotting potential', although, as noted previously, counts need to be severely depressed before clinical bleeding takes place. Conversely, a normal platelet count does not necessarily imply normal haemostatic function. Only the guidelines of the Ministry of Health and Welfare (MOHW), and the Ministry of Agriculture, Forestries and Fisheries in Japan go further in specifying that a platelet count and/or specific coagulation tests are required.

As far as the assessment of reticulocyte numbers is concerned, it is only the Japanese MOHW guidelines that specify that reticulocyte analysis should be performed. Many laboratories at the present time prepare slides for retrospective reticulocyte analysis and these are only examined if it is subsequently found necessary to investigate the mechanism behind erythrocyte changes. Such 'manual' reticulocyte counting is time-consuming and notoriously imprecise. The use of techniques based on flow cytometry is currently allowing routine reticulocyte analysis to gain acceptance. This has lead to more closely defined background ranges for reticulocytes to be established. Moreover, it permits the more sensitive assessment of the up- or downregulation of erythropoiesis, simply by examining the routine blood sample. However, such techniques for reticulocytes have the disadvantage of requiring expensive equipment, and this makes the cost per test relatively high.

6.5.2 *Testing for Haemolysis*

Where haemoglobin breakdown exceeds background levels as a result of intravascular (or extravascular) haemolysis, it is possible to confirm that this is the cause of a lowered erythrocyte count. In intravascular haemolysis, free haemoglobin is released into the plasma and bound to haptoglobin. The complex is carried to the liver where the catabolism of haem takes place. Plasma haemoglobin will therefore be elevated during intravascular haemolysis, plasma haptoglobin will be depleted, and unconjugated plasma bilirubin will be raised.

Some catabolism of the haem molecule also takes place within renal tubular epithelial cells, with the deposition of ferritin and haemosiderin. When the tubular epithelial cells are sloughed off into the urine, the presence of intracellular iron may be demonstrated by Perls' Prussian blue method in chronic haemolytic conditions.

6.5.3 *Examination of the Bone Marrow Smear*

This is considered a definitive test where peripheral blood changes have occurred. However, to screen bone marrow effectively, it is necessary to perform a full myelogram (i.e. the classification of all identifiable cell types by lineage and stage of development), and comment fully on morphological abnormalities and cellular distribution. This is very time-consuming, so an often-adopted substitute is simply to perform a myeloid:erythroid (M:E) ratio and an assessment of cell morphology. The M:E ratio is the ratio of the number of myeloid (granulocytic) lineage cells to the number of erythroid lineage cells. The limitation of carrying out only a M:E ratio is that an increased value may be caused by either a myeloid hyperplasia or an erythroid hypoplasia (or vice-versa) and in addition, a simultaneous up- or downregulation of *both* lineages together will give normal values [12]. Another disadvantage is that the M:E ratio alone cannot give an accurate impression of cellularity. The most important information to come from the examination of the marrow smear is the morphological assessment of precursor cells. A peripheral blood reticulocyte count will indicate whether an anaemia is due to the suppression of erythropoiesis (a non-regenerative anaemia), or if destruction of red cells is compensated for by increased erythropoiesis (a regenerative anaemia). Examination of the histological marrow section is the standard screen for assessment of cellularity. However, where a quantification is needed, the contents of one of the long bones can be flushed into saline and a cell count performed. Checking a histological section of the spleen extramedullary erythropoiesis, whilst being subjective and rather insensitive due to the non-homogeneous distribution of erythroid cells in the spleen, is nevertheless an important method of providing additional information on blood changes in rodent pathology.

Cytochemical methods are of use in differentiating abnormal or immature cells (e.g. in leukaemia) in the marrow or peripheral blood, whereas features identified with Romanowsky staining do not allow further classification. In broad terms, 'myeloid' markers such as peroxidase, Sudan black B and chloroacetate esterase react strongly in granulocytes, weakly in monocytes and not at all in lymphocytes. T lymphocytes are identifiable by focal positivity for α-naphthyl acetate esterase and acid phosphatase, both enzymes giving diffuse reactions in monocytes and weak reactions in B lymphocytes.

6.5.4 *Coagulation Testing*

To detect abnormalities of coagulation, two primary screening tests are employed in the laboratory. Stimulation of the *extrinsic* pathway of coagulation (Figure 6.5) is effected *in vitro* by the addition of a tissue extract (usually of brain) to citrated plasma. Recalcification of the plasma by the addition of calcium chloride then allows coagulation to proceed to fibrin formation. The time taken to the formation of a visible clot is known as the prothrombin time (PT), and is proportional to the concentration of coagulation factors present. It is of interest to note that beagles which are homozygous for factor VII deficiency have a markedly extended PT.

However, heterozygote beagles with levels of factor VII which overlap the normal range, may be more difficult to identify. *In vitro* stimulation of the *intrinsic* pathway is achieved by the addition of a fine particulate suspension (e.g. kaolin or silica) to citrated plasma, followed by phospholipid and calcium. The resultant coagulation time is known variously as the activated partial thromboplastin time (APTT), the partial thromboplastin time with kaolin (PTTK), the kaolin–cephalin clotting time (KCCT), or simply the partial thromboplastin time (PTT).

A basic coagulation screen should consist of both a PT and an APTT. Since most of the major liver-synthesized coagulation factors are involved in the extrinsic pathway, the PT is also a good test of liver function. Fibrinogen, a useful component of a co-agulation screen, may also be measured simultaneously by some coagulation analysers.

Because of the large volumes of blood required for coagulation tests, it is only possible to perform coagulation screens at interim bleeds in larger animals, not in rodents. A useful test for smaller animals is the modified thrombotest [13]. Platelet function testing, such as the response to aggregating stimuli (e.g. ADP, collagen, adrenaline) is beyond the scope of most laboratories in routine preclinical testing, due to the amount of labour involved. However, such tests may be relevant where antiplatelet compounds are being developed.

6.5.5 In vitro *Haematotoxicity*

The direct assessment of the toxicity of compounds to bone marrow may be made by culturing marrow cells *in vitro* and measuring the inhibition of the growth of morphologically recognizable colonies such as BFU-E, CFU-E and CFU-GM (Figure 6.1). The inhibition of colony growth with novel compounds has been shown to correlate well with *in vivo* haematotoxicity [14]. For example, it was found that significant inhibition of BFU-E growth *in vitro* was paralleled by anaemia in dosed animals; however there was evidence that the *in vitro* assay may be more sensitive than results obtained *in vivo*. As *in vitro* tests may be performed reasonably quickly (in about a week) such assays are becoming important in the screening of novel anticancer and antiviral compounds, where a dose-limiting marrow toxicity is a well-recognized hazard.

When novel compounds are formulated for intravenous infusion to patients, it is necessary to assess the effect of the direct contact of the formulation on the blood. In these assays, a range of suitable dilutions of the formulation are incubated with whole blood or plasma. Effects on plasma (e.g. flocculation, coagulation) are then evaluated, and haemolysis of the whole blood mixture is assessed photometrically after centrifugation. If a weak positive result is seen at high concentrations of the formulation, an allowance must be made as this situation would not be likely to persist longer than a few seconds *in vivo*, before dilution in the circulation occurred [15].

6.5.6 *Sources of Preanalytical Variation*

Many uncontrolled variables may conspire to make the interpretation of haematological data difficult if these variables are superimposed upon toxic effects. If, for example, due to budgetary, space, or other constraints, control groups are not used (e.g. as occurs in some acute studies), the following factors must be borne in mind.

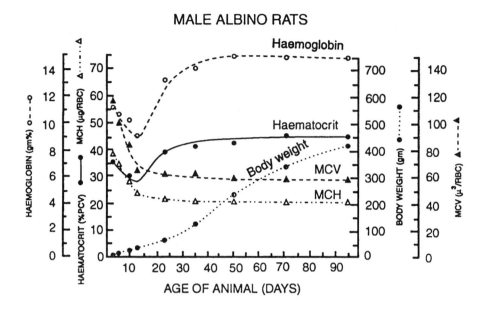

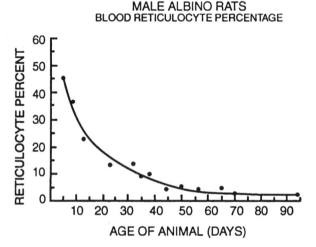

Figure 6.6 Effect of age on selected haematological parameters in male Sprague–Dawley rats. Central blood samples (from aortic puncture or decapitation) were analysed with a Coulter S analyser or by manual counting (reticulocyte analysis). Reproduced with permission from [17].

Strain differences Extrapolation of data from one strain of laboratory animal to another may be inappropriate. For instance, there is considerable variation in baseline leucocyte counts in different rodent strains [16].

Age differences Many haematological parameters vary with age and are in a state of flux, particularly when toxicological investigations are performed in young (post-weaning) animals (Figure 6.6). Comparing pre-treatment with post-treatment data in the same group of animals may therefore not be scientifically valid.

Venepuncture site variation   Cell counts are generally higher in the peripheral circulation [18] than in centrally-sampled blood which may be obtained from rodents at autopsy. Therefore, blood values from samples obtained at different sites may not be comparable.

Order of sample collection   Blood samples for coagulation studies should always be collected first, to reduce the effects of tissue activation. However, where skin puncture is used to obtain a capillary blood sample, the first drop should be wiped away as it will contain excess tissue factor and therefore give a shortened coagulation time. It has also been found that cell counts in samples taken from rodents at autopsy decrease rapidly during the period of sampling. For example, the total leucocyte count may be reduced by 50 per cent or more between a sample taken promptly (i.e. 10 to 15 s after death) and one taken 60 s later [18].

Diurnal variation   Counts of certain cell types exhibit a diurnal periodicity, which may complicate data interpretation if bleeding is not standardized to the same time each day. For example, in rodents, reticulocyte counts fall in the afternoon, reflecting reduced marrow mitotic activity. Daily rhythms are also seen in counts for neutrophils, lymphocytes and eosinophils, reflecting natural corticosterone levels.

Excessive venesection   Experimental design sometimes fails to take account of the effects of blood volume depletion if there is a need to remove many samples for diverse analyses (clinical chemistry, pharmacokinetics, etc). The cumulative effect of excessive sampling may be to induce blood loss anaemia, with depleted iron stores.

Anaesthesia   As explained earlier (Section 6.2.1), anaesthesia has a relaxing effect on the spleen, causing increased splenic pooling of peripheral cells. The net effect of this is to reduce erythrocyte, leucocyte and platelet counts in peripheral blood.

6.6   Conclusions

Blood is a tissue which is very vulnerable to a wide range of toxic insults (Table 6.1), and the effects may be far reaching and grave. The fact that examination of the blood is one of the central pillars of toxicity studies recognises this fact.

To a large extent, toxicity to the bone marrow can be assessed by peripheral blood measurements. Marked haematological changes at all dose levels would indicate that a drug would not be a suitable candidate for development. However, the sensitivity of haematological measurements is increasing constantly with the development of micro-automated methods. As a result, it should be recognized that subtle but significant treatment-related changes may come to light which have little clinical relevance. An example of this is the very narrow distribution of the MCV in rats, and this may lead to intergroup differences of under 1 per cent becoming statistically significant. It is therefore necessary to be aware of the limitations of the extreme precision of some haematological measurements, and to be familiar with the distribution of such values in the experimental animal population.

However, there has in recent years been an exponential increase in the body of knowledge surrounding the control of growth and differentiation of primitive haematopoietic cells. This has lead and will inevitably lead in the future to the development of assays which can pinpoint toxic lesions at the molecular level, and it may ultimately be possible to offer such assays routinely, using very small blood volumes and automated blood analysers.

At present it is possible to detect haematotoxicity in laboratory species and extrapolate to man for the classes of drugs where these effects are dose limiting, e.g. cytotoxic agents. Some of the *in vitro* culture assays now in use are accurately predictive for haematotoxicity *in vivo* for laboratory species, and these *in vitro* assays will undoubtably become more commonplace in the future. It will therefore become imperative that those wishing to understand the mechanisms of toxic effects on blood cells will need to become familiar with the interpretation of these assays and their extrapolation to man.

It is to be hoped that in addition to detecting the frequently-seen dose-related and reversible haematotoxic effects, models and screens of toxicity will be developed that will indicate whether a candidate compound has the potential to cause idiosyncratic bone marrow failure or other blood dyscrasias. When this occurs, ethical issues will be raised which will need to be confronted. Any regulatory framework governing testing for haematotoxicity will need to take account of all such questions.

References

1. BÖTTINGER, L.E. and WESTERHOLM, B. (1973) Drug-induced blood dyscrasias in Sweden, *British Medical Journal*, **3**, 339–343.
2. TESTA, N.G. and GALE, R.P. (1988) *Hematopoiesis: Long Term Effects of Chemotherapy and Radiation*, New York: Marcel Dekker.
3. BERGER, J. (1985) Experimentally induced toxic-haemolytic anaemia in laboratory rats following phenacetin administration, *Folia Haematologica*, **112**, S. 571–579.
4. IRONS, R.D. (1991) Blood and bone marrow, in HASCHEK, W.M. and ROUSSEAUX, C.G. (Eds) *Handbook of Toxicologic Pathology*, pp. 389–419, San Diego: Academic Press.
5. HAWKEY, C.M. (1991) The value of comparative haematology studies, *Comparative Haematology International*, **1**, 1–9.
6. SMITH, C.A., ANDREWS, C.M., COLLARD, J.K., HALL, D.E. and WALKER, A.K. (1994) *Color Atlas of Comparative, Diagnostic and Experimental Haematology*, London: Wolfe Publishing.
7. VACHA, J. (1983) Red cell life-span, in AGAR, N.S., and BOARD, P.G. (Eds) *Red Blood Cells of Domestic Mammals*, pp. 67–132, Amsterdam: Elsevier.
8. DAVIE, E.W., FUJIKAWA, K. and KISIEL, W. (1991) The coagulation cascade: initiation, maintenance and regulation, *Biochemistry*, **30**, 10363–10370.
9. ANDREWS, C.M., SPURLING, N.W. and TURTON, J.A. (1993) Characterisation of busulphan-induced myelotoxicity in $B_6C_3F_1$ mice using flow cytometry, *Comparative Haematology International*, **3**, 102–115.
10. HALL, R.L. (1992) Clinical pathology for preclinical safety assessment: current global guidelines, *Toxicologic Pathology*, **20**, 472–476.
11. EDWARDS, C.J. and FULLER, J. (1992) Notes on age-related changes in differential leucocyte counts of the Charles River albino SD rat and CD1 mouse, *Comparative Haematology International*, **2**, 58–60.
12. BROWN, G. (1991) The left shift index: a useful guide to the interpretation of marrow data, *Comparative Haematology International*, **1**, 106–111.
13. GODSAFE, P.A. and SINGLETON, B.K. (1992) The use of the whole blood thrombotest time (1/51) as a routine monitor of vitamin K-dependent blood coagulation factor levels in the rat, *Comparative Haematology International*, **2**, 51–55.

14. DELDAR, A. and STEVENS, C.E. (1993) Development and application of in vitro models of hematopoiesis to drug development, *Toxicologic Pathology*, **21**, 231–240.

15. SALAUZE, D. and DECOUVELAERE, D. (1994) In vitro assessment of the haemolytic potential of candidate drugs, *Comparative Haematology International*, **4**, 34–36.

16. ROE, F.J.C. (1994) Historical histopathological control data for laboratory rodents: valuable treasure or worthless trash?, *Laboratory Animals*, **28**, 148–154.

17. DAVIS, J.R. and AVRAM, M.J. (1978) Developmental changes in δ-aminolevulinic acid dehydratase activity and blood reticulocyte percentage in the developing rat, *Mechanisms of Ageing and Development*, **7**, 123–129.

18. SMITH, C.N., NEPTUN, D.A. and IRONS, R.D. (1986) Effect of sampling site and collection method on variations in baseline clinical pathology parameters in Fischer-344 rats, *Fundamental and Applied Toxicology*, **7**, 658–663.

Additional Reading

ARCHER, R.K. and JEFFCOTT, L.B. (1977) *Comparative Clinical Haematology*, Oxford: Blackwell Scientific.

EASTHAM, R.D. and SLADE, R.R. (1992) *Clinical Haematology*, 7th Edn, Oxford: Butterworth-Heinemann.

FISHER, J.W. (1992) *Biochemical Pharmacology of Blood and Bloodforming Tissues*, Berlin: Springer-Verlag.

JAIN, N.C. (1993) *Essentials of Veterinary Hematology*, Philadelphia: Lea and Febiger.

JONES, T.C., WARD, J.M., MOHR, U. and HUNT, R.D. (1990) *Monographs on Pathology of Laboratory Animals: Haemopoietic System*, Berlin: Springer-Verlag.

Clinical pathology testing in preclinical safety assessment (1992) *Toxicologic Pathology*, **20**, No. 3, Part 2.

Toxicologic pathology of the hematopoietic system (1993) *Toxicologic Pathology*, **21**, No. 2.

7

The Immune System

JOSEPH G. VOS, IAN KIMBER, C. FRIEKE KUPER, HENK VAN LOVEREN AND
HENK-JAN SCHUURMAN

7.1 Introduction

It is well established that each individual has an intrinsic capacity to defend itself against environmental pathogens. The host defence system, including the immune system, serves the body by the neutralization/inactivation/elimination of potential pathogens such as bacteria and viruses. The immune system also functions in preventing the uncontrolled growth of cells which may form a neoplasm (tumour). It has a specific branch, in which lymphocytes and antibodies provide the specificity for recognition and subsequent reactivity towards antigens, and a non-specific branch, which can initiate effector reactions itself or upon stimulation by antigen-specific components.

Immunotoxicology has been defined as:

> The discipline concerned with the study of the events that can lead to undesired effects as a result of interaction of xenobiotics with the immune system. These undesired events may result as a consequence of: (1) a direct and/or indirect effect of the xenobiotic (and/or its biotransformation product) on the immune system; or, (2) an immunologically-based host response to the compound and/or its metabolite(s), or host antigens modified by the compound or its metabolites [1].

When the immune system acts as a passive target of chemical insults, the result can be a decreased resistance to infection, certain forms of neoplasia, or immune disregulation/stimulation exacerbating allergy or autoimmunity. Immunodeficiency states and severe immunosuppression, as can occur in transplantation or cytostatic therapy, have been associated in particular with increased incidences of opportunistic infections. Exposure to immunosuppressive environmental chemicals may be expected to result in more subtle forms of immunosuppression which may be difficult to detect. These may lead to an increased incidence of infections such as influenza or the common cold. In those instances where the xenobiotic is recognized by the immune system, a specific immune response may develop resulting in allergy or autoimmunity. The distinction between immunosuppression and allergy is to a certain extent artificial. Some compounds like heavy metals are able to exert a direct toxic effect on the immune system as well as stimulating allergic responses. It should be noted that chemicals are able to induce allergic responses in susceptible individuals without perturbation of the immune system other than that caused by antigenic stimulation.

One of the first comprehensive reviews of xenobiotics that affect immune reactivity in laboratory animals was published in 1977 by Vos [2]. Since then, a number of textbooks and conference proceedings dealing with experimental and clinical immunotoxicology have been published [3–10]. Also, initiatives have been taken regarding the development and validation of methods for assessment of immunotoxicity and a number of compounds have been identified that manifest toxicity to the immune system (Table 7.1) [11]. A number of tiered approaches to immunotoxicity testing have been proposed [12–15]. With respect to man, only scant epidemiological data on immunotoxicity, indicative of suppression or altered resistance to infection and tumours, have been published. Such studies are rare and their interpretation often does not permit unequivocal conclusions to be drawn, due for instance to the uncontrolled nature of exposure. Immunotoxicity assessment in rodents, with subsequent extrapolation to man, forms the basis of decisions regarding hazard and risk.

Descriptions of histology, spontaneous pathology and chemically induced morphological alterations of lymphoid organs and tissues are found in textbooks and review articles [16–24]

Table 7.1 Examples of compounds that are immunotoxic for man or rodents

Chemical	Immunotoxicity	
	Rodent	Man
2,3,7,8-tetrachlorodibenzo-*p*-dioxin	+	+
Polychlorinated biphenyls	+	+
Polybrominated biphenyls	+	+
Hexachlorobenzene	+	unknown
Lead	+	unknown
Cadmium	+	unknown
Methyl mercury compounds	+	unknown
7,12-dimethylbenz[a]anthracene	+	unknown
Benzo[a]pyrene	+	unknown
Di-*n*-octyltindichloride	+	unknown
Di-*n*-butyltindichloride	+	unknown
Benzidine	+	+
Nitrogen dioxide and ozone	+	+
Benzene, toluene and xylene	+	+
Asbestos	+	+
Dimethylnitrosamine	+	unknown
Diethylstilboestrol	+	+
Vanadium	+	+

Source: [11]

7.2 Anatomy, Histology and Physiology

7.2.1 *Overview of Lymphoid Organs*

Components of the immune system are present throughout the body. The lymphocyte compartment is found within lymphoid organs (Figure 7.1). Phagocytic cells of the monocyte/macrophage lineage, called the mononuclear phagocyte system (MPS), occur in lymphoid organs and also at extranodal sites, such as Kupffer cells in the liver, alveolar macrophages in the lung, mesangial macrophages in the kidney and glial cells in the brain. Polymorphonuclear leucocytes (PMNs) are present mainly in blood and bone marrow, but accumulate at sites of inflammation.

Lymphoid organs can be classified as primary or central (antigen-independent) or secondary or peripheral (antigen-dependent) organs. The bone marrow, which is not discussed further in this chapter, and the thymus are primary lymphoid organs. Secondary lymphoid organs include lymph nodes, spleen, and lymphoid tissue along secretory surfaces such as the gastrointestinal and respiratory tracts, the so-called mucosa-associated lymphoid tissue (MALT). In addition the skin is an immunologically active and important organ.

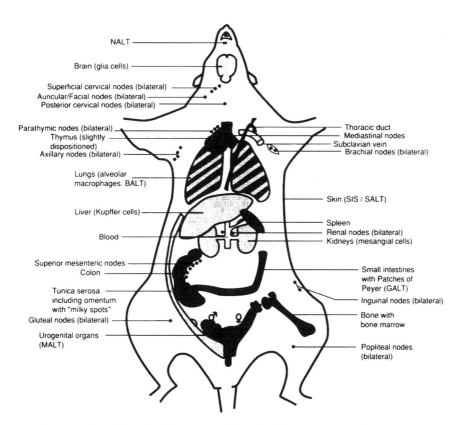

Figure 7.1 Overview of lymphoid organs and tissues in the rat. Lymphoid organs are presented in black, mucosal lymphoid tissue is presented in dark grey and the mononuclear phagocyte system is shown in light grey.

7.2.2 *Thymus*

The thymus is a bilobed organ located in the mediastinum, anterior to the major vessels of the heart. Each lobe consists of smaller lobules, that have the same architecture, with a subcapsular and outer cortical area, a cortex and a medulla. The supporting stroma consists of reticular epithelium. The cortex is densely packed with small-sized lymphocytes and the medulla contains medium-sized lymphocytes at a lower density. Macrophages occur in both cortex and medulla, and in the medulla, interdigitating dendritic cells are also found. The main function of the thymus is the processing of immature precursor pre-T-lymphocytes from the bone marrow into immunocompetent T (thymus-dependent) cells. This process comprises a number of steps. In the most immature stage, cells are found as large lymphoblasts in the outer cortex. Thereafter, lymphocytes localize in the cortex as small cells with scanty cytoplasm. Finally, cells are present in the medulla as medium-sized lymphocytes. During this process the cells express the antigen-recognizing unit (T-cell receptor) on their surface. All recognition specificities that are encoded in the genome are expressed initially and then a selection is made. T lymphocytes recognize antigen in the context of self major histocompatibility complex (MHC) antigens. Only precursor cells displaying this capacity and which, in addition, fail to react with autoantigens, are selected. Epithelial cells and interdigitating dendritic cells mediate this selection. If not selected, the cell dies by a mechanism of suicide or apoptosis. Histologically, apoptosis is recognized by the presence of condensed, sometimes fragmented nuclei, that can be found in phagocytic macrophages (so-called tingible body macrophages or 'starry-sky' macrophages). After selection, the immunologically competent lymphocytes leave the thymus and home to peripheral lymphoid organs.

The basic architecture of the thymus is not a fixed histological entity. Its features depend on the age and hormonal status of the individual. A 'normal' architecture can be expected only during the late gestational period until young adulthood. Thereafter, the thymus starts to involute and declines in immunological importance.

7.2.3 *Lymph Nodes*

For the return of tissue interstitial fluid to the blood circulation there is a finely branched lymph vessel system (lymphatics), with at regular intervals, lymph nodes. The main function of lymph nodes is to filter pathogens from the afferent lymph and they are the site of initiation of primary immune reactions. The afferent lymphatics penetrate the lymph node capsule and connect with the subcapsular sinus which in turn connects with the cortical and medullary sinuses. The lymph leaves the node via the efferent lymphatic(s) at the hilus and drains into other lymph nodes or directly via the thoracic duct into the blood, in the rat via the left subclavian vein. Blood vessels are connected to the node at the hilus. The various lymph node compartments include the outer cortex with follicles and interfollicular areas, the inner cortex or paracortex and the medulla with medullary cords and sinuses. Interfollicular areas/ paracortex (T-lymphocyte areas) are differentiated from follicles (B-lymphocyte areas) by the presence of postcapillary venules, through which lymphocytes enter the parenchyma. Follicles are spherical structures, mostly found immediately underneath the capsule, that consist of accumulations of small cells (primary follicle, resting state), or a pale-stained centre with large lymphoid cells (centrocytes, centroblasts) and tingible body macrophages surrounded by a mantle with small-sized lymphocytes (secondary follicles, activated state).

The major route of entry for antigens and pathogens, either free or processed by so-called veiled cells, is via the afferent lymph. From there, antigen moves to the paracortex, where interdigitating dendritic cells (the tissue equivalent of the veiled cell) present antigen to T cells and initiate the immune response. In follicles, antigen is presented to B cells, with help from T lymphocytes and/or their soluble products. The major site of immune effector reactions is the medulla, where macrophages, granulocytes, activated T cells and plasma cells are localized.

Lymph node morphology is dynamic and related directly to the nature and extent of antigenic stimulation. After stimulation, the node increases in size within a relatively short period (days). In the case of B-lymphocyte reactions, hyperplasia in follicles is seen (e.g. after bacterial infection); in the case of T-cell reactions, the interfollicular areas or paracortex becomes enlarged by hyperplasia of T cells (e.g. after viral infection), with activation of the high-endothelial venules. After termination of the reaction, the lymph node eventually regains its normal (resting) size.

7.2.4 Spleen

The main immunological function of the spleen is to guard the vascular compartment of the body. It has enormous phagocytic activity and generates (T-cell independent) IgM-class antibodies, especially to blood-borne antigens. There are no lymphatics in the spleen. The organ has two main compartments, the red pulp and white pulp. The red pulp consists of blood-filled sinusoids and the cords of Billroth, containing macrophages, lymphocytes and plasma cells. Macrophages perform an important function in blood cell clearance (e.g. of old red blood cells) and in phagocytosis. The filter function is made possible by the direct contact, unobstructed by blood-vessel walls, between phagocytic cells and blood-borne particles, facilitated by the large blood supply. In rodents the red pulp contains nests of haemopoiesis (megakaryocytes and normoblasts).

At any one time about a quarter of the body's total lymphocyte population is found within the splenic white pulp, which consists of a central arteriole surrounded by the periarteriolar lymphocyte sheath (PALS), a T-cell area. The outer PALS contains B cells and plasma cells. Adjacent follicles contain B cells. Around the PALS and follicles is a corona of B cells, called the marginal zone; this region is identified readily, especially in rats, as it contains medium-sized cells, that after histological staining appear larger and paler than small-sized lymphocytes in other areas of the white pulp. The marginal zone generates IgM-class antibody responses that do not directly require T-cell help (e.g. to polysaccharide antigens of encapsulated bacteria). This function is unique to the spleen.

7.2.5 Mucosa-Associated Lymphoid Tissue (MALT)

The digestive, respiratory and urogenital tracts contain lymphoid tissue which is organized into non-encapsulated structures of diffuse collections of lymphocytes. These lymphoid structures (Peyer's patches) occur in the small intestine, the appendix and the large intestine (gut-associated lymphoid tissue, GALT). Lymphoid tissue along the bronchi is called bronchus-associated lymphoid tissue (BALT) and in the oro- and nasopharyngeal region, nasal-associated lymphoid tissue (NALT). As these mucosal lymphoid tissues share structural and functional characteristics and are strongly interrelated, their common designation is 'mucosa-associated lymphoid tissue' (MALT). The major function of MALT is to initiate immune responses. Activated lymphocytes pass on to draining lymph nodes, and, after recirculation via the blood stream, return to the mucosal tissue. The histological organization of MALT is like that of lymph nodes, with B-cell (follicles) areas and interfollicular T-cell areas. There are no afferent lymph vessels or a medulla, because pathogens can enter directly through the covering epithelial layer and the immunological reaction is transferred quickly to the draining lymph node. Outside lymphoid structures, plasma cells and natural killer cells are present in the epithelial lining, in the interstitium and in the lamina propria.

About half of the body's lymphocytes are located at any one time in MALT and the capacity for antibody synthesis is about one and a half times that of the internal lymphoid system. The response in MALT is devoted primarily to the generation of IgA-antibody responses. After stimulation and recirculation, B cells home as IgA-producing plasma cells underneath the covering epithelium. The IgA antibodies are transported subsequently across the epithelium, e.g. in salivary and gastrointestinal secretions. Their main function is to prevent the entry of potentially pathogenic substances into the body, a specific antigen-exclusion function whereby the epithelium is coated with 'antiseptic paint'.

7.2.6 *Skin Immune System (SIS) or Skin-Associated Lymphoid Tissue (SALT)*

The principal physical function of the skin is that of providing a barrier. The immunological function of the skin is the induction of immune responses to antigens encountered at the external surface of the body. Important in this process are epidermal Langerhans cells, which are the equivalent of interdigitating dendritic cells in lymph nodes, and veiled cells in lymph, and have antigen-presenting functions. There are epidermotropic recirculating T-lymphocyte subpopulations. In the epidermis of rodents there is a special T cell, the so-called dendritic epidermal T cell. Keratinocytes can synthesize cytokines upon activation, thereby influencing T-cell differentiation and haematopoiesis. In the dermis, T cells and macrophages are present especially in the papillary part. In the connective tissue of the dermis, T cells, macrophages, mast cells, endothelial cells and dendritic cells are found, in common with connective tissue at other locations in the body. Finally there are skin-draining lymph nodes.

7.3 Biochemical and Cellular Mechanisms of Toxicity

7.3.1 *Immunosuppression*

Effective host resistance is dependent upon the functional integrity of the immune system, which in turn requires that the component cells and molecules which orchestrate immune responses are available in sufficient numbers and in an operational form. By analogy with congenital and acquired human immunodeficiency diseases, chemical-induced immunosuppression may result simply from a reduced number of functional cells. The absence, or reduced numbers, of lymphocytes may have profound effects on immune status. Loss may occur following exposure to cytotoxic or cytostatic drugs and chemicals, secondary to changes in the generative lymphoid organs, due to altered compartmentalization or from the induction of apoptosis. Normal immune effector function and homeostatic regulation of the immune response is dependent upon a variety of soluble products, known collectively as cytokines, which are synthesized and secreted by lymphocytes and by other cell types. Cytokines have pleiotropic effects on immune and inflammatory responses. Cooperation between different cell populations required for the developing immune response, the regulation of antibody responses, the accumulation of immune cells and molecules at inflammatory sites, the initiation of acute phase responses, the control of macrophage cytotoxic function and many other processes central to host resistance are influenced by, and in many cases are dependent upon, cytokines acting individually or in concert. Changes in the availability of cytokines, resulting directly from perturbation of synthesis and/or secretion or directly from a loss of producing cells, can have profound effects on the integrity of immune function. Although the nature of the initial lesions induced by many immunotoxic chemicals have not yet been elucidated, there is increasing information available regarding the immunobiological changes which result in depression of immune function.

7.3.2 *Allergy*

Allergy may be defined as the adverse health effects which result from the stimulation of specific immune responses. In the context of immunotoxicology, it is allergy resulting from the stimulation of immune responses to chemicals and drugs that are of interest. Allergic reactions may take a variety of forms and these differ with respect to both the underlying immunological mechanisms and the tempo in which the reactions can be elicited. Four major types of allergic reactions have been recognized: type I, or immediate-type hypersensitivity reactions, which are effected by IgE antibody and where symptoms are manifest within minutes of exposure of the sensitized individual. Type II hypersensitivity reactions result from the damage or destruction of host cells by antibody to an antigen on a cell or tissue component. In this case symptoms become apparent within hours. Type III hypersensitivity reactions, or Arthus reactions, also are antibody mediated, but against soluble antigen, and result from the local or systemic action of immune complexes. A general feature is vasculitis. Type IV, or delayed-type hypersensitivity reactions are effected by T lymphocytes and normally symptoms develop 24 to 48 h following exposure of the sensitized individual (Figure 7.2).

The types of chemical allergy of greatest relevance to the immunotoxicologist are contact sensitivity, or skin allergy, and allergy of the respiratory tract.

Contact hypersensitivity

A large number of chemicals are able to cause skin sensitization. Following topical exposure of a susceptible individual to a chemical allergen, a T-lymphocyte response

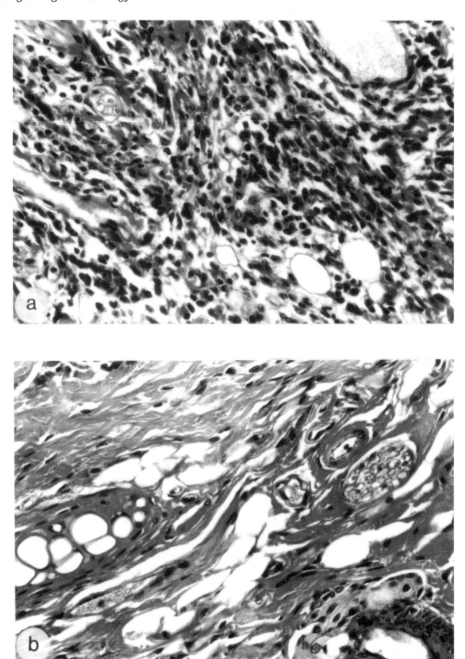

Figure 7.2 Delayed-type hypersensitivity (DTH) reaction to ovalbumin in rat earskin. Note the presence of a mononuclear cell infiltrate in the dermis of an immunocompetent animal (a) and the absence of a DTH-reaction in an immunodeficient (athymic) rat (b).

is induced in the draining lymph nodes. In the skin the allergen interacts (directly or indirectly) with epidermal Langerhans cells which transport the chemical to the lymph nodes and present it in an immunogenic form to responsive T lymphocytes. Allergen-activated T lymphocytes proliferate, resulting in clonal expansion. The individual is now sensitized and will respond to a second dermal exposure to the same chemical with a more aggressive immune response, resulting in allergic contact dermatitis. The cutaneous inflammatory reaction which characterizes allergic contact dermatitis is secondary to the recognition of the allergen in the skin by specific T lymphocytes. These lymphocytes become activated, release cytokines and cause the local accumulation of other mononuclear leucocytes. Symptoms develop some 24 to 48 h following exposure of the sensitized individual and allergic contact dermatitis therefore represents a form of delayed-type hypersensitivity. Common causes of allergic contact dermatitis include **organic chemicals** (such as **2,4-dinitro-chlorobenzene**), **metals** (such as **nickel** and **chromium**) and **plant products** (such as **urushiol** from poison ivy).

Respiratory hypersensitivity

Respiratory hypersensitivity is usually considered to be a type I hypersensitivity reaction. However, late phase reactions and the more chronic symptoms associated with asthma may involve cell-mediated (type IV) immune processes. The acute symptoms associated with respiratory allergy are effected by IgE antibody, the production of which is provoked following exposure of the susceptible individual to the inducing chemical allergen. The IgE antibody is distributed systemically and binds, via membrane receptors, to mast cells which are found in vascularized tissues, including the respiratory tract. Following inhalation of the same chemical, a respiratory hypersensitivity reaction will be elicited. Allergen associates with protein and binds to, and cross-links, IgE antibody bound to mast cells. This in turn causes the degranulation of mast cells and the release of inflammatory mediators such as histamine and leukotrienes. Such mediators cause bronchoconstriction and vasodilation, resulting in the symptoms of respiratory allergy: asthma and/or rhinitis. Chemicals known to cause respiratory hypersensitivity in man include **acid anhydrides** (such as **trimellitic anhydride**), some **diisocyanates** (such as **toluene diisocyanate**), **platinum salts** and some **reactive dyes**.

7.3.3 Autoimmunity

Autoimmunity can be defined as the stimulation of specific immune responses directed against endogenous 'self' antigens. Induced autoimmunity can result either from alterations in the balance of regulatory T lymphocytes or from the association of a xenobiotic with normal tissue components such as to render them immunogenic: 'altered self'. A variety of chemicals and drugs, in particular the latter, have been found to induce autoimmune-like responses [7].

7.4 Morphological Responses to Injury

7.4.1 Introduction

The dynamic nature of the immune system renders it particularly vulnerable to the toxic effects of xenobiotics (Tables 7.2 and 7.3). Conversely, this dynamic nature provides a significant regenerative capacity. When only leucocyte populations are

Table 7.2   Immunotoxicity of some agents

Agent	Effect	Target organ
Steroid hormones	Immunosuppression (oestrogens, via oestrogen receptors) Immunostimulation (androgens)	Thymus: cortical depletion, apoptosis, phagocytosis
Halogenated aromatic hydrocarbons	Immunosuppression, via Ah-receptor	Thymus: cortical depletion
Hexachlorobenzene	Immunostimulation (rat)	Spleen: B-cell hyperplasia Lymph nodes: increase in high endothelial venules
Organotin compounds	Immunosuppression, cytotoxic, antiproliferation	Thymus: cortical depletion
Heavy metals	Immunosuppression Immunomodulation/hypersensitivity	Multiple sites, dependent on the target of hypersensitivity
Drugs	Immunomodulation: various forms of hypersensitivity following immune response to drug determinants or drug-altered self components	Multiple sites, dependent on the target of hypersensitivity
Cyclosporine	Immunosuppression, via cyclophilin/calcineurin complex Autoimmunity, pseudo-graft-versus-host reaction	Thymus: medullary reduction
Cytostatic drugs (azathioprine, 5-fluorouracil)	Antiproliferative effect	Bone marrow: cytopenia Lymphoid organs: lymphocyte depletion, particularly in thymic cortex
Irradiation	Antiproliferative effect, interphase death of lymphocytes Immunomodulation/tolerance induction	Bone marrow: cytopenia Lymphoid organs: lymphocyte depletion
UV-B light	Immunomodulation, induction of suppressor cells	Skin: decrease of Langerhans cells
Oxidant air pollutants	Immunosuppression	Lung: influx of macrophages (O_3), pneumocyte alteration

affected, the lymphoid organs are restored within 3 to 4 weeks. When leucocyte stem cells in the bone marrow are affected (e.g. after sublethal irradiation), regeneration does not occur. Regeneration may include an overcompensation reaction, such as evidenced by an increased thymus weight and extramedullary haematopoiesis in spleen.

A decrease in cellularity or a depletion of lymphoid cells in the lymphoid organs, including blood, is often the first sign of immunotoxicity by xenobiotics. Effects on the framework result mostly in degeneration, ending in atrophy and fibrosis. Alternatively, framework cells and leucocytes may persist, but are unable to

Table 7.3 Sensitivity of cell populations in the thymus to toxic compounds

Cells	Location	Compound
Lymphocytes:		
Immature lymphoblasts	Outer cortex	Some organotin compounds
		2,3 ,7,8-tetrachlorodibenzo-*p*-dioxin
Small-sized cells	Cortex	Glucocorticosteroids
		Cytostatic drugs (e.g. azathioprine)
Intermediate-sized cells	Medulla	Ammonia caramel (THI)
Epithelial cells	Cortex	2,3,7,8-tetrachlorodibenzo-*p*-dioxin
	Medulla	Cyclosporine
		FK-506
Dendritic cells	Medulla	Cyclosporine
		FK-506
Macrophages	Cortex	Ammonia caramel (THI)

function, e.g. to secrete biologically active mediators, an aspect of toxicity that is not identified readily by histology and may require assessment of immune function. Inflammation (leucocyte cell infiltration and tissue destruction) is induced when toxicity results from allergy, as an immune response to the chemical, or from the stimulation of autoimmunity. Generally, inflammation occurs outside lymphoid organs, e.g. in skin, lungs, kidneys and joints, while in the lymphoid organs, hyperplasia of lymphoid cells can be a main feature. Inflammation can also result from non-immunological toxic mechanisms such as the irritation of skin and mucosal layers by xenobiotics, but this is outside the scope of this chapter and is not described in the following sections. Hyperplasia and neoplasia of lymphoid cells and framework tissue can be the long-term result of immunotoxic damage.

Importantly, endogenous factors, such as stress, nutritional status, sex hormone balance and age, can influence lymphoid organ histology and may hamper the interpretation of effects observed in toxicity studies.

7.4.2 Depletion/Atrophy/Regeneration

The compounds mentioned below illustrate the histological appearance of lymphoid organ depletion and atrophy. Despite the diversity in the underlying mechanisms of toxicity, a wide variety of tissue responses does not exist. However, detailed observation in the context of the histophysiology of lymphoid organs will often show subtle differences in response and provide clues to the underlying immunotoxic mechanisms.

Steroid hormones

Examples include alteration of sex steroid hormone balance in pregnancy and the increase in glucocorticosteroid levels during acute stress. Experimental treatment with sex steroid hormones like **oestradiol** and glucocorticosteroid drugs such as **dexamethasone** lead to a similar pattern of lymphocyte depletion and lymphoid organ atrophy. Pregnancy in rodents results in radical, but reversible, changes in lymphoid organs. After an initial rise in thymic weight in early pregnancy, involution begins with lymphocyte cell death in the cortex, leading to cortical thymocyte depletion. Histologically, cell death is associated with apoptotic bodies and lymphocyte phagocytosis by macrophages ('starry-sky' macrophages). Remarkably, large lymphoblasts in the outer cortex remain relatively unaffected. Acute stress in rodents similarly induces thymic involution. Changes in the cortex progress within a few days from lymphocyte phagocytosis ('starry-sky' appearance) to lymphocyte depletion. A reversed pattern of lymphocyte density then emerges, with a higher cellular density in the medulla than in the cortex. In man, histologically defined stages in thymic involution after acute disease correlate with the time course (up to 4 days) of acute stress observed in rodents. Following thymic involution, depletion of T cells in peripheral organs can occur, e.g. a reduced cellularity in the splenic PALS.

Organotin compounds

These compounds are used widely as pesticides, as preservatives of wood, paper, textiles and leather, in heat/light protection of PVC plastics and in antifouling paints. Various organotin compounds, such as **dibutyl-** and **dioctyltin chloride** and **tributyltin oxide** have been shown in rodents to be T-cell immunotoxicants, resulting in suppression of thymus-dependent immune responses [25]. Thymus atrophy is a sensitive parameter of exposure to these compounds. Histologically, there is depletion of large lymphoblasts located in the outer cortex, resulting in an inverse pattern of lymphocyte density in the cortex and medulla. This depletion is due to a direct toxicity to immature thymocytes. Starry-sky macrophages are not prominent, unlike those observed in corticosteroid-induced thymic atrophy. The thymus atrophy is rapidly reversible even resulting in an overshoot reaction. After prolonged exposure to organotin compounds, lymphopenia occurs and thymus and lymph node weights are reduced. The reduction in peripheral lymphoid organs affects particularly the T-cell compartment, such as the PALS in spleen and the paracortex in lymph nodes.

Dioxin

Halogenated aromatic hydrocarbons are well known environmental pollutants. Among the most immunotoxic is **2,3,7,8-tetrachlorodibenzo-*p*-dioxin (dioxin, TCDD)** [26]. **TCDD** causes profound effects on the thymus and peripheral lymphoid organs. As a result, cell-mediated and humoral immunity is compromised. Flow cytometry reveals that the thymic atrophy is due to a reduction in cortical-type thymocytes (CD4/CD8 double positive cells, Figure 7.3). Subsequent to thymic changes, T-cell areas in peripheral lymphoid organs become depleted after exposure to dioxins. The loss of lymphocytes in the thymic cortex caused by **TCDD** may result from changes in the status of thymic epithelial cells, rather than from direct toxicity to the lymphoid compartment. One proposal is that **TCDD** causes terminal differentiation of epithelial cells such that they are no longer able to support the functional maturation and selection of T lymphocytes. By electron microscopy, a higher incidence of electron-dense epithelial cells has been observed, which indicates an increased differentiation of electron-lucent cells that

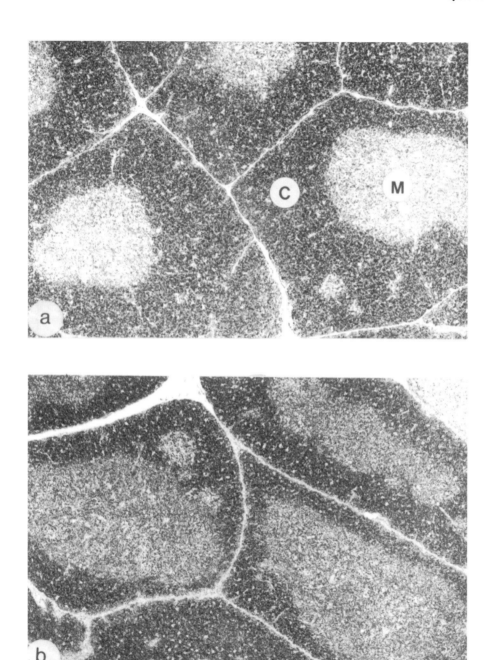

Figure 7.3   Thymus of control and TCDD-treated rat, 4 days following single oral exposure to 25 μg/kg body weight. (a) Control thymus with cortex (C) and medulla (M); (b) thymus of TCDD-treated animal showing atrophy of the cortex; (c) flow cytometric analysis of treated animals (shaded bar) in comparison with controls showing a significant reduction in cells with an immature phenotype (CD4/CD8 double positive cells) and no effect on cells with a more mature phenotype (CD3 high population). After: [42].

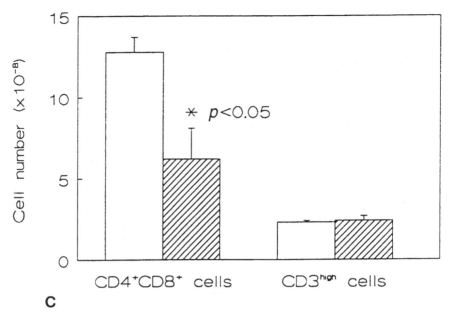

Figure 7.3 *Continued*

normally form the major epithelial component [27]. This indicates that the epithelial compartment can be a target for toxicity, which confirms data from *in vitro* experiments. **TCDD** appears to act primarily through a cytosolic aryl hydrocarbon (Ah) or TCDD receptor, which is present in relatively high concentration on thymic epithelium, although it is possible that some immunotoxic effects of this chemical are Ah-receptor independent.

Ammonia caramel

The compound **2-acetyl-4(5)-(1,2,3,4-tetrahydroxybutyl)imidazole (THI)** is used as a food colour additive, caramel colour III. **THI** induces a rapid reduction of B and T lymphocytes in peripheral blood and reduced lymphocyte numbers in the spleen and lymph nodes. In the thymus a decrease in the cortex over medulla ratio is seen. Moreover, a remarkable increase in cell density is observed in the medulla, caused by an increase of medullary thymocytes, in particular CD4 positive cells. Also, macrophages in the thymic cortex lose the expression of a phenotypic marker (recognized in the rat by the monoclonal antibody ED2). This loss of a cell surface antigen may be related to a diminished emigration of lymphocytes from the thymus into the periphery, resulting in immune suppression [28].

Cytostatic and immunosuppressive drugs

The cytostatic and immunosuppressive drug **azathioprine** produces atrophy of the thymus with histological features similar to those seen following exposure to organotins. In peripheral lymphoid organs, lymphocyte depletion of T-cell-dependent areas is observed. Another example is **5-fluorouracil**. Within 4 days of a single-dose exposure, a complete depletion of the bone marrow and the thymic cortex occurs. Subsequent recovery is almost complete by day 16, at which time there are many mitotic figures in the thymus indicative of a renewed functional activity. Thereafter the recovery shows an overshoot and the thymus weight can reach a value of about twice the 'normal-for-age' value. Changes in the spleen start at day 11 with a depletion in the PALS that is maximal at day 14, at which time the white pulp is hardly identifiable. Later on, the white pulp regains its original architecture, but with persistent low cellular density of the PALS. In the red pulp, increased haematopoiesis can be seen during the recovery of the bone marrow. This example illustrates the different changes that occur within various lymphoid organs with time after exposure and subsequent recovery.

Cyclosporine is a drug that is used widely as an immunosuppressant for organ transplantation and in the treatment of certain autoimmune diseases. In contrast to the above-mentioned effects on the thymic cortex, **cyclosporine** affects the thymic medulla [22]. There is a decrease of medullary interdigitating dendritic cells and more mature medium-sized lymphocytes. The outer medulla area is densely packed with small-sized cortical thymocytes and in effect there is a 'cortification' of the medulla. These changes are seen during continuous treatment and are reversible. About 2 to 3 weeks after discontinuation of treatment, a full recovery of the thymus is observed. The disappearance of interdigitating dendritic cells has been related to a disturbance in intrathymic selection of relevant (precursor) T cells, resulting in the emergence of autoimmune phenomena upon withdrawal of treatment.

UV-B light

The main effects of **UV-B** exposure are on Langerhans cells in the skin. It is suggested that these effects play a crucial role in the induction of immunosuppression by **UV light** [29]. The changes include a decrease in numbers of Langerhans cells and a change in their morphology and antigen-presenting function. After exposure, the cells are unable to present antigen in the normal way and the subsequent induction of T-cell differentiation is blocked. Keratinocytes are also affected by **UV light** and start to produce cytokines that influence immune reactivity. Finally, mast cells are directly influenced by **UV-B**, as these cells are present just beneath the basement membrane of the epidermis. Changes are dependent upon the dose of **UV-B** light. A low dose inhibits mast cell degranulation and this effect may underly the positive effect of **UV-B** exposure on patients with eczema or atopic dermatitis.

7.4.3 Hyperplasia/Hypersensitivity/Autoimmunity

Hexachlorobenzene (HCB)

HCB is a highly persistent environmental chemical that has been used in the past as a fungicide. Presently, emissions into the environment may occur due to its use as a chemical intermediate or as a by-product in chemical processes. **HCB** represents a well-characterized example of an agent which causes lymphoid hyperplasia in the rat. Prominent changes are the increase in weights of the spleen and lymph nodes. Histopathologically, the spleen shows hyperplasia of B lymphocytes in marginal zones and follicles. Lymph nodes are activated as shown by the appearance of secondary follicles and an increase in the number of high-endothelial venules in T-dependent areas (Figure 7.4). High-endothelial-like venules are also induced in the lung, in particular in Lewis strain rats (Figure 7.5). In addition, macrophage accumulations are found in lung alveoli. In function studies, cell-mediated immunity was enhanced and to

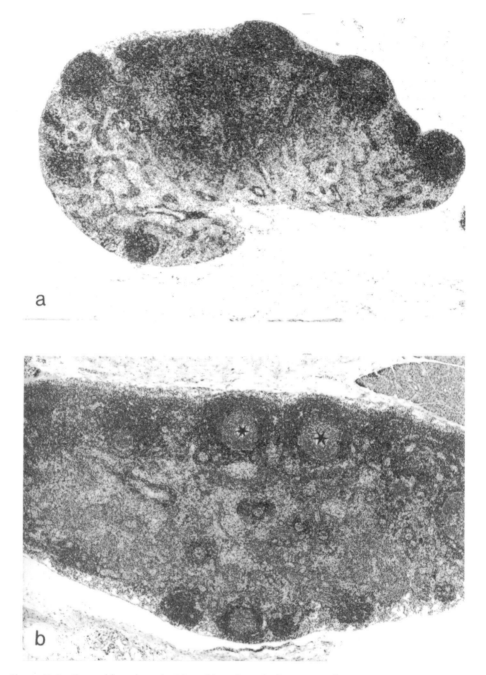

Figure 7.4 Control lymph node (a) and lymph node from a rat after exposure to hexachlorobenzene (b) showing activation as demonstrated by follicles with germinal centres (asterisks). There is also an increase of high-endothelial venules in the paracortex that cannot be seen clearly at this magnification.

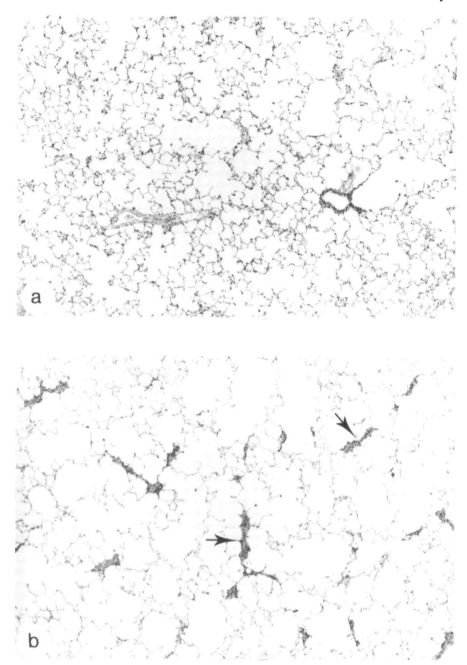

Figure 7.5   Control lung (a) and lung from a Lewis strain rat following hexachlorobenzene exposure (b) showing vessels with an appearance of high-endothelial venules (arrows).

an even larger extent an increase in humoral immunity was noted. More recent studies indicate that the immunostimulatory effect of **HCB** in the rat may be related to autoimmunity. Wistar rats treated with **HCB** produce antibodies to autoantigens: IgM, but not IgG, levels against single-stranded DNA, native DNA, rat IgG (representing rheumatoid factor), and bromelain-treated mouse erythrocytes (that expose

223

phosphatidylcholine as a major autoantigen) were elevated. It is suggested that **HCB** activates a recently described B-cell subset committed to the production of these autoantibodies and associated with various systemic autoimmune diseases [30].

Metal ions

Metal ions can initiate hypersensitivity reactions [5]. Examples are **nickel (Ni)**, **beryllium (Be)**, **mercury (Hg)**, **lead (Pb)** and **chromium (Cr)**. The delayed-type hypersensitivity response, with infiltration by lymphocytes and macrophages, apparently reflects a T-lymphocyte response towards the metal salt. Occupational exposure to **Be** can result in a hypersensitivity pneumonitis with pulmonary granuloma formation (berylliosis). The granulomatous hypersensitivity reaction reflects a T-cell reaction to the metal.

Adverse reactions induced by heavy metals can also be secondary to immune-complex formation. An example is **mercuric chloride ($HgCl_2$)**-induced glomerulonephropathy in the Brown Norway rat. This strain is peculiar among rats, by producing glomerulonephritis after $HgCl_2$ administration due to local fixation of autoantibody to the glomerular basement membrane and subsequent inflammation (Figure 7.6). Similar to the immune-complex glomerulonephritis in other rat strains after $HgCl_2$ exposure, histology of glomeruli shows infiltration by polymorphonuclear granulocytes. The interference by $HgCl_2$ in the balance of immunoregulatory T cells in the Brown Norway rat results in polyclonal stimulation of B lymphocytes that subsequently start to produce autoantibodies to the glomerular basement membrane. This interference in immune function is evident not only from the autoimmune kidney lesion, but also from changes in the spleen and lymph nodes. Spleen weight is increased markedly, and histologically, an expansion of follicles and marginal zones, resulting from lymphocyte hyperplasia, is observed. The PALS is either relatively unaffected or shows some decrease in cellularity.

Isocyanates

Some isocyanates, e.g. **toluene diisocyanate**, induce allergic respiratory disease, also diagnosed as occupational asthma, with bronchial obstruction and bronchial hyperreactivity. Most commonly, they are immediate-onset reactions although late-onset reactions do occur. Histology shows accumulation of leucocytes in the bronchial mucosa, mucus production, epithelial damage and connective tissue increase.

Drugs

Tissue damage following drug treatment or abuse can be the consequence of a direct effect of the drug on cell metabolism (e.g. hepatotoxic and nephrotoxic effects). Allergic or autoimmune reactions are characterized by direct immunological responses to drug determinants or drug-altered self components. The list of drugs and other xenobiotics that can elicit immune responses resulting in immunopathological changes is ever-increasing and is not discussed in detail here [5,7]. Most of the chemicals involved are low-molecular-weight compounds (100 to 500 Da) that act as haptens and need to be coupled to endogenous carrier proteins to become immunogenic. The elicitation of an immune reaction depends largely on the capacity of the compound to form immunogenic hapten−carrier conjugates with endogenous

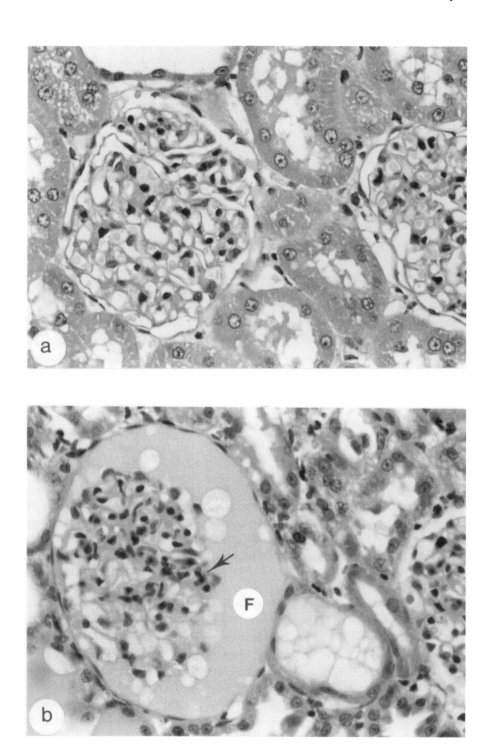

Figure 7.6 *Continued*

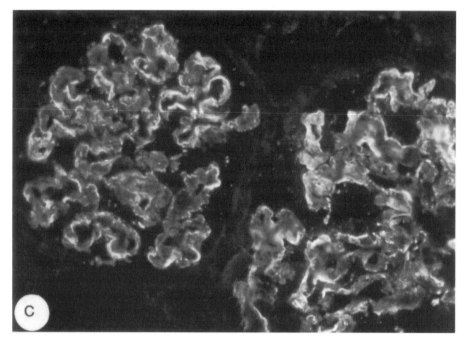

Figure 7.6 Autoimmune reaction in kidney of Brown Norway rat after HgCl$_2$ injections. Light microscopy of control kidney (a) and kidney of treated animal showing inflammatory cells (arrow) in the glomerulus, and as a result of this glomerulonephritis the appearance of protein-rich fluid (F) in Bowman's space (b); immunofluorescence microscopy of treated kidney showing the presence of immunoglobulin deposits along the glomerular capillary walls (c).

proteins. In the subsequent immune response, the compound in the native, unconjugated form serves as the target.

The pathological manifestations of drug hypersensitivity vary widely and include systemic anaphylaxis, haemolytic anaemia, serum sickness, vasculitis, urticaria, contact dermatitis, hepatitis and nephritis. Haemolytic anaemia results from different mechanisms including attachment of the drug to erythrocytes with subsequent antibody binding (e.g. **penicillin** and **cephalosporin**), attachment of drug-anti-drug antibody immune complexes after complement fixation to C3b receptors of the erythrocyte (e.g. **phenacetin** and **quinine**), and modification of self antigen with autoantibody generation and fixation to the cell (e.g. the Rhesus [Rh] antigen modified by *α*-**methyldopa**). In the latter mechanism, the drug itself is not directly involved in the antibody–erythrocyte reaction. This mechanism is very common in drug-induced allergy and antibodies in this situation are often directed to the Rh antigen. Another example of an autoimmune lesion due to drug exposure is **halothane** hepatitis, in which halothane-altered liver cells form the target of hypersensitivity reactions.

7.4.4 Neoplasia

Haematopoietic cell tumours, most frequently emerging in lymphoid organs, include leukaemias (in bone marrow or blood) and lymphomas (in lymphoid organs or extranodal tissue). Tumours of parenchymal cells in lymphoid tissues include thymoma (thymic epithelial cells), haemangiosarcoma (endothelial cell tumour, mainly in spleen and lymph nodes), and tumours of mesenchymal cells such as splenic sarcoma. Tumours of the MPS or tissue macrophages and tumours of mast cells can occur at various locations in the body; these are designated as histiocytic lymphoma (also called fibrous histiocytoma or histiocytic sarcoma), and mastocytoma (mast cell sarcoma), respectively [18, 21, 23].

Viruses capable of inducing neoplasia

Lymphotropic viruses cause leukaemias and lymphomas. Examples in man include **Epstein–Barr virus** (EBV) causing Burkitt-type lymphoblastic lymphoma, and **human T-lymphotropic virus type 1** (HTLV-1) causing T-cell leukaemia and lymphoma. Examples in the mouse are **Abelson murine leukaemia virus** and **radiation leukaemia virus**, both of which cause thymic lymphomas. Murine leukaemia viruses can also induce leukaemia in the rat. Virus-induced lymphoid malignancies are associated frequently with chromosomal translocations and oncogene activation.

Irradiation

Ionizing irradiation and **UV-B** light can induce lymphoma in mice and rats. The mouse is generally more susceptible to radiation-induced lymphoproliferative disease than the rat. Because of the immunosuppressive effects of these types of radiation, a role for oncogenic viruses in the aetiology of these tumours cannot be excluded.

Carcinogenic chemicals

A number of chemicals induce lymphoma and leukaemia. Examples include: **methylcholanthrene** in mice; the antitumour drug, **4(5)-(3,3-dimethyl-1-triazeno)imidazole-5(4)-carboxamide**, and the immunosuppressive drug **azathioprine** in Sprague–Dawley rats; **alkyl-nitrosourea** compounds and **alkylbenz[a]anthracenes** in Sprague–Dawley and Fischer rats. **Urethane** induces thymoma in Buffalo and Fischer rats.

Diet

Tumours of lymphoid cells may also be induced by dietary factors. For example, a **magnesium-deficient diet** has been associated with thymic lymphomas in Sprague–Dawley rats. This deficiency may underlie the genesis of lymphoma by the **alkyl-nitrosamide** compounds.

Immunological reactions

Atypical immunological reactions such as (pseudo)-graft-versus-host disease, in which there is lymphocyte stimulation under conditions of a marginally functional immune system, can result in lymphoproliferative disease. This type of induced lymphoid neoplasm has a predilection for the thymus, since developing T cells undergo proliferation in the thymus during generation of immune competence.

The status of immunodeficiency

This has been related to tumourigenesis. This relationship is based on the phenomenon of 'immune surveillance' that assumes a continuous guarding and elimination of potentially neoplastic (e.g. uncontrolled proliferating) cells in the body by the immune system. The importance of immune surveillance has been confirmed for antigenic tumours such as those induced by chemical carcinogens, viruses and ionizing or UV radiation. The relevance of immune surveillance in neoplasia has also been supported by epidemiological studies, which show an increased incidence of some forms of malignancy in patients with immunodeficiency, e.g. in organ transplant patients receiving immunosuppressive drugs.

7.5 Testing for Toxicity

7.5.1 *Methods*

A wide variety of methods for assessment of immune function is available for most species used in toxicity studies. A cornerstone of immunotoxicity testing in rodents is histopathological examination of lymphoid organs, particularly for those xenobiotics where the immune system is a passive target [20, 23, 24]. We survey here some morphological techniques used in the analysis of lymphoid tissue.

Tissue sampling

To obtain an acceptable overview of lymphoid organs, representative tissue from primary and secondary organs and internal/external sites should be sampled. The whole body and a selection of organs are weighed. In sampling lymph nodes, a selection is made dependent upon the route of exposure. For instance, lymph nodes draining the mucosa are invariably in a stimulated state due to intake of antigen via food and inhaled air. Conversely, popliteal and axillary lymph nodes are often not stimulated and thus provide information about the resting state of the immune system. Bone marrow is collected from the femur and/or the sternum and either processed into histological sections (with or without decalcification) or processed as cell preparations to provide information on cellularity. GALT requires processing into a so-called 'Swiss-roll' before fixation.

Conventional histology

The most frequently employed method is fixation in 10 per cent buffered formalin, paraffin embedding and staining of 6 μm-thick sections with haematoxylin and eosin. Changes in tissue architecture and the morphology of cells in various compartments of the lymphoid organs and tissues can be examined in this way. The detection of chemically induced effects can be enhanced by the use of additional stains, such as Giemsa, for improved cell morphology, reticulin for organ structure and methyl green pyronin for cells with high levels of protein production, e.g. plasma cells. For better cytomorphological detail (e.g. for the examination of bone marrow) semi-thin sections (about 1 μm) are prepared using harder embedding media than paraffin, such as the plastic glycol methacrylate.

Immunohistochemistry

This is used for the immunological phenotyping of cells (e.g. helper T cells and cytotoxic T lymphocytes) using specific antibodies against cell membrane markers, the study of cytoplasmic antigens (e.g. immunoglobulins or lysozyme), or the assessment of immune-complex components in inflammatory lesions. Cell surface antigens, which are present only in small amounts, are best preserved in frozen tissue sections. Mild acetone or methanol fixation permits the preservation of both tissue architecture and antigenicity of the markers analysed. For most cytoplasmic markers, formalin-fixed paraffin sections may be used. In particular, fixation with formalin containing mercuric chloride (sublimate) offers good preservation of intracellular antigens. A wide variety of immunohistochemical procedures use enzymatic (e.g. peroxidase) detection reactions or either gold or fluorochromes (e.g. FITC) as labelling substances.

Electron microscopy

This is used to study subcellular morphology. For optimal preservation of cellular architecture and avoidance of artefacts, rapid fixation of tissue in special fixatives such as a mixture of glutaraldehyde and paraformaldehyde is required. To achieve rapid penetration of the fixative, the specimen should be sectioned (quickly) into small pieces (1 to 2 mm) before fixation; *in vivo* perfusion with the fixative is recommended.

Hybridohistochemistry (in situ hybridization)

The analysis of DNA and RNA segments has only recently been introduced into toxicological pathology. The method can be performed on tissue sections using DNA or RNA probes complementary to the gene segment under study combined with immunochemical and/or enzymatic detection. DNA segments can be analysed in formalin-fixed tissue sections, whereas RNA is visualized primarily on frozen tissue sections. In cases where localization is not required, DNA and RNA segments can be detected with greater sensitivity in tissue digests using spot blots. Also Southern and Northern blotting are used for the detection of DNA and RNA, respectively. The polymerase chain reaction (PCR) is important; this technique is based upon the strong amplification of the segment to be analysed using DNA polymerase and primers complementary to the DNA segment of interest. Recently, a modified PCR has become available for use on tissue sections, the so-called '*in situ* PCR method'. In the toxicology setting, hybridohistochemistry for DNA and RNA segments has found application in the detection of modified DNA segments (mainly in genotoxicity). RNA analysis has found application in studies on cytokine and growth factor expression. Interference by toxic substances in such processes has been demonstrated for **steroid hormones** and **organotin compounds**.

Cell suspension analysis

Organ cell suspensions are used to determine total nucleated cell counts as well as differential cell counts. Quantitative assessment of lymphocyte populations can be performed readily by analytical flow cytometry. Lymphoid cells are isolated from tissues by mechanical disaggregation. Enzymatic digestion (e.g. by collagenase) can be used for the isolation of cells that are more adherent to the tissue matrix, such as macrophages. For immunophenotyping of cells in suspension, flow cytometry combines the simultaneous detection of cell size and (one or more) immunolabelling signals and thereby provides an important quantitative supplement to the information provided by histological analyses.

In vitro assays

These have recently assumed greater importance in assessment of immunotoxicity. *In vitro* experiments are not generally used in the screening of compounds for potential immunotoxicity. Their main value is in studies of immunotoxic mechanisms. *In vitro* studies also enable evaluation of immunotoxicity in man. Results of *in vitro* studies with human and animal cells, in combination with *in vivo* data of animal studies may be of particular help in predicting the human response to the compound under investigation.

7.5.2 *Immune Suppression/Stimulation;* In vivo *Approaches*

In evaluating the toxicity of a compound in animals, most regulatory authorities require, following an initial evaluation of acute toxicity, multidose testing according to the OECD guideline No. 407 (Repeated Dose Oral Toxicity–Rodent: 28-day or 14-day study). Subsequent to guideline No. 407, proposals have been made for follow-up studies in cases where there is an expectation of longer exposure, or in cases where there is a suspicion of toxicity based upon structural similarity with other known immunotoxicants. These include 90-day oral toxicity studies, chronic studies, or reproduction studies. Although these guidelines include examination of more parameters of the immune system than does guideline No. 407, it is questionable whether potential immunotoxicity is addressed adequately. Tiered approaches have therefore been proposed.

Tiered approaches

A tiered approach can be used to make a suitable selection from the overwhelming numbers of assays available. Generally, the objective of the first tier is to identify potential immunotoxicants. If potential immunotoxicity is identified, a second tier of testing is performed to confirm and characterize further the changes observed. Third-tier investigations include special studies on the mechanism of action of the compound. In such studies, *in vitro* assays are of great value (e.g. to elucidate the pathophysiological behaviour of cells in suspension under the influence of the toxic compound, or the interactions with humoral mediators of the immune system). Such studies can be extended using molecular biological techniques to evaluate the effect on gene expression at the RNA level. *In vitro* studies also offer the opportunity to perform comparative studies using human tissue.

Two examples of tiered approaches are described. The first was developed in 1980 at the National Institute of Public Health and the Environment, The Netherlands, and has been updated regularly [12, 13]. It is based on OECD guideline No. 407, and therefore performed in the rat using at least three dose levels; the maximum tolerated dose is used as the high dose. Immunotoxicity is evaluated such that other manifestations of toxicity are not compromised. There is no immunization or challenge with an infectious agent. The first tier comprises general parameters including conventional haematology, serum immunoglobulin concentrations, bone marrow cellularity, weight and histology of lymphoid organs (thymus, spleen, lymph nodes, MALT), flow cytometric analysis of spleen cells and possibly immunophenotyping of tissue sections. This approach has been used for the immunotoxic evaluation of pesticides [31]. Out of 18 pesticides that were selected at random, 7 showed no, or only marginal, effects. Six chemicals (including **hexachlorobenzene**) exhibited immunotoxicity at similar dose levels to those which caused toxic effects on other organ systems, and 5 chemicals (including **tributyltin oxide**) exhibited immune parameters as the most sensitive parameter of toxicity. Lymphoid organ assessment proved to be an accurate indicator of immune toxicity for 7 of these 11 chemicals, but was not informative for the other materials. Thus, in this tiered approach, the evaluation of lymphoid organs represents a valuable parameter in the identification of potential immunotoxicants.

The US National Toxicology Program has developed a tiered approach, originally in mice, that is linked closely with the standard protocol for subchronic oral toxicity and carcinogenicity studies [14]. Routinely, a 90-day exposure period is adopted, but 14- and 30-day exposure periods have also been used, at dose levels that have no effect on body weight or other toxicological endpoints. Thus, compounds are identified for which the immune system represents the most sensitive target organ system. Tier one includes conventional haematology; lymphoid organ weight; cellularity and histology of the spleen, thymus and lymph nodes; *ex vivo* splenic IgM-antibody plaque-forming cell assay following sheep erythrocyte immunization; *in vitro* lymphocyte proliferation after stimulation with mitogens and allogeneic cells; and an *in vitro* assay for natural killer (NK) cell activity. In an adapted form of this approach, 51 different chemicals were evaluated that had been selected on the basis of structural relationships with previously identified immunotoxic chemicals [15]. The splenic IgM plaque-forming cell response and cell surface marker analyses showed the highest accuracy for identification of potential immunotoxicity. Lymphoid organs proved to be comparatively insensitive parameters, presumably due to the low exposure concentrations used.

7.5.3 *Allergy*

The phenomenon of contact sensitization was investigated first in the guinea pig and until recently this has been the species of choice for predictive testing. Many guinea pig test methods are available, the most frequently employed being the guinea pig maximization test and the occluded patch test of Buehler. Although details vary, the principles of guinea pig sensitization testing are common to all methods. Animals are exposed to the test material by topical or intradermal administration, or by a combination of both. In the more sensitive assays, such as the guinea pig maximization test, adjuvant (Freund's complete adjuvant) is used to potentiate immune responses to the test material. Control animals are treated identically but with the relevant vehicle alone. Subsequently, test and control guinea pigs are challenged with a subirritant concentration of the chemical and responses measured as a function of erythema and/or oedema provoked at the site of contact. Skin sensitizing potential is determined usually from the percentage of test animals exhibiting a measurable challenge-induced cutaneous reaction. Such guinea pig tests have been used widely and have served toxicologists well as a means of identifying and classifying skin sensitizing chemicals. However, guinea pig methods are not without limitations and in recent years there has been proposed a variety of alternative murine test methods [32]. In 1986, Gad and his colleagues [33] described the development and validation of a mouse ear swelling test (MEST). In this method, skin sensitizing activity is determined by measurement of challenge-induced increases in the ear thickness of previously sensitized animals. Despite the use of a rigorous induction procedure, the sensitivity of the MEST has been questioned. More recently a modified version of the method, the non-invasive mouse ear swelling assay (MESA), has been reported [34] which, unlike the MEST, does not require the use of adjuvant and which employs instead mice fed on diets rich in vitamin A, a potentiator of cell-mediated immune function.

Other approaches to the analysis of changes which characterize the elicitation phase of contact hypersensitivity have been proposed. Included here is evaluation of the mononuclear cell infiltration associated with dermal hypersensitivity reactions. In addition, it may be possible in some instances to measure systemically the local elicitation of cutaneous responses. Thus, contact hypersensitivity has been shown to result in increased serum concentrations of interleukin 6, acute phase proteins and histamine [32].

Another strategy is to measure events induced during the sensitization, rather than elicitation, phase of contact allergy, following first exposure to the test material. The induction phase of skin sensitization is characterized by lymphocyte activation and proliferation in lymph nodes draining the site of exposure. The murine local lymph node assay seeks to identify chemicals with the potential to cause contact sensitization on the basis of this response [35]. Mice are exposed topically to the test material and proliferative responses provoked in draining lymph nodes measured by incorporation of radiolabelled thymidine. This method has been the subject of extensive comparisons with guinea pig tests, and of interlaboratory validation exercises, and has been found to offer a viable alternative for predictive testing [36].

Guinea pig tests and newer approaches developed in mice, such as ear swelling tests and the local lymph node assay, provide the toxicologist with the tools to assess skin sensitization hazard. The situation with respect to sensitization of the respiratory tract is very different. There are, as yet, no well-validated or widely accepted methods available for the identification of chemical respiratory allergens.

The progress that has been made in the development of animal models for the investigation of chemical respiratory allergy has been achieved primarily in the guinea pig. Of particular importance has been the contribution made by Karol and her colleagues [37]. Guinea pigs sensitized by inhalation are challenged with the same chemical in the form of a hapten–protein conjugate. It has been demonstrated also that significant changes in pulmonary function can be provoked in dermally sensitized guinea pigs by inhalation challenge with the free chemical [38]. Such methods are both costly and time-consuming and require the use of sophisticated inhalation facilities together with the instrumentation necessary to monitor changes in respiratory function. Recently, a tiered approach to investigating respiratory sensitization potential in guinea pigs has been proposed in which the first step is analysis of physicochemical properties and the second, measurement *in vitro* of reactivity with protein [39]. The third and fourth tiers measure, respectively, the ability of the chemical to induce antibody responses following repeated subcutaneous injection and to elicit changes in the breathing pattern of sensitized animals following intratracheal instillation. Attractive as this approach is, it has to be borne in mind that chemical allergens other than those capable of causing sensitization of the respiratory tract will form stable associations with protein and stimulate antibody reponses. Progress has been made with guinea pig models. However, their cost at present prohibits the routine use of inhalation methods in the context of predictive testing.

An alternative approach described recently is the mouse IgE test, a method in which respiratory sensitizing potential is measured as a function of changes induced in the serum concentration of IgE following topical exposure of mice to the test material. To date, those chemicals which are contact allergens, but which are known or suspected not to cause sensitization of the respiratory tract, have been found not to stimulate a substantial increase in serum IgE. In contrast, confirmed chemical respiratory sensitizers induce elevated concentrations of this immunoglobulin in mice [40].

7.5.4 *Autoimmunity*

There are a number of experimental animal models of human autoimmune diseases. Such models comprise both spontaneous pathology, such as systemic autoimmune phenomena in the $(NZB \times NZW)F_1$ mouse or MRL/*lpr* mouse, and autoimmune phenomena induced by experimental immunization with a cross-reactive autoantigen. These models are applied widely in the preclinical evaluation of immunosuppressive drugs. Very few studies have addressed the potential of these models for assessment of whether a xenobiotic exacerbates induced, or congenital, autoimmunity. **Hexachlorobenzene**, which produces immunostimulation in rats, has been tested in a rat model of experimental allergic encephalomyelitis induced by immunization with guinea pig myelin and in the rat model of H37RA adjuvant-induced arthritis. The severity of encephalomyelitis was enhanced strongly, whereas the arthritis was suppressed. This example illustrates that this chemical has immunotoxic effects that are biologically relevant and also that models of autoimmunity are an important aspect of immunotoxicity testing.

The popliteal lymph node assay in mice [41] is based upon the hyperplasia (increase in weight) of lymph nodes in graft-versus-host reactions or pseudo-graft-versus-host reactions, and has been modified to assess the immunomodulatory potential of drugs. The test substance is injected subcutaneously into one hind footpad, and the contralateral side is either untreated or inoculated with vehicle alone. Comparison of popliteal lymph nodes from both sides allows the effect of the test drug to be measured. Apart from differences in weight, histological evidence of *in vivo* immunostimulatory activity can be discerned. These pseudo-graft-versus-host reactions with follicular hyperplasia have been documented in mice for drugs such as **diphenylhydantoin**, **D-penicillamine** and **streptozotocin**. A positive outcome in this assay is considered to correspond with the potential of drugs to produce autoimmunity in man. The assay is not universally applicable, however, due primarily to false-negative results. Some drugs, such as **procainamide**, are known to cause autoimmune-like responses in man, but are negative in the assay. This is presumably attributable to pharmacokinetic factors and may be minimized by testing metabolites.

7.6 Conclusions

7.6.1 *Extrapolation of Immunotoxicity in Animals to Man*

Assessment of immune status in man is performed mainly using peripheral blood (serum or plasma for humoral substances like immunoglobulins/antibodies and complement, and blood mononuclear cells for lymphocyte subset composition and function). These investigations usually derive from methods used to investigate patients suspected of congenital or acquired immunodeficiency disease. Such approaches are revised regularly by national and international committees, and are not discussed in detail here. They require modification when used in screening of cohort populations for suspected immunotoxicity. The strategy in screening for immunotoxic effects after (accidental) exposure to environmental pollutants or other toxicants is much dependent on circumstances. The identification of immunotoxicity of a particular xenobiotic in man is extremely difficult and often impossible, due largely to the presence of various confounding factors of endogenous or exogenous origin that influence the response of individuals to toxic damage. The identification of potential immunotoxic xenobiotics is presently undertaken primarily in controlled studies in rodents and other experimental animals. *In vivo* exposure studies present, in this regard, the optimal approach to estimate the immunotoxic potential of a compound. This is due to the multifactorial and complex nature of the immune system and of immune responses. *Ex vivo* and *in vitro* studies are of increasing value in the elucidation of mechanisms of immunotoxicity. Based upon data in rodent immunotoxicity studies, a subsequent extrapolation to man is attempted. In risk assessment, the no-effect level can be based on parameters determined in relevant models, such as host resistance assays and *in vivo* assessment of hypersensitivity reactions and antibody production. Usually a factor of 10 is applied in the extrapolation of data from experimental animals to the human, and an additional factor of 10 for differences in susceptibility between individuals. A further safety factor can be used to compensate for the high sensitivity of the developing immune system *in utero*, in cases where data are not available on peri- or postnatal animal exposure. The relevance of this approach to risk assessment requires confirmation by studies in man. Such studies should combine the identification and measurement of the toxicant, epidemiological data and immune status assessments.

References

1. BERLIN, A., DEAN, J., DRAPER, M.H., SMITH, E.M.B. and SPREAFICO, F. (Eds) (1987) *Immunotoxicology*, Dordrecht: Martinus Nijhoff Publishers.
2. VOS, J.G. (1977) Immune suppression as related to toxicology, *CRC Critical Reviews in Toxicology*, **5**, 67–101.
3. DAYAN, A.D., HERTEL, R.F., HESELTINE, E., KAZANTIS, G., SMITH, E.M. and VAN DER VENNE, M.T. (Eds) (1990) *Immunotoxicity of Metals and Immunotoxicology*, New York: Plenum Press.
4. DEAN, J.H., LUSTER, M.I., MUNSON, A.E. and KIMBER, I. (Eds) (1994) *Immunotoxicology and Immunopharmacology*, New York: Raven Press.
5. DESCOTES, J. (1986) *Immunotoxicology of Drugs and Chemicals*, Amsterdam: Elsevier.
6. GIBSON, G.G., HUBBARD, R. and PARKE, D.V. (1983) *Immunotoxicology*, London: Academic Press.

7. KAMMÜLLER, M.E., BLOKSMA, N. and SEINEN, W. (Eds) (1989) *Autoimmunity and Toxicology. Immune Dysregulation Induced by Drugs and Chemicals*, Amsterdam: Elsevier Science Publishers.

8. MILLER, K., TURK, J.L. and NICKLIN, S. (Eds) (1992) *Principles and Practice of Immunotoxicology*, Oxford: Blackwell Scientific Publishers.

9. NEWCOMBE, D.S., ROSE, N.R. and BLOOM, J.C. (Eds) (1992) *Clinical Immunotoxicology*, New York: Raven Press.

10. Subcommittee on Immunotoxicology (1992) *Biologic Markers in Immunotoxicology*, Washington DC: National Academy Press.

11. IPCS (1986) *Immunotoxicology. Development of Predictive Testing for Determining the Immunotoxic Potential of Chemicals. Report of a Technical Review Meeting*, London, November 3–5.

12. VOS, J.G. (1980) Immunotoxicity assessment: screening and function studies, *Archives of Toxicology*, Suppl. **4**, 95–108.

13. VAN LOVEREN, H. and VOS, J.G. (1988) Immunotoxicological considerations: a practical approach of immunotoxicity assessment in the rat, in DAYAN, T.D. and PAINE, A.J. (Eds), *Advances in Applied Toxicology*, pp. 143–163, London: Taylor and Francis.

14. LUSTER, M.I., MUNSON, A.E., THOMAS, P.T., HOLSAPPLE, M.P., FENTERS, J.D., WHITE, K.L., LAUDER, L.D., GERMOLEC, D.R., ROSENTHAL, G.J. and DEAN, J.H. (1988) Methods evaluation. Development of a testing battery to assess chemical-induced immunotoxicity: National Toxicology Program's guidelines for immunotoxicity evaluation in mice, *Fundamental and Applied Toxicology*, **10**, 2–19.

15. LUSTER, M.I., PORTIER, C., PAIT, D.G., WHITE, K.L., GENNING, C., MUNSON, A.E. and ROSENTHAL, G.J. (1992) Risk assessment in immunotoxicology. I. Sensitivity and predictability of immune tests, *Fundamental and Applied Toxicology*, **18**, 200–210.

16. GOPINATH, C., PRENTICE, D.E. and LEWIS, D.J. (1987) The lymphoid system, in *Atlas of Experimental Toxicological Pathology*, pp. 122–137, Boston: MTP Press.

17. GREAVES, P. (1990) *Histopathology of Preclinical Toxicity Studies: Interpretation and Relevance in Drug Safety Evaluation*, Amsterdam: Elsevier.

18. JONES, J.C., WARD, J.M., MOHR, U. and HUNT, R.D. (Eds) (1990) *Hemopoietic System, ILSI Monograph*, Berlin: Springer-Verlag.

19. KRAJNC-FRANKEN, M.A.M., VAN LOVEREN, H., SCHUURMAN, H.-J. and VOS, J.G. (1990) The immune system as a target for toxicity. A tiered approach of testing, with special emphasis on histopathology, in DAYAN, A.D., HERTEL, R.F., HESELTINE, E., KAZANTIS, G., SMITH, E.M. and VAN DER VENNE, M.T. (Eds), *Immunotoxicity of Metals and Immunotoxicology*, pp. 241–264, New York: Plenum Press.

20. KUPER, C.F., SCHUURMAN, H.-J. and VOS, J.G. (1994) Pathology in immunotoxicology, in BURLESON, G., MUNSON, A. and DEAN, J. (Eds), *Modern Methods in Immunotoxicology*, New York: Wiley.

21. MOHR, U., DUNGWORTH, D.L. and CAPEN, C.C. (Eds) (1992) *Pathobiology of the Aging Rat*, Vol. 1, Washington DC: ILSI Press.

22. SCHUURMAN, H.-J., VAN LOVEREN, H., ROZING, J., VAN DIJK, A. and VOS, J.G. (1990) Cyclosporin and the rat thymus. An immuno-histochemical study, *Thymus*, **16**, 235–254.

23. SCHUURMAN, H.-J., KRAJNC-FRANKEN, M.A.M., KUPER, C.F., VAN LOVEREN, H. and VOS, J.G. (1991) Immune system, in HASCHEK, W.M. and ROUSSEAUX, C.G. (Eds), *Handbook of Toxicologic Pathology*, pp. 421–487, San Diego: Academic Press.

24. VOS, J.G. and KRAJNC-FRANKEN, M.A.M. (1990) Toxic effects on the immune system, rat, in JONES, T.C., WARD, J.M., MOHR, U. and HUNT, R.D. (Eds), *Hemopoietic System, ILSI Monograph*, pp. 168–181, Berlin: Springer-Verlag.

25. PENNINKS, A.H., SNOEIJ, N.J., PIETERS, R.H.H. and SEINEN, W. (1990) Effect of organotin compounds on lymphoid organs and lymphoid functions: an overview, in DAYAN, A.D., HERTEL, R.F., HESELTINE, E., KAZANTZIS, G., SMITH, E.M. and VAN DER VENNE, M.T. (Eds), *Immunotoxicity of Metals and Immunotoxicology*, pp. 191–207, New York: Plenum Press.

26. VOS, J.G., VAN LOVEREN, H. and SCHUURMAN, H.J. (1991) Immunotoxicity of dioxin: immune function and host resistance in laboratory animals and humans, in GALLO, M.A., SCHEUPLEIN, R.J. and VAN DER HEIJDEN, K.A. (Eds), *Banbury Report 35: Biological Basis for Risk Assessment of Dioxins and Related Compounds*, pp. 79–93, Cold Spring Harbor Laboratory Press.

27. DE WAAL, E.J., SCHUURMAN, H.J., RADEMAKERS, L.H.P.M., VAN LOVEREN, H. and VOS, J.G. (1993) Ultrastructure of the cortical epithelium of the rat thymus after *in vivo* exposure to 2,3,7,8-tetrachlorodibenzo-*p*-dioxin (TCDD), *Archives of Toxicology*, **67**, 558–564.

28. HOUBEN, G.F., VAN DEN BERG, H., KUIJPERS, M.H.M., LAM, B.W., VAN LOVEREN, H., SEINEN, W. and PENNINKS, A.H. (1992) Effects of the color additive Caramel Color III and 2-acetyl-4(5)-tetrahydroxybutyl-imidazole (THI) on the immune system of rats, *Toxicology and Applied Pharmacology*, **113**, 43–54.

29. GOETTSCH, W., GARSSEN, J., DE GRUIJL, F.R. and VAN LOVEREN, H. (1993) UV-B and the immune system: a review with special emphasis on T-cell mediated immunity, *Thymus*, **21**, 93–114.

30. SCHIELEN, P., SCHOO, W., TEKSTRA, J., OOSTERMEIJER, H.H., SEINEN, W. and BLOKSMA, N. (1993) Autoimmune effects of hexachlorobenzene in the rat, *Toxicology and Applied Pharmacology*, **122**, 233–243.

31. VOS, J.G. and KRAJNC, E.I. (1983) Immunotoxicity of pesticides, in HAYES, A.W., SCHNELL, R.C. and MIYA, T.S. (Eds), *Developments in the Science and Practice of Toxicology*, pp. 229–240, Amsterdam: Elsevier Science Publications.

32. KIMBER, I. and DEARMAN, R.J. (1993) Approaches to the identification and classification of chemical allergens in mice, *Journal of Pharmacological and Toxicological Methods*, **29**, 11–16.

33. GAD, S.C., DUNN, B.J., DOBBS, D.W., REILLY, C. and WALSH, R.D. (1986) Development and validation of an alternative dermal sensitization test: the mouse ear swelling test (MEST), *Toxicology and Applied Pharmacology*, **84**, 93–114.

34. THORNE, P.S., HAWK, C., KALISZEWKI, S.D. and GUINEY, P.D. (1991) The noninvasive mouse ear swelling assay. I. Refinements for detecting weak contact sensitizers, *Fundamental and Applied Toxicology*, **17**, 790–806.

35. KIMBER, I. and WEISENBERGER, C. (1989) A murine local lymph node assay for the identification of contact allergens. Assay development and results of an initial validation study, *Archives of Toxicology*, **63**, 274–282.

36. KIMBER, I. and BASKETTER, D.A. (1992) The murine local lymph node assay: a commentary on collaborative studies and new directions, *Food and Chemical Toxicology*, **30**, 165–169.

37. KAROL, M.W. (1992) Occupational asthma and allergic reactions to inhaled compounds, in MILLER, K., TURK, J. and NICKLIN, S. (Eds) *Principles and Practice of Immunotoxicology*, pp. 228–241, Oxford: Blackwell Scientific Publications.

38. BOTHAM, P.A., RATTRAY, N.J., WOODCOCK, D.R., WALSH, S.T. and HEXT, P.M. (1989) The induction of respiratory allergy in guinea-pigs following intradermal injection of trimellitic anhydride: a comparison with the response to 2,4-dinitrochlorobenzene, *Toxicology Letters*, **47**, 25–39.

39. SARLO, K. and CLARK, E.D. (1992) A tier approach for evaluating the respiratory allergenicity of low molecular weight chemicals, *Fundamental and Applied Toxicology*, **18**, 107–114.

40. DEARMAN, R.J., BASKETTER, D.A. and KIMBER, I. (1992) Variable effects of

chemical allergens on serum IgE concentration in mice. Preliminary evaluation of a novel approach to the identification of respiratory sensitizers. *Journal of Applied Toxicology*, **12**, 317–323.

41. GLEICHMANN, E., VOHR, H.-W., STRINGER, C., NUYENS, J. and GLEICHMANN, H. (1989) Testing the sensitization of T cell to chemicals. From murine graft-versus-host (GVH) reactions to chemical-induced GVH-like immunological diseases, in KAMMÜLLER, M.E., BLOKSMA, N. and SEINEN, W. (Eds), *Autoimmunity and Toxicology. Immune Dysregulation Induced by Drugs and Chemicals*, pp. 364–390, Amsterdam: Elsevier.

42. DE HEER, C., VERLAAN, A.P.J., PENNINKS, A.H., VOS, J.G., SCHUURMAN, H.-J. and VAN LOVEREN, H. (1994) Time course of 2,3,7,8-tetrachlorodibenzo-*p*-dioxin (TCDD) induced thymic atrophy in the Wistar rat. *Toxicology and Applied Pharmacology*, **128**, 97–104.

8

The Musculoskeletal System

RUTH M. LIGHTFOOT

8.1 Introduction

The musculoskeletal system comprises a large part of total body mass and weight but examination of this system during the conduct of routine toxicology studies is relatively cursory. This reflects the fact that induced lesions of muscle, cartilage and bone are an uncommon event compared with the frequency with which changes are observed in organs such as the liver or kidney, and that metabolic activation is not believed to be a feature of the musculoskeletal system. Detailed examination of the musculoskeletal system is not generally performed at necropsy, and bone in particular does not lend itself to macroscopic examination, although joints can be easily incised and examined at necropsy. Considerable information can be gained from the examination of sections of muscle, bone and joints stained with haematoxylin and eosin (H and E), but closer investigation and special techniques are required to demonstrate the dynamic nature of these tissues.

The complex nature of bone lesions, particularly those that relate to altered mineral homeostasis, require a sound understanding of the biology of bone. Likewise, an understanding of muscle metabolism and fibre distribution are essential to an appreciation of the effects of sample selection upon the outcome of toxicity testing. The following discussions attempt to provide an insight into these concepts.

This chapter is divided into two sections: (Section A) Skeletal Muscle and (Section B) Bone, Cartilage and Joints, with a general conclusion.

Section A: Skeletal Muscle

8.2 Anatomy, Histology and Physiology

Skeletal muscle is formed from the primitive mesoderm of the embryo. Many primitive myoblasts fuse to form a single muscle cell, or myofibre, which is therefore a large elongated multinucleated cell. In some muscles the myofibre may extend the whole length of a muscle with insertion into a tendon at either end resulting in a cell several centimetres long. Myofibre size and population numbers vary according to the need of the muscle for fine co-ordinated movement and by factors such as gender, exercise and age, being generally greater in young active males. These factors, in conjunction with the myocyte's unique internal contractile structure, enable skeletal muscle to produce both powerful movements of the skeleton, and fine, co-ordinated movements of the hands.

8.2.1 Myofibres

A transverse section of muscle reveals many eosinophilic polygonal myofibres in cross-section. Bundles of myofibres are grouped into muscle fascicles with small amounts of connective tissue in between. Many small myofibre nuclei are visible, arranged around the periphery of the cell (Figure 8.1) immediately underneath the cell membrane, or sarcolemma. A basement membrane (external lamina) lies around the external surface of the sarcolemma and surrounds the cell. The remainder of the cell constitutes the abundant eosinophilic cytoplasm (sarcoplasm), which is filled predominantly by the fibrils and filaments of the contractile apparatus along with other cell organelles such as mitochondria and sarcoplasmic reticulum. A longitudinal H and E section reveals many long cylindrical cells parallel to each other which may show the faint cross-striations formed by the filaments of the contractile apparatus. Phosphotungstic acid haematoxylin (PTAH) stained sections are often prepared to show this in better detail.

8.2.2 Myofibres and Myofilaments

The complete structure of the contractile apparatus of the skeletal myofibre can only be visualized fully by electron microscopy. Longitudinal sections show regular alternating light or dark bands and lines formed by overlapping thick and thin

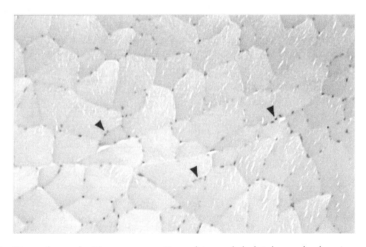

Figure 8.1 Normal muscle. Transverse section of normal skeletal muscle showing polygonal myofibres with many small peripheral myofibre nuclei (arrowheads).

myofilaments. Regular repeating units of light and dark bands form sarcomeres which are laid end-to-end to form a myofibril approximately 1 µm in diameter, and aligned side-to-side with sarcomeres in adjacent myofibrils. The thick filaments are composed of myosin molecules which are present in different isoforms in different types of skeletal muscle, according to the function or developmental state of that muscle, and the thin filaments are predominantly composed of actin molecules but also contain troponin and tropomyosin molecules. The Z band is the point of demarcation between adjacent sarcomeres and is the point of attachment for thin actin filaments. The light I (isotropic) bands lie either side of the Z band and contain the thin filaments, whereas the dark A (anisotropic) bands forming the centre of the sarcomere contain the thick myosin filaments (Figures 8.2 and 8.3). The amount of overlap between the actin and myosin filaments at the edge of the A band depends on the state of contraction of the sarcomere. Desmin, a filamentous protein, links the myofibrillar system to the myofibre cytoskeleton to maintain cell shape.

Mitochondria are prominent within the myofibre and lie between the myofibrils. The sarcoplasmic reticulum of the myofibre is analgous to the endoplasmic reticulum of many other cell types and ramifies around the myofibrils. A system of transverse T tubules formed by invagination from the sarcolemma also branches around the myofibrils and the two tubular systems join together at the junction of the A and I bands. The sarcotubular complex formed by these two systems is an important link in the process by which a nervous impulse results in muscular contraction.

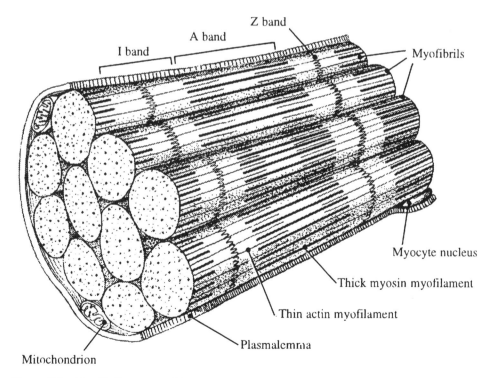

Figure 8.2 Myofibril structure. Diagrammatic representation of the internal structure of the myofibre. Bundles of myofilaments are arranged into myofibrils which almost completely fill the sarcoplasm. The arrangement of the thick and thin filaments to form sarcomeres, Z lines and A and I bands is shown.

241

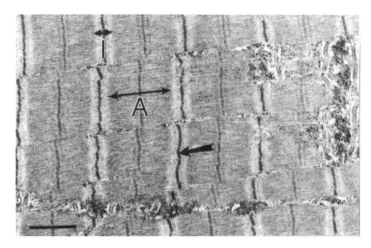

Figure 8.3 Myofibril structure. Electron micrograph of myofibrils in longitudinal section. Z lines (arrow), and A and I bands are shown. Bar marker equivalent to 1 μm. (Reproduced by kind permission of G. Ainge.)

8.2.3 *Myofibre Typing*

The different muscle fibres in the body have been subclassified in various ways which generally reflect their metabolic function and their type of activity. Some muscles are predominantly one fibre type whereas others are a mixture, particularly in man. Table 8.1 is a simplified summary of the most frequently used terminology and the type of metabolic activity in the different fibre types. Type II fibres are sometimes further subdivided into types IIA, IIB and IIC but it is likely that the subdivisions are arbitrary and that a spectrum of type II fibres exists.

The myofibre type distribution in adult skeletal muscle is controlled by the neural supply from spinal nerves to a muscle, since all myofibres innervated by one motor neuron will be the same type, and the type is determined by the motor neuron. Interruption of that nerve supply by trauma, disease or surgical intervention can result in the selective loss or atrophy of one fibre type in a muscle that may

Table 8.1 Classification of fibre types in skeletal muscle

Classification criteria	Type I	Type II
Colour	Red	White
Myoglobin content	High	Low
Rate of contraction	Slow	Fast
Rate of fatigue	Slow	Slow/fast
Type of metabolism	Oxidative	Glycolytic/oxidative
Concentration of myofibrillar ATPase	Low	Intermediate/high
Concentration of mitochondrial enzymes	High	High/low
Types of muscles containing a preponderance of this fibre type	Postural, sustained activity	Active, short bursts of activity
Example of muscle containing a preponderance of this fibre type	Rat soleus, diaphragm	Rat long digital extensor, chicken pectoral

originally contain a mosaic of all fibre types. Re-innervation of the damaged muscle can produce a change of fibre type since this is controlled by the innervating neuron, and so the myofibre pattern and distribution within a muscle can change. Also, some muscle toxicants may act selectively on one fibre type because of the different metabolic pathways present, and so it can be of value to the pathologist when investigating the possible origin of a muscle lesion to identify the fibre type and distribution in a muscle sample. Traditional histochemical methods using myosin ATPase at controlled pH and NADH-tetrazolium reductase (NADH-TR) reactions in frozen sections are valuable, but immunocytochemistry can also identify the different myosin isoforms present in different fibre types (Figure 8.4).

8.2.4 Myofibre Contraction

Contraction of skeletal muscle occurs when the thick and thin myofilaments slide across each other to increase the area of overlap at the edges of the A band. This decreases the length of the sarcomeres and therefore the length of the muscle. The overlap gradually increases by the continual formation and breaking of cross-links between the thick and thin filaments. This energy-dependent process is 'fuelled' when myosin ATPase releases energy from ATP provided by oxidative phosphorylation in type I fibres, and anaerobic glycolysis in type II fibres. The stimulus for contraction occurs when an incoming nerve impulse depolarises the sarcolemma and T-tubule system. The close relationship of the sarcoplasmic reticulum with the T-tubule system allows the depolarization 'message' of the T tubule to result in the release of calcium from the sarcoplasmic reticulum into the sarcoplasm. Increased sarcoplasmic calcium initiates thick-to-thin myofilament cross-binding and hence sarcomere shortening. The process ends when the sarcoplasmic reticulum retrieves calcium from the sarcoplasm.

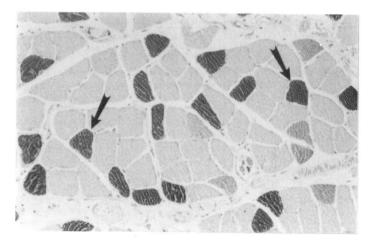

Figure 8.4 Myofibre typing. Transverse section of rat soleus muscle. Immunogold method for fast myosin with silver staining. The majority of fibres in the rat soleus muscle are slow type I fibres and therefore do not label. A few scattered fast (type II) fibres show intense staining (arrows).

243

8.3 Biochemical and Cellular Mechanisms of Toxicity

8.3.1 *Local Toxicity*

Skeletal muscle toxicity can arise from local or systemic effects. The local muscle degeneration caused by intramuscular injection of some antibiotics (**penicillin, streptomycin**), analgesics (**pentazocine**) and local anaesthetics (**bupivacaine, lignocaine**) are well known. Injection of xenobiotics into the rabbit sacrospinalis muscle may be used as a sensitive predictor for local irritancy.

8.3.2 *Systemic Toxicity*

Systemic skeletal muscle toxicity can be categorized according to the site of action of the agent, although the morphological result of that toxicity may not vary in the same manner.

Neurogenic toxicity

Interruption of the neural supply to muscle can produce complete muscle atrophy and, depending on the site of the lesion, loss of use of a limb. However, xenobiotics that interfere with the neural supply commonly do so by interfering with transmission of the impulse at the neuromuscular junction by the neurotransmitter acetylcholine (ACh). This may impair muscle function resulting in weakness, or may trigger hyperexcitability producing tremors or fasciculations (fine tremors). Acetylcholinesterase inhibitors such as the organophosphates **paraoxon** [1] and **parathion**, and carbamates such as **pyridostigmine** [2] and **physostigmine**, are well known for their potential to cause persistent muscle weakness and fasciculations via impaired neuromuscular transmission, and produce morphological changes in the muscle, probably either as a result of accumulation of high levels of ACh at the motor nerve terminal or hyperexcitability and increased contractile activity of the muscle itself. The precise effect appears to be exposure-dependent and although type I fibres are most susceptible to damage, the type I-rich diaphragm is more vulnerable than the purely type I masseter and soleus muscles of the rat [3].

Imparied sarcolemmal function

The sarcolemma may be subjected to increased excitability resulting in muscle cramping (myotonia) or muscle weakness, as a result of altered blood potassium levels. **Clofibrate** and other drugs such as **pravastatin, lovastatin** and **simvastatin** that lower plasma cholesterol levels have been linked with skeletal myotonia and myofibre necrosis, with interstitial oedema and inflammatory infiltration in man and rats. Type II glycolytic fibres are predominantly affected but the mechanism for this is uncertain and may be the result of impaired sarcolemmal synthesis and altered chloride permeability [4], or altered lipid or carbohydrate metabolism [5]. *In vitro* exposure of neonatal rat skeletal myotubes suggests that the differential toxicity of these agents is linked to the degree of inhibition of 3-hydroxy-3-methylglutaryl coenzyme A reductase (HMG CoA reductase) [6]. Increased membrane excitability may also be the cause of myotonia and myofibre damage caused by **salbutamol,**

clenbuterol and **cimetidine**. Carboxylic ionophores, typified by **monensin**, may interfere with ion pumps. **Amphotericin** and **azathioprine** increase potassium loss by the kidney and produce muscle weakness with muscle necrosis.

Microtubule disruption

Drugs such as **colchicine** and **vincristine** disrupt the microtubules of the cell cytoskeleton. These agents produce profound changes in the peripheral nervous system by this mechanism and in skeletal muscle, myopathic changes and muscular weakness may be related to impaired microtubular function within the myofibre with consequent effects upon the contractile apparatus. Type I fibres are preferentially affected [7].

Lysosomal myopathies

The amphiphilic cationic drugs such as **amiodarone, chlorphentermine, chloroquine, tamoxifen** and **chlorcyclizine** form stable intracellular drug-lipid complexes which resist normal lysosomal degradation. This causes a generalized phospholipidosis characterized by accumulation of undegradable phospholipid membranous material in lysosomes in many cell types. At prolonged or high doses, muscle weakness is associated with the accumulation of membranous material in sarcoplasmic lysosomes, although others have suggested that the skeletal muscle damage is independent of the generalized phospholipidosis and the result of a direct effect on the sarcolemma. Muscle atrophy occurs with administration of **L-** or **D- thyroxine** to rabbits and it has been suggested that this may be the result of effects upon the lysosomal enzymes cathepsin B and D.

Mitochondrial myopathies

Agents such as **2,4-dinitrophenol** that uncouple oxidative metabolism produce so-called ragged red fibres in type I fibres. Ultrastructurally this is characterized by aggregation of abnormal mitochondria containing inclusions adjacent to the sarcolemma. The effects of the antiviral agent **zidovudine** appear to be similar by electron microscopy, but are somewhat controversial since the muscular weakness and myofibre degeneration presumed to be the result of this change undoubtedly occur in patients with human immunodeficiency virus (HIV) infection undergoing treatment with **zidovudine**, but whether this is wholly attributable to **zidovudine** is unclear. *In vitro* studies with **zidovudine** implicate defects in mitochondrial enzyme activity and DNA replication or RNA transcription [8, 9].

Altered vascular supply

Vasoactive agents such as **imipramine, serotonin** and **adrenaline** produce damage in type I fibres and also in some type II fibres dependent upon oxidative metabolism. This effect has been attributed to infarction and ischaemia. The vasodilatory agent **dipyridamole** produces proliferation of the capillary bed in skeletal muscle.

Altered protein synthesis

The muscular weakness and atrophy associated with use of corticosteroids such as **betamethasone** and **dexamethasone** in man and animals are well recognized. There is selective atrophy of type II fibres with preservation of the postural type I fibres, probably due to decreased protein synthesis, although at high doses protein degradation is also increased. Concurrent administration of anabolic steroids and B vitamins can prevent this process in rats. A similar atrophic effect occurs in protein deficiency through malnutrition.

Net loss of skeletal muscle proteins due to disturbed protein synthesis also occurs with **ethanol** exposure in man and animals [10].

Growth hormone and anabolic β_2-adrenergic agonists such as **clenbuterol** and **salbutamol** produce an increase in muscle mass (hypertrophy) via increased protein synthesis without cell proliferation, leading to increased myofibre length and size. **Clenbuterol** also increased the proportion of glycolytic type II fibres at the expense of oxidative type II fibres, and increased the muscle DNA and RNA content [11].

Teratogenesis

There are very few reports of induced skeletal muscle lesions in the fetus or neonate. The adenine agonist **6-mercaptopurine** produces a muscular dystrophy-like lesion in the neonatal rat but only when administered to the dam during the prenatal period. This agent has immunosuppressive properties and interferes with the synthesis of DNA and RNA. *In vitro* studies show selective toxicity to myotubes, with inhibition of myotube formation [12]. Arthrogryposis is a congenital rigidity of the joints which may be due to muscle hypoplasia and denervation atrophy leading to lack of limb movement *in utero*. **Tubocurarine** causes this lesion in the rat, probably as a result of paralysis of the fetus, and many plants such as *Veratrum californicum* may also produce this defect in herbivores.

Carcinogenesis

Intramuscular or subcutaneous injection of chemical carcinogens such as some **nickel**, **cobalt** and **cadmium** compounds results in malignant tumours (rhabdomyosarcoma) of skeletal muscle.

Table 8.2 summarizes the extensive range of agents that cause muscle toxicity and gives examples of the types of lesions that may be induced, including agents such as **triethyltin sulphate** for which the mechanisms of action are poorly understood.

8.4 Morphological Responses to Injury

The term myopathy is used to indicate any pathological process occurring in skeletal muscle, but the range of morphological responses to injury exhibited by skeletal muscle is limited and not often indicative of the nature of the injury. Any discussion of morphological responses of skeletal muscle to injury must first recognize the possible occurrence of artefact in inappropriately manipulated samples, in order to differentiate this from some of the subtle alterations of early myopathies. In order to evaluate fully a muscle sample, and to differentiate artefact

Table 8.2 Induced lesions of skeletal muscle

Toxic agent	Type of agent	Species	Nature of effect
Paraoxon, DFP*	Organophosphate cholinesterase inhibitors	Rat	Necrosis
CPMF⁺	Organophosphate cholinesterase inhibitor	Monkey	Degeneration, necrosis, mineralization
Pyridostigmine, physostigmine	Anticholinesterase carbamate	Rat	Necrosis, leucocytic infiltrates, altered motor endplates
Monensin, maduramicin and others	Carboxylic ionophore agents: coccidiostatic agents and growth promoters	Mouse Dog Sheep	Granular degeneration and necrosis, regeneration
PD123244-15, clofibrate	Cholesterol-lowering agents	Rat	Necrosis and regeneration
N-methylated phenylenediamines	Industrial chemicals, hair dyes	Rat	Necrosis
Sodium diatrizoate	Iodinated contrast medium	Man	Necrosis, no inflammation
Vincristine sulphate, azathioprine	Chemotherapeutic agent	Rat	Impaired function by direct effect on contractile apparatus
		Man	Muscle fibre degeneration
Adriamycin	Anthracene antibiotic	Rat	Muscle fibre lysis, lipid droplet accumulation
Aminocaproic acid	Fibrinolytic agent	Man	Necrosis, regeneration, myoglobinuria
Amiodarone, chloroquine, tamoxifen	Amphiphilic cationic agents	Rat	Generalized phospholipidosis with involvement of skeletal muscle
Quinine, plasmocid, emetine, chloroquine	Antimalarial agents	Rat	Polyfocal necrosis, mitochondrial swelling, actin filament destruction
Triethyltin sulphate, triethyltin bromide	Fungicides, bactericides, molluscicides, stabilizers	Rat	Muscle cores in type I fibres of soleus muscle
2,4-dinitrophenol	Oxidative phosphorylation uncoupler	Rat	Ragged red fibres and mitochondrial inclusions
Zidovudine	Antiretroviral agent	Man, Rat	Mitochondrial myopathy
Methysergide	Antimigraine agent	Man	Mitochondrial inclusions
Acrylamide	Plasticizer	Rat	Atrophy
6-Mercaptopurine	Adenine agonist	Fetal rat	Atrophy, fibre splitting
Clenbuterol	β-adrenergic agent	Dog, Rat	Myofibre hypertrophy and necrosis
Salbutamol	β-adrenergic agent	Rat	Myofibre hypertrophy and necrosis
Cassia occidentalis seeds	Plant toxin	Horse	Segmental necrosis
Hornet venom	Animal toxin	Man	Disturbance of transverse T-tubule system
Stonefish venom	Animal toxin	Mouse	Irreversible muscle cell depolarization and muscle fibre degeneration
Nickel, cobalt, cadmium	Chemical carcinogens	Rat	Rhabdomyosarcoma

DFP*, diisopropylfluorophosphate;
CPMF⁺, cyclohexylmethylphosphonofluoridate.

from lesion, it is advisable that both transverse and longitudinal sections are prepared.

8.4.1 *Atrophy*

Muscle atrophy is a reduction in myofibre size occurring as a result of a drug-induced reduction in protein synthesis, malnutrition, or loss of use following disruption of neural supply or trauma requiring orthopaedic immobilization of a limb. In transverse section this appears as myofibres with a decreased diameter, a more irregular outline, and an apparent increased prominence of myofibre nuclei and inter-myofibre connective tissue. The reduction in myofibre size is due to a reduction in bulk of cell organelles, particularly the myofibrils. In advanced lesions, adipose tissue may replace atrophic fibres. Early diffuse atrophy could require careful comparison with unaffected muscle to recognize a slight effect, but drug- or malnutrition-induced atrophy and neurogenic atrophy arising from a partial lesion may produce atrophy of one fibre type only, in a muscle containing a mixed population of fibre types.

Atrophy of type II fibres occurs spontaneously in ageing rats but it is conceivable that, in the hindlimbs particularly, this could be a secondary response to age-related spinal nerve root degeneration since drug-induced exacerbation of age-related peripheral neuropathy in the rat also intensifies skeletal muscle atrophy.

8.4.2 *Hypertrophy*

Muscle hypertrophy is an increase in myofibre size achieved by addition of more sarcomeres and myofibrils to the contractile apparatus. Satellite cell proliferation to incorporate more myotubes into the myofibre may also be responsible for the size increase (see Regeneration, Section 8.4.5). This can be a response to increased work load or a direct effect of drugs with anabolic potential. Compensatory hypertrophy may also be recognized as a local response to atrophy. The muscle sample may appear normal in transverse section and morphometric techniques may be required to identify hypertrophy. Longitudinal splitting of hypertrophied myofibres can occur, possibly as an adaptive response of the myofibre to increased work load. Drug-induced hypertrophy may be most readily identified macroscopically in the hindlimbs (Figure 8.5).

8.4.3 *Dystrophy*

The term muscular dystrophy was originally proposed for progressive muscular diseases due to 'faulty nutrition', but the term is now generally reserved for many characteristic disorders that share similar pathological alterations and have a genetic basis. Muscular dystrophy is uncommon in laboratory animals, but muscular dystrophies have been recognized in inbred mouse strains (129/Re, mdg), the hamster and mink, with myofibre destruction and atrophy present in early life and only abortive attempts at regeneration.

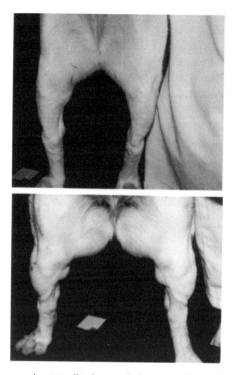

Figure 8.5   Muscle hypertrophy. Hindlimb muscle hypertrophy in the laboratory beagle. The upper photograph illustrates a control animal whereas the animal in the lower photograph had received treatment with a β-adrenergic agent. (Reproduced by kind permission of S. Damment.)

8.4.4   *Degeneration and Necrosis*

Reversible degeneration leading to irreversible necrosis or recovery may occur in skeletal muscle in response to a wide variety of agents (see Table 8.2). The sequence of events observed has resulted in descriptions of several different morphological types of degeneration which may reflect a particular aetiology, but generally the terms are not pathognomic. In any muscle showing evidence of degeneration or necrosis, the change may be 'segmental', that is, only parts or segments of the long myofibre may be affected.

Hyaline degeneration

In hyaline degeneration, the affected parts of the myofibre appear swollen and have more intense eosinophilic staining properties with conventional H and E sections (Figure 8.6). The cross-striations may also be indistinct. This is probably the most common type of degeneration observed in skeletal muscle. If necrosis ensues, the sarcoplasm in affected areas of the myofibre may appear paler but homogeneous, and a macrophage response rapidly occurs to remove necrotic sarcoplasm (Figure 8.7). Given the relative bulk of the sarcoplasm, the macrophage response may be dramatic. An 'empty' segment of sarcolemma and external lamina remains and regeneration may follow.

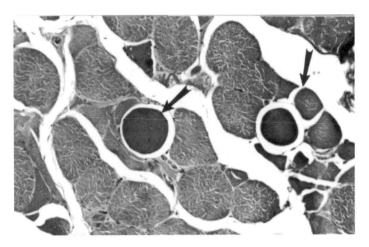

Figure 8.6 Hyaline degeneration. Transverse section of muscle showing hyaline degeneration. Affected fibres (arrow) demonstrate a more circular profile, increased staining intensity and cytoplasmic homogeneity.

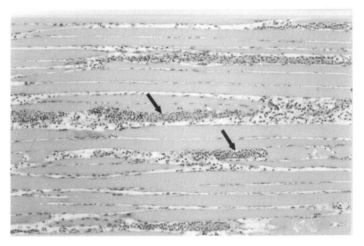

Figure 8.7 Hyaline degeneration. Longitudinal section of muscle showing an intense macrophage response in individual myofibres. The sarcoplasm has been completely removed by the infiltrating phagocytic cells (arrows). Note that adjacent myofibres are unaffected since this myopathy was segmental in distribution.

Granular degeneration

Granular degeneration, as its name suggests, is a form of degeneration in which the myofibre sarcoplasm takes on a granular basophilic appearance. This type of degeneration is associated with nutritional myopathies and extensive sarcoplasmic mineralization commonly follows.

Discoid degeneration

Discoid degeneration is thought to be typical of ischaemic muscle degeneration and is characterized by separation at the Z bands along the length of the myofibre into clumps or 'discs' of sarcomeres. Myofibre nuclei disappear and necrosis ensues. Agents that interfere with vascular supply rarely produce such a severe lesion, but this type of degeneration has been encountered as a result of thrombosis occurring at the site of cannulation of a major vessel, leading to complete occlusion of the vessel.

Fatty degeneration

Fatty degeneration is an unusual occurrence but may occur following granular degeneration and can be induced in skeletal muscle in response to agents such as **adriamycin**. In the mouse, this produces an increase in numbers of lipid droplets in the sarcoplasm with occasional myofibre destruction.

8.4.5 Regeneration

The regenerative capacity of sketal muscle is extensive and is greatly facilitated by the fact that many degenerative conditions of the myofibre are segmental in distribution. It is therefore possible for the muscle cells to replace only those parts that are affected, and to see necrosis and regeneration occurring concurrently. The ability to regenerate is reliant upon the preservation of the external lamina and sarcolemma to maintain a framework for the repair process and the presence of a reserve population of highly resistant, undifferentiated satellite cells which lie between the sarcolemma and the external lamina but cannot be distinguished from myofibre nuclei in conventional histology sections. After necrotic sarcoplasmic debris have been removed, satellite cells proliferate to produce myoblasts which fuse to form multinucleate myotubes. The myotube is then inserted into the 'empty' area of the myofibre and bridges the gap between sarcomeres either side of the lesion (Figure 8.8). The myotube is readily identified in regenerating muscle in longitudinal section since the immature nuclei are larger and form a row in the centre of the cell, and the myotube sarcoplasm is basophilic because of the higher levels of RNA

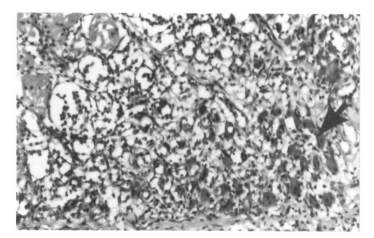

Figure 8.8 Myofibre regeneration. Transverse section of muscle showing necrotic myofibres undergoing phagocytic digestion (left of the photograph) with many 'empty' circular profiles composed of an external lamina and sarcolemma remaining (centre photograph). At the right, repopulation by small multinucleate myotubes is occurring (arrow).

present during synthetic activity. During regeneration of the myofibre, the myosin isoforms expressed by that muscle change and follow the sequence of myosin isoform expression that occurs during embryonic through to juvenile development. Expression of immature myosin isoforms by regenerating adult muscle can be demonstrated by immunocytochemistry.

In the event of more severe degeneration and complete loss of the myofibre, replacement fibrous and adipose tissue may be laid down between surviving myofibres.

8.4.6 Inflammatory Muscle Disease

Spontaneous inflammatory muscle disease is not common in laboratory animals, but eosinophilic myositis affecting primarily the temporal and masseter muscles of the beagle may be infrequently encountered. This is characterized by widespread infiltration of eosinophilic granulocytes and myofibre degeneration, accompanied by severe pain and swelling. The aetiology of this condition is unclear but may be an immunological response to a muscle protein. Various migrating parasites may cause localized muscle inflammation, e.g. *Toxoplasma gondii*, *Neospora caninum*.

8.4.7 Metabolic Myopathies

Muscle lesions have been reported in rats fed diets deficient in **vitamin D**, **magnesium** and **potassium**. Glycogen storage diseases, such as acid maltase or phosphofructokinase deficiencies, and lipid storage diseases such as carnitine deficiency are inherited diseases in man, but relatively few corresponding lesions are recognized in laboratory animals. Myofibre glycogen accumulation has been reported due to deficient lysosomal glucosidase activity in the mouse and rat.

8.4.8 Central Core Myopathy

Central core disease occurs in man where the majority of muscle fibres contain a central core composed of either hypercontracted sarcomeres or by proliferation of sarcotubular elements. Similar drug-induced lesions have been observed in laboratory rodents.

8.4.9 Proliferative Lesions of Skeletal Muscle

Spontaneous tumours of skeletal muscle, particularly benign tumours, are a very rare occurrence in laboratory species. Rhabdomyosarcoma, the malignant form of skeletal muscle tumour occurs very occasionally in the rat and hamster. The lesion is usually very infiltrative and the cells are typically very pleiomorphic. Multinucleate cells and cells with bizarre nuclei are seen. In well-differentiated neoplasms, PTAH staining may identify cross-striations, but often definitive diagnosis is based upon electron microscopic demonstration of some constituents of the sarcomere and immunocytochemical demonstration of markers of skeletal muscle differentiation, such as desmin and myosin isoforms.

8.5 Testing for Toxicity

8.5.1 *Microscopy*

Although it is generally impractical to examine all but a few skeletal muscles at necropsy, and fewer still by microscopy, ideally, skeletal muscle evaluation would comprise examination of several muscles exhibiting the various fibre types. The hindlimb of the rat is ideal for this purpose, since single- and mixed-fibre type populations exist in the soleus, long digital extensor and gastrocnemius muscles. In practice, however, many toxicological experimental protocols include only the examination of a defined section of skeletal muscle containing a mixture of fibre types such as the biceps femoris or gastrocnemius, and biochemical evaluation of peripheral blood for altered muscle-specific enzyme levels. Stains to demonstrate connective tissue (Masson trichrome), cross-striations (PTAH), lipid vacuoles (Sudan IV) and central cores (periodic acid Schiff) can be useful. Ideally, frozen sections are required for enzyme histochemical (ATPase, NADH-TR) and immunohistochemical analysis (fast myosin). Morphometric techniques to measure fibre diameter and numerical fibre type distribution may be useful adjuncts to microscopy.

8.5.2 *Biochemical Evaluation*

Biochemical analysis of blood for indications of myotoxicity is generally to evaluate creatine kinase (CK) levels. Injury to the myofibre allows the MM isoform of this enzyme to leak into the blood. The peak levels of serum CK may, however, occur rapidly and be overlooked in a standard protocol with defined sampling times. Other enzymes such as serum aspartate transaminase (AST), serum alanine transaminase (ALT) and lactate dehydrogenase (LDH) may also be increased but are not specific to muscle injury. Serum troponin T and myosin heavy-chain fragment levels have been evaluated as delayed markers for rhabdomyolysis in man and are able to detect rhabdomyolysis occurring up to 12 days previously. Urinary myoglobin measurement is also an indicator of muscle damage and myoglobin appears in the urine when plasma levels exceed 9 to 12µmol.

8.5.3 *Electrophysiology*

Electromyography involves recording the electrical activity generated in muscle fibres and can distinguish between drug-induced alterations in neuromuscular transmission and a primary neuropathy.

8.5.4 In vitro *Investigation*

Cultures of embryonic, fetal or adult myoblasts can be initiated and maintained *in vitro*, and, under the appropriate conditions, will fuse to form myotubes and muscle fibres. These cultures are useful for biochemical evaluation of the effects of adding xenobiotics to the culture medium but are not yet known to be of reliable predictive value for risk *in vivo*.

Section B: Bone, Cartilage and Joints

8.2 Anatomy, Histology and Physiology

The skeletal system is comprised of a number of specialized connective tissues that together provide a weight-bearing and protective framework for the attachment of skeletal muscles and protection of internal organs. In addition, bone acts as a large mineral reserve and bone marrow within the centre of many bones plays a major role in haematopoiesis. The skeletal system is part of the locomotor system and acts as a system of levers and pivots around which the skeletal muscles contract and relax to provide movement, or locomotion, of the different body parts. The principal connective tissue types that form the skeletal system are bone and cartilage, which between them allow for the formation and growth of all bones in the body, and the formation of joints at pivotal points between apposing bones. Dense fibrous connective tissue forms tendons which provide strong attachments between bone and skeletal muscles, and produces ligaments which provide stabilization around and within many of the more mobile joints. The cells that form these specialized connective tissues are all derived from primitive mesenchymal cells which have differentiated along diverging pathways but which possess the common ability to produce a specialized extracellular matrix that determines the mechanical properties and histological appearance of specialized connective tissue.

8.2.1 Cartilage and Bone Structure

Three types of cartilage are present at different sites, depending on the need for structural support, joint rigidity or mobility, or bone growth. They differ only in the fibre composition of the extracellular matrix. Elastic cartilage occurs in the external ear and larynx, and fibrous cartilage forms the joints between the spinal vertebrae, for example, which are relatively immobile. Hyaline cartilage is present in the synovial joint located at the ends of long bones such as the femur and humerus, and also plays an important role in bone formation and growth. The characteristic appearance of cartilage is of nests of adult cells (chondrocytes) entrapped within lacunae in a substantial matrix, which appears amorphous by conventional light microscopy but which is composed of a ground substance (proteoglycans) and collagen fibres (Figure 8.9).

Bone is formed in the immature skeleton by two different methods. The flat bones of the skull and jaw are formed within primitive mesenchymal tissue (intramembranous ossification), whereas the long bones of the limbs form by endochondral ossification within an existing hyaline cartilage template. Mature bones are composed of an outer layer (cortex) of dense compact bone laid down in concentric lamellar bundles (Haversian systems), and an inner layer of irregular cancellous (trabecular) bone which partially fills the marrow cavity of the long bones (Figure 8.10). Both types of bone are composed of cells (osteocytes) in lacunae surrounded by a substantial matrix (osteoid). Mineralization of the matrix by deposition of calcium hydroxyapatite and calcium phosphate occurs to produce rigid, weight-bearing mature bone. Compact lamellar bone grows and is remodelled comparatively slowly during adult life. Cancellous trabecular bone, however, can be laid down and mineralized comparatively quickly during juvenile growth and in special circumstances such as fracture repair. Bone growth in the juvenile skeleton occurs by continued endochondral ossification within the hyaline cartilage of epiphysial growth plates located between the shaft (diaphysis) and the end of the long bone that forms a joint (epiphysis). The area of new bone growth and remodelling immediately adjacent to the epiphyseal growth plate is known as the metaphysis.

Mature bone receives its blood supply from nutrient arteries that penetrate the compact bone of the cortices and branch into many small vessels that course along

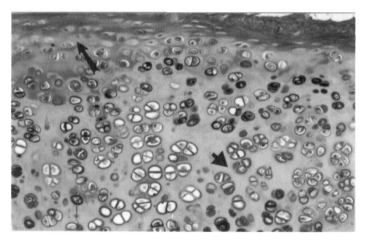

Figure 8.9 Normal cartilage. Longitudinal section through cartilage of the distal rib in a rat. Nests of lacunae in a homogenous matrix contain chondrocytes with large prominent nuclei (arrowhead). Immature chondroblasts are located peripherally (arrow). Many 'empty' lacunae are present in which the artefactually shrunken chrondrocyte is not in the plane of section shown.

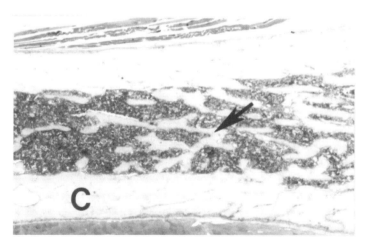

Figure 8.10 Normal compact and trabecular bone. Longitudinal section through the femur of a rat. Compact cortical bone is shown around the periphery of the femur (C), with islands of trabecular bone transecting the marrow cavity (arrow).

the centre of each Haversian system in Haversian canals to supply all osteocytes within that system. Branches of nutrient arteries also form sinusoids within the bone marrow that allow for exchange of nutrients with osteocytes within trabecular bone that have only irregular partial Haversian systems. Cartilage, however, has no blood supply, and depends on acquiring nutrients from surrounding tissues via the ground substance of the matrix. This limits the thickness of cartilage but also protects cartilage from blood-borne insult.

8.2.2 *Bone and Cartilage Formation*

Bone and cartilage are both formed from progenitor cells that differentiate into immature cells known as osteoblasts and chondroblasts, respectively. These cells undergo cell division and secrete copious matrix, resulting in the mature osteocyte or chondrocyte. Numbers of osteoblasts along with osteoprogenitor cells and fibroblasts remain as a reserve population for further growth in a tough fibrous membrane surrounding bone (periosteum). Similarly, chondroblast populations remain in areas towards the periphery of cartilage (perichondrium). Bone undergoes remodelling throughout life in response to the need for further growth and weight bearing, and since it also acts as a large reservoir for minerals such as calcium and phosphate, should be regarded as a very dynamic tissue with constant laying down of new bone and matrix mineralization, balanced by resorption of matrix and release of minerals throughout life. This resorptive function is a property of large multinucleate cells known as osteoclasts which secrete the enzymes and organic acids necessary for releasing the mineral and organic components of the matrix. Osteoclasts are generally found along the junction between the inner surface of bone and the bone marrow, a layer known as the endosteum.

8.2.3 *Mineral Homeostasis*

Mineral deposits in bone, and blood levels of calcium and phosphate, are closely regulated in order to produce a state of equilibrium whereby dietary intake is sufficient to achieve normal bone mineralization and blood mineral levels are controlled within a set range. At times of dietary insufficiency, disease, or increased demand for minerals such as during pregnancy and lactation, the mineral reserves in bone may be mobilized to meet the increased demand. This process is achieved by the relative stimulation or inhibition of osteoblast and osteoclast activity. These cells are regulated by systemic factors such as parathyroid hormone (PTH), the thyroid hormone calcitonin, and calcitriol (1,25-dihydroxycholecaliferol), a vitamin D metabolite. However, the importance of local effects of cytokines and growth factors is increasingly recognized, with the possibility that autocrine regulation is a significant influence. The osteocyte may play a role in release of minerals from bone, but the osteoclast is largely responsible for the process of bone resorption. PTH may increase the number and activity of osteoclasts but their stimulation may be largely due to the influence of PTH-activated osteoblasts which exert their effect by physical or paracrine means. The sex hormones, oestrogen and testosterone, and growth hormone influence bone growth in the juvenile, and falling levels of oestrogen postmenopause are known to affect bone density adversely.

8.2.4 *Joint Structure and Function*

Joints in the body have different structures according to the need for mobility or rigidity. For example, the joints between the bones of the skull are formed from dense fibrous tissue only, and are gradually replaced by bone in the maturing juvenile when body growth ceases. Fibrocartilage forms the relatively immobile joints of the sternum and also forms the cushioning intervertebral discs which connect adjacent spinal vertebrae. The synovial joint connects bones which require a high degree of mobility and flexibility and a typical example is the stifle joint between the femur and tibia. The synovial joint is so called because of the synovial membrane which lines the inner surface of the joint except over the ends of the bones themselves, which are covered by hyaline cartilage. The synovial membrane's functions include secretion of synovial fluid into the joint space to lubricate and cushion the joint, and removal of debris from the joint space by phagocytosis within the synovial cells. Stability of the stifle joint is provided by intra-articular cruciate ligaments and meniscal cartilages, collateral ligaments outside the joint, and a tough fibrous joint capsule.

8.3 Biochemical and Cellular Mechanisms of Toxicity

The mechanisms of bone, cartilage and joint toxicity can be categorized similarly according to whether they are local or systemic effects, according to the site of action, and also whether the effect is primary or secondary. Many induced abnormalities of bone growth and matrix result from dietary deficiencies or excess, which are manipulated in order to investigate mechanisms of disease in man.

8.3.1 *Local Toxicity*

Local bone toxicity is now known to occur secondary to the implantation of orthopaedic prostheses in fracture repair, for example. Orthopaedic prostheses may contain **titanium–aluminium–vanadium** or **chromium–cobalt–molybdenum** alloys. A zone of degenerate bone often forms around the implant and is thought to be responsible for the loosening of some implants. The zone of degenerate bone is likely to be the result of bone lysis around the implant site initiated by the metallic components of the prostheses. Corrosion of the implant also continually changes the biochemical environment of the tissue surrounding the implant to favour bone resorption [13]. *In vitro* investigations using bone progenitor cells have demonstrated adverse effects of these alloys on osteoblast differentiation.

Local toxicity in joints has been induced by intra-articular injection of many agents in an attempt to mimic human joint disease and produce animal models for the investigation of novel therapeutic agents. Injection of **polysaccharides** or **Congo red** dye induces proliferative changes in the synovial membrane. Overt arthritis has been induced by intra-articular injection of **sodium iodoacetate**, **formaldehyde** or **histamine**. Corticosteroids such as **triamcinolone**, which have been injected into joints to relieve inflammation, may also initiate degenerative changes in joint cartilage and bone. Immune-mediated arthritis may be induced by intra-articular injection of foreign protein antigenic agents such as **bovine serum albumin** or **type**

II collagen. Morphologically comparable arthritis has been produced by intra-articular injection of non-immunogenic agents such as **zymosan** and **amphotericin**. **Zymosan** is thought to activate prostaglandin-dependent inflammation and interleukin-1-dependent decreased cartilage proteoglycan synthesis [14].

8.3.2 Systemic Toxicity

Relatively few examples exist of primary bone and cartilage toxicity and in even fewer examples is the mechanism of toxicity fully understood. The following descriptions attempt to categorize skeletal toxicity according to the specific primary mechanisms that are currently recognized, and the traditional terminology applied to diseases of bone is alluded to where necessary and described in further detail under 'Morphological Responses to Injury', Section 8.4. It is inevitable that this classification will be somewhat artificial and oversimplified since many mechanisms are interlinked. For example, an agent that induces decreased bone mass may do so *via* altered matrix mineralization, increased osteoclastic bone resorption or impaired production of new bone by osteoblasts. In practice, given the dynamic interrelationships between the processes of bone deposition and resorption, it is likely that very few agents act upon just one facet of this process in isolation. This is also exemplified by the fact that a low dose of vitamin D is required to prevent abnormal bone growth, but higher doses can induce excessive deposition of osteoid. Complex or multifactorial aetiologies are particularly relevant when considering the influence of trace elements upon bone mass, where several different effects have been attributed to excess of one particular trace element, and some studies have considered the effects of one trace element in isolation without recognizing the interactions of the trace elements themselves *in vivo*.

Altered vascular supply

The complex vasculature of bone is not conducive to macroscopic or microscopic examination and, therefore, relatively little is known about the systemic effects of xenobiotics upon this system. Non-traumatic necrosis of bone (osteonecrosis) is a recognized complication of high-dose **corticosteroid** therapy, **alcohol** consumption, and some lipid disorders in man. The common mechanism is thought to be the appearance of circulating lipid particles in the bloodstream, which impair circulation to the affected bone.

Defective matrix formation

Defective mineralization of the osteoid matrix of bone is a relatively common effect observed with the administration of some toxic agents and also occurs following dietary manipulation of vitamin and mineral levels. Defective mineralization (osteomalacia) may lead to a condition of increased amounts of unmineralized matrix (hyperosteoidosis). Dietary deficiency of **vitamin D, calcium** or **phosphorus** all lead to reduced matrix mineralization. **Aluminium** overloading in dialysis patients and **aluminium** given by intraperitoneal injection in the rat, lead to accumulation of increased amounts of osteoid around the cartilage of the epiphyseal growth plate, and deposits of **aluminium** can be identified in this area. Chronic use of anticonvulsant drugs such as **diphenylhydantoin** may lead to abnormal matrix mineralization by induction of hepatic enzymes leading to altered vitamin D metabolism. **Fluoride** excess leads to reduced matrix mineralization and osteocyte loss. **Lead** is known to inhibit skeletal development and deposit in areas of bone formation and resorption, but the mechanism of **lead** toxicity in bone is largely undetermined, although it is thought to involve disrupted matrix mineralization with consequent impaired osteoclastic resorption of the lead-containing matrix [15]. **Cadmium** may have a similar effect, and interferes with hydroxyapatite formation *in vitro*.

Abnormalities of cartilage matrix are well known in association with the use of the quinolone antimicrobials such as **nalidixic acid**, which produces matrix rarefaction (chondromalacia) with chondrocyte loss in the joint cartilage, particularly the head of the humerus and the stifle joint, and especially in the laboratory beagle. Ultimately this may lead to severe erosion of synovial joint cartilage and extensive inflammation. Chondromalacia also occurs with the use of **cyclophosphamide** and **methotrexate** through impaired synthesis of the fibrous component of cartilage matrix.

Reduced bone or cartilage mass

A decrease in bone mass (osteoporosis) is a clinically recognized condition, and can arise through any of the following mechanisms; osteoblast inhibition, osteoclast stimulation and impaired division of bone progenitor cells. In practice, it is likely that a combination of these mechanisms interact.

Osteoblast inhibition is probably the main mechanism by which **vitamin A** and **retinoids** (derivatives of vitamin A) reduce bone formation, particularly in the long bones, leading to bone fractures and reduced longitudinal growth as a consequence of premature growth plate closure (Figure 8.11). Retinoid assays *in vitro* also suggest

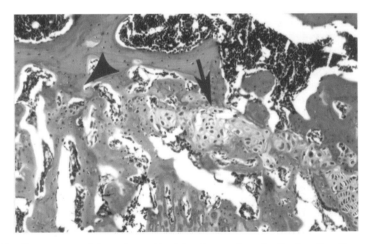

Figure 8.11 Premature epiphyseal growth plate closure. Longitudinal section through metaphyseal region of tibia from a rat treated by gavage with 60 mg/kg body weight per day of retinoic acid for 14 days. Fragments of disorganized epiphyseal growth plate remain (arrow) but the majority of the growth plate has been bridged and replaced by trabecular bone (arrowhead). (Reproduced by kind permission of M. Blades.)

some stimulation of osteoclast activity. **Aluminium** and **cadmium** also probably adversely affect bone formation by inhibiting osteoblast activity as well as reducing matrix mineralization.

Enhanced osteoclast activity has been demonstrated by some agents such as **corticosteroids** that produce a reduction in bone mass (osteoporosis), although this is only one facet of their mechanism of toxicity. Deficiencies of **vitamin A**, **protein** and **calcium** are all also thought to stimulate bone resorption by osteoclasts. **Magnesium** is known to enhance bone turnover through stimulation of osteoclastic function. **Corticosteroids** and **cyclophosphamide** also impair division of bone progenitor cells, contributing to the osteoporosis of chronic therapy.

Cartilage atrophy is associated with chronic administration of the anticonvulsant agents **sodium valproate** and **diphenylhydantoin**. Reduced chondrocyte numbers and decreased cartilage thickness occur at specific sites in young rats.

Increased bone mass

Increased bone mass can be described as either hyperostosis, osteosclerosis, osteolathyrism, or osteopetrosis depending upon the aetiology and nature of the increase and the clinically recognized condition, although the terms are imprecise and occasionally used interchangeably. Increased bone mass described as osteosclerosis most commonly arises as a result of osteoclast inhibition.

Specific inhibition of osteoclast activity is a function of the **bisphosphonate** group of compounds, such as **pamidronate** and **tiludronate** [16], by reducing the capacity of osteoclasts to secrete into the resorption space and favouring their detachment from bone matrix. These compounds were developed primarily to counteract age-related bone loss and typically result in reduced bone modelling at the epiphyseal plate in growing animals, with persistence of immature bone within the marrow cavity (osteosclerosis), and an increase in the amount of mineralized trabecular bone in adults. Under certain conditions of use, however, some compounds may also suppress bone growth and matrix mineralization, resulting in accumulation of increased amounts of unmineralized matrix as described above. Varying toxic effects upon bone are reported with **zinc** toxicity, but **zinc** is a potent inhibitor of osteoclast activity *in vitro* and abolishes the stimulatory effect of PTH [17]. **Zinc** also appears to regulate secretion of calcitonin from the thyroid gland.

The effects of **oestrogenic agents** and the anti-oestrogenic agent **tamoxifen** upon bone mass appear to contradict each other, and the extent to which the actions of oestrogen upon bone are mediated by oestrogen receptors remains unclear. In women, **oestrogen** is thought to protect the skeleton by inhibiting bone resorption, and in the rat oestrogen also increases bone mass by stimulating cancellous bone formation. Oestrogens such as **diethylstilboestrol** and **oestradiol** also produce increased bone mass characterized by dense thick trabeculae of bone in the metaphysis due to osteoclastic inhibition. However, inhibition of bone resorption has also been reported with use of the anti-oestrogenic agent **tamoxifen** in mice. This may be because **tamoxifen** also acts as a partial oestrogen agonist, but recent studies have indicated that **tamoxifen** strongly inhibits bone resorption that is stimulated by vitamin D analogues and which is therefore independent of oestrogenic activity [18]. A pure oestrogen antagonist, **ICI 182 780**, reduces cancellous bone volume in the rat, adding weight to the theory that the protective effect of **tamoxifen** upon bone mass is mediated by mechanisms other than oestrogenic activity.

The effects of non-steroidal anti-inflammatory drugs (NSAIDs) on bone are well known. **Acetylsalicylic acid**, **naproxen** and **ibuprofen** all enhance bone formation, and **flurbiprofen** has been shown to decrease the number of osteoclasts in the rat tibia model, although **flurbiprofen** itself has an equivocal effect on bone formation [19]. These agents inhibit the formation of cyclo-oxygenase products, which are known to represent a major regulatory step in bone destruction.

The synthetic prostaglandin analogue **misoprostol** has been associated with proliferation of bony tissue in the marrow cavity of the femur in mice (hyperostosis). Other prostaglandins have produced similar effects in the dog and rat. The mechanism for this effect is unclear, but **prostaglandin E_2** increases the frequency of remodelling of bone with an imbalance favouring bone formation. **Calcitonin** produces a diffuse increase in cortical bone thickness in rats and rabbits.

Osteolathyrism is a specific condition of bone in which bone deformity and shortening occur with marked proliferation of bone beneath the periosteum to form bony masses (exostoses). The underlying mechanism is thought to be inhibition of collagen cross-linking in bone matrix. This condition is induced by seeds of the plant *Lathyrus odoratus* and by lathyrogenic agents such as **aminopropionitrile**.

Replacement of normal cortical and medullary bone by dense trabecular bone is a condition described in man as osteopetrosis, in which failure of normal bone resorption by osteoclasts occurs, due to a deficiency of osteoclasts and lack of response to vitamin D and its analogues. Comparable lesions occur in transgenic and mutant mice and rats [20] but drug-induced osteopetrosis has not been recorded.

Secondary mechanisms of bone toxicity

Stimulation of osteoclastic resorption of bone is an effect mediated by PTH in response to falling blood calcium levels. This process normally maintains blood mineral homeostasis but under certain conditions can result in excessive absorption of matrix minerals leading to a condition described as 'fibrous osteodystrophy'. Therefore, any agent that induces hyperparathyroidism may induce fibrous osteodystrophy, particularly when excessive PTH secretion is the result of phosphate retention induced by renal failure.

Studies of the effects of **thyroxine (T_4)** on bone indicate that thyroid hormones are a requirement for normal bone turnover. Hyperthyroid animals show increased mineral formation and bone turnover rates, whereas hypothyroidism results in a marked reduction in osteoid and an increase in trabecular bone [21]. Therefore, agents which affect thyroid function have the potential to affect bone turnover, and **propylthiouracil** which is used in the treatment of hyperthyroidism in man produces decreased bone turnover in the rat.

Inflammatory lesions

The occurrence of xenobiotic-induced arthritis in the laboratory animal is often part of the experimental process of developing a reproducible model for the study of arthritis in man. The local induction of arthritis by intra-articular injection of various agents has been discussed earlier, but other agents induce arthritis after systemic administration, either by immune or non-immune mechanisms.

Immune arthritis is often induced experimentally by injection into the footpad of natural **adjuvants** containing heat-killed microorganisms or their cell wall components within an oily vehicle, and has also been recorded following subcutaneous or intravascular injection of a muramyl peptide immunostimulant **muroctasin** in the dog and rat. It can also occur as a side-effect of treatment with **trimethoprim** or **sulphadiazine**. Synovitis, with synovial hyperplasia, villus formation and periosteal new bone formation are characteristic findings that may be due to deposition of circulating immune complexes which provoke a chronic inflammatory reponse.

Non-immune arthritis has followed the administration of various agents such as **alkyldiamine** and **6-sulphanil-aminoindazole**. The pathogenesis of these lesions is largely unknown but probably involves cartilage matrix degradation and loss, with subsequent extensive arthritis. Arthritis can also be induced in **adrenalectomized** or **hypophysectomized** rats treated with **prolactin** and **growth hormone**.

Secondary mechanisms of joint toxicity

The most common cause of secondary joint toxicity in man is altered renal excretion of urate leading to hyperuricaemia and deposition of monosodium-urate crystals within connective tissues, particularly cartilage. A diagnostic feature is the presence of urate crystals within synovial fluid. Xenobiotics which alter urate excretion include diuretics such as **frusemide**, and the immunosuppressant **cyclosporine**.

8.3.3 *Teratogenesis*

Abnormalities of the skeletal system are a relatively common teratogenic effect in the rodent and range from minor changes such as absence of part of a digit to extensive spinal defects. The Skeletal Variant Assay System in the CD-1 mouse recognizes 88 morphological changes in the mouse skeleton, and the effects of different treatment regimes with six established skeletal teratogens upon this assay have been reviewed [22].

The drug **thalidomide** is probably one of the best-known skeletal teratogens and produces reduction deformities (absence of part or all of the extremities) by interference with limb bud development in man, primates and the rabbit. **Retinoic acid** and **cadmium** may also produce limb bud abnormalities in rodents and *in vitro* studies using **retinoic acid** suggest that impaired chondrogenesis and myogenesis play a significant role. Physiological levels of **retinoic acid** are essential for normal skeletal development, but high levels of **retinoic acid** also interfere with craniofacial development and vertebral ossification. **5-fluorouracil** induces hindlimb abnormalities and cleft palate in the rat by mechanisms that are not understood fully but include altered cell cycle progression. *In vitro* hindlimb explants from the rat treated with **5-fluorouracil** show deficits in protein and DNA content [23].

Anomalies of the digits are induced in rodents by **acetazolamide, cyclophosphamide** and **cytosine arabinoside** amongst other xenobiotics. The effects of **cytosine arabinoside** can also be enhanced by exposure to **microwave irradiation**.

Defects of the axial skeleton, such as spina bifida resulting from incomplete neural tube closure, occur spontaneously in most species but have also been induced in rodents by **vincristine** and **actinomycin D**.

The anticonvulsant drug **valproic acid** produces defects throughout the skeletal system of the rat, characterized by generalized underossification and abnormal vertebrae and ribs. Supernumerary ribs are a common occurrence in teratology studies and are an established effect of treatment of the rat with **aspirin**, but may be the result of a developmental delay rather than a true teratogenic effect [24]. **Ethylene glycol monoethyl ether** increases the incidence of various skeletal anomalies.

8.3.4 *Carcinogenesis*

The development of spontaneous tumours of bone and cartilage is an uncommon event in laboratory animal species. **Ionizing radiation** induces malignant bone tumours (osteosarcoma) in man and laboratory rodents, and the radioisotope **americium-241** produces malignant bone and cartilage tumours (chondrosarcoma) in the laboratory beagle.

Alkylating agents, polycyclic hydrocarbons, nitrosamines, nitrosoureas, acronycine, vinyl chloride and **aniline dyes** have all been used to induce bone tumours in laboratory animals in attempts to reproduce a model for study of osteosarcoma in man. **Acronycine** also induced osteosarcomas in tissues other than the skeleton.

Table 8.3 summarizes some of the types of compounds that induce skeletal toxicity and the nature of the effect they induce.

8.4 **Morphological Responses to Injury**

The morphological responses of bone to injury are generally discussed in most texts with reference to the terminology of clinical disease in man; that is, osteoporosis, osteomalacia and so on. The lesions induced in the skeletal system of laboratory animals do not necessarily fall into the same morphological categories but an understanding of the typical morphological changes that can occur, and that are well characterized, is useful in the interpretation of the effects induced by novel xenobiotic compounds.

8.4.1 *Degenerative Lesions of Bone*

The morphological changes associated with the degenerative metabolic diseases of bone are summarized below.

Osteomalacia

Osteomalacia is characterized by defective matrix mineralization leading to an excess of unmineralized matrix (hyperosteoidosis) which interferes with endochondral bone formation. Macroscopic enlargement of the growth plate area can be seen in the osteomalacic rat due to overgrowth of poorly mineralized matrix in the metaphysis. This is the result of failure of the epiphyseal plate cartilage cells to disintegrate during the normal process of endochondral ossification, producing irregular masses

Table 8.3   Induced lesions of bone, cartilage and joints

Toxic agent	Type of agent	Species	Nature of effect
Bone			
Methotrexate	Cytostatic agent	Rabbit Man	Bone growth suppression Osteoporosis
Corticosteroids	Anti-inflammatory agents	Man Rat	Osteoporosis Impaired division of bone progenitor cells Enhanced osteoclast activity
Diphenylhydantoin, phenobarbital	Anticonvulsants	Man	Osteomalacia by hepatic enzyme induction and increased catabolism of 25-hydroxyvitamin D
Lead, cadmium	Trace elements	Rat	Disruption of mineralization during growth
Ti, Cr, Co, Mo, Ni, Fe ions	Orthopaedic prosthetic implant	Man	Impaired osteoblast differentiation and osteogenesis *in vitro*. Periprosthetic osteolysis *in vivo*
Vitamin A	Essential vitamin	Rat	Fractures due to reduced bone formation via osteoblast inhibition. Premature growth plate closure
Oestrogen	Hormone	Rat	Decreased resorption of metaphyseal trabeculae, decreased bone length
Pamidronate	Bisphosphonate	Dog	Increased bone mineralization
Lathyrus odoratus seeds	Lathyrogenic plant toxin	Rat	Inhibition of cross-linking of collagen molecule leads to bone deformity
Americium-241, beryllium salts	Radioisotope	Dog Rabbit	Osteosarcoma, fibrosarcoma, chondrosarcoma of bone
Methylmercuric chloride	Heavy metal	Fetal rat	Incomplete formation of fetal ossification centres, in sternum, pelvis
5-Fluorouracil	Chemotherapeutic agent	Fetal rat	Growth retardation, hindlimb defects
Tobramycin	Aminoglycoside antimicrobial	Rat/Man	*In vitro* decreased osteoblast replication
Zinc, cadmium	Trace elements	Rat	*In vitro* osteoclast inhibition
Cartilage and joint			
Cyclophosphamide, methotrexate	Chemotherapeutic agents	Rat Man	Cartilage matrix degradation
Aluminium derivatives	Trace metal	Rat Rabbit	Synovial proliferation, loss of cartilage proteoglycan
Pipemidic acid, ciprofloxacin	Quinolone carboxylic acid analogue antimicrobial agents	Mouse Dog	Chondrocyte loss, matrix degeneration, articular cartilage erosion
Frusemide, ethacrynic acid	Diuretics	Man	Arthritis via altered uric acid metabolism
Isoniazid	Antibiotic	Man	Polyarthralgia
Interleukin-1, TNF*	Cytokines	Rabbit	Cartilage matrix loss *in vivo* and *in vitro*

*TNF, tumour necrosis factor.

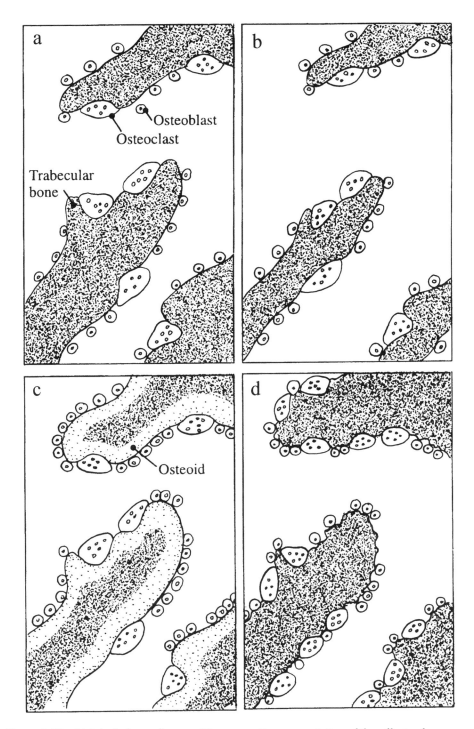

Figure 8.12 Metabolic bone diseases. Diagrammatic representation of the effects of metabolic bone diseases. (a) Control (normal trabecular bone). (b) The effects of osteoporosis are shown, with a decrease in trabecular bone mass. (c) Osteomalacia with defective matrix mineralization results in accumulation of unmineralized osteoid matrix on the surface of trabecular bone. Osteoblasts may be more numerous. (d) Fibrous osteodystrophy results in increased turnover of bone with raised numbers of osteoblasts along the endosteum attempting to match the rate of resorption by osteoclasts.

of cartilage projecting into the marrow cavity. Osteoid matrix accumulates upon these cartilage remnants and upon trabecular bone with no evidence of mineralization, and increased numbers of osteoclasts and osteoblasts are present in these areas (Figure 8.12). Bone remodelling is also impaired and with time the normal lamellar bone of the bone cortices is replaced by unmineralized bone and osteoid accumulates beneath the periosteum and endosteum.

Osteoporosis

Decreased bone mass and thinning of bone trabeculae are the hallmarks of osteoporosis resulting in reduced complexity of the trabecular bone system (Figure 8.12). In man, where osteoporosis has been extensively studied, morphometric analysis demonstrates a reduction in the number of interconnections between the bony trabeculae and the presence of microfractures. The bone cortex also becomes thinned and compression fractures may occur.

Fibrous osteodystrophy

Fibrous osteodystrophy most commonly affects cortical bone more severely than trabecular bone, for reasons that are obscure. In the rat, the femur, humerus, vertebrae and cranial bones appear to be most susceptible whereas in the dog, the susceptibility of the mandible led to use of the term 'rubber jaw'. Increased osteoclastic resorption of bone produces thinned cortices and clusters of osteoclasts bore into and enlarge the Haversian canals of compact bone. In cancellous bone, osteoclasts 'tunnel' along the length of the trabeculae leading to trabecular atrophy, and the bone marrow becomes replaced by fibrovascular tissue containing many osteoprogenitor cells and osteoblasts which attempt to maintain the balance of bone formation and resorption (Figures 8.12 and 8.13).

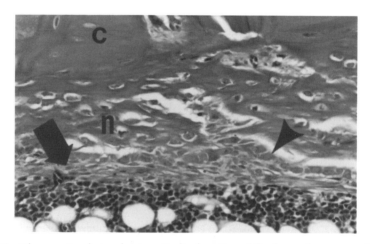

Figure 8.13 Fibrous osteodystrophy. Longitudinal section of the femur from a rat with endstage chronic renal disease and secondary hyperparathyroidism. The early lesion of fibrous osteodystrophy is shown. Many osteoblasts are clustered along the endosteum (arrowhead) and are laying down a layer of new bone (n) upon the existing cortical bone (c). The adjacent area of bone marrow has been replaced by a fibrous band of tissue containing osteoprogenitor cells (arrow).

Osteosclerosis

Osteosclerosis occurs spontaneously in the ageing female B6C3F$_1$ mouse and occasionally in the F-344 rat, as well as secondary to xenobiotic administration. The sternum appears to be most susceptible but the tibia and vertebrae may also show involvement. The marrow cavity becomes replaced by irregular trabecular bone beginning in the metaphysis, with proliferation of fibrous tissue on the surface of the new bone. The remodelling process may also involve the inner surface of cortical bone to a minor degree.

The increased medullary bone that accompanies osteoclast inhibition by **bisphosphonate** administration can be seen primarily in the sternum, rib and the long bone metaphyses. The lesion is characterized by the persistence of the new bone laid down upon the degenerating cartilage template produced by the epiphyseal growth plate. The remodelling of this bone that normally occurs to produce cortical bone at the periphery of the metaphysis, and trabecular bone elsewhere, is prevented, such that a considerable proportion of the marrow cavity may be replaced by immature bone (Figure 8.14). Osteoclasts may be numerous but their function is impaired.

Osteopetrosis

Osteopetrosis in man is characterized by filling of the marrow cavity of the long bones by immature unmodelled new bone, and mature trabeculae do not form.

Osteonecrosis

Bone necrosis has been recorded as a spontaneous event in laboratory animals either within the subarticular region or in the bone shaft as a consequence of impaired blood supply. Necrosis of the subchondral bone plate may be a feature of

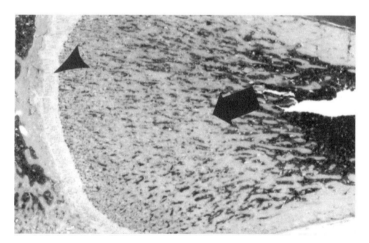

Figure 8.14 Osteosclerosis. Longitudinal section through the femur of a rat treated with a bisphosphonate for 16 days by the intraperitoneal route. An extensive area of the medullary cavity adjacent to the epiphyseal growth plate (arrowhead) has been replaced by dense trabecular bone (arrow). (Reproduced by kind permission of M. Blades.)

osteonecrosis in man irrespective of cause, and has also been seen associated with **adjuvant-induced arthritis** in the rat. The overlying cartilage may remain viable since it is avascular and derives its nutrition from synovial fluid. Many osteoclasts are attracted to the area to resorb the necrotic bone (Figure 8.15), although if the damage is not too extensive, some trabeculae remain to provide a scaffolding for repair.

8.4.2. Degenerative Lesions of Joints

Spontaneous lesions of the joints occur in ageing rats and mice and are characterized by degenerative changes in chondrocytes and matrix of the hyaline cartilage of synovial joints (chondromalacia). Xenobiotic-induced degenerative lesions have a similar appearance and may show a predisposition for specific joints. Special staining techniques demonstrate loss of cartilage matrix, and increased numbers of 'empty' cartilage cell lacunae suggest chondrocyte necrosis. The cartilage may develop 'blisters' and microfissures and undergo erosion, leading to degenerative changes in the underlying exposed bone. Chondrocyte and synovial cell proliferation (hyperplasia), and periosteal new bone formation may occur at the margins of the joint.

Degenerative lesions of articular or growth plate cartilage in the sternum or long bones occur frequently in ageing rats and are characterized by formation of cystic spaces containing material with mucinous characteristics.

8.4.3 Inflammatory Lesions of Bone and Joints

Spontaneous inflammatory lesions of bone (osteitis, osteomyelitis) are rare and likely to be secondary to joint disease or inflammation in surrounding tissues.

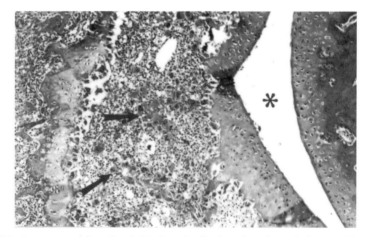

Figure 8.15 Immune-mediated arthritis. Longitudinal section through the tarsal joint of a mouse with adjuvant-induced arthritis. Necrosis of the subchondral bone has stimulated invasion by many osteoclasts to remove bone debris (arrows). The overlying cartilage is comparatively intact. (∗) joint space. (Reproduced by kind permission of H.R. Brown.)

Inflammation of the periosteum and underlying cortical bone is a relatively common event in ageing rats housed on wire mesh, and in conjunction with the extensive soft tissue and joint inflammation that also occurs, may lead to fusion (ankylosis) of the tarsal joint.

It is beyond the scope of this text to discuss the morphological changes occurring in immune-mediated and non-immune-mediated arthritis. Immune-mediated arthritis may be characterized only by synovitis with proliferation of the synovial cells, or it may lead to an exudative destructive lesion with vascular involvement leading to subchondral bone necrosis, severe degenerative changes in the joint and adjacent tissues, and collapse of the whole joint structure (Figure 8.15).

8.4.4 *Proliferative Lesions of Bone and Cartilage*

Proliferation of bone may be a feature of some degenerative and inflammatory diseases of the skeletal system and also a feature of fracture repair. Chondrocyte and synovial cell hyperplasia are both features, as discussed above, of degenerative or inflamatory joint disease.

Neoplastic proliferation of bone and cartilage results in a variety of benign and malignant tumours in man and animals. These tumours arise predominantly from osteoblasts/osteocytes and chondroblasts/chondrocytes but the classification of these tumours, particularly in man, is complex. The most common type of osteosarcoma, however, has prominent osteoid deposition with areas of osteoblast proliferation, but in other tumours areas of osteoclast-like cells also occur. Neoplasms of cartilage (chondroma, chondrosarcoma) are generally comprised of chondrocytes and matrix but areas of osteoid deposition may also occur.

8.5 Testing for Toxicity

8.5.1 *Microscopy*

The usual rationale in regulatory toxicity testing is to examine haematoxylin and eosin stained sections of part or all of the femur, the femoro-tibial joint and part of the tibia, in conjunction with the sternum. This allows the pathologist to assess areas of compact bone in the shafts of the long bones, epiphyseal growth plates and new bone in the metaphysis, trabecular bone, a synovial joint and fibrocartilage joints, and bone marrow. In order to produce these sections, the bone is usually first demineralized since it is generally too brittle to cut conventional sections. This process inevitably limits the amount of information to be gained about the mineral component of the bone matrix, but the organic component of the matrix is preserved. Histological stains such as haematoxylin and eosin combined with alcian blue can outline the spicules of calcified cartilage matrix upon which new bone is being deposited adjacent to the epiphyseal growth plate, and plane-polarized light will reveal the birefringent collagen fibres of the matrix. Ground thin sections of undemineralized bone can be produced to examine intact bone matrix, and stains such as Goldner's trichrome will demonstrate areas of unmineralized matrix. Histochemical stains such as alkaline phosphatase demonstrate osteoblasts, and lectin histochemistry can localize matrix proteoglycans.

8.5.2 *Morphometric Analysis*

The detailed study of bone morphology can be a useful adjunct to the examinations described above but because of the special techniques required, this is not usually incorporated into routine study design. It is beyond the scope of this chapter to describe these techniques in detail, but a brief outline is given below.

Examination of radiographs and undecalcified sections of bone can give useful information about bone remodelling and growth. Measurement of the rate of bone formation can be relatively simply achieved with the use of fluorochrome markers such as tetracycline, alizarin red S or calcein. Tetracycline is usually the marker of choice and is administered to the subject at two defined time points. The marker is incorporated into new areas of osteoid that are being laid down but not yet mineralized (osteoid seams) and its fluorescent properties will delineate two separate 'fronts' of osteoid formation in a subsequent bone biopsy or post-mortem sample. The distance between the two areas of labelling therefore gives an estimate of rate of bone formation.

8.5.3 *Biochemical Evaluation*

Plasma concentrations of calcium, phosphorus and alkaline phosphatase may alter in metabolic bone disease. Alkaline phosphatase is secreted by osteoblasts during osteoid synthesis and matrix mineralization, and levels are therefore generally higher in young animals. However, isoforms of this enzyme occur in other tissues such as the liver, and therefore the standard assay is not specific to bone metabolism. Radioimmunoassay for serum levels of PTH, calcitonin and calcitriol is feasible in several species of laboratory animals and serum levels of osteocalcin, a matrix protein expressed by differentiating osteoblasts, correlate well with bone growth.

Urinary calcium and hydroxyproline excretion may increase when osteoclastic bone resorption is increased. Hydroxyproline is an amino acid released during collagen degradation, as are peptides involved in cross-linking mature collagen (pyridinium cross-links) which are also excreted in urine during increased bone resorption.

8.6 **Conclusions**

Our knowledge of the pathology of the musculoskeletal system is expanding rapidly as the molecular basis for developmental control and normal function is gradually unravelled, and is matched by increasing opportunities for detailed investigation of morphology. Whilst the spectrum of pathological change encountered in the musculoskeletal system remains relatively unchanged, the understanding of physiology, mechanisms of disease and toxicity has grown and indicated how morphological and other investigations may be used to greater effect.

The musculoskeletal system is particularly accessible for examination during the in-life phase of toxicology studies, and alterations in behaviour and locomotion should lead the investigator to consider the possibility of musculoskeletal toxicity. Recent developments in clinical pathology offer more sensitive and accurate tests for monitoring muscle and bone integrity *in vivo* that may be incorporated into study design. The importance of careful sampling and observation in routine toxicological investigations should not be underestimated, however, and the restrictions enforced by limited sampling should also be appreciated.

References

1. WECKER, L. and STOUSE, M. (1985) Effects of chronic paraoxon administration on skeletal muscle fiber integrity, *Research Communications in Chemical Pathology and Pharmacology*, **49**, 203–213.
2. GEBBERS, J.O., LOTSCHER, M., KOBEL, W., PORTMANN, R. and LAISSUE, J.A. (1986) Acute toxicity of pyridostigmine in rats: histological findings, *Archives of Toxicology*, **58**, 271–275.
3. DE BLEECKER, J.L., VAN DEN ABEELE, K.G. and DE REUCK, J.L. (1992) Variable involvement of rat skeletal muscles in paraoxon-induced necrotizing myopathy, *Research Communications in Chemical Pathology and Pharmacology*, **75**, 309–322.
4. PIERNO, S., DE LUCA, A., TRICARIO, D., ROSELLI, A., NATUZZI, F., FERRANNINI, E., LAICO, M. and CARNERINO, D.C. (1995) Potential risk of myopathy by HMG-CoA reductase inhibitors: a comparison of pravastatin and simvastatin effects of membrane electrical properties of rat skeletal muscle fibers, *Journal of Pharmacology and Experimental Therapeutics*, **275**, 1490–1496.
5. SMITH, P.F., EYDELOTH, R.S., GROSSMAN, S.J., STUBBS, R.J., SCHWARTZ, M.S., GERMERHAUSEN, J.I., VYAS, K.P., KARI, P.H. and MACDONALD, J.S. (1991) HMG-CoA reductase inhibitor-induced myopathy in the rat: cyclosporine A interaction and mechanism studies, *Journal of Pharmacology and Experimental Therapeutics*, **257**, 1225–1235.
6. MASTERS, B.A., PALMOSKI, M.J., FLINT, O.P., GREGG, R.E., WANG-IVERSON, D. and DURHAM, S.K. (1995) *In vitro* toxicity of the 3-hydroxy-3-methylglutaryl coenzyme A reductase inhibitors, pravastatin, lovastatin, and simvastatin, using neonatal rat skeletal myocytes, *Toxicology and Applied Pharmacology*, **131**, 163–174.
7. DIGREGORIO, F., FAVARO, G. and FIORI, M.G. (1989) Functional evaluation of acute vincristine toxicity in rat skeletal muscle, *Muscle and Nerve*, **12**, 1017–1023.
8. MODICA-NAPOLITANO, J.S. (1993) AZT causes tissue-specific inhibition of mitochondrial bioenergetic function, *Biochemical and Biophysical Research Communciations*, **194**, 170–177.
9. d'AMATI, G. and LEWIS, G. (1994) Zidovudine causes early increases in mitochondrial ribonucleic acid abundance and induces ultrastructural changes in cultured mouse muscle cells, *Laboratory Investigation*, **71**, 879–884.
10. PREEDY, V.R., MARWAY, J.S., MACPHERSON, A.J. and PETERS, T.J. (1990) Ethanol-induced smooth and skeletal muscle myopathy: use of animal studies, *Drug and Alcohol Dependence*, **26**, 1–8.
11. REICHEL, K., REHFELDT, C., WEIKARD, R., SCHADEREIT, R. and KRAWIELITZKI, K. (1993) Effect of a β-agonist and a β-agonist/β-antagonist combination on muscle growth, body composition and protein metabolism in rats, *Archiv für Tierernahrung*, **45**, 211–225.
12. YANDER, G. and KAJI, H. (1984) Investigating the myopathic effects of 6-mercaptopurine on developing skeletal muscle cells *in vitro*, *Drug and Chemical Toxicology*, **7**, 177–192.
13. SHAHGALDI, B.F., HEATLEY, F.W., DEWAR, A. and CORRIN, B. (1995) *In vivo* corrosion of cobalt-chromium and titanium wear particles, *Journal of Bone and Joint Surgery*, **77**, 962–966.
14. GEGOUT, P., GILLET, P., CHEVRIER, D., GUINGAMP, C., TERLAIN, B. and NETTER, P. (1994) Characterization of zymosan-induced arthritis in the rat: effects on joint inflammation and cartilage metabolism, *Life Science*, **55**, PL321–326.

15. HAMILTON, J.D. and O'FLAHERTY, E.J. (1995) Influence of lead on mineralization during bone growth, *Fundamental and Applied Toxicology*, **26**, 265–271.
16. BONJOUR, J.P., AMMANN, P., BARBIER, A., CAVERZASIO, J. and RIZZOLI, R. (1995) Tiludronate: bone pharmacology and safety, *Bone*, **17**, 473S–477S.
17. MOONGA, B.S. and DEMPSTER, D.W. (1995) Zinc is a potent inhibitor of osteoclastic bone resorption *in vitro*, *Journal of Bone and Mineral Research*, **10**, 453–457.
18. VINK-VAN WIJNGAARDEN, T., BIRKENHAGER, J.C., KLEINEKOORT, W.M., VAN DEN BEMD, G.J., POLS, H.A. and VAN LEEUWEN, J.P. (1995) Antiestrogens inhibit *in vitro* bone resorption stimulated by 1,25-dihydroxyvitamin D3 and the vitamin D3 analogs EB1089 and KH1060, *Endocrinology*, **136**, 812–815.
19. WEBER, H.P., FIORELLINI, J.P., PAQUETTE, D.W., HOWELL, T.H. and WILLIAMS, R.C. (1994) Inhibition of peri-implant bone loss with the nonsteroidal anti-inflammatory drug flurbiprofen in beagle dogs. A preliminary study, *Clinical Oral Implants Research*, **5**, 148–153.
20. SUNDQUIST, K.T., JACKSON, M.E., HERMEY, D.C. and MARKS, S.C. (1995) Osteoblasts from the toothless (osteopetrotic) mutation in the rat are unable to direct bone resorption by normal osteoclasts in response to 1,25-dihydroxy-vitamin D, *Tissue and Cell*, **27**, 569–574.
21. ALLAIN, T.J., THOMAS, M.R., MCGREGOR, A.M. and SALISBURY, J.R. (1995) A histomorphometric study of bone changes in thyroid dysfunction rats, *Bone*, **16**, 505–509.
22. BECK, S.L. (1993) Additional endpoints and overview of a mouse skeletal variant assay for detecting exposure to teratogens, *Teratology*, **47**, 147–157.
23. SHUEY, D.L., BUCKALEW, A.R., WILKE, T.S., ROGERS, J.M. and ABBOTT, B.D. (1994) Early events following maternal exposure to 5-fluorouracil lead to dysmorphology in cultured embryonic tissues, *Teratology*, **50**, 379–386.
24. WICKRAMARATNE, G.E., 1988, The post-natal fate of supernumerary ribs in rat teratogenicity studies, *Journal of Applied Toxicology*, **8**, 91–94.

Additional Reading

GOPINATH, C., PRENTICE, D.E. and LEWIS, D.J. (1987) The musculoskeletal system and skin, in *Atlas of Experimental Toxicological Pathology*, pp. 156–166, Lancaster: MTP Press.

GREAVES, P. (1990) Musculoskeletal system, in *Histopathology of Preclinical Toxicity Studies*, pp. 143–186, Amsterdam: Elsevier.

GURLEY, A.M. and ROTH, S.I. (1992) Bone, in STERNBERG, S.S. (Ed.) *Histology for Pathologists*, pp. 61–79, New York: Raven Press.

HEFFNER, R.R. (1992) Skeletal muscle, in STERNBERG, S.S. (Ed.) *Histology for Pathologists*, pp. 81–108, New York: Raven Press.

LEININGER, J.R. and RILEY, M.G. (1990) Bones, joints, and synovia, in BOORMAN, G.A., MONTGOMERY, C.A. and MACKENZIE, W.F. (Eds) *Pathology of the Fischer Rat*, pp. 209–226, San Diego: Academic Press.

MCDONALD, M.M. and HAMILTON, B.F. (1990) Skeletal Muscle, in BOORMAN, G.A., MONTGOMERY, C.A. and MACKENZIE, W.F. (Eds) *Pathology of the Fischer Rat*, pp. 193–207, San Diego: Academic Press.

WOODARD, J.C. and JEE, W.S.S. (1991) Skeletal system, in HASCHEK, W.M. and ROUSSEAUX, C.G. (Eds) *Handbook of Toxicologic Pathology*, pp. 489–537, San Diego: Academic Press.

VAN VLEET, J.F., FERRANS, V.J. and HERMAN, E. (1991) Cardiovascular and skeletal muscle systems, in HASCHEK, W.M. and ROUSSEAUX, C.G. (Eds) *Handbook of Toxicologic Pathology*, pp. 539–624, San Diego: Academic Press.

9

The Nervous System

PETER BUCKLEY

9.1 Introduction

Scientific and public concern over the risk of neurotoxic damage from exposure to industrial chemicals and environmental contaminants has resulted in a renewed interest in the nervous system as a target for toxic injury. The magnitude of this concern can be gauged by the response of the regulatory authorities: many have issued, or are on the point of issuing, revised, more stringent guidelines for the assessment of neurotoxicity. These guidelines recommend that a thorough and specialized neurological examination, together with a more extensive neuropathological investigation, must be incorporated into any studies designed to detect neurotoxicity.

The nervous system has several unique anatomical and physiological features which make it exquisitely susceptible to toxic damage and to the consequences of this damage:

1 Neurons are dependent upon aerobic glycolysis for the production of the large quantities of high-energy phosphates which they require. Since neurons have no significant stored energy reserves, they must have a constant supply of glucose and oxygen to meet their energy requirements. In addition, many areas of the normal brain operate in an environment with a low oxygen tension. Thus any factor interrupting the supply of glucose or oxygen, even for a short period, may cause damage or death of the neurons.

2 Neurons have few enzymes which are able to metabolize xenobiotics, so that they may be more susceptible to the effects of toxins.

3 The nervous system has a high content of lipid, approximately half of which is contained in the myelinated nerve fibres. Many lipid soluble toxins are able to cross the blood–brain barrier, and will accumulate, therefore, in the nervous system, where they may remain within the lipids of the myelin for prolonged periods.

4 Neurons are the largest cells in the body, the axons of some cells being over 1 m in length in some species. Maintaining an ionic differential across the membrane

of such a large cell requires the expenditure of considerable amounts of energy. Furthermore, all of the materials required for the maintenance and nutrition of the axon are manufactured in the cell body, so these must be transported along the length of the axon. Other substances are transported in the opposite direction, towards the cell body. These transport processes are energy dependent. Any interference with cell metabolism, therefore, will lead to a rapid decline in axonal transport, followed by degeneration of the axon. Toxic chemicals may produce similar damage by blocking the mechanisms of axonal transport.

5 The neurons of the central nervous system are so specialized that they have lost the ability to undergo cell division. Therefore, any neurons within the central nervous system which are lost due to toxic damage, cannot be replaced.

6 Because of the complex integrated structure of the nervous system, and its control of vital biological functions, damage to even a small part of the system may lead to severe and diverse clinical signs or even to the death of the animal.

It is essential, therefore, that all novel substances are adequately tested to detect any evidence of neurotoxic potential. In order to design and conduct a satisfactory investigation it is important to understand the basic anatomy and physiology of the normal nervous system, to be aware of the problems inherent in examination of this system, and also to comprehend the range of biochemical and pathological changes which can occur. Before the relevance of any pathological findings which develop in such studies can be assessed in relation to the risk to man, it is essential to establish whether these findings are due to a direct toxic effect on the nervous system, or whether they are secondary to a toxic effect on non-neural tissue; only those substances producing direct injury to neural tissue should be classified as neurotoxic.

Before any meaningful interpretation of the results of such an investigation can be made, the problems associated with extrapolation of data from animals to man and from high-dose to low-dose exposure, must be appreciated. The study design must ensure that a dose−response curve can be constructed for any neurotoxic effects and that, whenever possible, a species is chosen in which the metabolism of the compound under examination is equivalent to that in man. Only by achieving these aims can a satisfactory risk assessment be made.

9.2 Anatomy, Histology and Physiology

Insufficient space precludes detailed descriptions of the gross and microscopic anatomy of the nervous system and of its physiology. Only those points which are essential to the understanding of the common pathological and toxicological changes will be described. More detailed descriptions can be found in the recommended texts [1−5].

The nervous system of all mammals has the same basic plan and physiological mechanisms, although some minor species variations do occur. For descriptive purposes the rat will be used as it is the species most commonly employed in toxicity testing.

9.2.1 *Anatomy*

Unlike most of the other organ systems, which are compact and readily identifiable on gross examination, the nervous system ramifies over the entire body and most parts can be revealed only by extensive and careful dissection, or by the use of a microscope. The distribution of nervous tissue, however, is not uniform throughout the body. In particular, there is a concentration along the midline axis within the bones of the cranium and the vertebral canal. These concentrations form the brain and spinal cord, respectively, and together are known as the central nervous system. The remainder of the nervous tissue constitutes the peripheral nervous system and consists of the cranial nerves, which emerge from the skull through tunnels or foramina in the bone, and the spinal nerves, which issue from the vertebral column through the intervertebral spaces.

On gross examination of the nervous system, areas of grey and white matter are visible: grey matter mainly consists of cell bodies, while white matter is mainly composed of myelinated nerve fibres. Within the central nervous system, grey matter occurs in layers or in more discrete areas, termed nuclei, and white matter as columns or tracts. In the peripheral nervous system, grey matter is in the form of circumscribed aggregations of neuronal cell bodies, the ganglia, or in more diffuse associations, termed plexuses. White matter exists as nerves, nerve roots or nerve trunks. Nerve fibres conducting impulses towards the central nervous system are known as afferent fibres, those conducting impulses away from the central nervous system as efferent fibres.

The central nervous system

In addition to the protection given by the bony casings, the central nervous system is protected further by layers of connective tissue, the meninges. The outermost layer, the dura mater, is composed of tough fibrous connective tissue. This overlies a thin connective tissue membrane, the arachnoid mater, from which extends a delicate network of fibres spanning a space, the subarachnoid space, through which the cerebrospinal fluid circulates. The innermost layer, the pia mater, is a thin, highly vascular membrane which closely invests the surface of the nervous tissue. Extensions of the pia and arachnoid membranes surround blood vessels as they enter and leave the central nervous system, producing perivascular spaces, the Virchow–Robin spaces, continuous with the subarachnoid space.

Embryologically the central nervous system arises from an infold of the ectoderm along the midline longitudinal axis. This infolding continues to form a tube, the neural tube. During subsequent development, the walls of this tube thicken so that the central canal becomes reduced in size. The cranial end of this tube undergoes exuberant differential growth to form the brain, while the remainder becomes the spinal cord.

The brain Initially three swellings arise, the forebrain (prosencephalon), the midbrain (mesencephalon) and the hindbrain (rhombencephalon). Coincidentally, the tube undergoes flexure, the forebrain bending ventrally in relation to the midbrain (the cephalic flexure) and the hindbrain bending upon itself in a dorsal direction (the pontine flexure). Further growth leads to differential thickening of the walls of the tube:

The hindbrain The flexing of the tube in the region of the hindbrain causes a widening and a flattening of the lumen which persists in the adult as the fourth ventricle. The dorsal part of the tube is stretched and becomes very thin over this flattened lumen, but the lateral and ventral walls undergo considerable thickening. That part of the hindbrain caudal to the pontine flexure (the myelencephalon) is the medulla oblongata which is continuous caudally with the spinal cord, but is distinguishable from it by its greater width and thin dorsal region. The part cranial to the pontine flexure becomes thicker ventrally, to form the pons, but, in addition, there is tremendous lateral swelling giving rise to two masses, the cerebellar hemispheres, which meet and fuse dorsally in the midline.

The midbrain   During development, the midbrain retains its tubular structure as the growth of the different parts is more equal. However, thickening of the lateral and ventral parts restricts the lumen to a very thin tube, the aqueduct, connecting the ventricles of the forebrain and hindbrain.

The forebrain   The caudal part of the forebrain (the diencephalon) grows less rapidly than that of the cranial part, and forms the hypothalamus, thalamus and subthalamus. The central canal becomes transformed into a vertical slit, the third ventricle. The cranial part of the forebrain (the telencephalon) undergoes exuberant growth to form the olfactory lobes, the limbic system and the cerebral hemispheres. The cavities of the cerebral hemispheres connect with the third ventricle through the interventricular foramina. In the rat, the surface of the cerebral hemispheres remains smooth (lissencephalic), but in the more highly evolved species, the surface is thrown into a series of complex folds (the gyri) separated by furrows (the sulci).

The spinal cord   The lateral walls of that part of the neural tube, destined to become the spinal cord, undergo thickening, so that the lumen becomes greatly compressed and forms the central canal. The inner region of the tube differentiates into grey matter, whereas the outer region becomes white matter, so that in transverse sections the spinal cord has a butterfly-shaped area of grey matter around the central canal, surrounded by white matter. The nerve fibres of the white matter are not arranged haphazardly but are assembled into functional units, the funiculi, such that, for example, all of the axons carrying impulses associated with pain are grouped together in a specific sector of the cord on either side. The thickness of the white matter layer increases towards the brain as more nerve fibres join the spinal cord at each intervertebral foramen.

Vertebrates retain the segmental arrangement of more primitive animals, each vertebra representing one bodily segment. Afferent and efferent fibres enter and leave the spinal cord in each segment through the intervertebral foramina. However, during development the vertebral column elongates to a much greater extent than the spinal cord. This results in two important anatomical features in the adult animal. First, as the spinal cord is connected to the brain cranially, the caudal extremity does not reach to the end of the vertebral canal. Second, each segment of the cord becomes progressively more out of line with its respective body segment, so that afferent and efferent fibres must pass caudally along the sides of the spinal cord before reaching their appropriate intervertebral foramen. In the rat, the spinal cord terminates at the level of the third or fourth lumbar vertebra, but in man the termination is at the level of the first or second lumbar vertebra. In carnivores it may extend to the end of the lumbar region, and in ungulates it reaches the mid-sacral region. However, beyond the point of termination, the vertebral canal is not empty but contains the nerve roots passing down the canal to their point of exit; these nerve roots are collectively known as the cauda equina.

The peripheral nervous system

The peripheral nervous system consists of peripheral nerves that extend out from the central nervous system to reach almost every part of the body. Each nerve may contain any combination of afferent or efferent fibres of either the somatic or autonomic systems, protected by layers of connective tissue. The cell bodies of these fibres lie within the central nervous system or within ganglia located at more peripheral sites.

Nerve fibres enter or leave the spinal canal through the intervertebral spaces in either the dorsal roots, which contain afferent fibres, or in the ventral roots, which contain efferent fibres (Figure 9.1). Each dorsal root contains a swelling, the dorsal root ganglion, which contains the cell bodies of the afferent nerve fibres. These roots first unite to form the spinal nerves but then branch again to form the peripheral nerves.

Functionally the peripheral nervous system may be divided into the somatic and autonomic nervous systems:

The somatic nervous system The somatic motor neurons which form this system lie either in the brain stem or in the ventral horn of the spinal cord (the upper and lower motor neurons respectively). Their axons pass directly from the spinal cord to the skeletal muscles which they innervate without forming synapses. Somatic motor neurons exit from the central nervous system at all levels, but are particularly numerous in the cervical and lumbar regions where they pass to the extensive muscle masses of the pectoral and pelvic limbs.

The autonomic nervous system The cell bodies of the neurons of the autonomic system lie within the grey matter of the brain stem or the spinal cord. The axons of these neurons leave the central nervous system in the cranial nerves, and also in the

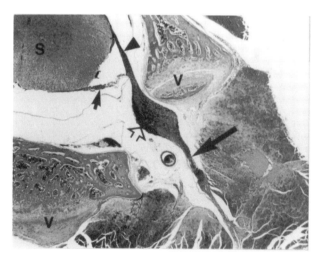

Figure 9.1 Intervertebral foramen. Transverse section of vertebral column (V) from a rat showing the origins of a spinal nerve (large arrow) from the spinal cord (S) as the dorsal (arrowhead) and ventral (small arrow) nerve roots, and a dorsal root ganglion (open arrow).

spinal nerve roots between, and caudal to, the major somatic outflows. These axons synapse within ganglia outside of the central nervous system. The autonomic fibres emerging in the cranial and caudal regions constitute the parasympathetic system and form synapses in ganglia close to the organs which they innervate, so that the postganglionic fibres are very short. In contrast, the autonomic fibres which exit from the spinal cord between the major somatic outflows and form the sympathetic system, synapse in ganglia close to the spinal cord within the sympathetic trunks.

9.2.2 *Histology*

The central nervous system

Histologically the central nervous system is composed of three distinct cell types: neurons, glial cells and the cells of blood capillaries:

Neurons

Despite variations in size and shape, all neurons have the same basic structure. The neuron consists of a cell body, or soma, composed of a centrally placed nucleus surrounded by cytoplasm, the perikaryon. Thin, branching cytoplasmic processes extend from the perikaryon and are of two types, dendrites or axons. Each neuron has one or more highly branched processes, the dendrites, which conduct impulses towards the cell body. The dendrites terminate in sensory receptors or form synapses with the axons of other neurons by means of short processes, the dendritic spines, which project from the surface of the dendritic membrane. In addition to the dendrites, each neuron has a single axon arising from a distinct area of the perikaryon, the axon hillock. The axon may branch also, each branch ending in a synapse with other neurons or effector organs (Figure 9.2).

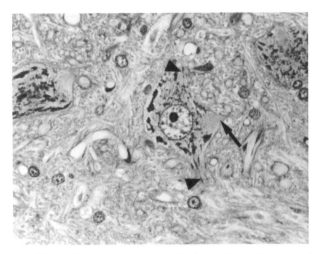

Figure 9.2 Nerve cell body (methacrylate embedded, toluidine blue stained). A lower motor neuron of the rat lumbar spinal cord showing the origins of the dendritic processes (arrowheads) and the axon hillock giving rise to the axon (arrow).

The fine structure of neurons resembles that of other actively metabolizing cells. The nuclei are generally large and rounded with completely dispersed chromatin and have prominent nucleoli. Aggregations of rough endoplasmic reticulum are conspicuous in the perikaryon and the dendrites, corresponding to the Nissl substance apparent in histological sections; the axon hillock and the axon itself are devoid of rough endoplasmic reticulum. Although a Golgi apparatus is present adjacent to the nucleus, smooth endoplasmic reticulum is not abundant. The cytoplasm of the dendrites, perikaryon and axon contain numerous vesicles, microtubules, microfilaments and mitochondria.

Glial cells

Four types of glial or non-neuronal cell are present within nervous tissue: astrocytes, oligodendrocytes, microglia and ependymal cells. Astrocytes, oligodendrocytes and ependymal cells arise from a common progenitor cell within the neural tube, the spongioblast, and constitute the neuroglia, but microglia originate outside of the nervous system from pluripotent stem cells in the haemopoietic tissue.

Astrocytes (Astroglia)　Astrocytes are the most numerous cell type in the central nervous system and play an important role in neuronal metabolism as well as providing mechanical support. Each astrocyte has numerous cytoplasmic processes which surround and support neurons and also terminate on the basement membranes of capillaries, forming an integral part of the blood–brain barrier. These processes also surround synaptic junctions and isolate them from adjacent neurons. Astrocytes are thus important in maintaining the microenvironment of the central nervous system, particularly the regulation of ion concentrations in the extracellular fluid. Furthermore, ultrastructural studies have shown that astrocytic processes may probe the cytoplasm of damaged, or even apparently normal neurons, phagocytosing cellular debris [6].

Two types of astrocyte are recognized: protoplasmic astrocytes, which occur mainly in the grey matter, have numerous freely branching cytoplasmic processes; fibrous astrocytes, which are found chiefly in the white matter, have very many long, unbranched processes. The processes of both types of astrocyte contain microfilaments. The principal constituent of the intermediate filaments is glial fibrillary acidic protein (GFAP), thus the cytoplasmic processes of astrocytes can be identified using the immunocytochemical demonstration of GFAP (Figure 9.3).

Oligodendrocytes (Oligodendroglia)　Oligodendrocytes have a variable histological appearance and cannot be reliably identified in sections stained by routine methods, although they may be noted lying in chains within the corpus callosum. Oligodendrocytes are best visualized using metallic impregnation techniques or immunostaining with antigalactocerebroside antibody.

Oligodendrocytes are responsible for the myelination of axons within the central nervous system and are the most abundant cell type in the white matter. Each oligodendrocyte may provide the myelin sheath for many axons. In the grey matter, oligodendrocytes provide support for unmyelinated axons and also form clusters of satellite cells around the cell bodies of neurons. The number of these satellite cells may increase in response to disease or toxic changes, a process termed satellitosis. As with astrocytes, oligodendrocytes may scavenge cell debris from the cytoplasm

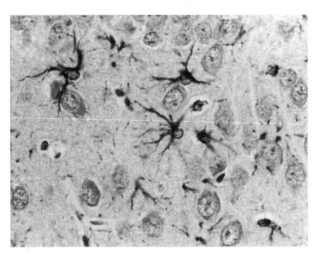

Figure 9.3 Astrocytes of rat hippocampus. Immunocytochemical staining of rat hippocampus for glial fibrillary acidic protein (GFAP), showing positive staining of astrocytic processes radiating from the astrocyte perikaryon.

of neuronal cell bodies and processes, and also contribute to the maintenance of the neural microenvironment.

Microglia   Microglia are small cells with irregularly shaped nuclei and scant cytoplasm which is arranged in fine, highly branched processes. The nuclear chromatin is coarsely clumped and lysosomes are abundant in the cytoplasm. They are most frequent around blood capillaries, between the endothelial cells and the neural tissue, but outside the basal lamina. In the normal central nervous system, microglia are few in number but, in response to tissue injury, may increase in number and transform into phagocytic cells. Although lacking some of the cell surface markers characteristic of macrophages in other tissues, microglia are part of the monocyte–macrophage series and many of the microglia within the nervous system are derived from the blood.

Ependymal cells   Ependymal cells are epithelial in nature forming a simple columnar or cuboidal epithelium which lines the ventricles of the brain and the central canal of the spinal cord. Cell membranes of adjacent cells are united by tight junctions. The luminal surface of the epithelial cells have cilia, which may assist in the circulation of cerebrospinal fluid, as well as microvilli, which probably have both secretory and absorptive functions. In the region of each choroid plexus, the ependymal cells overly a mass of thin-walled capillaries which project into the ventricles. Cerebrospinal fluid is actively secreted in these sites.

Capillaries and the blood–brain barrier

The endothelial cells of the capillaries of the central nervous system are connected by tight junctions. In addition, the cytoplasmic processes of astrocytes invest these capillaries. The result is a barrier to the passage of water-soluble and highly polar compounds from the blood into the central nervous system, with the exception of those compounds, such as amino acids, which are actively transported across the barrier into the nervous system. Although generally known as the blood–brain barrier, it is important to remember that this barrier is present also in the spinal cord and in the peripheral nervous system [7]. However, this barrier is not complete, certain areas, known as the circumventricular organs, having capillaries which lack tight junctions. These areas probably act as chemoreceptors and must, therefore, be outside of the blood–brain barrier, but this position also makes them especially vulnerable to toxic damage. In addition, the blood–brain barrier is incompletely developed at birth so that neonatal or premature animals are particularly susceptible to neurotoxins.

The peripheral nervous system

The peripheral nervous system is composed of a series of nerves which are distributed throughout the body in the connective tissue layers, generally in company with the blood vessels. These nerves consist of bundles of axons and dendrites, collectively known as nerve fibres, invested by protective layers of connective tissue. Each nerve fibre is associated with Schwann cells (neurolemma) which, like the oligodendrocytes of the central nervous system, provide mechanical and metabolic support and also, in myelinated fibres, form the myelin sheath. Several unmyelinated fibres may be found embedded in one Schwann cell, each fibre being surrounded by a thin layer of Schwann cell cytoplasm, but in myelinated nerve fibres, each Schwann cell provides myelin for only one fibre. The myelin is formed by the cytoplasmic processes of the Schwann cell wrapping themselves around the nerve fibre many times. Each nerve fibre is myelinated by a number of Schwann cells so that the myelin layer is discontinuous or segmental. These interruptions between the Schwann cells are known as the nodes of Ranvier. Schwann cells also form satellite cells around cell bodies of neurons within the peripherally situated ganglia. Like the glial cells of the central nervous system, Schwann cells have been shown to remove cell debris from neuronal cytoplasm.

9.2.3 *Physiology*

Normal functioning of the nervous system is dependent on the innate ability of neurons to express excitability. In the resting neuron, an ionic gradient is maintained across the cell membrane by an active process whereby Na^+ ions are extruded from the cell. This results in a potential difference across the cell membrane, the inside of the neuron being negatively charged in relation to the extracellular fluid. Any factor leading to an increase in the permeability of the cell membrane to Na^+ ions will allow an immediate influx of these ions into the cell, the charge inside the cell will become more positive and depolarization of the cell membrane will occur. If the stimulus to depolarization is sufficient, the depolarization will propagate along the nerve fibre resulting in the formation of an action potential. Generation of an action potential is an all or nothing response so that its magnitude is constant. Transmission of information, therefore, is reliant on changes in the frequency and regularity of the generation of action potentials. In myelinated fibres the depolarization is transmitted by saltatory conduction, the depolarization jumping along the axon to successive nodes of Ranvier; this form of conduction is more rapid than that which occurs in unmyelinated fibres. In unmyelinated fibres, the speed of conduction increases in proportion to the cross-sectional area of the fibre.

Restoration of the ionic differential follows the passage of the wave of depolarization as Na^+ ions are again extruded into the extracellular fluid, and the cell membrane is repolarized. In mammals, neurons rarely contact other neurons and cells directly so there is no uninterrupted passage of depolarization from one neuron to another. Between neurons, and between neurons and receptor cells, there are synaptic junctions in which transmission occurs by the release of a chemical. At a synapse, the presynaptic fibres are enlarged to form terminal boutons, otherwise known as synaptic knobs, which are separated from the membrane of the postsynaptic cell by a narrow space, the postsynaptic cleft. Within the terminal bouton are many mitochondria and membrane bound vesicles or granules, containing chemical transmitter. When an impulse arrives at the terminal bouton these vesicles or granules are released into the synaptic cleft, where they act at receptors on the postsynaptic membrane of the underlying cell. Some chemical transmitters are excitatory and when released in sufficient quantity cause depolarization of the postsynaptic cell, others are inhibitory and may prevent the postsynaptic cell from depolarizing. If repolarization or depolarization of the postsynaptic membrane is to occur, the chemical transmitter must be removed from the synaptic cleft or inactivated.

As a consequence of the structure and function of synapses, certain physiological effects are apparent, notably that there is a synaptic delay in transmission of an impulse and that conduction can only take place in one direction.

Each neuron may receive synaptic input from large numbers of other neurons. This input is both inhibitory and excitatory and only when there is an excess of excitatory input will the membrane of the neuron be sufficiently depolarized to initiate an action potential. This allows fine control over neuronal activity.

The different anatomical regions of the brain are associated with different functions: the cerebrum contains centres associated with perception, memory, learning and voluntary actions. Most of the sensory and motor-related pathways passing to the cerebral cortex synapse in the thalamus which acts as a processing centre for this information. The limbic system, containing the olfactory lobes, the hippocampus, the cingulate and dentate gyri, the amygdala, the stria terminalis and connections with the hypothalamus, is concerned with behaviour and the expression of emotion as well as memory and reproductive behaviour. The hypothalamus itself is responsible for the integration of the autonomic nervous system and for the control of endocrine functions. The cerebellum is concerned with the control and integration of muscular movements, and the maintenance of muscle tone and of equilibrium. The medulla oblongata contains the centres controlling the life-support systems, such as respiration, heart rate and blood pressure, but is also essential in activating the higher parts of the brain.

The brain may be divided also on a functional basis into various pathways containing cell groups and their axonal connections which utilize the same neurotransmitter. Five major pathways are recognized:

1 Cholinergic pathways of the basal part of the forebrain are concerned with memory, behaviour and mood, and those of the reticular formation of the brainstem influence the state of arousal and control sleep processes.
2 Noradrenergic pathways are restricted to the pontine and medullary regions but have connections with many regions of the central nervous system, including the

limbic system. These pathways are important in the regulation of fear and anxiety reactions, the sleep–wake cycle and the maintenance of vigilance.

3 Adrenergic neurons are confined to the caudal part of the hindbrain and the pathways are poorly understood. They are associated with control of respiration and blood pressure and also with the secretion of oxytocin and vasopressin.

4 Serotonergic pathways are found throughout the brainstem and regulate cardiovascular function, particularly cerebral blood flow, and control sleep processes.

5 Dopaminergic pathways are located in the mesencephalon and the hypothalamus. These pathways connect with the limbic system, influencing behaviour and emotions, and with the substantia nigra, controlling muscular movements. The hypothalamic branches regulate the release of prolactin.

Other neurotransmitters have been identified also, but have poorly documented functions. Some are associated with specific types of neuron, for example, γ-aminobutyric acid (GABA) which is the neurotransmitter for all of the inhibitory neurons throughout the central nervous system, and glutamate and aspartate which are associated with excitatory neurons.

9.3 Biochemical and Cellular Mechanisms of Toxicity

Much of the physiology and metabolism of the normal brain has not been fully elucidated. Thus, although the biochemical and cellular mechanisms of some neurotoxins are known, it should not come as a surprise to discover that the exact mechanisms by which many toxins cause damage to the nervous system are incompletely understood.

Considered at a cellular level, toxins may cause injury by a direct action on the neuron or, alternatively, the neuronal injury may be indirect, subsequent to toxic damage to other cell types or to a change in the environment around the neuron (Table 9.1). Direct acting toxins may cause damage by interfering with any of the components of the neuron, so that the mechanisms of toxicity are diverse. Similarly, the range of actions by which toxins indirectly cause neurotoxic damage is also extensive: the toxic effect may be in non-neuronal cells of the nervous system itself, or in cells remote from the nervous system.

The biochemical and cellular mechanisms of neurotoxicity may be classified in a number of ways, but the simplest is according to their toxic actions on the nervous system. However, it is important to remember that some neurotoxins may cause changes in more than one of these categories:

- Interference with aerobic metabolism (9.3.1)
- Interference with protein synthesis (9.3.2)
- Interference with intermediate metabolism (9.3.3)
- Changes to cellular membranes (9.3.4)
- Interference with neurotransmission (9.3.5)
- Disturbances of axonal transport (9.3.6)
- Damage to non-neuronal cells (9.3.7)
- Damage to capillaries (9.3.8)

Table 9.1 Chemicals associated with neurotoxicity

Site of action	Chemical	
Neuron	Methyl chloride	Trimethyltin
	Carbon monoxide	MPTP*
	Nitrites	Aluminium
	Hydrogen cyanide	Kainic acid
	Hydrogen sulphide	Domoic acid
	Methylmercury	Ricin
	Methyl alcohol	
Neurons of dorsal root ganglia	Doxorubicin	Cisplatin
Axon	γ-Diketones	Vinca alkaloids
	Acrylamide	Taxol
	β,β'-Iminodipropionitrile	Organophosphates
	Colchicine	Tetrodotoxin
	Local anaesthetics	Dichlorodiphenylethanes
Synapses	Nicotine	Botulinum toxin
	L-Glutamic acid	GABA-inhibiting organochlorines
	Domoic acid	Organophosphates
	Kainic acid	Carbamic esters
	Strychnine	Cocaine
Astrocytes	Ammonia	Methionine sulphoxamine
Oligodendrocytes, Schwann cells and myelin	Triethyltin	Tellurium
	Hexachlorophene	Lead
	Cuprizone	GABA-transaminase inhibitors
Ependymal cells	Amoscanate	
Vascular endothelium	Lead	Ethyl chloride
	Cadmium	Thiaminases
	Mercury	Mycotoxins

*1-methyl-4-phenyl-1, 2, 3, 6-tetrahydropyridine

- Neurocarcinogenesis (9.3.9)
- Developmental neurotoxicity (9.3.10)

9.3.1 *Interference with Aerobic Metabolism*

In man, the cerebral blood flow accounts for approximately 15 per cent of the cardiac output and, of the total oxygen consumption of the body, approximately 20 per cent is taken up by the brain. These figures are a reflection of the high metabolic requirements of neural tissues. The maintenance of large volumes of cytoplasm and extensive cell membranes, as well as the preservation and repetitive reinstitution of ionic gradients, means that the neuron has an exceptional requirement for high-energy phosphate bonds, even in the resting state. Formation of these high-energy bonds is dependent on glycolytic pathways. Since there is little storage of glycogen within the nervous system, neurons are reliant upon a continuous supply of oxygen and glucose. Any interruption to the availability of either oxygen or glucose, even for a relatively short period of time, can result in injury to the brain. The extent and distribution of the lesions will depend on the magnitude and duration of the deprivation and on the areas of the nervous system which are affected. Neurons in different anatomical sites vary in their susceptibility, the most vulnerable being those of the hippocampus, the deeper layers of the cerebral cortex, and the granule and Purkinje cells of the cerebellum. In addition, the degree of vascularization of the neural tissue is not uniform and the extent of collateral circulation and anastomoses between blood vessels varies, so that the effect of vascular impairment may be less severe in some areas. In general, white matter is less well vascularized than the grey matter, and glial cells are less sensitive than neurons to oxygen deprivation. However, in severe cases, glial cells will be affected also, particularly the oligodendrocytes, resulting in an inability to maintain the myelin sheath; extensive demyelination is a frequent sequel to the profound oxygen deprivation which occurs in **carbon monoxide** poisoning.

Hypoxia of the nervous system may be classified according to the underlying physiological mechanism, but with some toxins more than one mechanism may be involved:

Stagnant hypoxia   The central nervous system, or some portion of it, receives a reduced supply of blood (oligaemia) or is deprived of its blood supply completely (ischaemia). Stagnant hypoxia may arise due to cardiovascular toxicity, where there is a reduction in the cardiac output or a profound fall in arterial blood pressure, or when there is direct damage to the capillaries of the nervous system, as in **methyl chloride** toxicity.

Hypoxic or anoxic hypoxia   The low oxygen tension in the blood arises from a reduction in oxygen (hypoxia) or an absence of oxygen (anoxia) in the pulmonary alveoli. This may occur due to low levels of oxygen in the inspired air, to obstruction of the airways by physical or physiological changes, or to pathological processes in the lung preventing diffusion of oxygen across the alveolar walls.

Anaemic hypoxia   The hypoxia arises due to a diminished oxygen-carrying capacity of the blood. Except in cases of profound anaemia, the oxygen tension in the blood is generally sufficient to satisfy the demands of the nervous system. However, when there is interference with the ability of the blood to carry oxygen, as in **carbon monoxide** or **nitrite** poisoning, or in cases of intravascular haemolysis, extensive brain damage may occur.

Cytotoxic (histotoxic) hypoxia   Many tissue poisons block the respiratory enzymes so that oxygen cannot be utilized. **Hydrogen cyanide** and **hydrogen sulphide** act in this way by blocking cytochrome oxidase within the neuron. Oxidative phosphorylation is compromised and electron transfer from cytochrome oxidase to molecular oxygen is prevented.

Many situations which give rise to hypoxia, also result in hypoglycaemia. In addition, hypoglycaemia may follow excess or inappropriate insulin release. Since energy supplies in the nervous tissue are derived mainly from the oxidative metabolism of glucose, conditions of hypoglycaemia will cause damage similar to that which results from oxygen deprivation.

9.3.2 *Interference with Protein Synthesis*

Some neurotoxins exert their effect by blocking the synthesis of protein: this may occur in the nucleus or in the cytoplasmic organelles. Certain antineoplastic agents such as **doxorubicin** (adriamycin) and **cisplatin** (*cis*-dichlorodiammine platinum) [8] act on the nucleus, intercalating between the base pairs of the double-stranded DNA, preventing transcription and thus the production of RNA. Doxorubicin is unable to cross the blood–brain barrier, so that damage is restricted to areas outside of this barrier, most notably the dorsal root ganglia. However, if the blood–brain barrier is compromised, for example by the presence of inflammation or a tumour, the sites of toxic injury will be more widespread. **Ricin**, and some other lectins, and **methylmercury**, act directly on the rough endoplasmic reticulum, binding with ribosomal protein, and preventing protein synthesis. Initially there is loss of Nissl substance followed by neuronal death.

The effects of **methylmercury** intoxication are most evident in the granule cells of the cerebral cortex, the granular cell layer of the cerebellum and in the sensory neurons of the dorsal root ganglia. The mechanism of this predilection for injury to small neurons is unclear, but may be associated with an increased ability of larger cells to sequester the **methylmercury** within lysosomes, and thus prevent the binding of the toxin to the ribosomes.

9.3.3 *Interference with Intermediate Metabolism*

Many neurotoxins cause damage by interfering with metabolic processes within the neuron. Toxic damage may be apparent also in other tissues but the neuronal effects are generally more severe due to the high metabolic rate of the neurons and to the prominence of the clinical signs. The mechanisms of toxicity are diverse due to the wide range of metabolic processes affected.

Neuronal degeneration and necrosis within the basal ganglia, the cerebral cortex and the cerebellum occurs in man following exposure to **methyl alcohol**. Necrosis of retinal cells is also a prominent feature. Damage occurs due to a metabolic acidosis induced by the metabolism of the **methyl alcohol** to formic acid, but also results from histotoxic hypoxia caused by the inhibition of mitochondrial cytochrome oxidase by the formic acid.

Exposure to **trimethyltin** results in degeneration and necrosis of neurons within the limbic system, most notably in the hippocampus and in the pyriform cortex (Figure 9.4) [9, 10]. Affected cells show eccentricity of the nucleus and loss of Nissl substance, changes indicative of inhibition of protein synthesis, but no ultrastructural lesions are apparent in the rough endoplasmic reticulum or the ribosomes, the distinctive lesion being the accumulation of dense-cored vesicles in the neuronal cytoplasm. It appears that the target site for toxicity may be a region of the Golgi-associated smooth endoplasmic reticulum in which lysosomes are formed, this disturbance producing abnormalities in the subsequent processing of synthesized protein.

An extremely selective neurotoxicant is **1-methyl-4-phenyl-1,2,3,6-tetrahydropyridine** (**MPTP**), which produces a syndrome resembling irreversible Parkinson's disease [11]. Humans were affected when **MPTP** was present as a contaminant in batches of meperidine, manufactured illegally as a substitute for

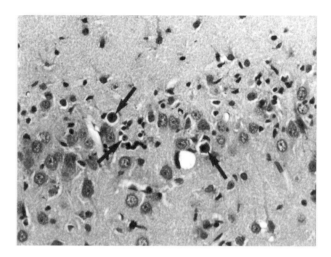

Figure 9.4 Neuronal necrosis. Necrotic neurons (arrows) in the hippocampus of a rat 1 week after the administration of a single intravenous dose of trimethyltin chloride (8 mg/kg body weight).

heroin. **MPTP** readily crosses the blood–brain barrier and enters cells of the central nervous system but is not itself toxic. Within astrocytes, **MPTP** is broken down by monoamine oxidase, to the pyridinium ion (MPP$^+$). This ion enters dopaminergic neurons of the substantia nigra by a system which is responsible normally for the uptake of dopamine. MPP$^+$ is a strong inhibitor of oxidative phosphorylation and neuronal death follows, leading to the characteristic symptoms of Parkinsonism: tremors, muscle rigidity and difficulties in initiating and terminating movements. The condition has been reproduced experimentally in primates and mice, but the rat is relatively refractory, possibly due to a reduced conversion of **MPTP** to MPP$^+$ within astrocytes.

9.3.4 Changes to Cellular Membranes

Any change in the structure of the cell membrane, or of the membranes of the cellular organelles, can alter ion homeostasis; this can have profound effects on the function of neurons. Toxins may restrict the movement of ions across membranes, preventing depolarization, or may increase the permeability of the membrane, leading to a state of partial or sustained depolarization. These changes may be reversible or permanent, and the mechanisms of the toxic action are diverse.

Local anaesthetics act on the membrane of the axon blocking the Na$^+$ ion channels and thus preventing depolarization and the passage of an action potential. The effect is transient. However, **tetrodotoxin**, a naturally occurring toxin of Tetraodontidae fishes and of some amphibians, produces a similar but irreversible blockage. The toxin prevents the inward movement of Na$^+$ ions that initiates depolarization, so that the membrane remains polarized. Another group of compounds, known as the **excitotoxic amino acids**, cause the neuron to remain in a state of persistent depolarization by opening ionic channels within cell membranes. The amino acid **L-glutamic acid** is an excitatory neurotransmitter in the central nervous system, but is itself neurotoxic when administered parenterally. Although it does not cross the blood–brain barrier readily, the neurons of the circumventricular organs, which lie outside of this barrier, are injured. However, certain analogues of glutamic acid, **domoic acid** (found in mussels contaminated with the diatom *Nitzschia pungens*) and **kainic acid** (found in certain types of seaweed), are not only more potent neurotoxins than glutamic acid but also cross the blood–brain barrier [12]. These toxins preferentially affect the dendritic processes and neuronal cell bodies, axons being spared. The site of action is the postsynaptic dendritic membrane, where glutamate receptors are situated, the neurotoxic amino acids inducing a continuous depolarization of the postsynaptic neuron. Ultimately this leads to the death of the neuron.

The **organochlorine insecticides** also cause toxicity by interfering with ionic movements across cell membranes and inducing a state of partial depolarization; the toxicity is characterized by uncontrolled excitatory activity. However, the different types of organochlorines have somewhat different modes of action [13].

Following the administration of **dichlorodiphenylethanes**, for example **dichlorodiphenyltrichloroethane (DDT)**, the axonal membranes remain in a state of partial depolarization after passage of an action potential, so that the nerve is extremely sensitive to further depolarizing stimuli.

The **cyclodiene, benzene** and **cyclohexane derived organochlorine insecticides** affect the central nervous system rather than the peripheral nervous system since they act as antagonists of GABA. Within the central nervous system, GABA induces the uptake of Cl^- ions by neurons, stabilizing the cell membrane. Antagonism of this effect, therefore, leads to a partial depolarization and an increased susceptibility to complete depolarization.

9.3.5 *Interference with Neurotransmission*

A large number of naturally occurring toxins, as well as many synthetic molecules, notably certain classes of pesticide, cause neurotoxicity by interfering with the processes of chemical transmission between neurons, or between neurons and other cell types, notably skeletal muscle cells. This interference may block either the transmission of impulses or result in accentuation of the neurotransmission, depending on the mechanism of action and on the type of synapse affected. The effect may be transient or permanent. Compounds with similar actions usually have similar chemical and structural properties, and act only on one particular type of synapse.

Mechanisms of action differ: some compounds act as agonists or antagonists to the chemical transmitter, while others act by preventing synthesis or release of the neurotransmitter, or by preventing its inactivation or resorption after release. Although these types of compound can produce marked clinical signs, pathological changes are not usually present.

Agonists to neurotransmitters **Nicotine**, a naturally occurring alkaloid of the tobacco plant, exerts its neurotoxic effect by binding to certain types of cholinergic receptors, the nicotinic receptors, at synapses in the central nervous system, the peripheral ganglia and the neuromuscular junctions, where it acts as an acetylcholine agonist. Clinical effects include sweating, tachycardia, elevated blood pressure and constriction of cutaneous blood vessels. The excitatory amino acid analogues, **domoic acid** and **kainic acid**, cause depolarization of postsynaptic neurons by acting as agonists of the excitatory neurotransmitter, glutamic acid.

Antagonists to neurotransmitters The alkaloid **strychnine**, isolated from the plant *Strychnos nux-vomica*, binds to receptors of postsynaptic membranes, antagonizing the hyperpolarizing action of glycine, an inhibitory neurotransmitter. This results in increased excitability of neurons and the precipitation of tonic convulsions in response to external stimuli such as loud noise or bright lights.

Antagonists to the release of neurotransmitters **Botulinum toxin** produced by the anaerobic bacterium *Clostridium botulinum*, induces a progressive muscular paralysis which terminates in death due to cessation of respiration. The toxin prevents the release of acetylcholine from cholinergic nerve endings by blocking the exocytosis of vesicles from the presynaptic axons of the peripheral nervous system. The molecule of the botulinum toxin is too large to cross the blood–brain barrier so that the neurons of the central nervous system are unaffected.

Prevention of the inactivation of neurotransmitters Both classes of **anticholin-esterase insecticides**, the esters of phosphoric or phosphorothioic acid and those of carbamic acid, have a common mode of neurotoxic action in that they bind to the active site of the acetylcholinesterase molecule. The destruction of acetylcholine at cholinergic nerve endings throughout the nervous system is thus prevented, resulting in continual stimulation of nerves and muscles. Binding of organophosphate esters with the acetylcholinesterase leads to the formation of a stable, unreactive complex, so that the enzyme inhibition may be considered irreversible. In the case of carbamate esters, however, the complex formed with the enzyme undergoes hydrolysis, followed by decarbamylation, so that free enzyme is released. The effects of carbamate ester toxicity are, therefore, transient and reversible [14, 15].

Prevention of the resorption of neurotransmitters **Cocaine** blocks the resorption of catecholamines at nerve endings, prolonging the effects of nerve stimulation. The addictive properties and the induction of euphoria are a reflection of the ability of **cocaine** to cross the blood–brain barrier.

9.3.6 *Disturbances of Axonal Transport*

In order to communicate over long distances, the neuron has developed extensive cytoplasmic processes. Although these processes are extremely attenuated, the total cell volume is still considerable and the volume of the axon may greatly exceed that of the cell body. The neuron must, therefore, maintain a considerable cellular volume and also transport intracellular materials over great distances. Since these processes are energy-dependent, any interference with cell metabolism may interfere with normal transport; interference with axonal transport mechanisms can lead to degeneration of the axon.

In common with other cells, neurons contain a cytoskeleton, composed of filaments (neurofilaments) and microtubules; the cytoskeleton is present both within the cell body and the cytoplasmic processes. The proteins which form this cytoskeleton are synthesized in the perikaryon and are then slowly transported along the axon at a rate of approximately 1 mm/day. Continual replacement of these structural proteins is essential for the maintenance of the axon. Other proteins are carried from the sites of synthesis in the cell body along the axon at a much faster rate of approximately 400 mm/day. This fast axonal transport is dependent on a supply of energy and is linked with a microtubule-associated adenosine triphosphatase. An intermediate rate transport system also exists, mainly involving the movement of cellular organelles, including mitochondria, at a rate of approximately 50 mm/day.

Movement of cell constituents occurs in both directions: anterograde, towards the periphery of the cytoplasmic processes, and retrograde, towards the cell body. The anterograde transport systems are the mechanism by which the cell maintains the axon, the retrograde movements probably supply the cell body with information on the functional status of the distal axon, thus providing some feedback control over axonal transport.

Degeneration of the axon will occur if it is physically transected or if the cell body is injured and no longer able to produce proteins. Distal portions of the axon will be affected initially but the degeneration will progress along the axon towards the cell body, giving rise to the process known as dying-back. However, some neurotoxins which act directly on the axonal transport systems, for example **γ-diketones**, **acrylamide** and **β,β′-iminodipropionitrile (IDPN)**, may induce initial damage at sites other than the periphery. The effect is one of chemical transection of the axon. Accumulations of neurofilaments and other cell constituents build up at the site of the damage (Figures 9.5 and 9.6). Initially, the myelin sheath remains intact as the axon retracts but, if the axon does not regenerate, the Schwann cells or oligodendrocytes will also undergo degeneration and the myelin sheath will be lost. Cross-linkage between neurofilament elements is postulated as the mechanism of toxicity [16, 17]. The site of the initial lesion appears to be a reflection of the potency of the neurotoxin to cause cross-linkages and also, therefore, of the dose regime: exposure to lower levels over an extended period will produce axonal swelling in a more distal location.

Microtubules are also the target for a group of neurotoxic alkaloids derived from plants. During transport of tubules along the axon there is a state of dynamic

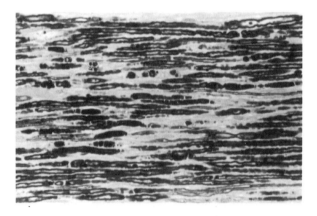

Figure 9.5 Acrylamide neurotoxicity (methacrylate embedded, toluidine blue stained). Longitudinal sections of the sciatic nerve of a rat treated with acrylamide by gavage, once daily for 21 days, at a dose level of 24 mg/kg body weight, showing axonal degeneration and secondary breakdown of myelin.

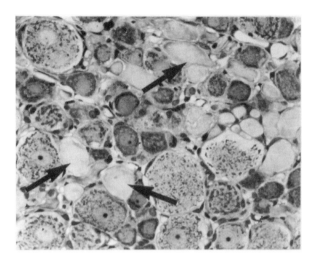

Figure 9.6 β,β'iminodipropionitrile (IDPN) neurotoxicity (methacrylate embedded, toluidine blue stained). Section of the gasserian ganglion of a rat treated with IDPN by gavage, once daily for 28 days, at a dose level of 100 mg/kg body weight, showing gross distension of the axons close to the neuronal cell bodies (arrows).

equilibrium between formed elements and the dissociated tubulin subunits. Interference with this equilibrium will disrupt axonal transport. **Colchicine** and the **vinca alkaloids** bind to the tubulin monomers preventing their association into tubules, whereas **taxol** stabilizes the microtubules preventing their dissociation into subunits: both are neurotoxic [18]. In cases of **colchicine** and **vinca alkaloid** toxicity, the axons undergo atrophy and there are few microtubules, but after exposure to **taxol**, excess numbers of microtubules are present. Axonal degeneration follows.

Apart from the acute neurotoxic effects of the **organophosphates**, some of the **organophosphorus esters (phosphates, phosphonates and phosphoramidates)** have the ability to induce a delayed-type of neurotoxicity, characterized by degeneration of axons some 7 to 10 days after exposure. The long, large diameter myelinated axons are the most susceptible to injury. Although the clinical syndrome is well characterized in man, following contamination of illicit alcohol with **tri-ortho-tolyl phosphate** and of cooking oils with **tri-ortho-cresyl phosphate**, and can be reproduced in animals, the hen and the cat being most susceptible, the mechanism of toxicity is not understood. Not all of the **organophosphate esters** which inhibit acetylcholinesterase induce delayed neurotoxicity, however, they all inhibit a membrane-bound neuronal, non-specific carboxylesterase known as the neuropathic target esterase, or neurotoxic esterase (NTE) [19]. This enzyme may be involved in lipid metabolism, but, although its inhibition gives a good indication of the ability of an **organophosphate** to induce delayed neurotoxicity, the role of NTE in its initiation remains unclear.

Administration of **aluminium** to primates over a prolonged period results in the accumulation of bundles of paired, helically wound filaments, the neurofibrillary tangles, within neuronal cell bodies, dendrites and proximal axons. The large neurons of the cerebral and cerebellar cortex are most severely affected. The tangles react with monoclonal antibodies to neurofilament antigens and the accumulation appears to be linked to decreased axonal transport. Affected neurons show atrophy of the dendritic processes and loss of synapses. The neurofibrillary tangles resemble those found in the human dementia syndromes, notably Alzheimer's disease, but there is little evidence that **aluminium** is involved in the aetiology of these syndromes.

The entry of **aluminium** into the central nervous system is not understood as it does not appear to cross the intact blood–brain barrier. However, there is some evidence for nasal absorption and also that **aluminium** itself increases the permeability of the blood–brain barrier [20].

9.3.7 Damage to Non-Neuronal Cells

The non-neuronal cells of the nervous system play an important role in the maintenance of the environment of the nervous tissue. Any damage to these cells, which results in a change in the environment, may lead to secondary neuronal injury. Damage to the cells may be direct or subsequent to damage in other tissues.

Astrocytes   Some cases of toxic damage to the liver may be associated with **hepatic encephalopathy**. The mechanism is not entirely understood, but is probably associated with elevated levels of ammonia in the blood. Normal astrocytes take up ammonia as a substrate for glutamine synthetase, an enzyme which converts glutamate into glutamine, but under conditions of ammonia excess the astrocytes may be damaged, leading to secondary neuronal changes with clinical signs of neurological injury [21]. Similar changes may occur in cases of **renal failure**.

Astrocytes may be affected directly by toxins also. **Methionine sulphoxamine** causes swelling of astrocytic cytoplasmic processes due to the accumulation of excessive quantities of glycogen granules. The ability of the astrocytes to control the environment of the nervous tissue is impaired, resulting in an elevation of the extracellular K^+ ion concentration, with persistent depolarization and death of neurons.

Myelinating cells (oligodendrocytes and Schwann cells)   The formation and main-tenance of myelin is an energy-dependent process which also requires structural proteins that are unique to the nervous system. Toxins may act directly on the myelin or on the cell bodies of the myelinating cell. **Triethyltin, hexachlorophene** [22] and **γ-aminobutyric acid-transaminase inhibitors** (e.g. **vigabatrin**) [23] cause the separation of myelin lamellae, resulting in intramyelinic oedema (Figures 9.7a and b). In the early stages, this may be reversible, but later there may be death of the myelinating cells and segmental demyelination. In severe cases, axonal degeneration follows. This degeneration may be associated with direct toxicity but is also probably a result of pressure on the axon from the swollen myelin. Both **triethyltin** and **hexachlorophene** are potent uncoupling agents of mitochondrial oxidative phosphorylation, but the mechanism whereby they cause toxicity is not clear. **Hexachlorophene** binds tightly to cell membranes, destroying any ionic gradients. It is possible that this binding occurs in the wealth of cell membrane which is the myelin sheath, leading to an osmotic oedema.

Peripheral demyelination follows exposure to **tellurium**, but in this form of

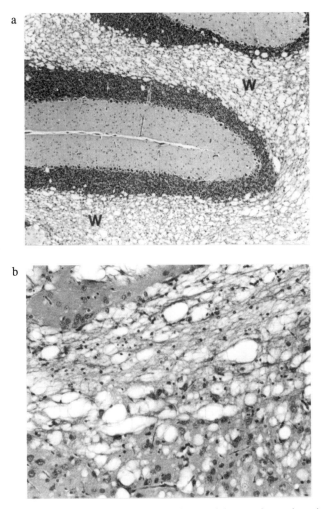

Figure 9.7 Hexachlorophene neurotoxicity. Oedema of the myelin in the white matter (W) of the cerebellum of a rat dosed orally with hexachlorophene for 28 days at a dose level of 35 mg/kg body weight: (a) shows the extent of the involvement of the white matter (low power), (b) shows the distension of the myelin sheaths (high power).

toxicity there is no intramyelinic oedema, damage being due to deranged lipid metabolism. Schwann cells show decreased synthesis of cholesterol and cerebrosides, both of which are constituents of myelin. However, levels of squalene, a precursor of cholesterol, rise, indicating that **tellurium** may interfere with the conversion of squalene to cholesterol. Schwann cells associated with the larger axons, and thus with the larger volumes of myelin, appear most vulnerable [24].

Segmental demyelination can result also from exposure to substances which are directly toxic to the myelinating cell. **Lead**, and the copper chelating agent **cuprizone** act in this way [25]. Although the mechanism of toxicity is unclear, with **cuprizone** it may be that the chelation of copper causes a deficiency of cytochrome oxidase activity which, in turn, reduces mitochondrial adenosine triphosphate formation resulting in cell death due to insufficient energy resources. The reason for the exquisite susceptibility of Schwann cells is not known. Remyelination may follow but this is always more rapid and more pronounced in the peripheral nervous system than in the central nervous system. During remyelination the number of myelinating cells involved is always greater than the number originally present, so that the internodal lengths are much shorter than normal. This may be a protective mechanism whereby each myelinating cell has a smaller volume of myelin to maintain.

Ependymal cells Reports of direct toxicity to ependymal cells are rare. However, exposure of rats to the potent antiparasitic drug **amoscanate** (4-isothio-cyanato-4'-nitrophenylamine) causes necrosis of ependymal cells adjacent to the choroid plexus of the lateral ventricles. Higher doses result in the erosion of the ventricular lining, astrocytic reaction and degeneration of the underlying neurons. It is suggested that the **amoscanate**, or a metabolite, penetrates the blood vessels of the choroid plexus to exert a toxic action on the adjacent ependymal cells. Ependymal cells are not known to proliferate in response to toxic substances [26].

Microglia Although microglia become activated when nervous tissue is damaged, no evidence for direct toxic effects is available.

9.3.8 *Damage to Capillaries*

Capillaries in the nervous system function as do those in other tissues, supplying oxygen and nutrients, as well as removing waste products. However, the transfer of many harmful substances from the blood into the neural tissue is prevented by the specialized structure of these capillaries. Thus toxic damage to the capillaries not only deprives the nervous tissue of oxygen and essential nutrients and allows the build up of potentially harmful metabolites, but may also expose the neurons to the direct action of the toxin by destroying the blood–brain barrier.

Exposure to a number of diverse substances, most notably **heavy metals (lead, cadmium, inorganic mercury), ethyl chloride, thiaminases** and **mycotoxins**, can cause vascular damage within the nervous system. Mechanisms of action vary but, generally, there is endothelial swelling with loss of vascular integrity, leading to oedema, extravasation of blood and proteins, and thrombus formation. Endothelial swelling may progress to necrosis resulting in massive oedema and haemorrhage which raise the intracranial pressure leading to further injury of neurons. This often presents as extensive necrosis of the brain.

The mechanism of **lead** neurotoxicity is poorly understood. In general, heavy metals destroy sulphydryl protein molecules which are important structural components of vessels, but a direct toxic action of **lead** on the neurons exacerbates the damage caused by endothelial dysfunction. Developing vasculature appears to be more sensitive to the effects of the **lead**, so that exposure of fetuses or newborn animals will produce more severe lesions [27].

9.3.9 *Neurocarcinogenesis*

Early studies with known potent carcinogens such as the polycyclic aromatic hydrocarbon derivatives, **benz[a]pyrene** and **3-methylcholanthrene**, failed to produce tumours of the central nervous system as the carcinogens did not cross the blood–brain barrier. However, inoculation of the carcinogen directly into the brain did yield tumours of the nervous system. Later, parenteral administration of **ethylnitrosourea (ENU)** and **methylnitrosourea (MNU)** was shown to elicit the formation of neurogenic tumours, including tumours of the central nervous system [28]. Since then a range of diverse neurocarcinogens has been identified, for example **acrylonitrile** and **ethylene oxide**.

In addition to the nature of the carcinogen, the age of the animal at the time of exposure is important in determining tumour yield. A single exposure of pregnant rats to **ENU** between days 12 and 20 of gestation induces a very high incidence of tumours of the nervous system in the offspring, but tumours cannot be induced by exposure prior to day 12 of gestation and the susceptibility declines up to the 30th day post-partum, when it is almost impossible to induce neurogenic tumours with a single dose of **ENU**. However, **MNU** is a more potent carcinogen than **ENU** in the adult rat, but repeated exposure is necessary to produce a high incidence of tumours.

9.3.10 **Developmental Neurotoxicity**

The nervous system of most species continues to develop after birth, so that abnormalities may occur if an animal is exposed to a toxin *in utero* or during the early neonatal period. However, the effect of exposure to a neurotoxin will depend on the stage at which the animal is exposed. The defects may be categorized according to the primary lesion:

Changes in the number of neurons   Any substance which interferes with mitosis or with DNA synthesis, for example **colchicine** or **methylmercury** will damage the proliferating cells of the nervous system. Early exposure results in a decrease in the number of neurons and a reduction in the volume of the affected part of the nervous system. Later exposure, when structures have already formed, will cause a reduction in the number of cells but this will be apparent as a reduced cell density and may not be accompanied by a decrease in the size of the affected area.

Changes in neuronal position and in neuronal connections   Damage to neurons at times of neuronal migration may lead to the prevention of migration, or to migration to the wrong area. Exposure to neuroteratogens may also interfere with neuronal connections, producing an increase or a decrease in the number of synaptic contacts. For example, **hypothyroidism** is associated with a decrease in the number of neuronal connections and exposure to **ethanol** *in utero* leads to a reduction in the number of dendritic spines, conditions associated with retarded mental development in the human [29].

Changes in non-neuronal cells   Injury to non-neuronal cells in the developing nervous system occurs in response to toxins as it does in the adult. Thus exposure to **methylmercury** can result in demyelination and exposure to **trimethyltin** can cause destruction of astrocytes [30]. Loss of astrocytes is particularly detrimental to the development of the nervous system as specialized astrocytes act as guides to the migrating neurons.

9.4 Morphological Responses to Injury

Many pathological changes within the nervous system are not generally evident upon gross examination. Frequently, therefore, identification of these changes is dependent on microscopic evaluation. The types of morphological changes exhibited by the neural tissues in response to toxic damage or disease are limited, and differ little from the pathological processes which occur in other tissues. However, before considering these morphological changes, it is important to be aware of the artefacts which are commonly encountered in histological preparations of neural tissues, and of the common spontaneous pathological changes which may interfere with the interpretation of lesions observed in neurotoxicity tests. Most of the artefacts associated with fixation can be prevented by the use of perfusion fixation.

9.4.1 *Artefacts*

Vacuolation of cells The presence of vacuoles in the cytoplasm or nucleus of neurons or within the myelin sheath is a frequent observation in sections of nervous tissue which have been processed in paraffin wax: the cell bodies of neurons in autonomic ganglia are often affected. This type of vacuolation must be distinguished from vacuolation due to toxic damage. The absence of any glial reaction and the lack of bilateral involvement of paired structures may be indicative of an artefactual change (Figure 9.8). Cytoplasmic vacuolation may also occur as a post-mortem artefact.

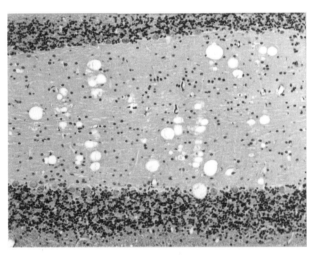

Figure 9.8 Artefactual vacuolation. A section of the cerebellum from an untreated rat, routinely processed in paraffin wax. There is extensive vacuolation of axons in the white matter.

Shrinkage artefacts In central nervous system tissue fixed by immersion, the Virchow–Robin spaces around the blood vessels are often disproportionately prominent due to differential shrinkage of the tissues. Clear pericellular spaces may be evident also around nerve cell bodies due to similar shrinkage artefact.

Dark neurons Even gentle handling of inadequately fixed nervous tissue may give rise to the phenomenon of dark neurons. These appear, generally in groups, as shrunken, deeply basophilic cell bodies, most noticeable in the hippocampus and cerebral cortex, and must be distinguished from necrotic neurons (Figure 9.9).

Disruption of myelin sheaths Inadequate fixation or a delay between fixation and processing of the tissues can result in degeneration of the myelin sheath with splitting of the myelin lamellae and the formation of myelin beads. This can obscure demyelination induced by a neurotoxin.

9.4.2 Spontaneous Lesions

Degeneration of individual nerve fibres This is a common age-related finding in the spinal cord, spinal nerve roots and peripheral nerves of male and female rats. The change is characterized by degeneration and fragmentation of the axon with swelling of the myelin sheath and the formation of myelin ovoids, often accompanied by an infiltration of macrophages [31].

Hydrocephalus Dilatation of the ventricular system is a not uncommon finding in the rat. Despite compression atrophy of the overlying brain tissue, clinical signs may be mild or absent. Secondary ependymal degeneration and oedema of the neural tissues adjacent to the ventricles may occur in severe cases.

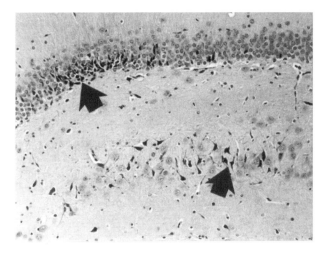

Figure 9.9 Dark neurons. A section from the brain of a rat, fixed by immersion in 10 per cent neutral buffered formalin, showing dark neurons (arrows) in the hippocampus and dentate gyrus.

Cerebellar hypoplasia　Hypoplasia of the cerebellum may arise spontaneously or as a result of exposure to viral infections, notably those due to the parvoviruses, during the period when the cerebellum is undergoing development, either *in utero* or in the neonatal period [32]. Affected animals show ataxia and muscle tremors, although the onset of these signs may be delayed. At necropsy, the cerebellum is small and the gyri poorly developed. Histological examination reveals disruption of the cerebellar granular cell layer with fewer neurons than normal being present (Figure 9.10);

Infections　Many viral, bacterial and parasitic infections of the nervous system can occur spontaneously and may be asymptomatic, leading to possible confusion on histological examination. A common finding in viral infections is a perivascular infiltration of lymphocytes within the Virchow–Robin spaces (Figure 9.11). Bacterial infections are associated with more acute inflammation, notably meningitis (Figure 9.12), or may take the form of abscesses, particularly when secondary to middle ear infections. Although rare in laboratory bred rats, parasitic infestations are common in rabbits, most notably due to *Encephalitozoon cuniculi* (Figure 9.13).

9.4.3　*Cellular Lesions*

Cellular lesions may involve the neurons themselves or the non-neural cells of the nervous system. However, it is essential to remember that because of the functional interdependence of these cells, changes in one cell type are generally followed by changes in other cell types. Toxic substances may act on the nerve cell body producing injury, or in severe cases, cell death. Death of the neuron also involves the loss of all of its cytoplasmic processes and the associated myelin sheath, and is irreversible: this type of injury is known as a neuronopathy. Alternatively, the toxic effect may begin in the axon, sparing the cell body, producing an axonopathy. In general, following the axonal decay, the associated myelin sheath will degenerate also. However, in myelinopathies, the myelinating cell, or the myelin itself, is the primary target of toxicity.

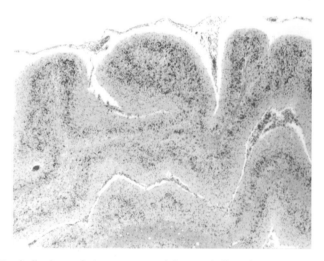

Figure 9.10　Cerebellar hypoplasia. A section of the cerebellum from a young rat which developed progressive ataxia 3 weeks prior to death. The cerebellum is deficient in neurons and lacks the strict laminar organization of the cerebellum from a normal rat.

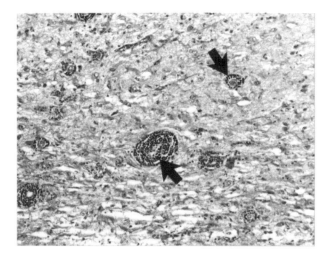

Figure 9.11 Perivascular cuffing. A section from the cerebrum of a rabbit which died from an unknown cause. The perivascular spaces are crowded with lymphocytes (arrows).

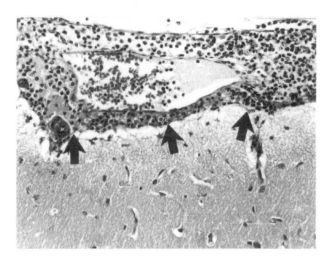

Figure 9.12 Acute meningitis. A section of cerebrum and meninges from a rat which died after receiving 15 daily oral doses of the immunosuppresive drug cyclosporin, at a dose level of 20 mg/kg body weight. The meningeal vessels are dilated and the meninges contain inflammatory exudate and neutrophils (arrows).

9.4.4 Neuronal Lesions

Neuronopathies

Initially a neuron may undergo a biochemical change without exhibiting any overt signs of altered morphology. However, if this change persists, or becomes more severe, cellular organelles will be damaged; this will be apparent on electron microscopic examination or may be evident on histological examination. Neurons damaged in this way may recover, leaving no evidence of previous injury, but if the lesion progresses, they will undergo further degeneration and may die.

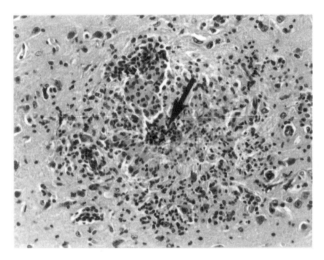

Figure 9.13 *Encephalitozoon* infection. A section of cerebrum from a rabbit showing infestation with the protozoal parasite *Encephalitozoon cuniculi*. The focal lesions contain a necrotic centre (arrow) which is surrounded by macrophage aggregations and inflammatory cells.

Initially, the cell body of the affected neuron shows minor evidence of injury, characterized by the process known as central chromatolysis (Figure 9.14). The nucleus shrinks and becomes eccentrically positioned within the soma. However, the nucleolus is often enlarged and shows condensation of granular and fibrillary components. In the cytoplasm, the Nissl substance is diminished and dispersed around the periphery of the perikaryon. These changes are indicative of a reduced synthesis of RNA in the nucleolus and a decrease in the formation of ribosomes, with

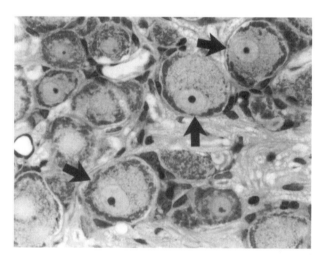

Figure 9.14 Central chromatolysis (methacrylate embedded, toluidine blue stained). A section from the dorsal root ganglion of a rat which had been dosed orally with acrylamide once daily for 21 days, at a dose level of 24 mg/kg body weight. Three neuronal cell bodies (arrows) show eccentrically placed nuclei and margination of the Nissl substance, the early signs of central chromatolysis.

a subsequent decrease in protein synthesis. Other cytoplasmic organelles, notably the Golgi apparatus and the smooth endoplasmic reticulum, become swollen: this may be evident in histological sections as cytoplasmic vacuolation.

In acute injury the neuron becomes necrotic without first exhibiting evidence of cell damage. This necrosis is characterized by retraction and increased eosinophilia of the cytoplasm and hyperchromasia and pyknosis of the nucleus (Figure 9.4).

Once the cell body is no longer able to function normally, axonal transport fails, resulting in degeneration of the axons and dendrites. Astrocytes adjacent to the damaged neuron undergo hypertrophy and hyperplasia. Oligodendrocytes or Schwann cells surrounding the cell body of the neuron, the satellite cells, may become reactive also and multiply, a process known as satellitosis; this may be a protective mechanism for the injured neuron. Microglia and also monocytes, which infiltrate the nervous tissue from the blood stream, become phagocytic and remove the dead cells. Evidence also exists that astrocytes may be responsible for removing some of the neuronal debris. In the central nervous system, lost neurons are replaced by the proliferating astrocytes, giving rise to a glial scar, but if extensive areas are involved, there may be liquefactive necrosis and resorption of the damaged tissue leaving an area of cavitation.

Axonopathies

When the primary site of the neurotoxicity is the axon, and the neuronal cell body is spared, the condition is classified as an axonopathy. Axonopathies may occur in both the central and peripheral nervous systems, but, whereas peripheral axons can regenerate, those of the central nervous system cannot.

Early investigations of toxic axonopathies concluded that the axonal degeneration began at the distal end of the axon and then progressed towards the cell body. This process was known as 'dying back'. However, more recent studies have shown that not all axonopathies arise in this way and, in many cases, the primary lesion does not develop at the distal extremity. The toxins block the systems of axonal transport producing a chemical transection of the axon. This results in disruption of the axon, and a series of characteristic changes known as Wallerian degeneration.

Transection of the axon, either by physical or chemical means, initiates a series of changes proximal and distal to the point of transection. The first change is the accumulation of cellular organelles, notably mitochondria, vesicles, filaments and, particularly in the distal segment, lysosomes, within axonal swellings either side of the transection. The distal portion of the axon, which is no longer supported by metabolites transported from the soma, rapidly degenerates and appears as a pale-staining line with a few granular remnants, inside an apparently normal myelin sheath. This axonal breakdown is more rapid in the peripheral nervous system than it is in the central nervous system. Macrophages appear within the myelin sheath and take up the axonal debris (Figure 9.15). The segment of the axon proximal to the transection may become atrophic also, due to the reduced synthesis of cytoskeletal elements in the perikaryon. Shortly after the axonal changes, the myelin sheath breaks down into short segments, or ovoids. These ovoids remain within the cytoplasm of the myelinating cell.

In the peripheral nervous system, if exposure to the toxic material is eliminated, the axon may regenerate. The Schwann cells in the portion of the axon distal to the transection begin to divide, but remain within the Schwann cell tube of the original axon. The dividing Schwann cells act as a guide for the axonal sprouts and also synthesize nerve growth factor which stimulates the axon to regrow.

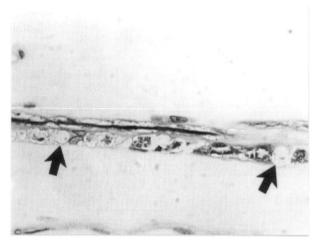

Figure 9.15 Axonal degeneration (methacrylate embedded, toluidine blue stained). A section of a teased preparation of the sciatic nerve from a rat which had received 0.5 mg/kg body weight per day of trimethyltin chloride orally for 28 days. A normal axon lies above a degenerate axon which shows loss of the axoplasm with disruption of the myelin sheath. Macrophages (arrows) are phagocytosing cell debris within the axon.

9.4.5 *Non-Neuronal Lesions*

Myelinopathies

Specific disorders in which there is primary degeneration of the myelin sheath without damage to the axon, are known as myelinopathies. However, due to the intimate association between the myelinating cell and the axon, secondary axonal degeneration may follow. Functionally, the demyelination results in impairment of the transmission of action potentials, and also in aberrant conduction of impulses due to the loss of electrical insulation between adjacent neurons.

The toxic damage may occur directly to the myelin itself or to the myelinating cell, leading to an inability to maintain the myelin. Direct damage to the myelin generally results in separation of the myelin lamellae, producing intramyelinic oedema (Figures 9.7a and b). In the early stages this may be reversible, but if the injury is severe or exposure to the toxin is prolonged, segmental demyelination will follow as the myelinating cells are destroyed. When the intramyelinic oedema is severe, there may be increased pressure on the axon causing atrophy, or, in the central nervous system, a generalized increase in intracranial pressure may develop leading to more extensive neuronal injury. Segmental demyelination may occur also as a primary toxic change due to direct toxic injury to the myelinating cell.

Macrophages, derived from microglia and entering the damaged area from the bloodstream, are responsible for the removal of most of the degenerate myelin. However, there is also evidence that Schwann cells, oligodendrocytes and astrocytes can take up some components of the myelin debris.

Remyelination occurs only to a limited extent in the central nervous system, but in the peripheral nervous system, in cases where the axon survives, it may be complete. Schwann cells divide and remyelinate the naked portions of the axon. However, the distances between nodes of Ranvier in the remyelinated sections of the axon are much shorter than those present prior to the injury. Sites of remyelination can thus be identified, particularly in teased fibre preparations, even when all other toxic damage has been repaired.

Changes in astrocytes

Astrocytes are less susceptible to damage than are neurons, but in cases of ischaemia or when exposed to neurotoxins, they may undergo reactive or degenerative changes. The first sign of degeneration is a swelling of the cell body, which becomes visible on one side of the nucleus, and this is followed by vacuolation of the cytoplasm. Cell processes disintegrate, a change known as clasmatodendrosis, and are phagocytosed.

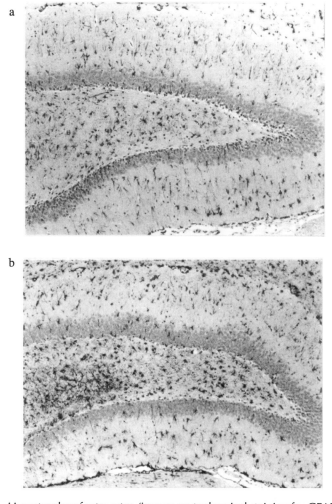

Figure 9.16 Hypertrophy of astrocytes (immunocytochemical staining for GFAP). Sections from the hippocampus of a control rat (a) and from a rat which had received a single intravenous injection of trimethyltin chloride (8 mg/kg body weight) 14 days previously (b). The section from the treated rat shows increased positive staining for GFAP due to an increased number of astrocytic processes which also stain more strongly for GFAP; there is little evidence of astrocyte proliferation.

The nucleus becomes pyknotic and the astrocyte dies. However, if the toxic insult is less severe, although the swelling of the cell body may be pronounced, the cytoplasmic processes are retained; these plump angular cells are called gemistocytic astrocytes. Recovery can occur with reduction to a normal size, but many changed astrocytes undergo necrosis.

In response to minor toxic insults or in response to neuronal damage, astrocytes may become reactive – the cell body and nucleus enlarge and new cytoplasmic processes form. Nuclear division frequently accompanies these changes but without separation of the cytoplasm so that multinucleate cells arise; however, some mitotic division may occur. Reactive cells stain more prominently with antibodies to glial fibrillary acidic protein (GFAP) since they contain increased quantities of neurofilaments (Figures 9.16a and b).

Microglial reactions

Microglia react rapidly to toxic injury, multiplying freely and becoming phagocytic. Many of these cells will be derived from monocytes entering the neural tissue from the blood stream. As microglia are less vulnerable than either neurons or the neuroglia, they are frequently seen in and around areas of necrosis. Lipid vacuoles are usually evident within the cytoplasm due to phagocytosis of myelin debris. Lipid-laden microglia, or gitter cells, may remain at the site of injury for some time, but gradually migrate to the blood vessels where they accumulate in and around the Virchow–Robin spaces.

9.5 Testing for Toxicity

Before a successful strategy can be derived for the detection of neurotoxicity, it is essential to formulate a satisfactory definition of what is meant by neurotoxicity. A simplistic definition of neurotoxicity is an adverse change in the structural or functional integrity of the nervous system that results from exposure to a chemical, biological or physical agent. However, caution must be exercised in the interpretation of the term 'adverse': some changes which may appear to represent adverse neurological effects are not important in terms of risk assessment. Only alterations which compromise the ability of the organism to function appropriately in its environment should be considered adverse. Whether a change is classified as adverse depends on several factors: the nature of the change (functional, behavioural, biochemical or morphological), the severity of the change and on whether the change is transient or persistent. Morphological changes such as neuronopathy, axonopathy and myelinopathy, even if mild and transient, would be considered adverse. However, the significance of other types of change is not as easily determined. For example, changes in biochemical parameters, such as the quantities of glial fibrillary acidic protein in the brain, particularly if transient, may not be of significance unless supported by evidence of other neurotoxic effects. Similar problems exist when assessing the significance of reversible functional or behavioural changes which are not associated with morphological abnormalities. It is also extremely important to differentiate between direct toxic effects on the nervous system and indirect or secondary effects, subsequent to toxic changes elsewhere in the body. Systemic toxicity, metabolic disturbances and reduced food and water intakes can all confound toxicity testing by causing signs indicative of neurotoxicity. In studies designed to detect neurotoxicity, the choice of dose level is, therefore, extremely important; the dose level should not exceed the maximum tolerated dose. To assist in the interpretation of any clinical and morphological changes, it is advisable to conduct neurotoxicity tests in association with conventional toxicity studies.

Only those substances which produce adverse effects by a direct action on the nervous system should be classified as neurotoxic: this designation is assisted by the use of a combination of functional, behavioural and morphological investigations.

Although conventional toxicity tests are able to detect neurotoxicity, many regulatory authorities consider that only neurotoxic effects associated with frank neuropathological lesions or overt neurological dysfunction can be detected using this type of study, and that the continued reliance on neuropathology as the main criterion for the evaluation of neurotoxicity may significantly underestimate the neurotoxic potential of a chemical. Consequently, many authorities have introduced, or are in the process of introducing, new guidelines specifically for the testing of chemicals for neurotoxicity (e.g. the Food and Drug Administration and the Environmental Protection Agency of the United States of America, the International Programme on Chemical Safety of the World Health Organization and the Organization for Economic Cooperation and Development). These are in addition to the specialized tests for organophosphates, which have been in existence for some time.

Most regulatory agencies recommend a structured or tiered approach. The first level is designed as a screen for the initial identification of chemicals that may be associated with neurotoxic effects. Conventional toxicity tests are adequate for this purpose, 28-day and 90-day studies to screen for potential adult neurotoxicity following short-term and more prolonged exposures, and reproduction and teratology studies to screen for potential neurotoxicity in the developing and mature offspring.

When there is no evidence of adverse effects on the nervous system and when the test substance shows no structure–activity relationship to known neurotoxicants, the substance can be regarded as not neurotoxic. However, if there is some evidence of adverse neurotoxic effects or some structure–activity relationship with known neurotoxins, further tests should be performed to characterize the neurotoxicity. These second tier tests should include a battery of behavioural and physiological tests to detect adverse changes in the primary functions of the mature and developing nervous systems, namely the cognitive, motor, sensory and autonomic functions, as well as a more extensive and detailed neuropathological evaluation.

If there is no evidence of adverse effects on the nervous system in the second tier studies, the substance can be regarded as not neurotoxic, but when adverse effects are identified the substance should be considered as a probable neurotoxicant. In such cases, third tier tests may be required. These should be designed to further characterize the adverse effects and to determine dose–response and dose–time relationships, and to estimate a no observed adverse effect level. Such tests may also include investigations into the mechanism of the toxic action and into the toxicokinetics of the substance; the nature of the investigations required must be determined on a case-by-case basis. Specialized techniques may include operant behavioural assessments, electrophysiology and *in vitro* studies, using brain slices, monolayers of cultured cells or cellular aggregations.

9.5.1 *Pathological Investigations in Neurotoxicity Studies*

Certain anatomical and physiological features of the nervous system ensure that the performance of a satisfactory and complete pathological examination is extremely difficult to achieve. First, the whole of the central nervous system is encased within bone and ensheathed by tough fibrous membranes, which prevent the adequate penetration of fixatives. Second, since there is little fibrous connective tissue within the substance of the brain and spinal cord, once these outer protective layers are removed, the nervous tissue is easily damaged by rough handling. Most of these difficulties can be overcome by using perfusion fixation: due to the extensive ramifications of the peripheral nervous system, whole body perfusion is essential to ensure successful fixation of all parts.

Histopathological examination of the whole of the nervous system is impractical. Furthermore, unlike the situation in the parenchymal organs, such as the liver and lung, in which examination of a few sections will, in general, give a representative picture of the whole organ, the intricate anatomy of the brain precludes this. As a minimum, the areas of brain specified by most of the regulatory organizations, namely the forebrain (including the basal ganglia), the centre of the cerebrum, the hippocampus, the midbrain, the cerebellum and pons, and the medulla oblongata must be examined. Examination of the spinal cord is also difficult, partly because of the variety of the different fibre tracts, but also because of its great length. Most protocols advise examination of the cervical and lumbar regions, but this may be inadequate. Both longitudinal and transverse sections should be examined, although oblique sections have the advantage over the traditional longitudinal section in that they permit examination of all white matter tracts and also the grey matter, yet still show relatively long segments of nerve fibres. Similarly, because of the extensive ramifications of the peripheral nervous system, it is feasible to examine only a small proportion of the whole. A further complication arises because structurally similar fibres within peripheral nerves have different functions, either motor or sensory. Most peripheral nerves, including the sciatic, which is the one most commonly examined owing to its size and accessibility, contain both sensory and motor fibres. Proximal sections of the sciatic nerve will, therefore, consist of a mixture of fibre types. However, some distal divisions of the sciatic are composed almost exclusively of one fibre type. For example, the tibial nerve contains mainly motor fibres, whereas the sural nerve has mainly sensory fibres; both transverse and longitudinal sections of these nerves should be examined routinely in all neuropathological investigations to ensure that there is no preferential injury to either motor or sensory fibres.

It must be remembered that many sections of non-neuronal tissue will contain nerve fibres, often both myelinated and unmyelinated, and these should be examined for the presence of lesions. Similarly, nerve cell bodies can be found in many tissues. Examination of the autonomic nervous system is dependent on this chance finding of cell bodies and axons as much of the system is not visible to the naked eye. However, a notable exception is the ganglion of the trigeminal nerve, the gasserian ganglion, which is readily dissected from the cranial cavity after removal of the brain. This structure should be examined specifically in all neurotoxicity studies. Similarly, dorsal and ventral root fibres and the associated dorsal root ganglia of the cervical and lumbar regions of the spinal cord should be sectioned. It should be remembered also that the special sense organs, namely the eye (including the optic nerves), the ear and the olfactory epithelium, are extensions of the central nervous system and must be examined whenever neurotoxicological evaluations are performed. Likewise, skeletal muscle must be included in the list of protocol tissues to avoid the possibility of abnormal locomotion due to muscular injury being ascribed to neurotoxicity.

The tissues of the central nervous system may be assessed adequately after routine processing in paraffin wax, followed by sectioning and staining with haematoxylin and eosin. This allows complete slices of brain to be examined. Unfortunately, most of the lipids of the myelin sheath are extracted by the solvents used in processing prior to paraffin embedding, so that it is difficult to assess the presence of any degenerative changes in the myelin. This can be overcome by the use of solochrome cyanin stain or luxol fast blue stain which demonstrate myelin sheaths. Alternatively, the tissue can be exposed to a 2 per cent solution of osmium tetroxide prior to processing.

Similar techniques may be used for the peripheral nervous system, but resin-embedding followed by staining with toluidine blue allows a much more detailed examination of the morphology. To demonstrate the myelin sheath, osmication prior to processing, or a modified luxol fast blue staining technique may be used. Both longitudinal and transverse sections of the nerves should be examined as some lesions are more apparent in one plane of section than the other.

Electron microscopic examination is of little value in routine neurotoxicity testing as the number of sections required would be too great: the chances of selecting an area affected by a lesion would be extremely small. However, electron microscopy is of great value in the investigation of a change identified and localized by light microscopy.

9.5.2 *Quantitative Techniques*

A number of quantitative techniques are available for the investigation of neurotoxicity. These include the estimation of indicators of neuronal injury, such as GFAP, in samples of brain [33]. Such assays can be performed on homogenized preparations of whole brain, or the sensitivity of the estimation can be increased by dissecting the brain into its anatomical components prior to performing the assay; this also gives an indication of the location of any toxic injury. Alternatively, immunocytochemically stained sections may be evaluated quantitatively using image analysis techniques to assess the degree of positive staining.

Certain aspects of neuropathological examination also lend themselves to quantification, particularly the examination of transverse sections of peripheral nerves, using resin-embedded thin sections, post-fixed in osmium tetroxide. The ratio of myelinated to unmyelinated fibres can be assessed as well as factors such as axonal area, the thickness of the myelin sheath and the ratio of axonal diameter to total fibre diameter [34].

When demyelination is suspected, or to assess the extent of any remyelination, teased fibre preparations are invaluable, as they allow the quantitative evaluation of internodal lengths. Whole fibres may be teased out from a nerve and examined unstained using Nomarski optics, or the fibres may be stained and examined by conventional microscopy (Figure 9.15).

9.5.3 *Risk Assessment*

The establishment of a risk assessment for a neurotoxic substance is, generally, dependent upon the setting of an allowable dose (exposure) by dividing the no observed adverse effect level (NOAEL) by uncertainty factors, which hopefully account for inter- and intraspecies differences resulting from the extrapolation of animal data to man. The reliability of this calculation can be increased by obtaining toxicity data from animal studies over a range of dose levels and in more than one species, to give a dose–response relationship and to show the shape of the dose–response curve. Ideally the species chosen should show similarities to man in the absorption, distribution and metabolism of the neurotoxin. An understanding of the mechanism of the toxic effect will assist also in any extrapolation. For risk assessment it is necessary to extrapolate from high-dose exposure to low-dose exposure at which no adverse effects are expected in humans [35].

Ultimately, reliable extrapolation from laboratory tests to man will require the understanding of structure–activity relationships, pharmacokinetic data and mechanisms of toxicity, but until these factors can be elucidated, risk assessment will be dependent upon the use of fixed-size uncertainty factors, which may be entirely inappropriate.

9.6 Conclusions

The survival of mammalian organisms is intimately linked to normal functioning of the nervous system, so even minor injury or dysfunction can have serious consequences. Despite intensive research, many aspects of the function of the normal nervous system are incompletely understood, and the mechanism by which a large number of neurotoxins exert their effects is entirely unknown. The protection of humans in the home, in the workplace and in the environment is thus difficult, as satisfactory risk assessments cannot be established.

Unfortunately the anatomical and physiological complexity of the nervous system makes it exquisitely susceptible to toxic injury, and this same complexity renders the performance of a satisfactory neurological examination extremely difficult. Only by combining a series of functional, behavioural and neuropathological investigations can the integrity of the nervous system be assessed adequately, and the potential of any novel compound to cause neurotoxic injury be evaluated; an understanding of the pathology of the nervous system is thus extremely important in both the design and interpretation of neurotoxicity studies.

Studies designed to detect neurotoxicity must answer certain questions in order to be of value in formulating a risk assessment for man:

- Is the neurotoxic effect direct or secondary to toxic damage in non-neural tissues?
- Is the neurotoxic effect transient or permanent?
- Is the neurotoxic effect due to functional or morphological changes?
- Does the neurotoxic effect show a dose–response relationship?

Furthermore, whenever possible, the metabolism of the compound under investigation in the species chosen for the study should resemble that in man. Only when these questions have been answered can a meaningful risk assessment for man be established.

Acknowledgements

I would like to thank all members of the Environmental Safety Laboratory at Colworth House for their help in the preparation of this chapter, particularly Andrew

Shaw for the photography and Linda Lea for her constructive comments on the manuscript.

References

1. ZEMAN, W. and INNES, J.R.M. (1963) *Craigie's Neuroanatomy of the Rat*, New York: Academic Press.
2. PETERS, A., PALAY, S.L. and WEBSTER, H. DE F. (1976) *The Fine Structure of the Nervous System. The Neurons and Supporting Cells*, Philadelphi0a: W.B. Saunders Company.
3. JENNETT, S. (1989) *Human Physiology*, Edinburgh: Churchill Livingstone.
4. SPENCER, P.S. and SCHAUMBURG, H.H. (Eds) (1980) *Experimental and Clinical Neurotoxicology*, Baltimore: H.H. Williams and Wilkins.
5. JONES, T.C., MOHR, U. and HUNT, R.D. (Eds) (1988) *Monographs on Pathology of Laboratory Animals Sponsored by the International Life Sciences Institute: Nervous System*, Berlin: Springer-Verlag.
6. CAVANAGH, J.B., NOLAN, C.C. and BROWN, A.W. (1990) Glial cell intrusions actively remove detritus due to toxic chemicals from within nerve cells, *Neurotoxicology*, **11**, 1–12.
7. RECHTHAND, E. and RAPOPORT, I.S. (1987) Regulation of the microenvironment of peripheral nerve: role of the blood–nerve barrier, *Progress in Neurobiology*, **28**, 303–343.
8. TOMIWA, K., NOLAN, C. and CAVANAGH, J.B. (1986) The effects of cisplatin on rat spinal ganglia: a study by light and electron microscopy and by morphometry, *Acta Neuropathologica* (Berlin) **69**, 295–308.
9. CHANG, L.W. (1986) Neuropathology of trimethyltin: a proposed pathogenetic mechanism, *Fundamental and Applied Toxicology*, **6**, 217–232.
10. O'SHAUGHNESSY, D.J. and LOSOS, G.J. (1986) Peripheral and central nervous system lesions caused by triethyl- and trimethyl-tin salts in rats, *Toxicologic Pathology*, **14**, 141–148.
11. LANGSTON, J.W., FORNO, L.S., REBERT, C.S. and IRWIN, I. (1984) Selective nigral toxicity after systemic administration of 1-methyl-4-phenyl-1,2,5,6-tetrahydropyridine (MPTP) in the squirrel monkey, *Brain Research*, **292**, 390–394.
12. TRYPHONAS, L. and IVERSEN, F. (1990) Neuropathology of excitatory neurotoxins: the domoic acid model, *Toxicologic Pathology*, **18**(2), 165–169.
13. JOY, R.M. (1982) Chlorinated hydrocarbon insecticides, in ECOBICHON, D.J. and JOY, R.M. (Eds) *Pesticides and Neurological Diseases*, pp. 91–150, Boca Raton, Florida: CRC Press.
14. ECHOBICHON, D.J. (1982) Organophosphorus insecticides, in ECHOBICHON, D.J. and JOY, R.M. (Eds) *Pesticides and Neurological Diseases*, pp. 151–203, Boca Raton, Florida: CRC Press.
15. ECHOBICHON, D.J. (1982) Carbamic acid ester insecticides, in ECHOBICHON, D.J. and JOY, R.M. (Eds) *Pesticides and Neurological Diseases*, pp. 205–233, Boca Raton, Florida: CRC Press.
16. GRAHAM, D.G., ANTHONY, D.C., BOEKELHEIDE, K., MASCHMANN, N.A., RICHARDS, R.G., WOLFRAM, J.W. and SHAW, B.R. (1982) Studies of the molecular pathogenesis of hexane neuropathy. II: Evidence that pyrrole derivatization of lysyl residues leads to protein crosslinking, *Toxicology and Applied Pharmacology*, **64**, 415–422.
17. CHOU, S. and HARTMANN, H.A. (1965) Electron microscopy of focal neuroaxonal lesions produced by β–β′-iminodipropionitrile (IDPN) in rats. I. The advanced lesions, *Acta Neuropathologica*, **4**, 590–603.
18. ROYTTA, M. and RAINE, C.S. (1986) Taxol-induced neuropathy: chronic effects of local injection, *Journal of Neurocytology*, **15**, 483–496.

19. ABOU-DONIA, M.B. and LAPADULA, D.M. (1990) Mechanisms of organophosphorus ester-induced delayed neurotoxicity: type I and type II, *Annual Review of Pharmacology and Toxicology*, **30**, 405–440.

20. BANKS, W.A. and KASTIN, A.J. (1983) Aluminium increases the permeability of the blood–brain barrier to labelled DSIP and β-endorphin: possible implications for senile and dialysis dementia, *Lancet*, **ii(8361)**, 1227–1229.

21. NORENBURG, M.D. (1981) The astrocyte in liver disease, in FEDEROFF, S. and HERTZ, L. (Eds) *Advances in Cellular Neurobiology*, pp. 304–352, London: Academic Press.

22. LAMPERT, P., O'BRIEN, J. and GARRETT, R. (1973) Hexachlorophene encephalopathy, *Acta Neuropathologica*, **23**, 326–333.

23. YARRINGTON, J.T., GIBSON, J.P., DILLBERGER, J.E., HURST, G., LIPPERT, B., SUSSMAN, N.M., HEYDORN, W.E. and MARLER, R.J. (1993) Sequential neuropathology of dogs treated with vigabatrin, a GABA-transaminase inhibitor, *Toxicologic Pathology*, **21**, 480–489.

24. BOULDIN, T.W., SAMSA, G., EARNHARDT, T.S. and KLIGMAN, M.R. (1988) Schwann cell vulnerability to demyelination is associated with internodal length in tellurium neuropathy, *Journal of Neuropathology and Experimental Neurology*, **47**, 41–47.

25. SUZUKI, K. and KIKKAWA, Y. (1969) Status spongiosus of the central nervous system and hepatic changes induced by cuprizone, *American Journal of Pathology*, **54**, 307–325.

26. KRINKE, G., GRAEPEL, P., KRUEGER, L. and THOMANN, P. (1983) Early effects of high-dosed absorbable amoscanate on rat brain, *Toxicology Letters*, **19**, 261–266.

27. POWELL, H.C., MYERS, R.R. and LAMPERT, P.W. (1982) Changes in Schwann cells and vessels in lead neuropathy, *American Journal of Pathology*, **109**, 193–205.

28. KOESTNER, A. (1990) Characterization of *N*-nitrosourea-induced tumours of the nervous system: their prospective value for studies of neurocarcinogenesis and brain tumour therapy, *Toxicologic Pathology*, **18**, 186–192.

29. ABEL, E.L., JACOBSEN, S. and SHERWIN, B.J. (1983) *In utero* ethanol exposure: functional and structural brain damage, *Neurobehavioural Toxicology and Teratology*, **5**, 139–146.

30. PAULE, M.G., REUHL, K., CHEN, J.J., ALI, S.F. and SLIKKER, W. Jr. (1986) Developmental toxicology of trimethyltin in the rat, *Toxicology and Applied Pharmacology*, **84**, 412–417.

31. BERG, B.N., WOLF, A. and SIMMS, H. (1962) Degenerative lesions of spinal roots and peripheral nerves in aging rats, *Gerontologia*, **6**, 72–80.

32. KILHAM, L. and MARGOLIS, G. (1966) Spontaneous hepatitis and cerebellar 'hypoplasia' in suckling rats due to congenital infections with rat virus, *American Journal of Pathology*, **49**, 457–475.

33. O'CALLAGHAN, J.P. (1991) Quantification of glial fibrillary acidic protein: comparison of slot-immunobinding assays with a novel sandwich ELISA, *Neurotoxicology and Teratology*, **13**, 275–281.

34. BROXUP, B.R., YIPCHUCK, G., MCMILLAN, I. and LOSOS, G.J. (1990) Quantitative techniques in neuropathology, *Toxicologic Pathology*, **18**, 105–114.

35. GAYLOR, D.W. and SLIKKER, W. Jr. (1990) Risk assessment for neurotoxic effects, *Neurotoxicology*, **11**, 211–218.

10

The Endocrine System

MARY J. TUCKER

10.1 Introduction

The endocrine system is the second major regulatory system of the body, after the neurological system, and it has two main components. The classic endocrine organs include the pituitary, thyroid, parathyroid and adrenal glands, the islets of Langerhans in the pancreas, and the ovary and testis. The diffuse endocrine system consists of cells dispersed, either singly or in small groups, in various non-endocrine organs such as the gastrointestinal tract. These diffuse endocrine cells and the reproductive organs are discussed elsewhere and this chapter will be confined to the classic endocrine organs.

The endocrine glands regulate the function of other organs and tissues by secreting hormones directly into the blood which carries them to specific target cells that bear the appropriate hormone receptors. The glands have complex control systems which include the neurological systems common to all tissues but also unique negative feedback controls. These are very sensitive systems which respond rapidly to changes in hormonal homeostasis. The secretion of hormones is cyclical and may show a marked circadian pattern. Spontaneous diseases or toxic effects in the endocrine system are expressed as hyperfunction or hypofunction with associated perturbation of the target organs. The changes are dependent on the continuous stimulation of the trophic hormone and are reversible if this ceases. Generalized toxic effects on all the endocrine organs do not occur in animals, but effects on specific organs, and occasionally on more than one, are not uncommon in toxicity testing.

A chemical which overrides the negative feedback and produces constant stimulation of the target organ may result in hyperplasia, or tumours, of the target cell in long-term studies; this is particularly true in the rat, which has a highly sensitive endocrine system. All strains of rat have a high incidence of spontaneous neoplasia in the pituitary gland, but spontaneous tumours in the thyroid and adrenal glands vary markedly with the strain; tumours are rare in all strains in the parathyroid gland and the islets of Langerhans. The majority of rat endocrine tumours are benign and many appear to be non-secretory. Similar post-mortem material is not available from man, so it is not possible to compare the incidence of benign endocrine

311

tumours, but two of the most common tumours in humans, those of prostate and breast, are hormonally dependent tumours. The rat is one of the species normally used in standard toxicology studies and carcinogenicity bioassays, and the frequent spontaneous abnormalities in some of the endocrine organs increases the problem of assessing the risk to man of any toxicological findings. The mouse, which is the other species normally used in the carcinogenicity bioassay has, by comparison, far fewer spontaneous endocrine abnormalities and they are difficult to induce in almost all strains. Dogs and primates are rarely used in long-term studies but appear in short-term studies to have a lower sensitivity to endocrine effects compared with the rat.

Standard histological techniques such as staining with haematoxylin and eosin (H and E) do not distinguish specific cell types, but the relatively recent development of antibodies to many hormonal peptides has provided a means of characterizing specific cells within the organs and also of measuring hormone levels in the blood.

10.2 The Pituitary Gland

10.2.1 Anatomy, Histology and Physiology

The pituitary gland (hypophysis) lies below the brain in the sella turcica of the sphenoid bone. Blood is supplied from the hypophyseal arteries which originate from the internal carotid arteries and the blood then drains into the hypophyseal portal veins of the anterior lobe of the pituitary. Histologicaly, several separate areas can be identified (Figure 10.1). The anterior lobe (adenohypophysis) includes the

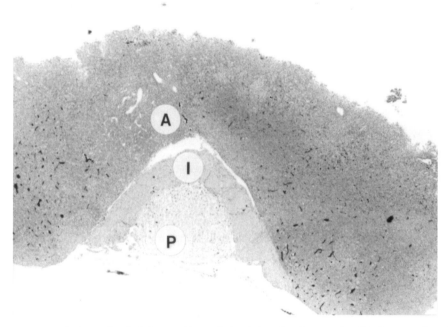

Figure 10.1 Pituitary gland of the rat. Normal gland showing the anterior (A), intermediate (I) and posterior (P) lobes.

pars distalis and the pars intermedia, and the posterior lobe (neurohypophysis) includes the pars nervosa. The size and position of these lobes and the distribution of the cell types within them varies with different species, but in the rodent the major areas are readily identified by their different histological structures. The hormones secreted by the pituitary are listed in Table 10.1. The pars distalis is the largest part of the pituitary and in sections stained with H and E can be seen to be comprised of polygonal or polyhedral cells separated by sinusoidal structures (Figure 10.2). Three types of cells can be identified: basophils, acidophils and chromophobes which constitute 10, 40 and 50 per cent of the total population, respectively. The acidophils which are eosin positive, and can also be stained with orange G, produce growth hormone (GH) and prolactin (PRL); these hormones stimulate the growth of other

Table 10.1   Hormones produced by the pituitary gland

Anterior lobe (Adenohypophysis)
Pars distalis: Thyroid stimulating hormone (TSH, thyrotrophin)
                 Prolactin (PRL)
                 Luteinizing hormone (LH)
                 Follicle stimulating hormone (FSH)
                 Adrenocorticotrophic hormone (ACTH, corticotrophin)
                 Growth hormone (GH)
                 Melanocyte stimulating hormone (MSH)

Posterior lobe (Neurohypophysis)
Pars nervosa: Oxytocin
                 Antidiuretic hormone (ADH, vasopressin)

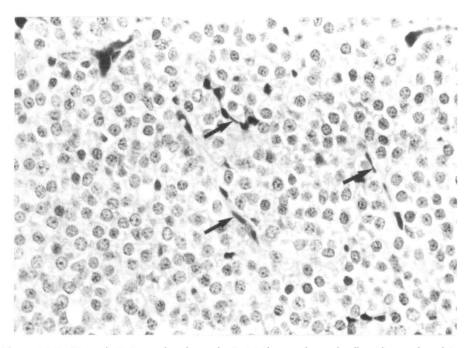

Figure 10.2   Normal pituitary adenohypophysis. Uniform polygonal cells with round nuclei and clear cytoplasm separated by vascular channels (arrows).

tissues (bone and muscle, and mammary gland, respectively). In the actively metabolizing phase, these cells may contain few of the secretory granules which stain with eosin and may, therefore, appear chromophobic. Adrenocorticotrophic hormone (ACTH, corticotrophin) is produced by cells which may be basophilic (haematoxylin positive) or chromophobic. Thyroid stimulating hormone (TSH, thyrotrophin) and the gonadotrophic hormones, luteinizing hormone (LH) and follicle stimulating hormone (FSH) are glycoproteins produced by basophils which stain positively with periodic acid Schiff. Chromophobic cells also include undifferentiated stem cells which have the ability to differentiate to specific secretory cells when required.

Immunohistochemical stains can be used when accurate estimations of specific cell populations or identification of the cell type in a tumour are required (Figure 10.3). The majority of the cells in the pars intermedia are chromophobic cells which produce ACTH and melanocyte stimulating hormone (MSH). The pars nervosa consists of nerve fibres and blood vessels with supporting tissue. It is concerned with the secretion of two hormones, oxytocin and antidiuretic hormone (ADH, vasopressin). These hormones are manufactured within the hypothalamus and travel down the connecting nerve fibres to be released in the pars nervosa. The cells concerned with the production of the peptide hormones, ACTH, MSH, GH and PRL have a well-developed endoplasmic reticulum (ER) with many ribosomes and a prominent Golgi apparatus to facilitate intracellular transport and storage of secretory granules. GH cells have many round, dense-cored, secretory granules, up to 350 nm in size, while PRL cells have larger ovoid granules up to 900 nm. LH and FSH cells have fewer, small granules up to 300 nm and abundant dilated rough ER. These membrane-limited granules represent aggregations of hormone. The signal for

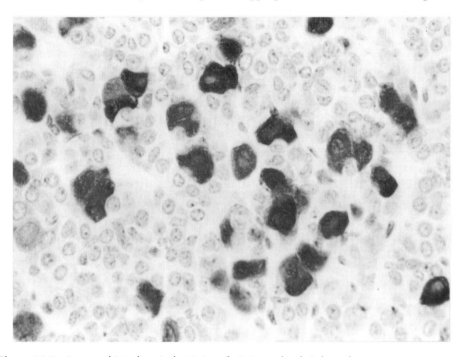

Figure 10.3 Immunohistochemical staining of pituitary gland. Enlarged, immunohistochemically stained, TSH-secreting cells.

secretion causes the granules to congregate at the cell periphery where the hormone-containing core is fragmented, extruded into the perivascular space and the hormone is then transported into the blood capillaries. A detailed description of the histology, immunocytochemistry and ultrastructure of the pituitary gland has been given by Osamura [1].

Each type of endocrine cell in the adenohypophysis is controlled by another hormone produced in the hypothalamus. Those hormones which stimulate other endocrine organs (e.g. TSH, ACTH, LH and FSH) are all stimulated by a releasing hormone and inhibited by the hormones produced by the target tissue. For example, thyrotrophin releasing hormone (TRH) stimulates the pituitary to secrete TSH; this in turn stimulates the thyroid gland to produce the hormone thyroxine, and the elevation of levels of this hormone in the blood inhibits the production of TRH in the hypothalamus. The three other cell types which do not stimulate target organs to produce a hormone (i.e. PRL-, GH- and MSH-secreting cells) are stimulated and inhibited by separate stimulating and releasing hormones produced in the hypothalamus, but this is not clear in the case of MSH. These complex interrelationships are summarized in Table 10.2. In contrast to the adenohypophysis, the two hormones of the neurohypophysis are synthesized by neurons in the

Table 10.2 Hormones of the hypothalamus and pituitary, and their target tissues

Hypothalamus	Pituitary	Target	Hormone
TRH	TSH	Thyroid	Thyroxine
GnRH	LH/FSH	Gonad	Oestrogen/androgen
CRH	ACTH	Adrenal	Corticosterone/cortisol
GHRH	GH	Various	
SS[a]	↓GH	Various	
TRH	PRL	Mammary	
Dopamine[b]	↓PRL	Mammary	
?[c]	MSH	Melanocytes	
?[c]	↓MSH	Melanocytes	

TRH:	Thyrotrophin releasing hormone
TSH:	Thyroid stimulating hormone (thyrotrophin)
GnRH:	Gonadotrophin releasing hormone
LH:	Luteinizing hormone
FSH:	Follicle stimulating hormone
CRH:	Corticotrophin releasing hormone
ACTH:	Adrenocorticotrophic hormone (corticotrophin)
GHRH:	Growth hormone releasing hormone
GH:	Growth hormone
SS:	Somatostatin
PRL:	Prolactin
MSH:	Melanocyte stimulating hormone

[a] SS functions as a GH release inhibiting factor.
[b] Dopamine functions as a PRL release inhibiting factor.
[c] The existence of hypothalamic releasing hormones controlling MSH release is in doubt.
↓ Inhibition of hormone release.

hypothalamus, oxytocin in the paraventricular nucleus and ADH in the supraoptic nucleus; they are transported to the pars nervosa via the axonal processes of the neurons and released into the circulation. Oxytocin produces contraction of uterine muscle and ejection of milk in lactation; it has no known function in the male and no diseases due to excess or deficiency have been identified. ADH is transported to the kidney where it binds to specific receptors on the epithelial cells of the distal tubules and collecting ducts. Its action is to increase water absorption. The hypothalamic control of oxytocin and ADH secretion is from neural input by higher centres within the brain. There are many subtle differences between species in the function and activity of the pituitary hormones and it is important that the endocrine function of all the laboratory animals and man are understood if the risk factors, of the endocrine perturbation seen in toxicity studies, are to be assessed.

10.2.2 *Biochemical and Cellular Mechanisms of Toxicity*

Toxic changes in the pituitary gland are chiefly related to effects on a single cell type. Such a change may be induced by the adverse effect of a chemical on the target organ which then removes the negative feedback control. The initial response is a rapid release of the secretory granules in the specific pituitary cell. After several days the cells will become enlarged (hypertrophic) due to the expansion of the cell cytoplasm and organelles (rough endoplasmic reticulum [RER], mitochondria, Golgi apparatus), increasing hormone synthesis in response to the increased demand. If the demand continues for weeks, the specific cell will also increase in number (hyperplasia) by cell division and recruitment of undifferentiated stem cells. The cells may also become vacuolated and the nucleus displaced. Hypertrophy and hyperplasia of thyrotropes in the pituitary can be induced in rats by **thyroidectomy**, **iodine deficiency** and by numerous chemicals which have antithyroid activity such as **propylthiouracil** [2], **amitrole** and **2,4-diaminoanisole**; and in dogs treated with **sulphonamides**. These compounds induce large 'thyroidectomy' cells, which have dilation and ballooning of the RER; few secretory granules are present due to their rapid discharge. Prolonged treatment with such chemicals will result in their appearance of 'exhausted' thyrotropes, which are intensely vacuolated with small dense nuclei. **Pyridoxine deficiency** in the rat causes a decreased serotonin secretion from the hypothalamus, a reduction in TSH and thyroxine levels, and degranulation of the pituitary thyrotropes. Diffuse hyperplasia of GH cells has been reported in dogs treated with **progestogens** and **oestrogens** [3]. This exemplifies one species difference in the pituitary function of laboratory animals. In dogs, **progestogens** produce tumours of the mammary gland because, in the dog, GH is the hormone which stimulates mammary gland activity and progestogens increase GH release [4]. In the rat, progestogens do not have this effect because mammary gland function is controlled by PRL, which is not increased by the administration of progestogens.

In the rat and man, PRL secretion by the pituitary is controlled by an inhibiting factor, dopamine. Therefore, chemicals which inhibit dopamine production in the rat, such as **bromocriptine**, may produce hyperplasia and tumours of PRL-secreting cells in the pituitary gland and atrophy of the intermediate lobe [5]. **Oestrogen** administration is a reproducible method of inducing pituitary tumours in the rat; it has been suggested that this could be a direct effect of oestrogens on the pituitary, as oestrogen receptors have been identified in pituitary cells. **PRL** also appears to be toxic to the dopamine-producing neurons in the hypothalamus; thus the increasing levels of **PRL**, which occur in the rat after reproductive cycling ceases, may be the cause of the high incidence of spontaneous pituitary tumours in the female rat. **Oestrogens** can produce hyperplasia of MSH cells in the hamster [6]. The pesticide **chlordecone** inhibits the release of pituitary gonadotrophin which is thought to be the cause of this compound's reproductive toxicity in animals and man. Castration, or chemically induced gonadal atrophy, may increase the number of gonadotrophin secreting basophils of the pituitary and the cells may then develop vacuolation and a displaced nucleus to give the typical signet ring appearance of castration cells. The hyperplasia of all the above mentioned cell types is reversible.

Metals have been shown to produce pituitary toxicity [7]; **selenium** is directly toxic to pituitary cells but the mechanism is not known. **Lead** has been shown to produce a significant reduction of GH levels in rats, although pituitary GH levels were not affected, indicating an effect on release mechanisms. **Cisplatin** affects release of PRL and LH from the pituitary in rats and is consequently embryotoxic in reproductive studies. The compound **bis(tributyltin) oxide** is unusual in increasing pituitary LH secretion, and decreasing TSH also, by a direct effect on the pituitary. Pituitary tumours are readily induced by sustained and uncompensated hormonal derangement alone (administration of **oestrogens**, **progestogens**, **dopamine antagonists**), less readily by **radiation** or chemicals alone, but most effectively by a combination of hormonal derangement and radiation or carcinogenic chemicals [8]. In the rat, **high levels of protein** in the diet promote the development of pituitary adenomas.

10.2.3 Morphological Responses to Injury

Chemicals accumulate in the pituitary gland infrequently, hence the wide range of necrotic, degenerative and regenerative changes which are encountered in organs such as the liver or kidney, do not occur. Histological changes are relatively few. Increased or decreased numbers of specific cell types can be identified by appropriate immunohistochemical staining. Hyperplasia of thyrotropes occurs in rats after prolonged treatment with **antithyroid compounds** or feeding **iodine-deficient diets**. PRL-secreting cells are increased in rats, mice, dogs and non-human primates treated with **oestrogens**. In sections stained with H and E, vacuolation may be seen after hyperstimulation of any of the cells subjected to negative feedback. Infarction of the adenohypophysis has been reported in rats treated with **hexadimethrin** and widespread vacuolation with apoptosis at this site has been seen in cynomolgus monkeys treated with an **anticancer agent**. Spontaneous tumours of the adenohypophysis of the pituitary gland are common in all strains of rat and are chiefly prolactinomas; although invariably benign tumours, they frequently cause death due to compression, or local invasion, of adjacent brain tissue. Hyperplasias and adenomas (Figure 10.4) may be single or multifocal and in sections stained with H and E are invariably chromophobic, although a small number may be acidophilic. The distinction between hyperplasia and adenoma is somewhat arbitrary. Hyperplastic areas tend to be composed of small uniform populations of cells similar to, but slightly larger than, those in surrounding tissue; adenomas are less well organized, the cells may vary considerably in shape and size with nuclei of varying size, with prominent nucleoli, and increased mitotic activity.

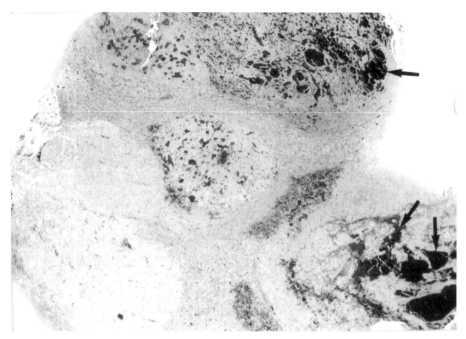

Figure 10.4 Pituitary adenoma in the rat. Large multifocal tumour with angiomatous areas (arrows).

Immunohistochemical staining demonstrates that most of the tumours in the rat are PRL secreting.

10.3   The Adrenal Glands

10.3.1   *Anatomy, Histology and Physiology*

The adrenal glands are paired organs, each located on either side of the anterior poles of the kidneys. In some species, such as the dog, they have a flattened shape. They are supplied with blood from branches of the aorta, and from the phrenic, renal and lumbar arteries which form a vascular plexus. The glands are divided into two distinct areas, the cortex which occupies two-thirds of the gland, and the medulla which comprises the remaining third (Figure 10.5). In man, the adrenal is divided into head, body and tail and the medulla is not present in the tail of the gland.

The cortex is characterized histologically by three separate regions but these are not always clearly identified, for example in the rat. The gland is enclosed by a thin fibrous capsule and immediately below this is the zona glomerulosa that is composed of small cells which comprise 15 per cent of the cortex. Below this is the largest zone, the zona fasciculata, which comprises 70 per cent of the cortex. Here the cells are arranged in cords separated by small capillaries. The inner part of the cortex, the zona reticularis, contributes the remaining 15 per cent of the cortex, and is composed of similar cells to the zona fasciculata and, therefore, may be difficult to distinguish as a separate area. The ultrastructure of the cortex shows that the cells have many lipid droplets which contain cholesterol, the basic steroid precursor. The droplets are close to the smooth

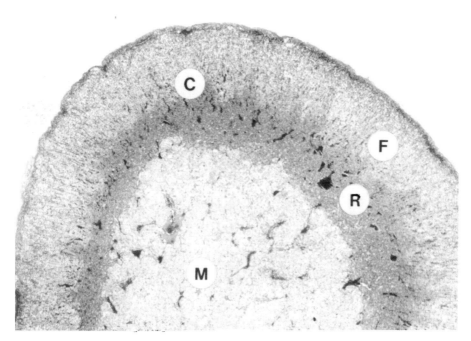

Figure 10.5   Adrenal gland of the rat. Central medulla (M) and outer cortex (C) with distinct zonas fasciculata (F) and reticularis (R).

endoplasmic reticulum (SER) and the mitochondria; all the cells of the zona glomerulosa show less SER than those of the other two zones, and the cells of the zona reticularis have fewer lipid droplets. A detailed description of the ultrastructure of the cortex has been given by Capen *et al.* [9]. The adrenal medulla is composed chiefly of regular polyhedral chromaffin cells separated by fine vascular channels. The cytoplasm is extensive and more basophilic than the cortical cells, and ultrastructurally shows RER, a Golgi apparatus, mitochondria and, unlike the cells of the cortex, scattered secretory granules. In addition, the medulla has scattered ganglion cells.

All of the hormones produced by the cortex are steroids. They are not stored in any significant amount and, therefore, the cells must synthesize the steroids continually to maintain homeostasis. When released into the circulation they are bound to plasma proteins, which is a reversible affinity, to allow the steroid to interact with its target receptor. The zona glomerulosa produces mineralocorticoids under the influence of the renin–angiotensin system. The mineralocorticoids control ion transport by epithelial cells, particularly kidney cells, conserving sodium and increasing potassium loss. When renin is released from the juxtaglomerular apparatus of the kidney glomerulus, it changes a plasma precursor to angiotensin I, which is hydrolysed to angiotensin II and further modified to angiotensin III. These enzymes promote the synthesis of aldosterone in the zona glomerulosa and have a negative feedback control on renin production.

The zonas fasciculata and reticularis produce the glucocorticoids which elevate blood sugar and promote gluconeogenesis from the breakdown of proteins. They also suppress inflammation by effects on lymphoid cells. The secretion of glucocorticoids and, to a much lesser extent aldosterone, is increased by ACTH from the pituitary and decreased by a negative feedback of the glucocorticoids, such as cortisol, to the pituitary and hypothalamus. The zona reticularis also produces small quantities of the sex steroids progesterone, oestrogen and androgen. The adrenal medulla is concerned with the synthesis of the catecholamines, adrenaline and noradrenaline, and the control of the secretion of these chemicals by chromaffin cells is via the neurological components of the medulla.

10.3.2 *Biochemical and Cellular Mechanisms of Toxicity*

The adrenal glands are the most frequently affected of the endocrine organs in toxicity studies. It is not within the scope of this chapter to describe the numerous adrenal toxins in any great detail, but they have been reviewed elsewhere [10]. Toxic agents include those compounds which act directly on the gland and also those whose effects require the production of toxic metabolites. It is widely recognized that many compounds which are metabolized in the adrenal cortex may result in the formation of metabolites which have much greater activity than the parent compound.

The zona glomerulosa is least affected by toxic injury but compounds which produce electrolyte imbalances, such as the diuretic **furosemide**, may cause hypertrophy of this site. Another example is the diuretic **spironolactone** which acts on the kidney by inhibiting the binding of aldosterone to the mineralocorticoid receptors; this compound also has direct effects on the adrenal cortex, reducing the cytochrome P-450 content [11]. **Spironolactone** produces a characteristic degenerative change, the eosinophilic 'spironolactone bodies' in the cells of the zona glomerulosa [12]. Atrophy of the zona glomerulosa has been reported after treatment with compounds which decrease aldosterone production, such as the angiotensin-converting enzyme (ACE) inhibitor **captopril**. Necrosis of the zona glomerulosa is rare but has been seen with **hexadimethrin**; this compound liberates histamine from mast cells and this is implicated in arteriolar spasm and infarction.

Carbon tetrachloride (CCl_4) is another compound which requires metabolic activation and produces cortical lipidosis and necrosis. CCl_4 is covalently bound to adrenal microsomal protein and its effects are greater in the inner cortex (zona reticularis), which is the location of the necrotic lesions. The other two zones of the cortex are affected by various classes of chemicals. **Short-chain aliphatic compounds** frequently produce necrosis by mechanisms not fully defined. It is thought that embolization of medulla cells into cortical capillaries may damage the vascular system of the cortex, with resultant epithelial necrosis. Administration of **ACTH** causes cortical hypertrophy due to an increase in the size of the cells and the induction of hyperaemia of the cortex.

Many xenobiotics produce enlarged cortical cells with vacuolar, frequently lipid, degeneration. This is a reflection of impaired steroidogenesis with a resultant accumulation of precursors in the cortical cells. An example is **aminoglutethimide**, a compound which inhibits steroidogenesis by impeding the conversion of cholesterol to pregnenolone. The resulting lack of a negative feedback maintains a high ACTH secretion and the lipidosis reflects the storage of non-utilized steroid precursors. Administration of **oestrogens**, natural and synthetic, produces cortical hypertrophy by a similar mechanism. The accumulation of neutral fats in cortical cells can be of suffient quantity to cause tissue destruction or loss of function. Amphiphilic compounds such as **triparanol** and **chloroquine** cause widespread phospholipidosis of the cortex and this affects the functional integrity of the lysosomes which become enlarged and filled with myelin bodies. Other natural or synthetic steroids, such as **progestogens**, may cause marked supression of ACTH and, when prolonged, cause functional and morphological atrophy of the cortex in rats and dogs.

Proliferative lesions of the adrenal cortex are not common in most species; they may be induced by hormonal manipulation. For example, castration and **oestrogen** administration in the rat both produce cortical hyperplasia and adenomas. A few xenobiotics including the insecticides **parathion** and **tetrachlorovinphos** have produced adrenal cortical adenomas in the rat, and the androgen **testosterone** has induced cortical tumours in the hamster. Non-proliferative lesions of the adrenal medulla are rare in all species.

Focal necrosis has been reported after the administration of **cysteamine hydrochloride** and **pyrazole** to rats, and fatty change with **triparanol**. By contrast, spontaneous proliferative lesions are not uncommon in most rat strains and may be induced by several mechanisms; prolonged administration of **GH** will induce phaeochromocytoma in the rat. Compounds affecting sympathetic activity such as **reserpine** and **propylthiouracil** produce proliferation in the medulla, possibly by increasing neurogenic stimulation via the splanchnic nerve. Other xenobiotics inducing medullary proliferation include **synthetic retinoids**, some **neuroleptics**, and **sugar alcohols** such as **mannitol**. A variety of other causes have been postulated including excessive food intake and disruption of calcium homeostasis.

10.3.3 *Morphological Responses to Injury*

The range of morphological responses to injury in the adrenal gland is small. Necrosis is a relatively rare occurrence and may be zonal in distribution; CCl_4 causes necrosis in the zona reticularis since this is the zone with the highest level of cytochrome P-450 mono-oxygenases, the mediating components in this necrosis. The heparin antagonist **hexadimethrin** produces a haemorrhagic necrosis of the zona glomerulosa, while wedge-shaped areas of infarction in the zonas fasciculata and reticularis have been recorded with other xenobiotics. Hypertrophy and altered staining of the cells of one or more zones is the most commonly induced histological change. The cells may show a decrease in the amount of lipid and become more dense, with little distinction between the different zones. More frequently there is a marked increase in vacuolar degeneration which may be accompanied by single cell degeneration and minimal inflammatory cell infiltrates. Accumulation of lipid in the cortex may be in the form of fine vacuoles, coarse vacuoles which coalesce, or large ballooned cells which suggest rupture of cell membranes. **Triparanol** and other amphiphilic compounds produce marked phospholipidosis of the cortex, with cytoplasmic inclusions which have been shown to have the ultrastructure of multilamellar bodies. The cytoplasmic eosinophilic 'spironolactone bodies' of the zona glomerulosa have the ultrastructural appearance of concentric agranular membranes with central droplets of lipid. Cytoplasmic hyaline droplets have been induced by **hexadimethrin** and **aminoglutethimide**; cortical brown pigmentation (ceroid degeneration) has been observed in mice treated with **stilboestrol** and **propylthiouracil**.

Atrophy of the cortex occurs after depression of ACTH by **exogenous steroid** administration and results in a greatly reduced cortex (Figure 10.6) and loss of the

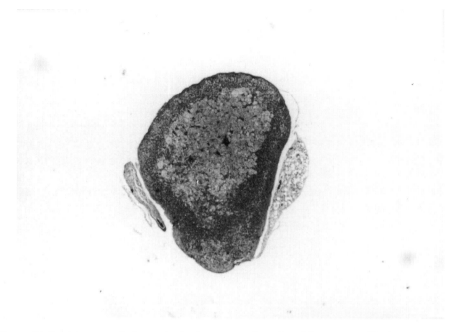

Figure 10.6 Adrenocortical atrophy in the mouse. Atrophy of the cortex with the normal cortex/medulla ratio of 2 : 1 reduced to 1 : 1.

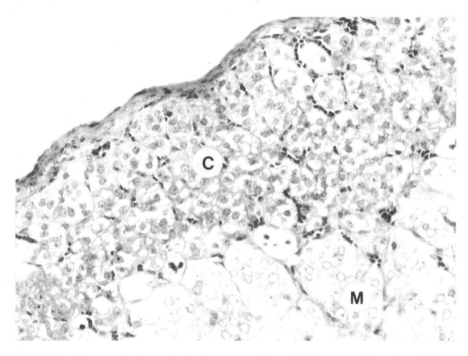

Figure 10.7 Adrenocortical atrophy in the mouse. Cortex (C) shows no distinction of the three cortical zones; medulla (M).

distinction between the zonas fasciculata and reticularis (Figure 10.7). Atrophy of the zona glomerulosa follows administration of the ACE inhibitor **captopril**.

Proliferative lesions in the cortex are nodular, and often multifocal, and may be distinguished from surrounding parenchyma only by subtle differences in tinctorial properties. Tumours may be encapsulated or distinguished only by zones of compressed cells, whereas malignant tumours are less well differentiated, with atypia and nuclear pleomorphism, and local invasion occurs as the chief criterion of malignancy and metastases are rare. In the adrenal medulla, hyperplastic areas are composed of smaller more basophilic cells with hyperchromatic nuclei and these areas may be single or multiple.

10.4   The Thyroid Gland

10.4.1   *Anatomy, Histology and Physiology*

The thyroid gland is situated below the cricoid cartilage and, in rodents, consists of two lateral lobes joined by an isthmus. In the dog, accessory thyroid tissue is common, most frequently located in the adipose tissue attached to the intrapericardial aorta. The basic structure of the gland includes two distinct cell types. The thyroid follicles vary in size, the larger follicles are at the periphery of the gland in the rat, and contain colloid, the stored form of thyroglobulin. In sections stained with H and E, the colloid is eosinophilic and is enclosed by the follicular epithelial cells; these may be cuboidal to columnar depending on the state of activity of the gland (Figure 10.8). Ultrastructurally, follicular cells have an extensive RER and a large Golgi apparatus

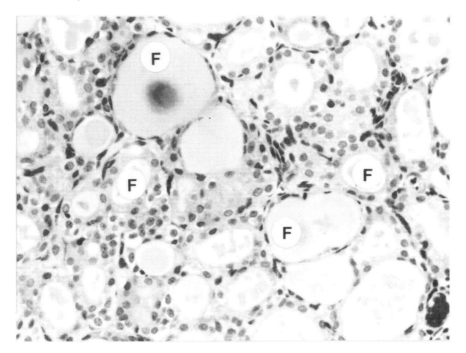

Figure 10.8   Normal thyroid gland of rat. Follicles (F) of varying size with differing height of follicular epithelium.

for the synthesis of thyroglobulin. The luminal edge of the follicular cell has numerous microvillar projections which are important in the process of hormone production. The second component of the thyroid is the C cell (parafollicular cell) which is named after its chief secretory product, calcitonin (CT). These cells lie within the thyroid follicles between the basal region of the follicular cell and the basal lamina, and the cells are concentrated in the centre of the thyroid lobes. Histologically the C cells have a clear cytoplasm and ultrastucturally they show membrane-bound secretory granules in which CT is stored. C cells also contain small quantities of other peptides including somatostatin and bombesin. All of these thyroid hormones can be demonstrated immunohistochemically.

CT is involved in the control of calcium and phosphorus levels and acts in concert with parathyroid hormone (PTH). PTH interacts with target cells in the bone, kidney, and, to a minimal extent, the intestine. CT inhibits osteoclastic osteolysis and consequently reduces the release of calcium from bone into the plasma. CT also decreases renal tubular absorption of phosphate. The levels of calcium and phosphorus in the plasma act as the negative feedback control on C-cell function.

The biosynthesis of the two thyroid follicular hormones (thyroxine or tetraiodothyronine [T_4], and triiodothyronine [T_3]) begins with the synthesis of the protein thyroglobulin by the ribosomes of the ER of follicular cells; the protein is then passed into the lumen of the follicles where it is bound to iodine, to form T_3 and T_4. These hormones are stored within the colloid until required. On receipt of a stimulus by TSH from the pituitary gland, the microvilli of the follicular cells extend into the colloid and a fragment of the protein is ingested, a process called endocytosis. Proteolytic enzymes then release T_3 and T_4 which diffuse out of the follicular cells into the rich network of interfollicular capillaries. Normally the thyroid produces more T_4 than T_3 and the latter is also formed by deiodination of T_4. Both hormones act on many different tissues in the body and have a similar function, although T_3 is the more biologically active form. Thyroid hormones are bound to protein in the plasma and are degraded, principally, by conjugation in the liver and excretion into the bile. The plasma half-life of T_4 in the rat is short (up to 24 h) compared with man (up to 9 days). This is due to the presence, in man, of the protein thyroxine binding globulin, which has a high affinity for thyroxine; the protein does not exist in the rat. The differences in plasma half-life are considered to be one of the reasons the rat, unlike man, is prone to develop thyroid tumours as a result of TSH stimulation.

10.4.2 Biochemical and Cellular Mechanisms of Toxicity

The thyroid gland is one of the most frequently affected endocrine organs but, as with the pituitary gland, it shows a very limited range of changes. The most frequent alteration is hypertrophy and hyperplasia of the follicular cells which can be caused by interference with any stage in the biosynthesis and metabolism of thyroid hormone. Direct antithyroid agents such as **propylthiouracil** and **methimazole** directly affect hormone synthesis by inhibiting the thyroid-peroxidase catalysed organification of iodide. The consequence is reduced T_3 and T_4 levels and sustained high levels of circulating TSH; the latter will cause follicular hypertrophy and hyperplasia and, after long-term exposure, tumours. Rats are more sensitive to this effect than mice, dogs or primates; the difference in sensitivity may be due to the differences in half-life of the thyroid hormones (which are much shorter in the rat) or to the responsiveness of follicular cells to TSH. Other compounds which interfere with this stage of biosynthesis include aniline derivatives such as **sulphonamides**, substituted phenols such as **resorcinol** and a miscellaneous variety of other chemicals. **Sulphonamides** interfere with iodine binding in many species, including rodents and the dog, but not in primates or man.

Toxicology studies in the last decade have demonstrated that an increase in the metabolism of thyroid hormones is another means of inducing hypertrophy of the thyroid in the rat. Many xenobiotics which are liver enzyme inducers increase the induction of the enzyme concerned with the liver metabolism of thyroid hormones, namely the conjugating enzyme uridine diphosphate glucuronyltransferase. In this way, xenobiotics may increase the excretion of the conjugated hormone into the bile. This is one of the major elimination routes in all species, but there are subtle differences between species and also between the sexes. Examples of compounds which affect thyroid function by this route include **phenobarbital** and **β-naphthoflavone**. In this case it is the negative feedback of low levels of T_3 and T_4 which stimulates increased TSH production, with consequent hypertrophy, hyperplasia and neoplasia. Such compounds can be considered indirect tumour-promoting agents. Another mechanism of inducing hypertrophy and cell proliferation is the inhibition of the enzymes which control the deiodination of thyroid hormones. Inhibition of the enzyme 5'-deiodinase reduces circulating T_3, increases TSH, while T_4 is unaffected or slightly elevated. An example of a compound which acts by this mechanism is the colour additive **erythrosine**, which in a carcinogenicity study in the rat produced thyroid tumours in males but not females.

Another type of change in the thyroid follicles is the deposition of various types of pigments associated with several different xenobiotic treatments (Figure 10.9). For

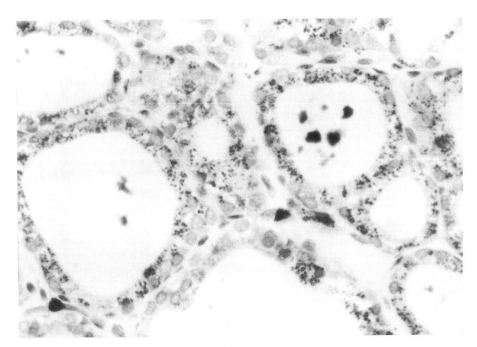

Figure 10.9 Thyroid gland of rat treated with a xenobiotic. Granular black pigment in follicular epithelial cells. Masson–Fontana stain.

example, the antibiotic **minocycline** produces a black discoloration of the thyroid in animals and man due to the accumulation of a substance, possibly a metabolite, in the RER and lysosomes [13]. Thyroid pigmentation is also produced by **synthetic vincamines** and **vitamin E deficiency**. This pigment may be melanin, lipofuscin or a metabolic derivative of the xenobiotic. As with **minocycline**, the pigment may remain in the thyroid for long periods after the cessation of treatment.

Irradiation of the thyroid gland with **iodine-131** causes a rapid loss of C cells, followed by a later proliferation to produce hyperplasia and tumours. **Excess vitamin D** in the diet can also produce C-cell tumours. It is thought that **vitamin D** or its metabolites affect the C cells directly rather than through effects on the feedback mechanism. **Diets high in protein** also facilitate the development of C-cell tumours and it is also a common spontaneous tumour of the ageing rat [14].

The incidence of spontaneous follicular tumours of the rat varies with the strain but they are not common in any strain. Hyperplasia and tumours of follicular cells may be induced in the rat by various means which have been reviewed [14]. Follicular tumours are seen more frequently in males than females and can be induced by **iodine-131 irradiation**, **TSH**, **iodine deficiency**, various genotoxic carcinogens such as *N*-methyl-*N*-nitrosourea, and any xenobiotic which increases the output of pituitary TSH.

10.4.3 *Morphological Responses to Injury*

The thyroid has a noticeably limited range of morphological changes that result from injury. Chronic thyroiditis has been reported in mice, rats and monkeys treated with **trypan blue**, **methylcholanthrene** and an immunosuppressive compound, **frentizole**. Pigment deposits in the thyroid can be demonstrated by various staining techniques such as Masson–Fontana (Figure 10.9). Exogenous administration of **thyroid hormones** will produce atrophy with loss of colloid and a flattened follicular epithelium; in monkeys follicular collapse and basophilia of follicular cells is a prominent feature. Changes in the gland resulting from **excess TSH stimulation**, whatever the cause of the stimulation, produces a gland composed of small follicles with little colloid, surrounded by hypertrophied follicular cells with basal nuclei, an extensive vacuolated cytoplasm, and an often basophilic colloid (Figure 10.10). Papillary projections into the lumina may be present and ultrastructurally the RER is dilated and surface microvilli blunted; some compounds may also produce cystic follicles. The colloid may become more basophilic than normal in severe hyperplasia and corpora amylaceae may be present. Regression of the hypertrophic and hyperplastic changes will occur after cessation of treatment with **antithyroid** compounds and with some, such as **methimazole**, necrosis and inflammation develop. Tumours of the thyroid gland can be derived from follicular cells or from C cells and both benign and malignant tumours may occur. Benign follicular tumours are well-differentiated tumours with recognizable follicular structures and colloid is often present; malignant tumours may also be well differentiated and diagnosis of malignancy is dependant on local invasion and distant metastases; less commonly the tumours may form solid masses of cells with a scirrhous reaction. Poorly differentiated follicular carcinomas may be distinguished from C-cell tumours by the absence of immunohistochemical staining for CT.

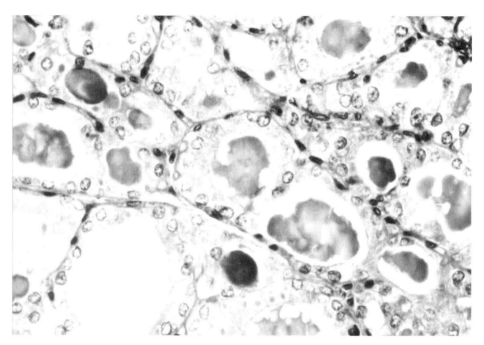

Figure 10.10 Hyperactive thyroid. The follicles are small and lined by a columnar epithelium with basal nuclei and basophilia of the colloid.

10.5 The Parathyroid Gland

10.5.1 *Anatomy, Histology and Physiology*

In most species there are two pairs of parathyroid glands, but rats have only one pair. They lie posterior to the thyroid gland with two at the upper and two at the lower pole. One or more glands may be intrathyroid, particularly in the rodent. In dogs, the glands lie in close proximity to the thyroid and their blood supply is from the cranial thyroid artery. Histologically, the parathyroids are primarily composed of chief cells which produce a single hormone, PTH. The cells show a range of secretory activity with the majority in a resting (inactive) stage. These inactive cells are cuboidal with a clear cytoplasm; ultrastructurally, they show few secretory granules and poorly developed organelles. The cytoplasm may have numerous lipid bodies and lipofuscin granules or glycogen particles: active chief cells show an increased electron density due to loss of glycogen and lipid bodies, and a closer proximity of organelles and secretory granules. Secretory granules in active cells remain sparse in the rat, but are numerous in the mouse. In man and some animal species, but not the rat, a second cell type, the oxyphil cell, is present. These cells are larger than chief cells with a more eosinophilic cytoplasm due to the large number of mitochondria, often with unusual shapes, present in the cytoplasm. The cells may be distributed singly or in small groups between the chief cells; absence or sparsity of secretory granules is thought to indicate a lack of function in hormone production.

PTH is a polypeptide with a molecular weight of 9500. The precursor is synthesized in the ribosomes of the RER which then passes to the Golgi apparatus where the active hormone is produced and packaged into secretory granules. It is stored within secretory granules except for occasions of great demand when it may be released directly from the chief cells without first being formed into secretory granules. In response to the appropriate signal, the secretory granules migrate to the periphery of the cells and liberate the hormone. The secretion of PTH is controlled by the serum level of calcium and to some extent, magnesium. It is the principal hormone concerned with the regulation of blood calcium and acts on target cells in the bone, kidney and intestine. Osteoblasts in bone have PTH receptors and, when stimulated by PTH, secrete products which stimulate the osteoclastic cells to increase resorption of bone with release of calcium. In the kidney, PTH receptors are located in the proximal convoluted tubules and stimulation causes decreased absorption of phosphorus and enhanced calcium absorption. PTH promotes the absorption of calcium from the gastrointestinal tract; this action is much slower than the effect of PTH on the kidney, and it does not occur in animals which are deficient in vitamin D. The kidney and liver are major sites for the degradation of the hormone.

10.5.2 *Biochemical and Cellular Mechanisms of Toxicity*

There are few reports of toxic effects in the parathyroid. Atrophic and degenerative changes are rare; the few records of inflammation of the gland include parathyroiditis in dogs and rabbits exposed to **ozone** [15]. Renal hyperparathyroidism is a relatively common spontaneous disease, particularly in the rat, but it does not progress to neoplasia. Severe renal disease causes hyperphosphaturia which lowers blood calcium and stimulates increased PTH

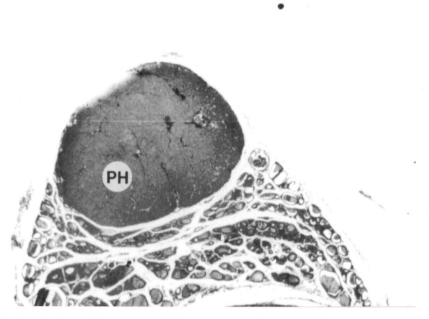

Figure 10.11 Parathyroid hyperplasia. Diffuse parathyroid hyperplasia (PH) in the rat secondary to severe renal disease.

secretion from chief cells, which are initially hypertrophied and then hyperplastic. Any xenobiotic which causes severe damage to the kidneys can cause this secondary effect in the parathyroid glands. Proliferative diseases of the parathyroid are not common. Chief cell adenomas have been produced by **irradiation** and low dietary levels of **vitamin D**. Cancers of other tissues which spread to, and destroy bone tissue, increase the release of calcium into the plasma and depress PTH secretion. Spontaneous tumours of the parathyroid are very rare in all species.

10.5.3 *Morphological Responses to Injury*

Parathyroiditis has been induced in rabbits and dogs exposed to **ozone**. The inflammation is lymphocytic and is accompanied by vasculitis. Degenerative changes in chief cells are very rare but **L-asparginase** has been reported to produce cytoplasmic, eosinophilic ovoid bodies in the chief cells of rabbits; ultrastructurally, there are autophagic vacuoles within the cells. Chief cells may increase or decrease in size depending on their stage of activity and may become vacuolated. Hyperplasia can be focal or multifocal and the areas are usually poorly demarcated, while diffuse hyperplasia involves a great enlargement of the whole gland (Figure 10.11).

10.6 The Islets of Langerhans

10.6.1 *Anatomy, Histology and Physiology*

In the pancreas of most species the islets of Langerhans comprise only 1 to 2 per cent of the organ, with the population of islets highest in the tail of the pancreas. The number of islets depends on the size of the pancreas, with small species such as the mouse having approximately 800, and man, 500 000. The lobules of the pancreas have single branches of the pancreatic artery and the islets are supplied by arterioles and drain from the sinusoids to a portal system of capillaries in the exocrine pancreas. The islets also contain fibrocytes and pericytes, to support the capillary channels, and autonomic nerve fibres which penetrate the secretory cells of the islets.

There are three major cell types in the islets. The most common are the insulin-producing β-cells which comprise about 80 per cent of the islets and are centrally located. The α-cells produce glucagon and comprise around 15 per cent, and the somatostatin-producing δ-cells about 4 per cent of the islets. These last two cell types are located at the periphery of the islets. The remaining 1 per cent includes cells which produce pancreatic polypeptide. In man, islets in the head of the pancreas contain more polypeptide-producing cells and almost no glucagon-secreting cells. Ultrastructurally, the insulin-secreting β-cells contain secretory granules about 300 nm in diameter with a large Golgi apparatus and numerous mitochondria. By contrast, glucagon-secreting α-cells have smaller secretory granules (250 nm) with a small Golgi apparatus, while in the δ-cells the secretory granules are larger than 300 nm. The different cell types are difficult to distinguish in sections stained with H and E (Figure 10.12), but are readily identified by immunohistochemical techniques.

The prime function of the islets is the control of glucose metabolism which includes complex biochemical processes beyond the scope of this discussion.

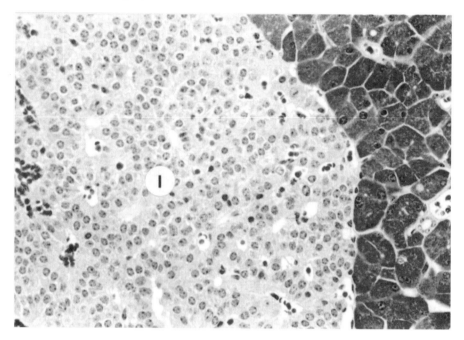

Figure 10.12   Normal pancreatic islet (I) in the rat. The cells are uniform with pale cytoplasm and small round nuclei.

However, briefly, all three hormones are concerned in this function: insulin promotes the uptake of glucose and the synthesis of glycogen, fat and protein in tissues throughout the body; glucagon promotes the production of glucose from hepatic glycogen and other gluconeogenic precursors; and somatostatin inhibits the secretion of insulin and glucagon.

10.6.2   Biochemical and Cellular Mechanisms of Toxicity

Changes in the islets are relatively uncommon and have been reviewed elsewhere [16]. The result of damage to the β-cells is the development of diabetes mellitus, a disease of defective carbohydrate metabolism with hyperglycaemia which, if uncontrolled, may be fatal. Xenobiotics such as **alloxan** and **streptozotocin** specifically destroy β-cells and cause nuclear pyknosis, loss of secretory granules, and vesiculation of the ER. These compounds are used to produce a model of diabetes in animals.

A range of compounds which have a piperidine or piperazine ring in their molecule (substituted at the 4 position), for example the antihistamine **cyclizine**, can produce a degenerative vacuolation of insulin-secreting cells in rats, but not in the dog, mouse or primate. The changes are characteristic of hypersecretion and are reversible. The consequence of prolonged hypersecretory changes is usually subsequent atrophy, failure of insulin secretion and clinical diabetes. A similar vacuolation of β-cells was seen in dogs treated with the synthetic progestogen **chlormadinone acetate** [4]. Necrosis of islet cells may also be produced by **oxine** and **dithizone** which form complexes with zinc (zinc is found in β cells in a complex with insulin), and a **zinc deficient diet** will also damage islet cells. Hypersecretion of glucagon has been reported with **cobalt salts** and **phenylethyldiguamide** but specific toxins to somatostatin-secreting δ-cells have not been identified. **Adrenal corticosteroids** produce hyperglycaemia which increases insulin production, and hypertrophy and hyperplasia of β-cells, particularly in the hamster [17].

Islet cell hyperplasia may be induced by a few xenobiotics including **cyproterone acetate** (in mice), and tumours have been induced by **alloxan** and **streptozotocin** treatment, but are otherwise rare.

10.6.3 *Morphological Responses to Injury*

Vacuolation of β cells is the most common morphological change seen in the islets. Atrophy of cells due to oversecretion has been recorded for glucagon-secreting cells in animals treated with **cobalt salts**. Ultrastructurally, the cells show dilatation of the RER, loss of secretory granules, hypertrophy of the Golgi and accumulation of granular material. An increase in the size or number of specific cell types may be quantified by immunohistochemical staining. Hyperplasia of insulin- and somatostatin-secreting cells has been reported in rats treated with **streptozotocin** and **alloxan**. Enlargement due to hypertrophy and hyperplasia may affect many, but not all, islets within a pancreas (Figure 10.13). Islet cell tumours are invariably solitary and well differentiated (Figure 10.14), and malignant tumours show local invasion.

10.7 **Testing for Toxicity**

Most effects on endocrine glands are discovered for the first time at necropsy, or even later at histological examination during routine toxicological studies. It is not

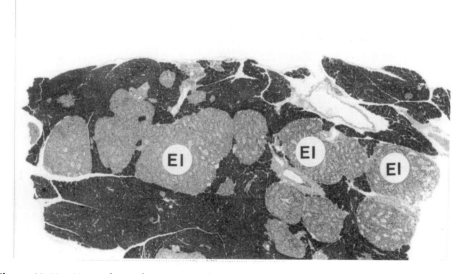

Figure 10.13 Hyperplasia of pancreatic islets. The hyperplasia does not affect all islets (EI, enlarged islet).

331

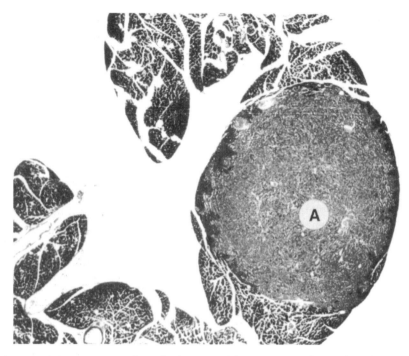

Figure 10.14   Pancreatic islet cell adenoma of the rat. Large solitary islet cell adenoma (A) compressing adjacent exocrine parenchyma.

common practice to routinely measure circulating hormone levels or to immunostain endocrine tissues, since these are time-consuming and expensive. Since the whole toxicology programme for safety evaluation of new chemical entities involves studies of increasing duration, it is possible to build into later studies more intensive examination of those organs where effects have been observed in earlier shorter-term studies. For example, a preliminary toxicological evaluation in the rat, of only 2 weeks duration, may produce histological evidence of thyroid hypertrophy. In the longer studies, required for submission to regulatory authorities, it would be possible to measure circulating levels of TSH and thyroid hormones, to weigh the glands, to sample some glands for the examination of ultrastructure by electron microscopy, and to examine the liver for evidence of increased degradation of the hormones. Alternatively, special investigative studies with much smaller numbers of animals can be set up to examine these features. *In vitro* methods, which include cell cultures from endocrine glands, may provide additional information on function. However, care must be taken to use appropriate cultures since there are differences in endocrine function between the species. The toxicologist must be aware of the possible significance of changes observed in the routine investigations in a toxicity study. These can include changes in organ weights; blood levels of electrolytes, lipid and protein; cardiac function; oestrous cyling and mating behaviour. Histological changes, often very minimal, can be good markers of endocrine dysfunction. The investigator must also understand that changes in the endocrine system may involve more than one organ and that effects may only evolve with time. Our rapidly increasing knowledge of receptors, signal transduction mechanisms, and the interactions between DNA and hormones, together with the availability of new methods of investigation such as immunochemical stains and assays, *in situ* hybridization, and methods of morphometric analysis, will be important to our future understanding of the endocrine system in all species and these techniques are likely to be obligatory tools for future toxicologists.

10.8 Conclusions

The endocrine system is concerned with the homeostasis of many functions within the body. At present our understanding of endocrine toxicology is confined to changes in the structure and function of these organs. In the future, however, the term endocrine system is likely to include the function of regulatory peptides and this will mean a much broader definition of the endocrine system and will necessitate a greater understanding of the molecular basis of control.

To extrapolate any effect to man requires a detailed understanding of the endocrine systems in the experimental animal, and man, since there are both marked and subtle differences in function. In man, investigation of endocrine abnormalities can provide individual data on the circulating levels of any hormone and can be followed over a period of time. Such information is not, and is not likely to be, available from experimental animals. The most difficult problems in risk assessment include effects on the hormones which are known to have different actions in different species, such as PRL and GH in rats and dogs, compared with humans. The roles of some hormones such as neuropeptides have not been defined precisely yet, even in man, and little or nothing is known about the mechanism of action of others. The same hormone may have different effects on different target tissues; an example is cystokinin which has different actions in the central and peripheral nervous system. Evaluation of the risk to man of endocrine tumours in rodents is also difficult, as in animals, unlike man, they are functionally silent or arise secondary to other factors rather than by direct hormonal stimulation.

Some effects can be predicted in animals, because of the known pharmacological action of some classes of drugs, but again caution should be the watchword of the toxicologist; not all **dopamine antagonists** and **synthetic oestrogens** produce pituitary tumours in rats, not all **ACE inhibitors** affect the adrenal glands. In toxicology, dose, bioavailibility, species and strain, significantly influence the actions of xenobiotics. More important are the unpredictable actions. The very high doses used in toxicity studies may produce effects which will not occur at the dose to be used in clinical practice; liver enzyme induction is an example. Enzyme induction may not occur in the liver of patients receiving therapeutic doses, but in animals the consequences of induction on hormonal homeostasis may be profound and prolonged effects may produce tumours.

Cost is of great importance in toxicology testing and it is vital to design studies that will maximize the data obtained in any one investigation. Endocrine toxicology is likely to expand significantly in the future and should increase our knowledge of this important regulatory system.

References

1. OSAMURA, R.Y. (1983) Pituitary gland, rat, in JONES, T.C., MOHR, U. and HUNT, R.D. (Eds) *Endocrine System*, pp. 121–129, New York: Springer-Verlag.

2. TAKAYAMA, S., AIHARA, K., ONODER, A.T. and AKIMOTO, T. (1986) Antithyroid effects of propylthiouracil and sulphonomethoxine in rats and monkeys, *Toxicology and Applied Pharmacology*, **82**, 191–199.

3. EL ETREBY, M.F., GRAF, K.J., GUNZEL, P. and NEUMANN, F. (1979) Evaluation of effects of sexual steroids on the hypothalamic pituitary system of animals and man, *Archives of Toxicology*, **Suppl. 2**, 11–39.

4. TUCKER, M.J. (1970) Some effects of prolonged administration of a progestogen to dogs, *Proceedings of the European Society for Study of Drug Toxicity*, Vol. **XII**, 228–238.

5. PASTEELS, J.L. (1970) Control of prolactin secretion, in MARTIN, C., MOTTO, M. and FRASCHINI, F. (Eds) *The Hypothalamus*, pp. 385–399, New York: Academic Press.

6. SALUJA, P.G., HAMILTON, J.M., THODY, A.J., ISMAIL, A.A. and KNOWLES, J. (1979) Ultrastructure of intermediate lobe of the pituitary and melanocyte stimulating hormone secretion in oestrogen-induced kidney tumours in male hamsters, *Archives of Toxicology*, **Suppl. 2**, 41–45.

7. WALKER, R.F. and COOPER, R.L. (1992) Toxic effects of xenobiotics in the pituitary gland, in ATTERWILL, C.K. and FLACK J.D. (Eds) *Endocrine Toxicology*, pp. 51–82, Cambridge: Cambridge University Press.

8. FURTH, J., NAKANE, P. and PASTEELS, J.L. (1976) Tumours of the pituitary gland, in TURUSOV, V.S. (Ed.), *Pathology of Tumours in Laboratory Animals*, Vol. 1, Part 2, *Tumours of the Rat*, pp. 201–238, Lyon: IARC Scientific Publications.

9. CAPEN, C.C., DeLELLIS, R.A. and YARRINGTON, J.T. (1991) Endocrine system, in HASCHEK, W.M. and ROUSSEAUX, C.G. (Eds) *Handbook of Toxicologic Pathology*, pp. 675–760, New York: Academic Press.

10. RIBELIN, W.E. (1984) The effects of drugs and chemicals on the structure of the adrenal gland, *Fundamental and Applied Toxicology*, **4**, 105–119.

11. SHERRY, J.H., FLOWERS, L., O'DONNELL, J.P., LaCAGNIN, L. and COLBY, H.D. (1986) Metabolism of spironolactone by adrenocortical and hepatic microsomes: relationship to cytochrome P-450 destruction, *Journal of Pharmacology and Experimental Therapeutics*, **236**, 675–683.

12. DAVIES, D.A. and MEDLINE, N.M. (1970) Spironolactone (aldosterone) bodies: concentric lamellar formations in the adrenal cortices of patients treated with spironolactone, *American Journal of Clinical Pathology*, **78**, 651–654.

13. TAJIMA, K., MIYAGAWA, J.-I., NAKAJIMA, H., SHIMIZU, M., KATAYAMA, S., MASHITA, K. and TARUI, S. (1985) Morphological and biochemical studies in minocyclin induced black thyroid in rats, *Toxicology and Applied Pharmacology*, **81**, 393–400.

14. NAPALKOV, N.P. (1976) Tumours of the thyroid gland, in TURUSOV, V.S. (Ed.) *Pathology of Tumours in Laboratory Animals*, Vol. 1, Part 2, *Tumours of the Rat*, pp. 239–272, Lyon: IARC Scientific Publications.

15. ATWAL, O.S. and PEMSINGH, R.S. (1981) Morphology of microvascular changes and endothelial regeneration in experimental ozone-induced parathyroiditis, *American Journal of Pathology*, **102**, 297–307.

16. FISCHER, L.J. and RICKERT, D.E. (1975) Pancreatic islet cell toxicity, *CRC Critical Reviews in Toxicology*, **4**, 231–282.

17. FRENKEL, J.K. (1983) Pancreatic islet cell hyperplasia, golden hamster, in JONES, T.C., MOHR, U. and HUNT, R.D. (Eds) *Endocrine System*, pp. 304–307, New York: Springer-Verlag.

The Respiratory System

JOHN R. FOSTER

11.1 Introduction

The respiratory tract has multiple functions, the most important of which is the efficient exchange of oxygen into and carbon dioxide out of the body. Imbalances in respiratory rate and gaseous exchange can lead to a number of life-threatening physiological disturbances, including respiratory and metabolic acidosis and alkalosis. The system has evolved a number of both physiological and biological mechanisms that limit the impact of external factors on the organ and subsequently on the body.

Along with the development of Western industrial society, man has become increasingly exposed to numerous respiratory pollutants including cigarette smoke, car exhaust gases such as oxides of nitrogen and sulphur, carcinogenic and fibrogenic chemicals such as asbestos and silica, and industrial gases such as sulphur dioxide and hydrogen sulphide to name but a few. The respiratory system is the major line of defence in preventing or ameliorating the effects of these chemicals that enter the body in inhaled air.

In situations where cellular damage is unavoidable, such as those that occur following ingestion of asbestos fibres, the cells of the respiratory tract have a highly developed capacity for regeneration and adaptation in response to damage, and hyperplasia and metaplasia are common responses of the respiratory tract mucosa to a number of chronic irritant stimuli, these changes acting to repair and protect the airways from further insult.

Because this system, unlike the other organ systems of the body, lies in a highly oxidative environment, the component cells also have well-developed antioxidant enzymes such as the glutathione S-transferase (GST) and superoxide dismutase systems. The lungs and upper respiratory tract also have respectable amounts of metabolic enzymes, both detoxifying and activating, which can target the system to xenobiotics entering the lung, either in inspired air or given systemically. Of the cells within the respiratory tract, the olfactory epithelium of the nasal turbinates and the Clara cells of the bronchiolar epithelium are particularly rich sites for these enzymes, and make such cells targets for metabolically activated toxins. Although generally regarded as being poorly endowed with metabolic capability, recent studies have shown that even the endothelial lining of the alveoli has elaborate mechanisms for metabolizing substances such as the vasoactive peptides angiotensin and prostaglandin.

11.2 Anatomy, Histology and Physiology

The respiratory apparatus can be divided conveniently into the upper respiratory tract, or conducting portion, and the lungs, which comprise the lower respiratory tract or respiratory portion.

11.2.1 *Upper Respiratory Tract*

Air enters the nasal cavity via the nostrils externally and the cavity itself is divided longitudinally by a cartilaginous central septum. Each side of the cavity is divided further into dorsal, middle and ventral meatus by two turbinate bones that project in a scroll-like fashion from the lateral wall of the cavity. The most dorsal scroll is known as the nasoturbinate, followed by the maxilloturbinate and finally the ethmoturbinate is the most ventral scroll in the nasal cavity (Figure 11.1 a to c). The floor of the nasal cavity has an additional pair of tubular structures known as the vomeronasal organ of Jacobsen.

The upper respiratory tract filters and moistens air prior to it entering the lungs and regulates heat loss during respiration. The olfactory region has the additional role of monitoring inspired odours for recognition of food, territory and friends. The epithelium of the upper respiratory tract is covered by a continuous layer of mucus which has clearly defined flow patterns. It is moved by the action of the cilia on the ciliated epithelium and, in the posterior regions of the nose, the mucus is moved in the opposite direction to the inspired air, this action being responsible for the scrubbing function of this part of the airway. Mucus is subsequently moved ventrally to the nasopharyngeal meatus from where it passes into the pharynx and hence is swallowed. The moistened surface of the nasal cavity is also thought to dissolve molecules and facilitate their detection by the olfactory neurons. The vomeronasal organ is more specifically involved in the detection of sex pheromones released during sexual behaviour.

The nasal cavity proper is lined by four major epithelial cell types: stratified squamous, transitional, respiratory and olfactory. Distribution of the epithelia is very species specific. In the rat, the stratified squamous epithelium lines the ventral meatus, the distal portion of the nasopharynx and the larynx. A region of transitional (non-ciliated) epithelium lies between the squamous and respiratory epithelium on the lateral wall of both the nasal cavity and the turbinates.

The respiratory epithelium is pseudostratified and is predominantly composed of a mixture of ciliated and non-ciliated epithelial cells. It lines the anterior part of the turbinates, the maxilloturbinates and the proximal nasopharynx. The proportion of ciliated to non-ciliated cells and the number of goblet cells contained within the epithelium differs considerably depending on the site within the nasal cavity. The lamina propria contains both mucous and serous glands which open directly onto the surface of the mucosa.

The olfactory epithelium is a pseudostratified neuroepithelium lining the posterior portion of the turbinates, being particularly abundant in the ethmoturbinates. The

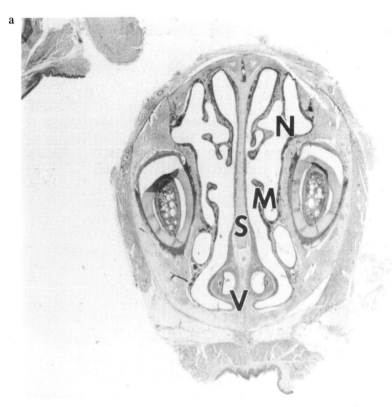

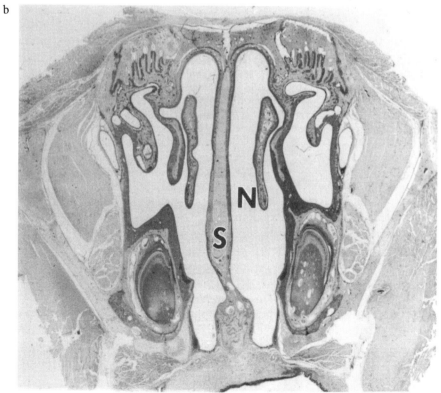

Figure 11.1 *Continued*

c

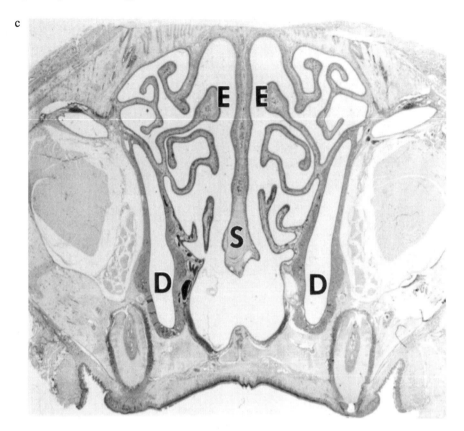

Figure 11.1   Transverse sections through the nasal passages of a rat (see Reference 35). Figure 11.1 (a) is a section through level I showing the nasoturbinates (N), the maxilloturbinates (M), the central septum (S) and the vomeronasal organ of Jacobsen (V); (b) is a section at level II showing nasoturbinates (N) and the central septum (S); (c) is a section through level III showing the location of the ethmoturbinates (E), the nasolacrymal ducts (D) and the central septum (S).

epithelium consists of three cell types, the sustentacular (supporting) cells, the sensory (neuronal) cells and the basal cells (Figure 11.2). Sustentacular cells are tall, non-ciliated, columnar cells with prominent apical branched microvilli and cytoplasm containing abundant smooth endoplasmic reticulum, a well-developed Golgi body and numerous mitochondria. They provide nutritional support for the sensory cells but they also contain large amounts of both phase I and II enzyme systems, which probably function by breaking down odour molecules following their detection by the sensory cells.

The sensory cells are bipolar neurons that lie between the sustentacular cells. The nuclei of the sensory cells are the most numerous in the mucosa and lie in the middle third of the epithelial layer. At their apical sides, a single dendritic process extends up to the luminal surface to form an olfactory vesicle which lies in contact with the luminal mucus and which has up to a dozen sensory cilia. The base of the sensory cell possesses an axon which passes through the basal lamina to join axons from other sensory cells and form non-myelinated nerve bundles, which are particularly conspicuous in the lamina propria. These axons synapse with neurons within the

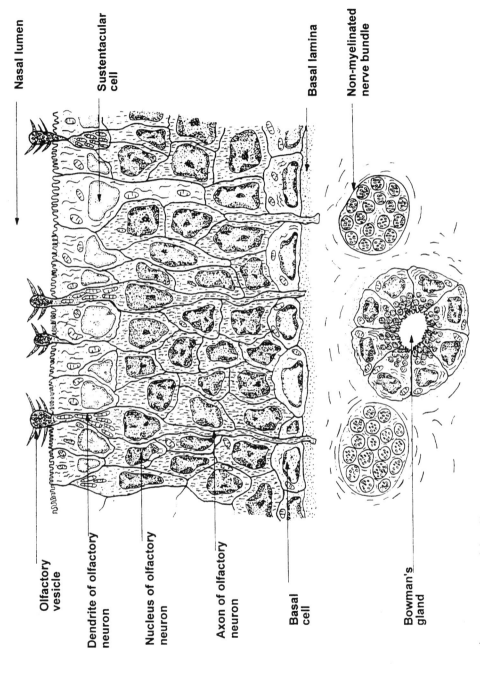

Nasal lumen

Sustentacular cell

Basal lamina

Non-myelinated nerve bundle

Olfactory vesicle

Dendrite of olfactory neuron

Nucleus of olfactory neuron

Axon of olfactory neuron

Basal cell

Bowman's gland

Figure 11.2   The organization of the olfactory epithelium.

olfactory bulb of the brain. Unlike other neurons in the adult mammalian body, the sensory neurons of the olfactory epithelium are able to regenerate, having a reported turnover time of approximately 30 days.

The third cell type present within the olfactory epithelium is the basal cell. This cell is considered to be a stem cell for the regeneration of both sustentacular and sensory cells. The lamina propria of the olfactory epithelium contains prominent nerve bundles, blood vessels and secretory glands known as Bowman's glands. The latter are mixed serous and mucous glands which discharge their secretion directly onto the surface of the olfactory epithelium via ducts that traverse the depth of the mucosa.

The trachea is the major conducting portion of the respiratory tract and is formed by a number of C-shaped cartilage structures with smooth muscle joining the loose ends. It is lined by a pseudostratified respiratory epithelium which in the rat consists primarily of ciliated cells and mucous cells. The underlying lamina propria is demarcated from the submucosa by an elastic membrane, and serous and mucous glands are variably present within the submucosa together with the cartilaginous rings. The glands are innervated by the parasympathetic and sympathetic branches of the autonomic nervous system and secretion is controlled via these inputs. The trachea is continuous with the larynx and bifurcates distally into two main branches or bronchi which enter the left and right lobes of the lung.

Species differences in anatomy

The anatomy of the region shows significant differences between species, with the most obvious being in the structure of the turbinates. These are relatively simple in man and the higher primates, whereas complex scrolling is observed in the rodents and the dog. These structural variations produce significant differences in the air flow of the respiratory tract and, whereas in rodents and the dog, air is directed into the upper half of the nasal passages, in man the air is confined to the lower regions of the nasal cavity. The anatomical differences are probably a reflection of the relative importance of olfaction amongst the various species.

Differences in the structure of the epiglottis and soft palate also mean that in species having close apposition of the two, oral respiration, bypassing the nasal cavity, cannot occur, whereas in higher primates and man, where the epiglottis and palate are relatively distant, oral respiration (facultative nose breathing) takes place naturally. Obligate nose breathing may assume great significance in inhalation studies in rodents where major toxic effects may be observed in the nasal cavity, whereas in those species able to undergo oral respiration, such as primates and man, the avoidance of extensive passage of the toxic chemical through the nose may not result in nasal toxicity.

11.2.2 Lower Respiratory Tract

The lower respiratory tract is represented by the lungs which lie in an airtight chamber, the thorax. The lungs are always made up of several distinct lobes and there is considerable interspecies variability in the total number of lobes present. The rat and mouse have one left lobe and four right lobes, whereas the dog and cat have three left lobes and four right lobes; man has two left lobes and three right lobes.

The trachea bifurcates to form the two bronchi, which progressively subdivide into increasing numbers of smaller bronchi and bronchioles until finally, as in the branches of a tree, the bronchioles open into the respiratory units proper, the alveoli. The outer surface of the lung is covered, in common with other organs, by a pleura composed of mesothelial cells.

The bronchi are morphologically similar to the trachea, although the number of cartilage rings in the submucosa become progressively less with decreasing bronchial diameter and are completely absent in the bronchioles. The lining epithelium is basically of tracheal type (pseudostratified) in the larger bronchi, but as the diameter decreases the number of goblet and serous cells diminish and the epithelial height decreases along with the number of submucosal glands. There are no submucosal glands in the bronchioles and the lining epithelium is simple columnar. The most distant branches of the bronchiolar tree are called terminal bronchioles and, in rodents and cattle, these end in alveolar ducts which are lined by alveolar epithelium and contain smooth muscle in the submucosa. These alveolar ducts then open directly into alveoli. In man, dogs and other species. the terminal bronchioles end in respiratory bronchioles which have a cuboidal epithelial layer and into which alveoli open directly.

The lining epithelium of the bronchioles is composed of a mixture of ciliated and non-ciliated or Clara cells (Figures 11.3 and 11.4). The co-ordinated beat of the cilia on the ciliated epithelial cells moves mucus away from the lower respiratory tract toward the pharynx where it is swallowed. Ciliary action is influenced by histamine and serotonin and ciliated cells have been shown to be exquisitely sensitive to injury by toxic inhalants such as **nitrogen dioxide, sulphur dioxide, ozone** and **cigarette smoke**. The cilia themselves show a remarkable propensity to regenerate rapidly following injury.

The non-ciliated or Clara cell of the bronchioles is a dome-shaped columnar epithelial cell which is present in varying numbers dependent on animal species and location in the bronchiolar tree, there being larger numbers in the respiratory regions

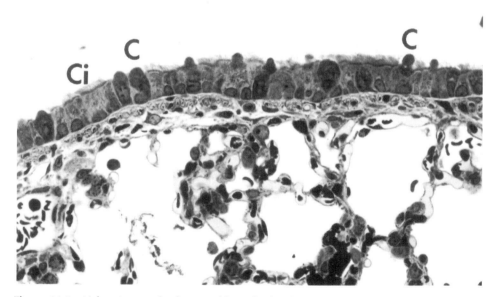

Figure 11.3 Light micrograph of terminal bronchiole of rat lung showing Clara cells (C) and ciliated epithelial cells (Ci). Epoxy resin embedded, toluidine blue.

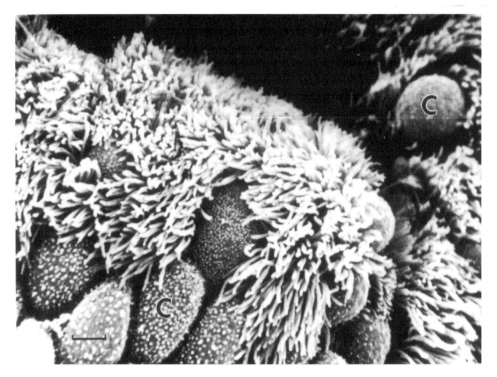

Figure 11.4 Scanning electron micrograph of bronchiolar region in the rat showing the Clara cells (C) and the complex relationship of the cilia from the ciliated epithelial cells. Scale bar indicates 10 *μ*m.

than in the larger bronchioles. The cells synthesize, store and secrete protein components of the extracellular lining of the bronchioles and they also have abundant smooth endoplasmic reticulum and a number of isoenzymes of the cytochrome P-450 and GST superfamilies.

Other minor cell types present in the bronchioles are neurosecretory cells (Kultschitzky cells), brush cells and basal cells. The basal cells are thought to represent the stem cell of the bronchiolar epithelium, while the neurosecretory cell has been shown to possess granules containing serotonin, calcitonin, bombesin or encephalin. The neurosecretory cells are sensitive to oxygen tension in the inspired air and have been shown to increase in numbers following prolonged hypotensive exposure regimes. The exact function of the brush cell is unknown.

The epithelial cells of the alveoli are the flattened, elongated alveolar type I cells, which have been estimated to cover some 90 per cent of the alveolar surface, and the cuboidal alveolar type II cells (Figure 11.5). The main function of the alveolar type I cell, together with the endothelium of the alveolar capillaries, is maintenance of the air–blood barrier and prevention of leakage of plasma proteins and fluid into the air spaces, whilst allowing free passage of oxygen. Type I cells have little metabolic capability even though metabolically activated chemicals such as **butylated hydroxytoluene** specifically target these cells [1].

The major function of the alveolar type II cell is the production and maintenance of pulmonary surfactant, which acts to decrease surface tension and prevent alveolar collapse. The cells contain characteristic lamellar bodies within which surfactant is

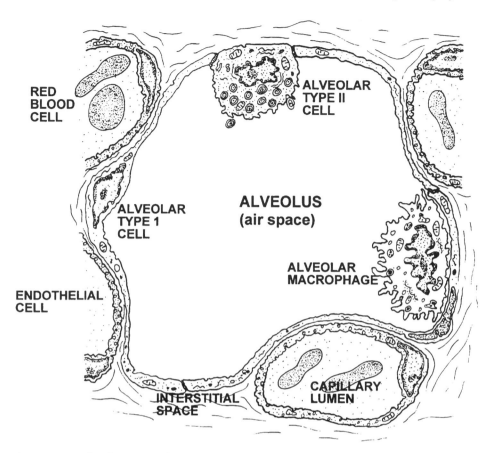

Figure 11.5 Alveolar region of the lung.

stored. The lamellar appearance of the inclusion bodies, as seen in the electron microscope, is due to their phospholipid composition (Figure 11.6). Surfactant is a lipoprotein rich in phospholipids, especially dipalmitoyl lecithin, and it completely coats all cell surfaces on the air side of the alveoli. Surfactant is not present in the alveolar lumen until birth, when a rapid discharge from type II cells into the lumen occurs. Surfactant ensures that on expiration some air is kept within the alveoli at all times. The type II cell is also thought to be the progenitor cell for the regeneration of both alveolar cell types following cytotoxicity. Type II cells can synthesize arachidonic acid metabolites and type IV collagen for basement membranes and are able to metabolize certain xenobiotics by virtue of their possession of drug-metabolizing enzymes.

A third major cell component of the alveolus, the alveolar macrophage, is most commonly found in the alveolar lumen and the interstitial spaces of the alveoli. Alveolar macrophages have a general morphology similar to macrophages from other parts of the body and they function in regulating the quality and quantity of surfactant, in defence against inhaled substances and, in common with their functions in other parts of the body, they are important regulators of inflammation and fibrosis. Specifically in the lung they are also a mainline defence against oxidant injury by gases such as **nitrogen dioxide**, **ozone** and hyperbaric **oxygen** and they

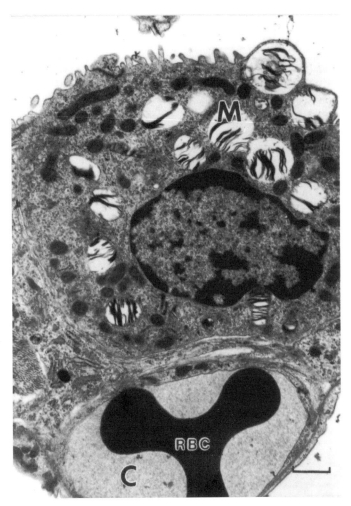

Figure 11.6 Transmission electron micrograph of type II alveolar cell from rat lung. The cell contains characteristic lamellar bodies (M). A red blood cell (RBC) is present in an alveolar capillary (C). Scale bar indicates 3.3 μm.

possess large amounts of antioxidant enzyme systems such as superoxide dismutase and glutathione peroxidase.

In addition to the epithelial component of the alveoli, there are also the endothelial cells of the alveolar capillaries. The endothelial cells of the alveolar capillaries function in the transport of gases, fluids and water and they possess all of the biologically active molecules found in endothelial cells throughout the body, i.e. vasoactive amines, prostaglandins, peptides, etc. Morphologically, they are elongated cells with large numbers of pinocytotic vesicles that function in the transcellular transport of macromolecules.

In addition to the major cell types of the lung, there are also large blood vessels, lymphatics, lymphoid tissue, nerves and varying amounts of fibrous tissue, but the reactions that these tissue components show under toxicological conditions in the respiratory system are similar to those expressed in other tissues and hence they will not be described further here.

11.3   Biochemical and Cellular Mechanisms of Toxicity

The vulnerability of the respiratory system to any particular toxicant depends on a number of factors. These include the route of administration of the toxicant, the chemistry of the toxicant itself, i.e. whether it is intrinsically toxic or whether it needs to be activated via biotransformation systems present in the different cells within the respiratory tract, and finally, the influence of other organs such as the liver and kidney in determining the dose or chemical species delivered to the lung.

11.3.1   *Route of Administration*

The respiratory system can receive toxic chemicals from one of two routes: the first route results in substances being presented to the tissue in inspired air, while the second is via the pulmonary vasculature in the blood, from chemicals that have entered the body systemically (see Figure 11.7, adapted from Cohen [2]). Although the inhalation route is the major one for toxins entering the lungs, the vascular entry of chemicals into the respiratory system can be a significant route for specific types of toxicity. This latter route is essentially a product of the lung's function as an excretory organ, particularly for organic chemicals which can partition from the blood into the expired air within the alveoli. The excretory role can assume

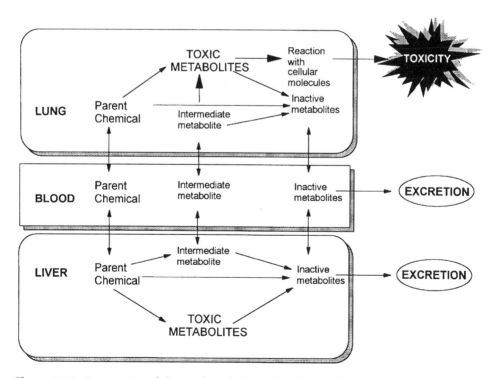

Figure 11.7   Presentation of chemicals to the lung. The 'intermediate' metabolite is one at a crossroads whereby further metabolism can either produce a toxic end product or alternatively metabolism via detoxification can occur.

importance in high-dose situations where normal metabolic and excretory pathways are exceeded such that increased amounts of parent compound are present in the vascular circulation [3].

11.3.2 *Chemistry of the Toxicant*

Just as there are two routes of entry for substances into the respiratory system, there are also two types of interaction that can occur following contact between the substances and the cells and tissues of the system. Interactions can be *direct*, whereby the substance is intrinsically toxic and will damage any cells with which it comes into contact by interfering directly with critical physiological processes. Examples are the oxidant gases such as **sulphur dioxide** and the **oxides of nitrogen**, vapours such as **methyl isocyanate** and **hydrochloric acid**, and particles such as **asbestos** and **quartz**. Toxicity due to direct acting pulmonary toxins will depend primarily on the chemical contacting the tissue and hence will tend to be non-specific. However, differences in sensitivity owing to the presence or absence of protecting systems such as antioxidants and/or functional properties of the cells, for instance those possessing uptake mechanisms, will lead to some cells exhibiting greater cytotoxicity than others even when direct acting substances are involved.

The second type of interaction is an *indirect* one whereby metabolic activation of the parent substance to a cytotoxic product will need to occur before cytotoxicity takes place. Toxicity resulting from the latter type of agent is almost always specific for the cell types possessing the appropriate activating enzyme systems. However, selectivity will be dependent on the toxin reaching the target population, and factors such as the solubility of the toxin in airway fluids and the presence or absence of susceptibility factors such as specific uptake systems and protector enzyme systems will significantly alter the specific cytotoxicity even of metabolically activated pulmonary toxins.

11.3.3 *Toxicity due to Direct-Acting Substances*

Particulates

The toxicity of inhaled **particles** is determined by their site of deposition within the respiratory system. Particles can enter the lung by three different interactions: by *impaction*, by *sedimentation* and by *diffusion*.

In determining the penetration of particles into the lung, a factor known as the aerodynamic diameter of the particle best represents the degree to which the particle will enter the system. The aerodynamic diameter is defined as the diameter of a unit density sphere having the same settling velocity as the particle in question, irrespective of its size, shape or density. It is calculated by taking into account both the density of the particle and its shape. These factors give the particle resistance within the transporting air. The aerodynamic diameter of a particle will determine whether it is deposited by impaction, sedimentation or diffusion.

Particles with an aerodynamic diameter of 5 to 30 µm are deposited in the nasopharynx and upper airways by *impaction* due to the high air velocity in these regions. Particles with an aerodynamic diameter of 1 to 5 µm will be deposited, by gravitational *sedimentation*, in the bronchial region of the respiratory system. Particles of less than 1 µm will reach the alveoli primarily by *diffusion*.

A fourth type of interaction is exemplified by **asbestos** and is termed *interception*, whereby specific cell types, in this case macrophages, phagocytose the particles because of the unique surface properties of the asbestos and thereby accumulate the particles within the lung. Although asbestos fibre length and diameter are important determinants for the site of deposition of the fibres within the tract, fibres up to 200 µm in length have been found to be respirable provided that their diameter did not exceed 3 µm.

Particles deposited in the upper airways will be removed by ciliary action, whereas those reaching the alveoli will be phagocytosed by alveolar macrophages which then leave the lung via the lymphatics. Particulates such as **quartz** are cytotoxic by virtue of their reaction with intracellular proteins and they invariably incite an inflammatory reaction. In those situations where continued damage occurs, fibrogenesis and ultimately pulmonary fibrosis will follow and is a feature of those particulates such as certain types of **silica** that have surface active properties. More inert particulates such as **titanium dioxide**, one of the so-called 'nuisance dusts', will result in passive accumulations of particle-filled macrophages without the accompanying cell death and fibrosis.

Vapours

Toxic vapours and gases may be taken up by tissues at all levels depending upon the solubility of the vapour in the mucous layer coating the cells of the respiratory system. This last property is an important determinant of the degree of penetration of the gas into the respiratory tract. For irritant vapours such as **methyl isocyanate**, the upper respiratory tract epithelium in the nasal cavity and trachea is the target by virtue of this being the first tissue with which the chemical comes into contact. In contrast, oxidant gases such as **nitrogen dioxide**, **oxygen** and **ozone** penetrate throughout the respiratory tract but have a predilection for the ciliated epithelial cells in the terminal bronchioles of the lung. This is probably because of the decreased thickness of the protective mucous layer at this point.

11.3.4 Toxicity due to Metabolic Activation

The metabolic basis for target cell toxicity depends upon the concentrations of activating and detoxifying enzyme systems and their respective cofactors. The presence of appropriate enzymes and the proximity of the nasal passages to entry of toxins are reasons for the target toxicity displayed by the rodent olfactory epithelium over the respiratory epithelium of the nasal passages. The respiratory tract metabolizes chemicals by a large number of different pathways including oxidative, reductive, hydrolytic and conjugation reactions. It is the balance of activating and deactivating enzymes and their cofactors which determine the cytotoxicity of a compound, and both phase I and phase II enzyme systems are present throughout the respiratory tract (Table 11.1).

The concentration of enzyme systems present in the lung as a whole and in different portions of the respiratory tract varies among different species, and whereas human lung has relatively low cytochrome P-450 levels compared with human liver, rodent lung and liver have comparable total amounts, even though the levels of specific isoenzymes differ between the two tissues. Figure 11.8 illustrates the differing concentrations of cytochromes P-450 between lung and nasal passages in several species.

Phase I enzyme systems

Mono-oxygenases High concentrations of specific isoenzymes of cytochrome P-450 have been immunolocalized in the olfactory epithelium, in Bowman's glands of the nasal cavity, and in Clara cells and type II cells of the bronchiolar and alveolar epithelium, respectively. Bronchoalveolar macrophages have also been shown to possess aryl hydrocarbon hydroxylase activity in addition to epoxide hydrolase and GST activity. Cytochromes P-450 are responsible for the bioactivation of a large

Table 11.1 Xenobiotic enzyme systems present in the respiratory tract

Phase I enzymes:
    Mono-oxygenases, e.g. cytochrome P-450s, flavin mono-oxygenases
    Dehydrogenases, e.g. alcohol dehydrogenase
    Hydrolases, e.g. epoxide hydrolase
    Esterases, e.g. carboxylesterases

Phase II enzymes:
    Glutathione S-transferases
    UDP-glucuronyl transferase

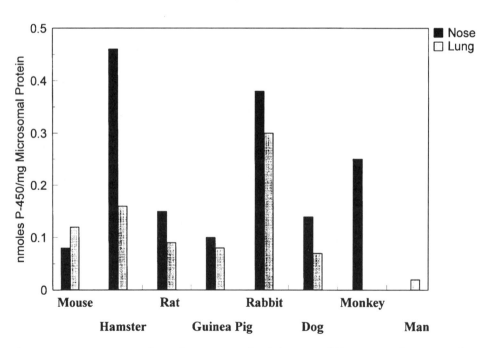

Figure 11.8 Comparison of cytochrome P-450 levels between different animal species and between the pulmonary and nasal compartments (adapted from [4]).

number of chemicals including **polycyclic aromatic hydrocarbons** and **nitrosamines**, and the tissues of the nasal cavity have been shown to be particularly susceptible to the carcinogenic action of **dimethylnitrosamine**. Table 11.2 gives examples of chemicals activated by P-450s that cause cytotoxicity and/or cancer in the respiratory tract.

Flavin-containing mono-oxygenases are found throughout nasal and lung tissue and are the second major mono-oxygenase group responsible for the metabolism of foreign compounds. They have been shown to metabolize *N,N*-**dimethylaniline** and **ethanthiol** to reactive intermediates. Although not as extensively studied as the cytochrome P-450s, it is generally acknowledged that their distribution in the respiratory tract is similar to that of the P-450s [4].

Dehydrogenases and hydrolases These include the enzymes alcohol and aldehyde dehydrogenase, carboxylesterases and epoxide hydrolase and they are found throughout the respiratory tract. Inhalation studies with **acetic acid, acrylate esters, glycol ether esters** and other esters have shown specific degenerative changes in the olfactory epithelium in the nose. Carboxylesterases, located within the nasal mucosa are thought to mediate this toxicity via hydrolysis of the inhaled esters. Bowman's gland and olfactory epithelial mucosa have been shown to be rich sites for carboxylesterases, while smaller amounts are present in the respiratory mucosa of the nose [4].

Both **formaldehyde** and **acetaldehyde** have been shown to be carcinogenic to the nasal cavity of rats on prolonged inhalation exposure. Tumours arise in the anterior and posterior part of the nasal cavity after **formaldehyde** and **acetaldehyde** exposure, respectively. Although differing water solubility between the two compounds has been cited as the explanation for the site differences in the development of tumours, regional differences in nasal metabolism are also thought to play a pivotal role in determining target susceptibility. Studies comparing biochemical and histochemical activities of acetaldehyde dehydrogenase between olfactory and respiratory tissues have revealed a five-fold difference in favour of the respiratory epithelium [4]. In contrast, the oxidation of formaldehyde is two-fold higher in the olfactory epithelium than in the respiratory epithelium, hence the

Table 11.2 Chemicals activated by cytochrome P-450 in the respiratory tract

Chemical	Target	Species
Dimethylnitrosamine	Nasal tissue	Hamster
Benzo(a)pyrene	Nasal cavity	Hamster/rat
1,3-butadiene	Lung	Rat/mouse
4-ipomeanol	Clara cell/type II cell	Mouse/rat
Butylated hydroxytoluene	Type I cell/endothelium	Mouse
Naphthalene	Clara cell	Mouse
Carbon tetrachloride	Clara cell/type II cell	Mouse
1,1-dichloroethylene	Bronchiolar epithelium	Mouse
p-xylene	Clara cell	Mouse
3-methylindole	Olfactory epithelium/Clara cell	Mouse
3-methylfuran	Clara cell	Rat/mouse
Bromobenzene	Clara cell	Rat/mouse
Trichloroethylene	Clara cell	Mouse

susceptibility of the latter to **formaldehyde** toxicity. For these two chemicals, therefore, the distribution of the respective enzyme systems correlates well with the known regional resistance to the toxic effects of inhaled **formaldehyde** and **acetaldehyde**.

Within the tracheobronchial tree, levels of xenobiotic metabolizing enzymes in general are relatively low in the upper regions with progressively higher concentrations present in the lower bronchioles, Clara cells having especially high levels of the majority of metabolizing enzymes, including aldehyde dehydrogenase, whereas the ciliated bronchiolar cells have low amounts. The relative amount of aldehyde dehydrogenase in different tissues within the respiratory tract [4] is shown in Figure 11.9.

Epoxide hydrolases have been found in both nasal and lung tissue and their substrates are the highly reactive epoxides that can be generated via the oxidative metabolism of specific xenobiotics. Generally these enzymes act to reduce the reactivity of these epoxides and hence neutralize their potential for interaction with tissue macromolecules. Exceptions exist, however, and the carcinogen **benzo(a)pyrene** is metabolized by epoxide hydrolase to a diol epoxide which is considered to be a proximate precursor of the carcinogenic chemical species generated from **benzo(a)pyrene**.

Different isoenzymes of particular families are known to activate/deactivate chemicals at different rates, so that even where total amounts of enzyme in an organ may be similar, the absence of specific isoenzymes can profoundly affect the resultant toxicity of a given chemical. This is adequately illustrated by **benzo(a)pyrene** which is extensively metabolized in the liver and poorly metabolized by the respiratory system even though both organs contain adequate amounts of cytochrome P-450, the enzyme system responsible for its metabolism.

Phase II enzyme systems

GSTs and uridine diphospate-(UDP-)glucuronyl transferases have been demonstrated in abundance throughout the respiratory tract [5, 6], with the olfactory epithelium

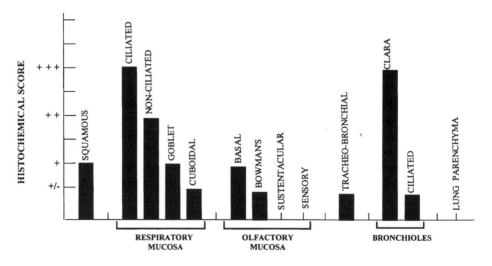

Figure 11.9 Relative distribution of aldehyde dehydrogenase activity between the various tissues of the upper and lower respiratory tract based on histochemical reaction [36].

and respiratory epithelium having the highest levels of GST-B and GST-C, respectively, in the nasal tissue. In the lung, Clara cells and ciliated bronchiolar epithelial cells have comparable levels of GST-B, GST-C and GST-E [7]. The immunohistological distribution of glucuronyl transferase enzymes has not been studied owing to the unavailability of antibodies to the enzymes.

These enzymes are generally associated with detoxification reactions but on occasions they are able to activate chemicals to cytotoxic/carcinogenic products. For example, the nasal carcinogen, **dibromoethane**, is thought to be activated via GST to form an episulphonium ion, the proximate carcinogen, following glutathione conjugation of the parent. No activating reaction has yet been demonstrated for the glucuronyl transferases and products of metabolism by these enzymes are generally acknowledged to be less toxic than the parent compound.

Inducibility of drug metabolizing enzymes in the respiratory tract

Ethanol and **acetone** have been reported to induce the protein levels of cytochrome P-450 2E1 in the olfactory mucosa of rabbits, while the polychlorinated biphenyl mixture, **Aroclor 1254**, has been shown to induce cytochromes P-450 1A2 throughout the nasal epithelium following systemic administration [6]. As in the liver, pulmonary cytochrome P-450s are inducible by chemicals such as the polycyclic aromatic hydrocarbon **3-methylcholanthrene**, while in contrast, **sodium phenobarbitone**, a potent hepatic enzyme inducer, does not induce pulmonary cytochrome P-450s. The type II alveolar cells and the Clara cells show greatest inducibility with **3-methylcholanthrene**. In contrast **Aroclor 1254** induced comparable amounts of cytochrome P-450 1A1 throughout the lower respiratory tract [6].

Genetic polymorphisms for drug metabolizing enzymes in the human population

Within the human population there are several examples of isoenzymes of P-450 that show genetic polymorphism. Cytochrome P-450 2E1 is one such example that has been related to differences in the incidences of lung cancer. P-450 2E1 is known to be responsible for the oxidation of *N*-nitrosamines present in tobacco smoke, and the current data suggest a link to lung cancer where extensive metabolizers for P-450 2E1 are more susceptible to developing cancer [7].

In addition to the polymorphism that has been found in the cytochrome P-450, a similar polymorphism has also been recognized in the GST isoenzyme GSTM1-1. It has been estimated that about 50 per cent of the human population totally lack this GST isoenzyme and a link has been postulated with subsequent susceptibility to developing lung cancer as a result of smoking, particularly that of adenocarcinoma [8]. Absence of the appropriate GST isoenzyme is thought to lead to increased levels of smoke-derived chemical species, possibly from polycyclic aromatic hydrocarbons, adducting to the DNA of the target cell population.

Species differences in drug metabolizing enzymes in the respiratory tract

There are considerable differences in the levels of xenobiotic enzyme activity in the same tissues from different animal species. Whereas in the rabbit, the ethmoturbinates have a higher capacity to metabolize *β*-**butyrolactone** than the liver or maxilloturbinates, in the rat, the liver has the highest capacity to metabolize the chemical. In the respiratory system of the rat, epoxide hydrolase, UDP-glucuronyl transferases and GSTs are generally present in higher quantities than levels of the potentially activating, cytochrome P-450 enzyme systems. However, regional differences in specific cellular content, such as the levels of cytochrome P-450s in the bronchiolar Clara cell, can significantly alter the resultant cytotoxicity and/or carcinogenicity of chemicals such as *p*-**xylene**, **naphthalene**, **trichloroethylene** and **methylene chloride** for these cells. Similarly in the olfactory epithelium the presence of high local concentrations of drug metabolizing enzymes is thought to be responsible for the selective toxicity of **3-methylindole** and **methyl bromide** for this tissue.

Development of metabolic tolerance

Several studies have demonstrated that low doses of cytotoxic chemicals such as **4-ipomeanol** or **butylated hydroxytoluene** protect against subsequent cytotoxic doses of the same chemical [9] and that chemicals that may cause cytotoxicity on initial exposure, on continued exposure at the same dose levels fail to show morphological damage. This development of refractiveness in the lung to an initially toxic compound has been termed 'tolerance'. It has been shown for chemicals such as **trichloroethlylene** [10], **naphthalene**, **methylene chloride** [11] and **4-ipomeanol** that require metabolic activation to a cytotoxic metabolite, and also for chemicals such as **ozone, oxygen** and **nitrogen dioxide** that act by other mechanisms [12]. The underlying cause of the tolerance may be different in each case, but evidence suggests both a selective loss of the isoenzyme responsible for activating the protoxin and an induction of conjugating or antioxidant systems such as GST enzymes, glutathione, superoxide dismutase and catalase [11, 13, 14].

11.4 Morphological Response to Injury

11.4.1 *Upper Respiratory Tract*

Methyl bromide, **3-methylindole** and **3-trifluoromethyl pyridine**, when given acutely, induce specific necrosis of the olfactory epithelium and Bowman's glands of the nasal turbinates, while respiratory epithelium throughout the nasal cavity remains unaffected. In contrast, **methyl isocyanate** damages the epithelial lining throughout the upper and lower respiratory tract. Typically, substances toxic for the nasal passages can impair mucociliary flow, alter airflow resistance, can irritate and produce necrosis of the nasal mucosa. This effect is normally manifest by the appearance of an exudate of proteinaceous material and cell debris in the nasal passages [15].

The immediate sequelae that result from acute exposure to a cytotoxic substance in the nose are similar to those in other organs and are observed as degeneration and necrosis of the affected tissue or cell type, inflammation and repair, and regeneration. An inflammatory response in the nose is referred to as rhinitis. In the olfactory region of the nasal turbinates, inflammatory cells are most commonly seen in the lamina propria, although intense intraepithelial inflammatory cell infiltration is common in the respiratory mucosa of the nasal turbinates. If the insult is severe, complete mucosal erosion and/or ulceration can occur. Olfactory mucosal damage, if severe, may be accompanied by atrophy of the nerve bundles present in the lamina propria with a corresponding loss of olfactory function [16].

With continued exposure there is generally adaptation to the toxin, which might present itself as a biochemical loss of an activating enzyme system, or a morphological transformation such as hyperplasia or metaplasia of a formerly simple ciliated epithelial lining. Both hyperplasia and metaplasia have the effect of reducing the cytotoxicity of a given chemical. The hyperplasia that occurs can be simple and seen as multifocal segmental increases in the epithelial cell layers, or it may be papillary where the proliferative epithelium grows out into the luminal cavity of the nose. Nodular hyperplasia can also occur whereby the proliferating epithelium grows down into the submucosa.

The degree of response is generally dependent on the severity of the insult and with chronic, mild irritation, goblet cell hyperplasia is commonly seen accompanying simple epithelial proliferations. Continued exposure to more severe irritants can induce epithelial proliferations that can develop into hyperplasia, metaplasia or most commonly, a mixture of both. Squamous metaplasia is seen in the anterior portions of the nasal cavity following chronic **formaldehyde** inhalation and is also commonly observed in the laryngeal epithelium of rats following exposure to aerosol formulations of various kinds [17]. Respiratory metaplasia of the olfactory epithelium is seen in rats chronically exposed to **ethyl acrylate** and **dibasic esters** and is thought to represent an adaptive response to chronic irritation. Respiratory metaplasia, goblet cell hyperplasia and squamous metaplasia are considered to be adaptive responses of the tissue which limit continued cell damage either by increasing the protective mucus layer over surviving cells (goblet), or by altering the susceptible cell population (squamous and respiratory). They are common responses to certain gaseous irritants such as **cigarette smoke, formaldehyde** and **ammonia**.

The olfactory epithelium itself is sensitive to a variety of inhaled and systemically administered toxicants such as **methyl bromide** and **3-trifluoromethylpyridine** (see Table 11.3), and following acute exposure responds by undergoing necrosis. Sensory and sustentacular cells are damaged and regeneration is accomplished via proliferation and maturation of the surviving basal cells. Studies with **methyl bromide** have shown that functional recovery of olfaction occurred before complete morphological reorganization of the epithelium was observed [16].

Chronic exposure to irritant gases such as **acetaldehyde** and **formaldehyde** induce hyperplasia and squamous metaplasia in the lining epithelium of the airways and the submucosal glands [18]. Similarly, **propylene glycol monomethyl ether acetate, dimethylamine** and **methyl isocyanate** also induce olfactory and, in the case of **methyl isocyanate**, respiratory epithelial damage in rodents. However, these chemicals only affect those regions of the olfactory epithelium that are in or adjacent to the main route of air passage through the nose, such that the specificity is a product of position rather than one of uptake or chemical activation.

Under conditions of chronic cell damage, regenerative cell division has to occur in order to replace cells killed by the chemical. During chronic regenerative cell replication there is a greater than normal chance of mutations becoming fixed in the proliferating cell population, derived from either the irritant chemical itself or from environmental carcinogens [19]. Hence, following continued exposure to certain chemicals, progression within the damaged epithelium can occur and neoplastic cell populations can arise. Such a situation is seen with chronic exposure of rats to

Table 11.3 Chemicals acutely cytotoxic to the nasal cavity (modified from [15, 37])

	Squamous epithelium	Respiratory mucosa	Olfactory mucosa
Acetaldehyde	–	+	+
Acrolein	–	+	+
Acrylic acid	–	–	+
Bis(chloromethyl)ether	–	–	+
1,2-dibromo-3-chloropropane	–	–	+
Dimethylamine	+	+	+
Ethyl acrylate	–	–	+
Formaldehyde	–	+	+
3-trifluoromethylpyridine	–	–	+
3-methylfuran	–	–	+
3-methylindole	–	–	+
Methyl bromide	–	–	+
N-nitosamines	–	–	+
Nickel sulphate	–	–	+
Phenacetin	–	–	+

chemicals such as **formaldehyde** and **acetaldehyde** where squamous cell carcinomas were observed following a 2-year exposure. Several examples of chemicals that induce nasal tumours are shown in Table 11.4 [20].

Neoplasms of the rat nasal cavity have been classified according to their proposed tissue of origin as adenomas, adenocarcinomas, carcinomas of various tissue types and esthesioneuroblastomas (olfactory neuroblastoma). The last are derived from the olfactory epithelium and possess neurosecretory granules which can be visualized using immunohistochemistry or electron microscopy. Spontaneous neoplasms of the nasal cavity are rare in laboratory rats and mice, although **nitrosamines**, when given either by inhalation or systemically, have induced esthesioneuroblastomas with smaller numbers of adenomas and adenocarcinomas in the nasal cavity of hamsters, mice and rats. **Phenacetin** has induced tumours in the nasal cavity of rats following lifetime administration. These have been described variously as squamous cell carcinomas, transitional cell carcinomas and adenocarcinomas, the latter appearing to be derived from the glands of the cavity.

11.4.2 *Lower Respiratory Tract*

Bronchi and bronchiolar region

The way in which a noxious chemical affects the lower respiratory tract is dependent on a number of often interconnected factors, with some chemicals being exquisitely specific for a single cell type while others ubiquitously damage cells throughout the system. A common acute response to non-specific irritation in the bronchi and bronchioles is an increase in mucus secretion from surface goblet cells, and on prolonged exposure, mucous cell metaplasia can occur in the lining epithelium. This type of response is seen following exposure to **ammonia** or **ozone**. The irritant action

Table 11.4 Chemicals inducing nasal tumours following lifetime exposure

Chemical	Species/strain	Route
1,2–dibromo-3-chloropropane	F-344 rat/B6C3F1 mouse	Inhalation
1,2-dibromoethane	F-344 rat	Inhalation
α-Epichlorhydrin	SD rat	Inhalation
Dimethylvinyl chloride	OM rat	Drinking water
1,2-ethoxybutane	F-344 rat	Inhalation
2,6-xylidine	F-344 rat	Diet
Propylene oxide	F-344 rat	Inhalation
Procarbazine	F-344 rat	Intraperitoneal
p-Cresidine	F-344 rat	Diet
Bis(cholromethyl)ether	F-344 rat	Inhalation/parenteral
Nitrosaminoketone	F-344 rat	Intraperitoneal
Formaldehyde	F-344 rat	Inhalation

of the chemical together with the excess mucus is able to provoke the autonomic innervation of the smooth muscles lying in the submucosa of the bronchioles and cause contraction and bronchiolar luminal constriction resulting in a chronic bronchitis. Mucous metaplasia is a hallmark of chronic bronchitis (Figure 11.10). The decreased airway luminal diameter, together with exfoliated damaged cells and excess mucus can obstruct the airways and induce further alveolar injury. The presence of debris in the bronchiolar and alveolar lumen can elicit an inflammatory response in both the interstitial tissue and the airways themselves. This generally involves neutrophils in the acute phase and mononuclear cells following chronic exposure to damaging chemicals and vapours.

Eosinophils are commonly present in varying numbers during both the acute and chronic inflammatory phases in the lung under a variety of pathological situations, but predominance of this cell type is indicative of a hypersensitivity reaction such as occurs in asthma.

In the absence of damage to the basement membrane, cellular regeneration will occur via proliferation of basal cells in the bronchi and bronchioles and via type II alveolar cell proliferation in the alveoli. If basement membrane damage occurs, a fibrinous exudate can be observed in the lumen of the airway and organization with luminal fibrosis or bronchiolitis obliterans will follow where complete occlusion of the airway occurs. Such obstruction can lead to alveolar injury and a local emphysema, whereby the alveolar lining wall becomes extremely attenuated following a gross extension of the alveolar sac.

Acute irritation, such as that produced by the oxidant gases **ozone, nitrogen dioxide** and **oxygen**, causes a pneumonitis which is limited to the central alveoli and the adjacent terminal bronchioles. The peripheral airways and larger bronchioles are generally much less affected. Within the bronchiolar epithelium the oxidant gases can target both the ciliated epithelial cells, causing deciliation and loss of ciliary clearance from the airways, and also the Clara cells lining the bronchioles. The toxicity shown with the oxidant gases is a product of oxidative damage and the selectivity of the cell degeneration observed is dependent on the differing amounts of antioxidant mechanisms in the cells at the time of exposure [21].

355

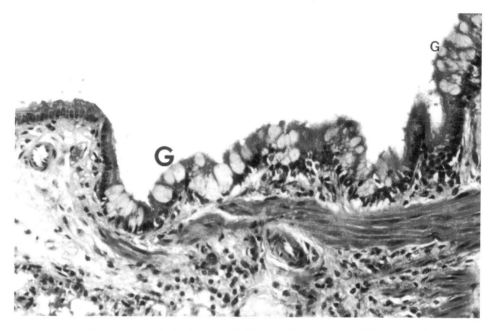

Figure 11.10 Mucous metaplasia of the epithelium (goblet cells, G) of the terminal bronchiole of a rat given a single 6-h inhalation exposure of spermidine and killed 9 days later.

Of the two cell types lining the bronchiolar mucosa, the Clara cell shows by far a greater degree of sensitivity to selective cytotoxicity than the ciliated epithelial cell. Hence chemicals such as ***p*-xylene, naphthalene, 3-methylindole, 4-ipomeanol** and a range of **chlorinated hydrocarbons** (Figure 11.11) all selectively damage the Clara cell following systemic administration or inhalation exposure [22]. These chemicals have in common their requirement for metabolic transformation to a cytotoxic metabolite, and the selective cytotoxicity to the Clara cell has been postulated to be by virtue of this cell having some of the highest levels of cytochrome P-450s in the respiratory tract [22].

Cigarette smoke produces goblet cell hyperplasia in the larger conducting airways, glandular hyperplasia, and conversion of mixed serous and mucous glands into predominantly mucus-secreting glands. Within the goblet cell metaplasia of the terminal bronchiolar region, mucous plugging and obstruction of the lumen can also occur. The mucous metaplasia, together with the inhibition of ciliary beat that smoking produces throughout the airways, is responsible for the cough and build-up of sputum seen in chronic smokers. Long-term partial or total restriction of the bronchioles can lead to gross enlargement of the bronchiolar lumen due to trapped inspired air, leading to fibrosis of the bronchial wall and the observation of bronchiectasis and emphysema in the lung parenchyma. Cigarette smoke contains large numbers of chemicals including **catechol, naphthalene, 1-methylindole, nitrosamines** [23] and **polycyclic aromatic hydrocarbons** such as **benzo(e)pyrene**, plus a variety of acidic components in the gas phase that include **formaldehyde, acrolein** and **acetaldehyde**. It is conceivable that the principal carcinogenic cause of cigarette smoking is the continual exposure of the bronchial epithelium to this wide variety of carcinogenic and chronic irritant agents.

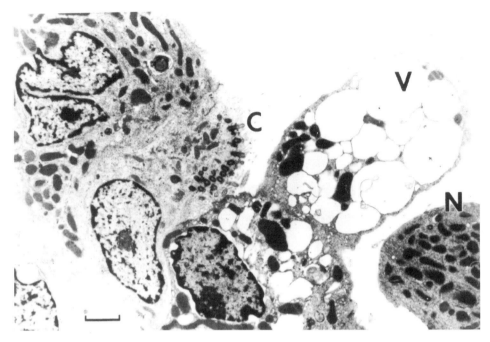

Figure 11.11 Transmission electron micrograph of the terminal bronchiolar region from a mouse given a single 6-h inhalation exposure of 2000 ppm methylene chloride and killed 18 h later. The photomicrograph illustrates the exquisite nature of the targeting of methylene chloride to particular populations of the Clara cells. V, vacuolated Clara cell; N, non-vacuolated Clara cell; C, ciliated cell. Scale bar indicates 6.6 μm.

Alveolar damage

Toxicants, whether inhaled or systemically arriving in the alveoli via the blood system, are able to affect both the alveolar epithelium and the endothelial cells of the pulmonary vasculature. The degree and specificity of the resulting damage is highly dependent on the toxin in question and while *O,O,S*-**trimethylphosphorothiolate** specifically damages the alveolar type I cell, **butylated hydroxytoluene** and **methylprednisolone** affect both the alveolar type I cell and capillary endothelial cells preferentially; **bleomycin** and **busulphan** induce damage throughout the alveolar epithelium, while **nitrogen dioxide** and **ozone** affect both the alveolar and terminal bronchiolar regions of the lung.

Necrosis of the alveolar epithelium by whatever cause is always accompanied by an acute inflammation (alveolitis) of varying severity and, if permitted, is followed by proliferation of the alveolar type II cells. The acute alveolitis accompanying cell necrosis is characterized by fibrin exudation and neutrophilic infiltration and, on prolongation will be followed by a predominantly mononuclear cell influx into the alveoli (Figure 11.12).

Proliferation of type II cells presents a morphological picture of alveoli lined by cuboidal epithelium (termed alveolar bronchiolization/epithelialization) and these changes are seen in rats during the recovery phase of inhalation studies with **oxidant gases**. If the extent of the damage is limited, maturation of the cuboidal type II cells occurs such that flattened type I cells are once again seen to line the resolved alveoli.

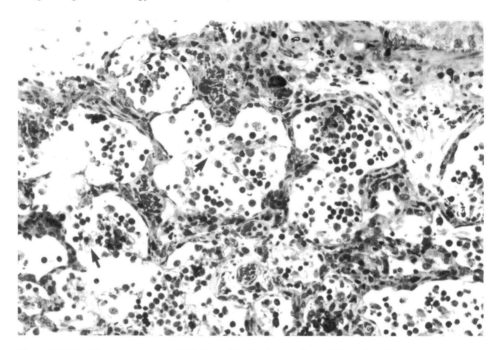

Figure 11.12   Severe pneumonitis induced in the lungs of rats infected with the bacterium *Klebsiella pneumoniae*. The micrograph shows the presence of fibrin strands within the alveoli (arrowhead) and a mononuclear and neutrophilic cell infiltration into the alveolar lumina and interstitium. Epoxy resin embedded, toluidine blue.

If the damage is very severe, complete resolution of the lesion will not occur and permanent loss of lung function results as the alveoli are replaced by an increased interstitial compartment with varying degrees of fibrosis (Figure 11.13). Whereas in man, pulmonary fibrosis is a common sequel to extensive lung damage, in rodents even extensive bronchopneumonia, that permanently removes functional respiratory units, such as that produced by the compound **spermidine** [24], resolves into a poorly fibrosing peribronchiolar and perivascular reaction. This example serves to illustrate the difficulty in producing a convincing rodent model of human lung fibrosis even under severe damaging conditions. Cholesterol clefts, often surrounded by a macrophage cell response, are commonly seen within the lung parenchyma under a variety of inflammatory conditions (Figure 11.14).

Damage to either the alveolar epithelium and/or the endothelium can result in increased vascular permeability and plasma leakage into the alveolar air space to produce alveolar oedema with an accompanying reactive inflammatory response (Figure 11.15). Oedema might present itself as perivascular, with expansion of the underlying interstitial tissue of blood vessels, or alveolar where expansion of the alveoli occurs. In both instances, associated lymphatics will show dilated lumens as they attempt to remove the excess lung fluid. *α*-**Naphthothiourea (ANTU)**, when given to rats at appropriate dose levels, induces a classic pulmonary oedema as a result of damage to the endothelial cells. **Oxygen, monocrotaline** and **4-ipomeanol** have also been shown to induce alveolar oedema via their action on both the alveolar epithelium and endothelium. One interesting example of a chemical which is specifically toxic to the endothelium of the alveoli is the pyrolizidine alkaloid

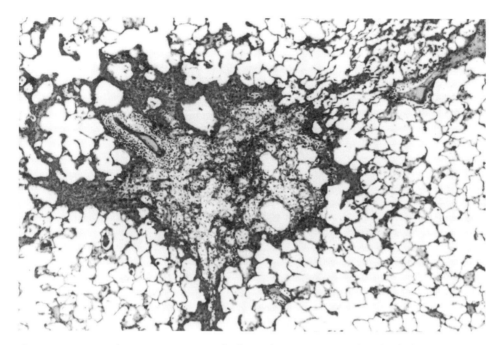

Figure 11.13 Resolving pneumonitis in the lung of a rat given a single 6-h inhalation exposure of spermidine and killed 14 days later.

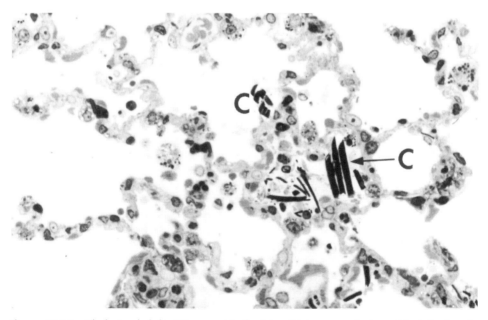

Figure 11.14 Cholesterol clefts (C) present in the interstitial spaces of rats accidentally dosed in their lungs with corn oil. Epoxy resin embedded, toluidine blue.

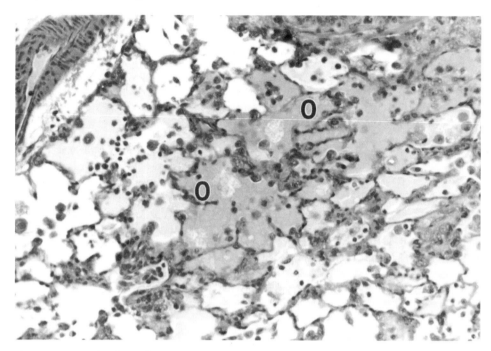

Figure 11.15 Alveolar oedema (O) present in the lungs of rats given a single 6-h exposure to spermidine and killed 2 days later.

monocrotaline, which has been shown to be metabolically activated in the liver to highly reactive pyrrolic derivatives that are then transported in the blood stream to the pulmonary vasculature where they induce damage.

The herbicide **paraquat** is accumulated selectively in the type I and type II alveolar cells and, on undergoing a continuous redox cycling reaction mediated by a microsomal NADPH-dependent oxidoreductase, generates a superoxide anion which ultimately, through the production of lipid peroxides, leads to cell death. The primary event in this instance is the accumulation of **paraquat**, and the selectivity of the toxicity for the type I and II alveolar cells is by virtue of their possession of a polyamine uptake system, through which **paraquat** enters the cell. Consequent to destruction of the alveolar epithelium, a neutrophilic alveolitis and pulmonary oedema develop, followed by an intra-alveolar and inter-alveolar fibrosis which results in complete destruction of the alveolar architecture. This may be severe enough to prevent adequate gas exchange and result in death of the affected subject.

Pulmonary fibrosis may be produced by a number of agents including **silica**, **asbestos** and the antineoplastic agent, **bleomycin**. Although in the case of toxins such as hyperbaric **oxygen, bleomycin** and **paraquat**, damage through the lung may be diffuse, and hence the resultant fibrosis is diffuse, with **silica, beryllium** and **asbestos**, fibrotic nodules form around the offending fibres and are observed focally throughout the lung parenchyma. Increased collagen deposition in the lung can be produced by a combination of increased production and decreased degradation, and fibrosis most commonly follows when disruption of the basement membrane of the alveolar epithelium has occurred. The fibrotic reaction is mediated by pulmonary macrophages via the production of cytokines such as leukotrienes and prostaglandins E_2 and I_2. Fibrosis and oedema may be accompanied by emphysema, whereby the elastin supporting structure of the alveoli becomes digested following protease release from damaged cells. This leads to breakdown of the normal alveolar structure and results in grossly expanded alveoli which tend to fibrose and inhibit efficient gas exchange across the alveoli. Emphysema is a common disorder following chronic inflammatory conditions such as those induced by **cigarette smoking** and **coal dust** inhalation. Deficiency in production of the antiprotease enzyme, α_1-antitrypsin, is considered to be instrumental in the progression of changes leading to emphysema.

Toxicity resulting in increased numbers of alveolar macrophages can be seen in the phospholipidosis group of diseases, best illustrated in experimental animal studies with amphipathic drugs such as **chlorphentermine**. Morphologically, the lung appears full of lipid-laden macrophages and the pathogenesis is related to the inhibition of lysosomal lipid breakdown by the drugs. The human disease of silicosis is found amongst slate workers and quarrymen, and is caused by the **silica** particles entering the lungs, being phagocytosed by alveolar macrophages which then die and release various cytokines which cause further phagocytosis, cell death, etc. A continuous cycling of these factors acts to trap the silica in the lung and potentiate the cycle of cell death, cell reaction and fibrosis. As with the drug-induced phospholipidoses, accumulations of lipid-laden alveolar macrophages are also commonly seen in this disease. Coal workers pneumoconiosis is a similar disease to silicosis, caused by ingestion of **coal dust**, and also results in pulmonary fibrosis and a permanent impairment in lung function.

Asbestosis is a chronic interstitial lung fibrosis that results from the inhalation of various forms of **asbestos** fibres during certain manufacturing processes. On inhalation of **asbestos** fibres of the required dimensions, the fibres are deposited in the bronchioles and proximal alveoli, generally through ingestion by macrophages. This results in the release of acid hydrolases from lysosomes which kill the macrophage. This sequence of phagocytosis and cell death is repeated and ultimately initiates a chronic inflammatory reaction which results in multinodular bronchiolar and alveolar fibrosis. The degree of toxicity varies considerably with the type of asbestos inhaled and whereas **amosite** is a relatively innocuous fibre, **chrysotile** is intensely fibrogenic. The magnesium content of the fibres is thought to be critical in determining the degree of fibrogenicity resulting from contact with these chemicals, with cytotoxicity being directly proportional to the amount of magnesium in the fibres. Asbestos fibres may be located within the fibrosed areas, with a minority acquiring a ferroprotein coating to become the so-called 'asbestos bodies' seen within sections of lung. It is generally regarded that such coated fibres are no longer harmful. The asbestos body is formed by macrophages that are thought to leave small cytoplasmic fragments around the fibre which they have failed to ingest.

Metals such as **cadmium**, **beryllium** and **cobalt**, and **fungi** and **cotton** also stimulate pulmonary fibrosis on inhalation. Cotton fibre pulmonary disease is known as byssinosis and is thought to be a product of an immune-mediated inflammatory disease. There are several important occupational diseases of the lung, the most common being listed in Table 11.5.

11.4.3 Cancer in the Respiratory Tract

Lung cancer in the human population is a leading cause of death in the 20th century. The majority of human cases of lung cancer originate in the bronchial epithelium and

Table 11.5 Some important occupational diseases of the lung

Agent	Disease	Predominant pathology
Silica	Silicosis	Nodular fibrosis
Coal	Coal worker's pneumoconiosis	Emphysema
Asbestos – general	Asbestosis	Interstitial fibrosis
Asbestos + smoking	Bronchogenic cancer	Bronchial neoplasia
Asbestos – crocidolite	Mesothelioma	Pleura/peritoneal neoplasia
Cadmium	Metal fume fever	Pulmonary oedema
Beryllium	Berylliosis	Beryllium granulomatous fibrosis
Fungi – mouldy hay	Farmer's lung	Granulomatous pneumonitis (acute exposure); interstitial fibrosis (chronic exposure)
Cotton fibres	Byssinosis	Allergic pneumonitis; interstitial fibrosis

of these approximately 50 per cent are the so-called oat cell or small cell lung carcinoma. Epidemiological data show an excellent link between this tumour type and **cigarette smoking** and the tumour is almost never seen in non-smokers. These cancers are hormonally active, secreting adrenocorticotrophic hormone, calcitonin, bombesin and serotonin and are thought to be derived from the neuroendocrine cells of the bronchial epithelium. Other risk factors for the development of these cancers in man include exposure to **radiation, uranium mining** and **asbestos** working [25]. Only one experimental situation exists that has resulted in a neuroendocrine cancer, and this is the **nitrosamine/hyperbaric oxygen** model in hamsters developed by Schuller *et al.* [26]. In contrast to the lower respiratory tract, human tumours of the upper respiratory tract are relatively rare, although both malignant and benign tumours do occur in the nasal cavity and have been linked to exposure to **hardwood dust** and to occupational exposure to **nickel** and **chromium** [27, 28].

Unlike the situation in man, bronchial tumours are universally rare in laboratory animals. In laboratory studies with F-344 and Wistar rats, chemically-induced tumours of the lungs are rare, while in contrast in mouse oncogenicity studies, the lung is the second most frequent site for the development of tumours [29]. The most common type of lung tumour found both spontaneously and induced by exposure of rodents to carcinogens occurs in the parenchyma as alveolar/bronchiolar adenoma (Figure 11.16). The cells may be arranged in a solid, glandular or papillary pattern and ultrastructurally they frequently show the morphology of type II alveolar epithelial cells. Carcinomas are also seen and are defined by local invasion and cellular pleomorphism; they may also show areas of necrosis. Although other types of pulmonary neoplasms are generally rare, inhalation studies with **cigarette smoke** in rodents induced increased incidences of squamous cell carcinomas in the periphery of the lungs. Various types of mesenchymal tumour can infrequently be observed in the lungs of laboratory animals and they include fibrosarcoma, leiomyoma and sarcomas.

Metastases from spontaneous lung tumours in laboratory rodents are seldom, if ever, seen, although chemically induced tumours showing a papillary or glandular growth pattern have been reported to exhibit a greater propensity for metastatic

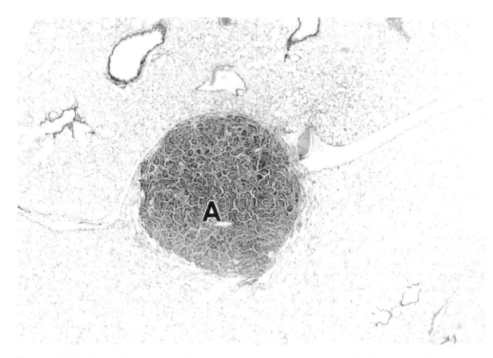

Figure 11.16 Bronchioalveolar adenoma (A) present in the lungs of mice given daily 6-h exposures to 2000 ppm methylene chloride for 12 months.

behaviour than do tumours showing other morphological phenotypes. Due to the fine capillary bed of the pulmonary vasculature, the lung provides a filtering system for metastases from distant tumours, and the presence of various types of sarcoma and carcinoma can be seen within the lung parenchyma under situations that produce malignant transformation within other organs such as the liver or lymphoreticular organs.

Pleural mesotheliomas in man are associated with exposure to **blue asbestos (crocidolite)** and these tumours are not known to be produced by exposure to any other environmental contaminant including smoking. After smoking, asbestos exposure has been estimated to be the next greatest risk of respiratory cancer in the human population. It has been shown that asbestos can act synergistically with smoking in increasing the risk of developing bronchial cancer and a positive correlation exists between the development of fibrosis and induction of bronchogenic cancer after asbestos exposure. The relationship does not hold for mesothelioma where even low-dose exposure to **crocidolite** has been found to carry significant carcinogenic risk. There is currently much debate about the dose−response relationships regarding asbestos and cancer, particularly with regard to non-occupational exposures such as those encountered in public building insulation schemes. Mesothelioma can be produced in laboratory animals by intrapleural injection of several mineral fibres including asbestos, but inhalation studies with asbestos have not been found to reproduce mesotheliomas reliably in rats. Mesotheliomas may show either epithelial or mesenchymal (fibroblastic) differentiation patterns and most frequently are exophytic growths into the mediastinum from a stalk on the lung surface. In contrast to the fibrogenesis of asbestos fibres, where the larger fibres are most fibrogenic, for the production of mesothelioma, the shorter, slimmer fibres have been found to be most potent since they are best able to reach the pleural surface to institute the mesothelial reaction.

11.5 Testing for Toxicity

In the whole animal, chemicals may prove toxic to the respiratory system either by inhalation in inspired air or via the pulmonary vasculature following systemic administration of chemicals. The anatomical and physiological differences between individual animal species in their respiratory apparatus include differing minute volume of ventilation, frequency of respiration, bronchial dimensions, arterial blood flow to the respiratory system and percentage of retention of the inhalant in the lung. These factors are independent of the physical and chemical properties such as solubility, diffusion coefficients and particle size of the toxicant itself, that will also influence its presentation to the lung. Hence, the complexities of both the physical properties of the test chemical and the biological properties of the respiratory system itself are great, and care is necessary to ensure that chemical testing for respiratory toxicity is done correctly.

In testing for respiratory toxicity there are two basically different protocols, one in which the toxicant is presented directly to the lung via inhalation exposure, while the second exposes the animal to the toxicant systemically by one or other of the acceptable routes of administration, e.g. oral, intraperitoneal, intravascular or subcutaneous.

11.5.1 *Inhalation Exposure*

The practicalities of undertaking an inhalation toxicology study have evolved over the last 20 or so years during which time the physics of aerodynamics, inhalation chamber design, generation of suitable atmospheres for test compound and development of whole body, nose only and head only systems have come to be understood [30]. In terms of exposure conditions, animals may be exposed in *whole body* inhalation chambers, or in *partial body* exposure systems (head only, nose only, lung only).

For *whole body* exposure, animals are housed in cages, in chambers containing the required atmosphere present as a dynamic system continuously recirculating through the exposure chamber. Although gases and vapours can be administered successfully in this way, several factors need to be borne in mind when embarking on whole body inhalation studies. If the compound is an aerosol, it may condense onto the animal's fur and be subsequently ingested when the animal cleans itself so that significant oral administration can also occur; also of relevance if the compound is particularly hazardous, such as a harmful gas, asbestos or a radioactive chemical, is that large volumes are generated in the exposure chamber and these will need to be removed safely at the termination of the experiment. Whole body inhalation systems are generally applied where large numbers of animals are to be exposed over extended periods of time or for lifetime studies. They are expensive but best represent the situation pertinent to human exposure conditions.

Head only or nose–mouth only systems will greatly reduce the potential for chemical contamination of the fur and hence help to prevent inadvertent oral exposure to condensed vapours. However, in both of these latter systems, the animals are tightly restrained for the duration of the exposure period and problems with stressing animals may become paramount if long-term exposure protocols are undertaken. Stress has been cited as a critical factor in increasing the acute inhalation toxicity of **carbon monoxide**.

For any of the systems, the toxicant is mixed with air to the required concentration and then administered to the animal. Considerable expertise is required both in designing the exposure procedure and in developing an appropriate system for delivering atmospheres to the animal in a respirable form while maintaining the physical and chemical properties found under normal exposure conditions. It is common for the inhalation toxicologist to collaborate with an aerosol engineer for advice in generating suitable atmospheres from particulates, gases and liquids. Once the required atmosphere has been generated, the concentration of toxicant delivered to the animal has to be monitored either continually or at intervals via a sampling port using a suitable method such as absorption spectrometry (UV, infrared, visible) or gas chromatography [31].

11.5.2 *Systemic Administration*

Although not generally considered part of the battery of testing for specific pulmonary toxins, the systemic route of administration is nevertheless an important way in which chemicals can reach the respiratory system. Hence chemicals administered orally, intraperitoneally, intravascularly and subcutaneously can, on occasion, produce highly specific lesions in the cells of both the upper and lower respiratory tract. **Paraquat, *a*-naphthylthiourea, butylated hydroxytoluene** and many anticancer agents such as **bleomycin** and **busulphan** can, on systemic administration, produce highly specific lesions in the lungs of both experimental animals and man.

11.5.3 **Ex Vivo/in Vitro *Systems***

Of significance in recent years has been the introduction of isolated perfused lung preparations [31] whereby acute responses to chemical and drug administration can be studied. The application of tissue slice technology to the lung, where sections of tissue are incubated with toxins *ex vivo*, has also proven to be instrumental in elucidating the mechanism whereby **paraquat** accumulates within the lung and so induces its characteristic toxicity [32].

Truly *in vitro* techniques have also been developed for studying the individual cell populations, and both bronchiolar Clara cell and alveolar type II cell cultures have been established to study the biological and biochemical responses in the target cell population in the absence of the pharmacokinetic and metabolic influences of the other cell populations in the lung [33, 34].

11.5.4 *Histological Considerations*

Because of the extremely complex structural organization of the respiratory tract, it is imperative that appropriate preparative and sampling procedures are adopted. In general, fixation of the nasal epithelium of the upper respiratory tract is by infusion of formalin via the trachea or nasopharyngeal duct in a direction anterograde to that of the inspired air, so that fixative flows out through the nares. Fixation of the lungs is generally by inflation via the trachea using a sufficient volume of fixative to inflate the lobes fully without over-distending them. A common protocol for rat lungs utilizes a 30-cm high-pressure line for the fixative with the solution being contained in a 20-ml syringe. Sampling of the lungs is generally by sections through each of the major lobes.

A recommended protocol for histopathological examination of the nasal cavity details fixation of the whole head, followed by decalcification and subsequent trimming. Sampling of the nasal regions requires care if all relevant target areas of the nares are to be sampled. An excellent review of histological techniques as applied to investigations of the nasal cavity is given in Uriah and Maronpot [35]. For trimming purposes, the nasal passages are divided into four levels referred to as level I to IV, and although sampling of all levels is not essential, it is to be recommended if all tissue types present in the nose are to be examined adequately (see Figures 11.1a to 11.1c).

It should also be borne in mind that any immunocytochemical technique used to study the distribution of the drug metabolizing enzymes, such as cytochrome P-450s and GSTs, may require special fixation and processing schedules other than those used for routine histology if the antigenicity of the respective proteins is to be maintained [36].

11.6 Conclusions

Lung-specific toxicity is a complex issue incorporating both inhalation and systemically derived toxins. Unlike the situation pertaining in most other internal organs, both direct and indirect toxins can exert their toxicity on the lung, the former via inspired air while the latter can be presented to the lung either in inspired air or via the systemic circulation. Testing for pulmonary toxicity is also complex, with inhalation exposures varying from the extreme of complexity using whole body inhalation chambers to the more simplified head or nose only systems. The histological make-up of the upper respiratory tract, in particular, is exquisitely dependent on the position at which the histological section is taken, and significant differences can be apparent between the anterior and posterior chambers of the nasal cavity alone. The presence or absence of activating and detoxifying enzyme systems are important determinants as to whether or not toxins exert their effects in a specific or a non-specific way, and significant differences in enzyme localization exist between the various cell types of the upper and lower respiratory tract. Of particular importance in the study of pulmonary toxicity, as it is in the study of mammalian toxicity in general, is a realization of the pivotal importance that target organ dosage and species differences can exert in the determination of whether or not a chemical which is dramatically toxic in one animal species proves to be so in man. Only by a thorough knowledge of the biochemical, pharmacological and histopathological processes involved in the toxic reaction can any meaningful extrapolation be made of the risk to man of contact with the toxin.

References

1. SMITH, L.L. and NEMERY, B. (1986) The lung as a target organ for toxicity, in COHEN, G.M. (Ed.) *Target Organ Toxicity*, Vol. II, pp. 45–80, Florida: CRC Press.

2. COHEN, G.M. (1990) Pulmonary metabolism of foreign compounds: role of metabolic activation, *Environmental Health Perspectives*, **85**, 31–41.

3. GREEN, T. and HATHAWAY, D.E. (1975) The biological fate in rats of vinyl chloride in relation to its oncogenicity, *Chemico-Biological Interactions*, **11**, 545–562.

4. DAHL, A.R. (1989) Metabolic characteristics of the respiratory tract, in MCCLELLAN, R.C. and HENDERSON, R.F. (Eds) *Concepts in Inhalation Toxicology*, pp. 141–160, New York: Hemisphere Publishing Corporation.

5. VAINO, H. and HIETANEN, E. (1980) Role of extrahepatic metabolism in drug disposition and toxicity, in JENNER, P. and TESTA, B. (Eds) *Concepts in Drug Metabolism*, pp. 251–284, New York: Marcel Dekker.

6. BARON, J., BURKE, J.P., GUENGERICH, F.P., JAKOBY, W.B. and VOIGT, J.M. (1988) Sites of xenobiotic activation and detoxification within the respiratory tract: implications for chemically induced toxicity, *Toxicology and Applied Pharmacology*, **93**, 493–505.

7. KATO, S., SHIELDS, P.G., CAPORASO, N.E., HOOVER, R.N., TRUMP, B.F., SUGIMURA, H., WESTON, A. and HARRIS, C.C. (1992) Cytochrome P-450 IIE1 genetic polymorphisms, racial variation and lung cancer risk, *Cancer Research*, **52**, 6712–6715.

8. KETTERER, B., HARRIS, J.M., TALASKA, G., MEYER, D.J., PEMBLE, S.E., TAYLOR, J.B., LANG, N.P. and KADLUBAR, F.F. (1992) The human glutathione S-transferase supergene family, its polymorphism, and its effects on susceptibility to lung cancer, *Environmental Health Perspectives*, **98**, 87–94.

9. WITSCHI, H.P. and HAKKINEN, P.J. (1984) The role of toxicological interactions in lung injury, *Environmental Health Perspectives*, **55**, 139–148.

10. ODUM, J., FOSTER, J.R. and GREEN, T. (1992) A mechanism for the development of Clara cell lesions in the mouse lung after exposure to trichloroethylene, *Chemico-Biological Interactions*, **83**, 135–153.

11. FOSTER, J.R., GREEN, T., SMITH, L.L., LEWIS, R.W., HEXT, P.M. and WYATT, I. (1990) Methylene chloride: an inhalation study to investigate pathological and biochemical events occurring in the lungs of mice over an exposure period of 90 days, *Fundamental and Applied Toxicology*, **18**, 376–388.

12. CRAPO, J.D., MARSH-SALIN, J., INGRAM, P. and PRATT, P.L. (1978) Tolerance and cross-tolerance using NO_2 and O_2 II. Pulmonary morphology and morphometry, *Journal of Applied Physiological Respiration and Environmental Exercise Physiology*, **44**, 370–379.

13. O'BRIEN, K.A.F., SUVERKROPP, C., KANEKAL, S., PLOPPER, C.G. and BUCKPIT, A.R. (1989) Tolerance to multiple doses of the pulmonary toxicant, naphthalene, *Toxicology and Applied Pharmacology*, **99**, 487–500.

14. MUSTAFA, M. and TIERNEY, D.F. (1978) Biochemical and metabolic changes in the lung with oxygen, ozone and nitrogen dioxide toxicity, *American Review of Respiratory Diseases*, **118**, 1061–1090.

15. GASKELL, B.G. (1990) Non-neoplastic changes in the olfactory epithelium—experimental studies, *Environmental Health Perspectives*, **85**, 275–289.

16. HURTT, M.E., THOMAS, D.A., WORKING, P.K., MONTICELLO, T.M. and MORGAN, K.T. (1988) Degeneration and regeneration of the olfactory epithelium following inhalation exposure to methyl bromide: pathology, cell kinetics and olfactory function, *Toxicology and Applied Pharmacology*, **94**, 311–328.

17. BURGER, G.T., RENNE, R.A., SAGARTZ, J.W., AYRES, P.H., COGGINS, C.R, MOSBERG, A.T. and HAYES, A.W. (1989) Histologic changes in the respiratory tract induced by inhalation of xenobiotics: physiologic adaptation or toxicity? *Toxicology and Applied Pharmacology*, **101**, 521–542.

18. BOGDANFFY, M.S. (1990) Biotransformation enzymes in the rodent nasal mucosa: the value of a histochemical approach, *Environmental Health Perspectives*, **85**, 177–186.
19. AMES, B.N. and GOLD, L.S. (1990) Too many rodent carcinogens: mitogenesis increases mutagenesis, *Science*, **249**, 970–971.
20. BROWN, H.R. (1990) Neoplastic and potentially preneoplastic changes in the upper respiratory tract of rats and mice, *Environmental Health Perspectives*, **85**, 291–304.
21. EVANS, M.J. (1984) Oxidant gases, *Environmental Health Perspectives*, **55**, 85–95.
22. BOYD, M.R. (1980) Biochemical mechanisms of chemically-induced lung injury: role of metabolic activation, *CRC Critical Reviews in Toxicology*, **7**, 103–176.
23. HECHT, S.S. and HOFFMAN, D. (1988) Tobacco-specific nitrosamines, an important group of carcinogens in tobacco and tobacco smoke, *Carcinogenesis*, **9**, 875–884.
24. FOSTER, J.R., SMITH, L.L., HEXT, P.M., BRAMMER, A., SOAMES, A.R. and WYATT, I. (1990) Target cell toxicity of inhaled spermidine in rat lungs, *International Journal of Experimental Pathology*, **71**, 617–630.
25. WITSCHI, H.P. (1990) Responses of the lung to toxic injury, *Environmental Health Perspectives*, **85**, 5–14.
26. SCHULLER, H.M., BECKER, K.L. and WITSCHI, H.P. (1988) An animal model for neuroendocrine lung cancer, *Carcinogenesis*, **9**, 293–296.
27. KLINTENBERG, C., OLOFSON, J., HELLQUIST, H. and SOKJER, H. (1984) Adenocarcinoma of the ethmoid sinuses: a review of 28 cases with reference to wood dust exposure, *Cancer*, **54**, 482–488.
28. HUEPER, W.C. (1966) Occupational and environmental cancers of the respiratory system, *Recent Results in Cancer Research*, **3**, 59–85.
29. HUFF, J., CIRVALLO, J., HASEMAN, J. and BUCHER, J. (1991) Chemicals associated with site-specific neoplasia in 1394 long-term carcinogenesis experiments in laboratory rodents, *Environmental Health Perspectives*, **93**, 247–270.
30. DORATO, M.A. (1990) Overview of inhalation toxicology, *Environmental Health Perspectives*, **85**, 163–170.
31. NIEMEIER, R.W. (1984) The isolated perfused lung, *Environmental Health Perspectives*, **56**, 35–42.
32. SMITH, L.L. and WYATT, I. (1981) The accumulation of putrescine into slices of rat lung and brain and its relationship to the accumulation of paraquat, *Biochemical Pharmacology*, **30**, 1053–1058.
33. DEVEREUX, T.R. (1984) Alveolar type II and Clara cells: isolation and xenobiotic metabolism, *Environmental Health Perspectives*, **56**, 95–102.
34. OREFFO, V.I.C., MORGAN, A. and RICHARDS, R.J. (1990) Isolation of Clara cells from the mouse lung, *Environmental Health Perspectives*, **85**, 51–64.
35. URIAH, L.C. and MARONPOT, R.R. (1990) Normal histology of the nasal cavity and application of special techniques, *Environmental Health Perspectives*, **85**, 187–208.
36. BOGDANFFY, M.S., RANDALL, H.W. and MORGAN, K.T. (1986) Histochemical localisation of aldehyde dehydrogenase in the respiratory tract of the Fischer-344 rat, *Toxicology and Applied Pharmacology*, **82**, 560–567.
37. MONTICELLO, T.M., MORGAN, K.T. and URIAH, L. (1990) Non-neoplastic nasal lesions in rats and mice, *Environmental Health Perspectives*, **85**, 249–274.

Additional Reading

BRODY, A.R. and DAVIS, G.S. (1982) Alveolar macrophage toxicology, *Mechanisms of Respiratory Toxicology*, **2**, 3–28.
FINKELSTEIN, J.N. (1990) Physiologic and toxicologic responses of alveolar type II cells, *Toxicology*, **60**, 41–52.
GARDNER, D.E., CRAPO, J.D. and MASSARO, E.J. (1988) *Toxicology of the Lung*, New York: Raven Press.

HOOK, G.E.R. (1984) Monograph on pulmonary toxicology, *Environmental Health Perspectives*, **55**, 1–416.

RICHARDS, R. (1990) Chemicals and lung toxicity – to study the agent or the disease? *Environmental Health Perspectives*, **85**, 3–151.

URIAH, L.C., MORGAN, K.T. and MARONPOT, R.R. (1990) Toxicologic pathology of the upper respiratory system, *Environmental Health Perspectives*, **85**, 161–352.

12

The Male Reproductive System

DIANNE M. CREASY

12.1 Introduction

There is increasing concern about the potential effects of environmental chemicals on the male reproductive system of man. Over the last 50 years the mean human sperm count has declined by more than 40 per cent, while the incidence of congenital reproductive tract deformities and testicular cancer has risen by up to fourfold [1]. While many chemicals have been shown to be male reproductive toxicants in laboratory animals, relatively few have been confirmed to be a problem in man [2]. The reasons for this are very likely to reside in the inherent problems of carrying out meaningful epidemiological studies in this delicate area of occupational health research. Apart from the fact that semen samples are not readily donated, there are few reliable parameters which can be used to quantify fertility. However, one of the best documented human testicular toxicants, **dibromochloropropane (DBCP)** which produced infertility in industrial workers exposed to this nematocide, also produces similar effects in rats, mice, rabbits and dogs at equivalent levels of exposure.

Successful functioning of the male reproductive system involves the complex, dynamic process of sperm production (spermatogenesis) carried out in the testis, the maturation and storage of sperm in the epididymis, the production and secretion of the nutrient-rich seminal fluid by the prostate and seminal vesicles and the effective delivery of these products into the female reproductive tract. Toxicants may directly damage the cellular processes involved in these functions or interfere with their hormonal or neural control mechanisms. In order to understand how these processes may be disturbed and how effects on one process affect another, it is essential to have a basic understanding of the normal structure and physiology of the male reproductive system.

Research in mammalian testicular physiology and toxicology has largely concentrated on the rat as a research model, thus providing a detailed picture of sperm production and regulation in this species. Since the process is essentially similar in most mammalian species, including man, most of the information in this chapter refers to the rat, but major species differences are pointed out where appropriate.

12.2   Anatomy, Histology and Physiology

12.2.1   *Introduction*

In most mammals the testes are situated in a scrotal sac outside the abdominal cavity to maintain the sperm-producing tissue a few degrees (2 to 7°C) lower than normal body temperature. Temperature regulation is critical for normal sperm development and is controlled partly by heat loss through the scrotal vasculature and also by a counter-current cooling mechanism for the incoming blood. The testis is made up of seminiferous tubules surrounded by interstitial tissue that is composed of a loose connective tissue containing the testosterone-producing Leydig cells, macrophages, lymph and blood vessels. The seminiferous tubules are lined by a stratified epithelium (seminiferous, germinal or tubular epithelium) which is made up of germ cells at various stages of development and Sertoli cells which provide structural and nutritional support for them. A fibrous capsule, the tunica albuginea, encloses these structures within the highly vascularized scrotal sac.

Figure 12.1 shows the overall relationship of the testes, excurrent duct system and the secondary sex organs. In the rat, 20 to 30 highly coiled seminiferous tubules open

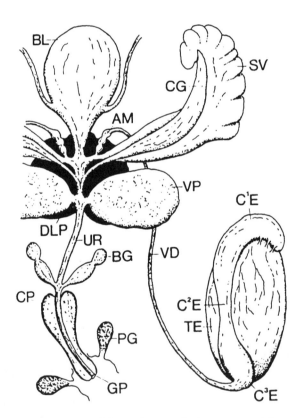

Figure 12.1   General organization of the male reproductive system of the rat. BL, bladder; SV, seminal vesicle; CG, coagulating gland; AM, ampulla; VP, ventral prostate gland; DLP, dorsolateral prostate gland; UR, penile urethra; BG, bulbourethral gland; VD, vas deferens; CP, corpus penis; GP, glans penis; PG, preputial gland; TE, testis; $C^1/C^2/C^3E$, caput/corpus/cauda epididymis.

into a small subcapsular sac-like space termed the rete testis. Sperm leave the testis via the efferent ducts which join to form the single coiled duct of the epididymis. The dumbell-shaped epididymis comprises the head (caput), the tail (cauda) and the narrow body (corpus) which joins the two. Although similar in cellular morphology, there are differences in function between the different portions of the epididymis. The vas deferens carries sperm from the epididymis to the seminal vesicle where it joins with the seminal vesicle duct to form the ejaculatory duct. This passes through the prostate and empties into the urethra. During ejaculation, the prostate, seminal vesicles and coagulating gland add their secretions to the sperm as it is propelled along this duct system. A final secretion from the bulbourethral gland is added into the penile urethra.

A pair of preputial glands lying between the skin and abdominal wall adjacent to the penis are also present in rodents. These secrete pheromonal substances directly onto the skin.

For a more comprehensive and detailed account of the normal structure and physiology of the male reproductive tissues the reader is referred to [3,4,5,6,7].

12.2.2 Cellular Components and Function

Testis

There are two morphologically and functionally distinct compartments in the testis, the tubular and the interstitial compartments (Figure 12.2). Spermatogenesis (gametogenesis) takes place within the tubules. This is a complex cellular process which requires a specialized microenvironment for its completion and also necessitates immunological isolation of its product, the antigenically 'foreign' haploid sperm. Both requirements are satisfied by the specialized features of the Sertoli cell which plays a key role in the seminiferous epithelium.

Sertoli cell Sertoli cells are somatic cells which enclose the germ cells in cytoplasmic sheets. They have a wide base which sits on the basal membrane of the tubule and cytoplasmic extensions which stretch to the luminal surface, enveloping germ cells in an amoeboid manner (Figure 12.2). The plasticity of the Sertoli cell membrane and its cell to cell junctions allows controlled movement of the germ cells through the depth of the tubular epithelium, thus providing a structural framework for the orderly process of spermatogenesis.

In addition to this structural role, the Sertoli cell produces metabolic substrates for the germ cells, secretes a variety of proteins and peptides involved in the regulation of spermatogenesis and also secretes the seminiferous tubular fluid required to maintain a patent lumen and to transport the newly formed sperm into the epididymis.

One other major function and feature of the Sertoli cell is to contribute to the permeability barrier between the interstitial compartment and the tubular compartment (blood–tubule barrier). This is accomplished largely by the presence of tight occluding junctions between adjacent Sertoli cells at a level above the spermatogonia, preventing intercellular access or egress of cells, fluids or substances (endogenous or xenobiotics) (Figure 12.2). Since there are no blood vessels or capillaries within the tubules, this means all nutrients, oxygen and any other endogenous or exogenous substances must enter through the Sertoli cell. This not only protects the sensitive meiotic germ cells from potentially harmful mutagenic

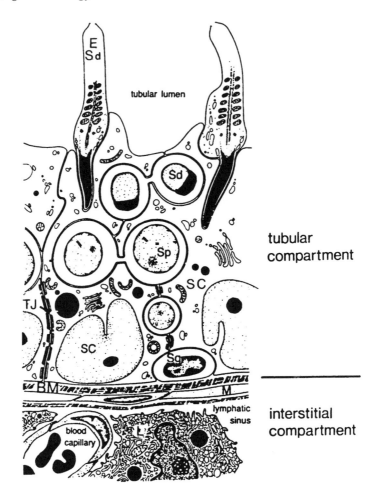

Figure 12.2   Arrangement of cells within the seminiferous tubule and in the interstitial tissue of the testis. The germ cells: spermatogonia (Sg), spermatocytes (Sp), round spermatids (Sd) and elongating spermatids (ESd) are arranged in layers and enveloped by the cytoplasm of the Sertoli cell (SC). Tight junctions (TJ) join adjacent Sertoli cells at a level above the spermatogonia. A basal membrane (BM) and peritubular myoid cells (M) separate the epithelium from the interstitial tissue comprising Leydig cells (L), blood vessels and lymphatics. Reproduced from Foster, 1988, *Physiology and Toxicology of Male Reproduction*, Lamb, J.C. and Foster, P.M.D. (Eds), Academic Press, with permission.

substances, but also prevents recognition of the novel surface antigens which develop as the cells progress through meiosis, by the host's immunological system.

Germ cells   Unlike the female where the main parts of gametogenesis, including meiotic division, occur during fetal development, spermatogenesis in the male is a continuous process throughout adult life (see Spermatogenesis, Section 12.2.3). The process is illustrated in Figure 12.3; essentially there are three different germ cell types: spermatogonia, spermatocytes and spermatids. Primitive stem cell spermatogonia undergo numerous mitotic divisions to form committed spermatogonia and the final mitotic division produces spermatocytes. These cells undergo the lengthy

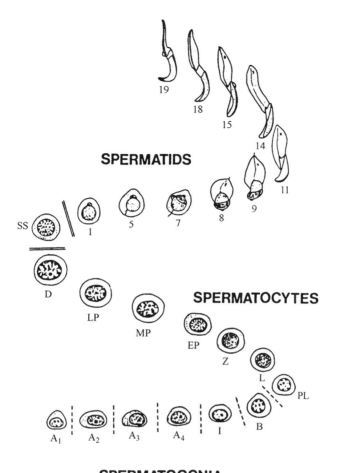

SPERMATIDS

SPERMATOCYTES

SPERMATOGONIA

Figure 12.3 Spermatogenesis in the rat. The stem cell spermatogonia undergo a number of mitotic divisions (----) to produce type A (A_1 to A_4), intermediate (I) and type B (B) spermatogonia. The final mitotic division produces spermatocytes which undergo the lengthy process of meiosis, including the stages of preleptotene (PL), leptotene (L), zygotene (Z), early, mid- and late pachytene (EP, MP, LP) and diplotene (D). The first meiotic reduction division (=) produces secondary spermatocytes (SS) and the second meiotic division (=) produces the haploid spermatids. The complex differentiation of the spermatid can be separated into 19 different steps (1 to19). Reproduced from Creasy and Foster, 1991, *Handbook of Toxicologic Pathology*, Haschek, W.A. and Rousseaux, C.G. (Eds), Academic Press, with permission.

process of meiosis, passing through preleptotene, where DNA replication produces tetraploid cells, followed by leptotene, zygotene, early, mid- and late pachytene, during which the chromosomes pair-up and become thicker. During diplotene and diakinesis the nucleus reaches its maximum size and the chromosomes become dispersed. The first meiotic division produces diploid secondary spermatocytes and the second meiotic division produces the haploid spermatids. The spermatids, without further division, undergo complex cellular remodelling to produce highly specialized spermatozoa (sperm) which are released into the tubular lumen. This remodelling process is called spermiogenesis and it can be separated into 19 different *steps* (1 to 19) on the basis of detailed morphological criteria [8, 9]. The remodelling begins with the development of the acrosome, a glycoprotein cap which forms around part of the nucleus and which is important for penetration of the ovum at fertilization. The nucleus becomes elongated and condensed and, with its acrosomal covering, becomes the head of the sperm. The volume of cytoplasm becomes greatly reduced and is rearranged to form the mid-piece and the tail of the sperm. A central flagellum which provides the motile force of the sperm, runs from the head through the mid-piece and tail, while tightly packed mitochondria in the mid-piece surround the flagellum and provide the necessary energy for motility.

The progeny from a single spermatogonial division remain in contact with one another via cytoplasmic bridges (Figure 12.2). This clone of cells represents a syncytium allowing rapid intercellular communication. This may play a role in maintaining synchrony during cellular development.

Peritubular myoid cells The main function of these cells is to provide a limiting layer around the seminiferous epithelium (Figure 12.2). The myoid properties of the cells allow for pulsatile contraction which is thought to be important in moving the sperm along the tubules to the rete testis. As a semipermeable cell layer, myoid cells also contribute to the blood–tubule barrier. However, poorly understood interactions between Sertoli cells and peritubular cells suggest other, as yet unknown, roles for these cells.

Leydig cells These are also known as interstitial cells and their prime function is the production of testosterone. They appear as clusters of plump cells with eosinophilic cytoplasm, positioned around the interstitial blood vessels (Figure 12.2). Their central role in endocrine control of reproduction and paracrine control of spermatogenesis is discussed below.

Efferent ducts, epididymis and vas deferens

The duct system of the reproductive tract is more than just a transport route from the testis to the penis, since it also acts as a storage reservoir and is critical in the maturation of the sperm (Table 12.1). When sperm are shed into the seminiferous tubule they show no progressive forward motility and are incapable of fertilizing an ovum. These properties are gained during passage through the head and body region of the epididymis, the mechanism of which is still poorly understood but involves alteration of sperm surface components, and minor changes in morphology and metabolism. Passage through the epididymis takes days or weeks depending on the species (5.5 days in man, 8.1 days in the rat, 14.1 days in the hamster) [10]. The sperm are stored in the tail of the epididymis, which explains the large diameter of the duct in this region. In immature animals or when sperm production is reduced, the diameter of the ducts of the cauda epididymis and the height of the epithelial lining changes to more-nearly resemble the head region of the epididymis.

Fluid reabsorption is another important function of the duct system. Tubular fluid is continuously produced by the Sertoli cells and almost totally reabsorbed by the caput epididymis. Secretion of a variety of substances including ions, glycoproteins, and small organic molecules such as carnitine, inositol and glycerophosphorylcholine occurs throughout the excurrent duct system.

Table 12.1 Components of the male reproductive tract of the rodent

Structure	Major functions
Testis	Production of spermatozoa from stem cells Testosterone production from Leydig cells
Efferent ducts	Transport of sperm from testis to epididymis
Epididymis	Modification of sperm enabling fertilization Storage of sperm prior to ejaculation Resorption of seminiferous tubule fluid Secretory function
Vas deferens/ ejaculatory duct	Transport of sperm from epididymis to urethra Secretory function
Prostate	Production of 15 to 30 per cent of seminal fluid Production of nutrient-rich, proteolytic fluid Aids in copulatory plug formation
Seminal vesicle	Production of 50 to 80 per cent of seminal fluid Production of nutrient-rich, alkaline fluid which neutralizes acidic vaginal fluid Aids in copulatory plug formation
Coagulation gland	Production of vesiculase for copulatory plug
Bulbourethral gland	Aids in copulatory plug formation
Preputial gland	Pheromone production

The vas deferens has a thick muscular wall for contraction and the epithelium is thrown into deep folds. Its main function is in the propulsion of sperm from the epididymis during ejaculation, but it also has secretory functions.

Secondary sex organs

An ejaculate is composed of sperm and seminal plasma, which is formed primarily by the secretions of the secondary sex organs and the excurrent duct system (Table 12.1). The composition of seminal plasma varies greatly between species, for example, fructose is produced as the major substrate for sperm glycolysis in most species but it is absent in the semen of others (dog and stallion). In some species, some of the secondary sex organs are absent, the dog for example having no seminal vesicles. In some species, removal of the seminal vesicle has no effect on fertility (boar and bull), in others it reduces fertility (rat), or may even cause sterility (hamster). Similarly, the importance of the prostate for fertility is unclear.

Coagulation of semen also varies markedly between species. In man, semen coagulates within 5 min of ejaculation and subsequently liquefies spontaneously. The semen of the bull and dog does not coagulate at all, whereas the semen of the rat and the guinea pig is composed of a fluid phase which contains the sperm followed by a solid phase which forms the copulatory plug. In man, the clotting factors are secreted by the seminal vesicles, while in the boar, a sialomucin from the bulbourethral gland interacts with seminal vesicle fluids to bring about coagulation.

In the rat, the coagulation enzyme, vesiculase, produced by the coagulating gland, converts procoagulase, secreted by the seminal vesicles, into coagulase. A factor secreted by the bulbourethral gland is also required. The overall significance of coagulation and liquefaction remains unclear.

For detailed information on the composition of the various secretions and on species differences, the reader is referred to [4].

Prostate   The anatomical arrangement of the prostate varies greatly with species. In rodents, it consists of a ventral portion and a dorsolateral portion which together encircle the urethra (Figure 12.1). Each portion secretes different proteins and responds differently to various prostatic toxicants.

The spherical glands of the prostate have a low cuboidal or columnar epithelium (depending on secretory activity) and are filled with a pale eosinophilic, sometimes flocculent secretory material. The prostatic secretion contributes 15 to 30 per cent of the volume of the ejaculate. It is rich in inositol, acid phosphatase, proteolytic enzymes, citric acid, zinc and polyamines, particularly spermine and spermidine. In man, proteolytic enzymes such as seminin and plasminogen activators, which are responsible for semen liquefaction, are also secreted.

Coagulating gland (anterior prostate)   This gland is derived from the prostate and lies adjacent to the seminal vesicles (Figure 12.1). It has a folded columnar epithelium and a secretory product similar in staining characteristics to the prostate. It secretes fructose and glucose in the rat and produces vesiculase, an enzyme which is required for copulatory plug formation in the rodent.

Seminal vesicles   These are paired, sac-like organs with an epithelium thrown into fronds projecting into the secretory lumen. The secretion is deeply eosinophilic and contributes 50 to 80 per cent of the ejaculate volume. In most species it is rich in prostaglandins, glucose, fructose (except in rodents where the coagulating glands secrete fructose), inositol, glycerophosphorylcholine, proteins and a large number of other components of which the physiological role is unknown. In the rodent, secretions of the seminal vesicles are important in copulatory plug formation.

Bulbourethral gland (Cowper's gland)   These small paired organs secrete a viscous sialomucin which is responsible for semen coagulation in boars, and clotting factors required for copulatory plug formation in rodents. In other species, the function of the secretion, which constitutes about 5 per cent of the ejaculate, is poorly understood but it may serve a lubricant function.

Preputial glands   These are modified sebaceous glands which produce a fatty secretion (possibly seven- and eight-carbon alcohols) and are associated with pheromone production in the rodent.

12.2.3   *Physiological Considerations*

Spermatogenesis

The cellular progression of spermatogonia into sperm takes about 56 days in the rat and 74 days in the human (timing is strain and species dependent) and comprises well-defined morphological changes combined with mitotic and meiotic cell divisions at predetermined time points [8, 9] (Figure 12.3).

Evaluation of the process within a tubular cross-section is complex because four generations of cells are progressing through spermatogenesis at any one time, and each generation of cells is continually changing its appearance with time (Figure 12.4). Each generation of cells, represented in the diagram as spermatogonia, spermatocytes, round spermatids and elongating spermatids, develop at a predetermined rate and in synchrony with one another, thus producing 'cell associations'. Fourteen different cell associations or *stages* have been defined for the rat (four of which are illustrated in Figure 12.4) and together, they comprise the *cycle of the seminiferous epithelium*. As the cells develop, they move up through the epithelium, being replaced by the next generation of basal stem cell spermatogonia and being shed as they reach maturity (stage VIII). Meiotic division of spermatocytes (stage XIV) produces a new population of spermatids, returning the tubule into the cell association which defines it as stage I. The entire epithelium of one tubule does not go through this process simultaneously; rather, a *wave* of spermatogenesis proceeds along the length of the tubule. Thus, the *cycle* of spermatogenesis is chronological, while the *wave* of spermatogenesis is linear.

The number of different cellular associations or stages that are recognizable, depends on the criteria used to identify morphological changes in the cell populations. In the case of the rat, the Leblond and Clermont classification [9], which is the most widely accepted, uses the detailed nuclear, acrosomic and cytoplasmic changes of the spermatid to identify 14 different stages which are numbered I to XIV. Nineteen different steps in the development of the spermatid (spermiogenesis) have been characterized and these are denoted by arabic numerals 1 to 19 (Figure 12.3). So, the *cycle* of the seminiferous epithelium is made up of *stages* of spermatogenesis which are identified by *steps* of spermiogenesis.

In the Sprague–Dawley rat, one cycle takes 12.9 days to complete and the time taken for a spermatogonium to complete development through to sperm release is 4 to 4.5 cycles, i.e. 52 to 56 days (the precise time depends on which spermatogonial mitotic division is used as the start point). The duration of the stages varies greatly, some being short (7 h for stage III) and some long (65 h for stage VII). The longer the duration of the stage, the more frequently it will be seen in histological tubular cross-sections, i.e. stage frequency is proportional to stage duration. Since the frequency of the different stages in a cross-section of testis is relatively constant for a given strain and species, alterations in stage frequency can be used to detect alterations in the kinetics of spermatogenesis [11].

Evaluation of testicular histology, therefore, requires an adequate knowledge of the various cellular associations to be expected in tubular cross-sections and an appreciation of the kinetics of spermatogenesis. For a practical and more detailed account of this complex subject see [8].

Spermatogenesis in the rat is essentially similar to other laboratory animal species and to man. However, the numbers of stages recognized and their timing differs significantly. In man, cross-sections of tubules contain more than one cellular association, making evaluation more difficult.

Endocrine and paracrine regulation

Overall control of testicular function occurs in the hypothalamus, which controls the release of pituitary hormones which then act on receptors in the Sertoli and Leydig

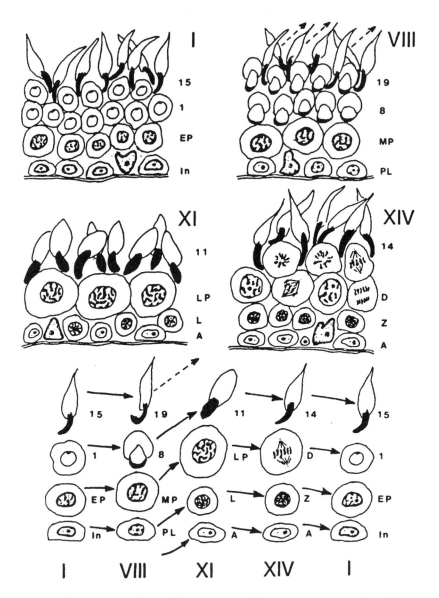

Figure 12.4 Cell associations for 4 of the 14 stages of the spermatogenic cycle of the rat (stages I, VIII, XI, XIV). Spermatogonia: A, type A; In, intermediate. Spermatocytes: PL, preleptotene; L, leptotene; Z, zygotene; EP, early pachytene; MP, mid-pachytene; LP, late pachytene; D, dividing spermatocyte. Spermatids: 1, 8, 11, 14, 15 and 19 – steps 1 to 19 of spermatid development. The tubular cross-sections (stages I, VIII, XI, XIV) show the arrangement of the cells within the seminiferous epithelium. The columns of cells at the base of the figure show the maturation of the cells during one spermatogenic cycle. Each generation of cells develops sequentially. During stage VIII the mature sperm are shed into the lumen (⌁) while a new generation develops from stem cell spermatogonia. As spermatocytes undergo meiotic division in stage XIV (D), they produce step 1 spermatids and the cell association returns to stage I to begin another cycle.

cells. Local (paracrine) regulation between cells in the testis provides a more sensitive co-ordination of cellular interactions and allows a rapid, fine-tuning of cellular function to changing requirements (Figure 12.5).

Follicle stimulating hormone (FSH)   FSH acts on the Sertoli cell, although in the adult surprisingly little is known about the effects of this hormone. In the immature testis, FSH initiates spermatogenesis and stimulates the production of tubular fluid, androgen binding protein (ABP, which binds and transports testosterone) and inhibin by the Sertoli cell. In the adult testis, most of these functions appear to be more responsive to testosterone than to FSH. Although the precise role of FSH in the adult testis is unclear, recent studies indicate a close interrelationship between FSH, testosterone and the Sertoli cell.

Luteinizing hormone (LH)   LH acts on the Leydig cell to stimulate testosterone production. The resulting testosterone has a local effect on the adjacent Sertoli cells and wide-reaching peripheral effects, not only on the secondary sex organs, but also on other androgen-responsive tissues such as muscle, bone, and skin. However, the levels of testosterone required within the testis to maintain spermatogenesis are much higher than normal circulating levels.

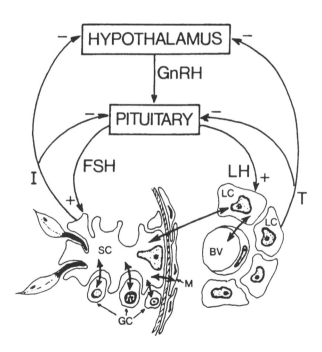

Figure 12.5   Endocrine and paracrine regulation of spermatogenesis. Gonadotrophin releasing hormone (GnRH) from the hypothalamus controls secretion of follicle stimulating hormone (FSH) and luteinizing hormone (LH) from the pituitary. FSH acts largely on the Sertoli cell (SC) with a negative feedback loop through inhibin (I). LH acts on the Leydig cell (LC) with testosterone (T) as the feedback inhibitor. Locally secreted peptides mediate regulatory pathways between Leydig and Sertoli cells, Leydig cells and endothelium of blood vessels (BV), Sertoli and germ cells (GC) and between Sertoli and peritubular myoid cells (M).

Paracrine regulation The cellular processes involved in spermatogenesis are complex and highly synchronized. Mitosis, meiosis, spermiogenesis, movement of cells through the epithelium, the release of sperm into the lumen and expulsion of tubular contents into the epididymis, are just a few of the processes which involve delicate regulation and co-ordination. Substances secreted by the Leydig cell, such as testosterone and opiates (e.g. β-endorphin), act on the Sertoli cell to cause secretion of a variety of products. Oxytocin is also secreted by the Leydig cell and acts on the peritubular cells to bring about contraction. A variety of potentially vasoactive substances are secreted by Leydig cells and interstitial macrophages and these may play a role in local vascular control. Regulatory substances secreted by the Sertoli cells include a mitogen which is thought to regulate spermatogonial mitosis, a meiosis-inducing and meiosis-inhibitory factor, plasminogen activator (which may be involved in movement of preleptotene spermatocytes through the Sertoli cell tight junctions) and many other peptides and substances. The precise roles of these paracrine hormones are still unknown, but most appear to be secreted at specific stages in the spermatogenic cycle to synchronize the different events which occur during the cycle [12]. The presence (or absence) of different germ cell types appears to be the controlling factor for this stage specificity. Thus, it is the germ cells which stimulate the Sertoli cells to produce their myriad of controlling factors. Loss or damage to germ cells, therefore, modifies the response of the Sertoli cell.

12.3 Biochemical and Cellular Mechanisms of Toxicity

12.3.1 *Introduction*

Although a large number of diverse agents are known to affect the male reproductive system (Table 12.2), the target site of toxicity is known for only a small proportion (Table 12.3), and the biochemical mechanism of toxicity is understood for even fewer. For general reviews covering male reproductive toxicants and their mechanisms of action see [5, 6, 7].

A major distinction can be made between agents which directly interfere with the cells involved in spermatogenesis, e.g. affect the sperm, germ cells or the Sertoli cells, and those which indirectly affect spermatogenesis or accessory sex organs through disturbance of endocrine or paracrine pathways. In addition, some agents injure or modify the function of the epididymis while others interfere with the complex neural control of ejaculation.

12.3.2 *Agents Causing Direct Damage to Sperm or Spermatogenesis*

Due to the interdependence of cells within the testis, pinpointing the initial site or sites of action of a chemical is difficult. Functional damage to Sertoli cells will rapidly affect the germ cell population which rely on the Sertoli cell for many metabolic and structural requirements. Conversely, the function and morphological appearance of the Sertoli cell is modified by its surrounding germ cell complement; if this is damaged or depleted, the Sertoli cell will respond. The same holds for the Leydig cell.

At the molecular level, mechanisms of cellular injury involve damage to macromolecules necessary for normal cell physiology, namely DNA, RNA, enzymatic proteins or structural proteins and membranes. As with any other tissue,

Table 12.2 Examples of agents reported to affect male reproduction

Therapeutic agents
Analgesics and antipyretics: phenacetin
Anticonvulsants: diphenylhydantoin
Antineoplastic drugs: antibiotics, alkylating agents, antimetabolites, vinca alkaloids
Antiadrenergic drugs: α- and β-blockers
Antinfective drugs: sulphasalazine, hexachlorophene
Antiparasitic drugs: chloroquine, niridazole
Diuretics: spironolactone, thiazides
Histamine and histamine antagonists: cimetidine
Hypoglycaemic drugs: chlorpropamide
Xanthines: caffeine, theobromine
Steroids: natural and synthetic androgens, oestrogens, progestins

Drugs affecting the central nervous system
Alcohol
Anaesthetics: halothane, nitrous oxide
Narcotic and non-narcotic analgesics: opiates
Neuroleptics: phenothiazine, amitryptaline
Tranquillizers: reserpine, monoamine oxidase inhibitors

Metals and trace elements
Cadmium, aluminium, boron, lead, mercury, nickel

Insecticides
Carbamates: carbaryl
Indane derivatives: aldrin, dieldrin, chlordane
Cholinesterase inhibitors: dichlorvos

Herbicides, fungicides and sterilants
2,4-dichlorophenoxyacetic acid (2,4-D), diquat, paraquat, dibromochloropropane, carbon
disulphide, ethylene dibromide, ethylene oxide, triphenyltin

Food additives and contaminants
Aflatoxin, cyclamate, monosodium glutamate, metanil yellow

Industrial chemicals
Polychlorinated hydrocarbons
Polycyclic aromatic hydrocarbons
Solvents: glycol ethers, benzene, hexane, toluene, carbon disulphide
Plasticizers: phthalate esters
Flame retardents: tris-(2,3-dibromopropyl) phosphate (TRIS)

Compiled from Klaassen, C.D., Amdur, M.O., Doull, J. (Eds), 1986, *Casaret and Doull's
Toxicology*, Third Edition, New York: Macmillan.

there are important factors which will determine or modify the toxic effect of the
chemical to the reproductive tract, including species and age of the animal and the
absorption, distribution, metabolism and excretion of the chemical.

Injury to DNA and RNA

This can result in the death of the cell when it attempts division (cytotoxic damage)
or in a heritable defect in the DNA which may have consequences if fertilization

Table 12.3   Examples of cell/site specific male reproductive toxicants

Target cell	Toxicant
Leydig cells	Acetaldehyde, ethanedimethane sulphonate
Sertoli cells	Phthalate esters, 2,5-hexanedione, dinitrobenzene
Spermatogonia	Busulphan, bleomycin
Spermatocytes	Glycol ethers, dinitropyrroles
Spermatids	Ethylmethane sulphonate, methyl chloride
Epididymal sperm	6-chlorodeoxyglucose, α-chlorhydrin
Epididymis	Methyl chloride

occurs (genotoxic damage). While damage to DNA frequently results in the death of the cell, a moderate amount of RNA injury may be reversible.

Cytotoxic damage   The large number of actively proliferating cells in the testis make it particularly sensitive to agents which damage DNA or interfere with its synthesis. Many cancer chemotherapeutic agents rely on damaging DNA for their activity and, therefore, invariably have some effect on spermatogenesis [13]. Within this group of chemicals are the alkylating agents such as **cyclophosphamide**, **cis-platinum**, **chlorambucil** and the intercalating antibiotics such as **actinomycin D**, **daunorubicin** and **adriamycin**. These agents covalently bind to the DNA strands preventing DNA replication and may also interfere with RNA synthesis. DNA repair enzymes may be able to repair this damage before division occurs, but the faster the cell cycle, the less time is available for repair.

Antimetabolites such as **cytosine arabinoside**, **methotrexate** and **5-fluorouracil** interfere with nucleotide incorporation during DNA and RNA synthesis. The microtubule disrupting agents **vinblastine** and **vincristine** affect spindle formation during division but also have a more general effect on microtubules in interphase cells (see below). **Radiation** and radiomimetic agents such as **bleomycin** produce reactive free radicals which interact with DNA, causing damage.

There is differential sensitivity between the various populations of dividing cells to these DNA damaging agents. The slow cycling stem cell spermatogonia are markedly more resistant to all cancer chemotherapeutic drugs than are the differentiated (committed) spermatogonia. Prezygotene stages of spermatocyte meiosis, where DNA synthesis occurs, are susceptible to some of these chemicals, but the later meiotic stages, including the two divisions, are resistant. This is probably explained by the protection afforded to postzygotene spermatocytes by the Sertoli cell tight junctions, preventing chemical access to these cells.

Genotoxic damage   As with genotoxicity of somatic cells, injury may reside at the DNA level where deletion, insertion or substitution of nucleotide bases during replication or repair results in point mutations. Alternatively, chromosomal breaks or rearrangements will produce chromosomal aberrations, while alterations in chromosome numbers may result in aneuploidy or polyploidy. To date, all germ cell mutagens have been shown to be somatic cell mutagens but the reverse is not always the case. For a mutagen to be genotoxic to germ cells, it must first gain access to these cells.

Genotoxic damage to the germ cell may allow fertilization but result in death of the conceptus; the dominant lethal test detects such damage. Reciprocal translocations of chromosome fragments which do not interfere with fertility of the parent or viability of the fetus but result in reduced or lack of fertility in the F_1 generation, are tested for using the heritable translocation test. Aneuploidy or polyploidy, which can be seen in chromosome spreads, can result in developmental abnormalities such as Down's syndrome in man. Although the effects of **radiation** exposure on male germ cells has caused much controversy in recent years, there is no proven instance of genetic disease arising from induced mutation of germ cells in humans. However, experimental data indicate a potential risk from a variety of chemicals, e.g. paternal chronic exposure to low doses of **cyclophosphamide** results in preimplantation or postimplantation losses and congenital malformations in rats. Also, **methylmethane sulphonate** and **ethylmethane sulphonate** produce genetic damage in the mid- to late-stage spermatids and spermatozoa of mice, giving rise to dominant lethal mutations.

Injury to enzymes and metabolic processes

Each of the cell types within the testis has very different metabolic processes and requirements. In many cases, this is probably the basis for the differential susceptibility of testicular cells to different toxicants. By using *in vitro* techniques with individual or mixed cell cultures or by using isolated tubules, the effects of many toxicants on protein secretion, energy metabolism and enzyme activities have been examined. Although changes are often observed, the relationship of these changes to the critical biochemical lesion responsible for toxicity *in vivo* is unknown.

The Sertoli cell is perhaps the most metabolically active cell in the testis, secreting large numbers of different proteins and providing energy precursors for the surrounding germ cells as well as the seminiferous tubule fluid for sperm transport. It has been suggested as the target cell for a wide variety of testicular toxicants, generally on the basis of early morphological changes. Using isolated tubules, **1,3-dinitrobenzene (DNB)** has been shown to alter the secretion of up to 15 different proteins by the Sertoli cell, decreasing some and increasing others in a stage-specific manner [14]. Chemically induced alteration in the proteins secreted by the Sertoli cell is a frequently encountered observation but as yet, the identity and functions of most of these proteins is largely unknown, as is the significance of their altered secretion. ABP is perhaps the best characterized protein and can be measured *in vivo* and *in vitro*. It is sometimes used as a marker of Sertoli cell function. Secretion into the tubular lumen and also into the interstitial compartment occurs, leading to entry of ABP into the blood. With a number of testicular toxicants including **phthalate esters** and **irradiation**, an initial increase in serum ABP is followed by a prolonged decrease in circulating levels, the significance of which is unclear.

The effects of toxicants on energy metabolism in isolated germ cells or on the production of lactate and pyruvate from glucose by Sertoli cells in culture has been investigated. Using **glycol ethers**, which affect pachytene spermatocytes, the active metabolite has been shown to inhibit lactate production by cultured Sertoli cells and inhibit the germ-cell specific isozyme of lactate dehydrogenase (LDH-C4). Since spermatocytes depend on lactate and pyruvate produced by the Sertoli cell as their energy source, these effects may play a role in the aetiology of the lesion. In contrast, phthalate esters which appear to act on the Sertoli cell have been shown to increase lactate in cultured Sertoli cells while decreasing testicular glucose and fructose levels *in vivo*. Increases in lactate production by Sertoli cells in culture have also been reported with **DNB, gossypol, 2,5-hexanedione, DBCP, cadmium** and **lead**. Such changes, along with the inhibition of succinic dehydrogenase in Sertoli cell mitochondria (**phthalate esters** and **DNB**), suggest interference with glycolysis and the Kreb's cycle but, as with alterations in protein secretion, their relevance to the critical biochemical lesion is unknown.

Inhibition of energy pathways in sperm has been identified as the biochemical lesion for some testicular toxicants. The site of inhibition may be glycolysis or the Kreb's cycle, for example *a*-**chlorhydrin** and **6-chlorodeoxyglucose** which reduce ATP levels, or **DBCP** which inhibits postglycolytic reactions. Inhibition of energy production results in reduced sperm motility and decreased capacity for reaching the egg.

Injury to structural proteins and membranes

The orderly process of spermatogenesis is dependent on the spatial arrangement of the germ cells within the tubular epithelium. The movement of cells from a basal to an adluminal position and the release of the mature spermatids into the lumen is a function of the microtubules and microfilaments which maintain the structural shape of the Sertoli cell and the complex specialized junctions between the Sertoli and germ cells. The importance of Sertoli cell shape to the integrity of the seminiferous epithelium is demonstrated by the effects of microtubule disrupting agents such as **colchicine** and **vinblastine** on the rat testis [15]. Apart from their effects on spindle formation during mitosis and meiosis, they cause depolymerization and loss of Sertoli cell microtubules. Effects on the Sertoli cell include sloughing of apical processes with associated germ cells into the tubular lumen, and basal accumulation of smooth endoplasmic reticulum vesicles. In less severe lesions produced in other species, the disruption of microtubules in the Sertoli cell prevented movement of the elongating spermatids to an apical position, thus disrupting normal spermiation, and caused abnormalities to the head and acrosome of developing spermatids, structures which are closely associated with Sertoli cell microtubules.

Other cytoskeletal components such as micro- (actin) filaments and intermediate filaments are also important to the function of the Sertoli cell. Disruption of actin filaments with **cytochalasin D** affects the specialized junctions between Sertoli cells, causing focal impairment of the blood–tubule barrier as well as disruption of Sertoli–germ cell junctions, causing loss of adherence and malorientation of germ cells.

A number of chemicals including **2,5-hexanedione, acrylamide** and **organophosphorus esters** exhibit selective toxicity for the nervous system and the testis. Intermediate filament disruption has been suggested as the mechanism of action which links these toxic effects [16].

Phthalate ester-induced lesions share many similarities in their pathogenesis with those of **2,5-hexanedione** and the microtubule depolymerizing agents. Since disruption of microfilaments has been demonstrated in Sertoli cells exposed to **phthalate esters** in culture, cytoskeletal effects may play an important part in the mechanism of action for these toxicants also.

Defective sperm function in humans has been linked with increased levels of plasma membrane lipid peroxidation induced by the production of high levels of reactive oxygen species [17]. Although this is an idiopathic condition in humans, the potential exists for xenobiotics to enter epididymal fluid and chemically induce reactive oxygen species, as can be demonstrated using the **ionophore A23187** [17].

12.3.3 *Agents Causing Indirect Damage Through Hormonal or Neural Mechanisms*

Endocrine, paracrine and neural control of reproductive function covers a very wide range of potential targets for toxicological injury. The hypothalamic–pituitary–gonadal axis is the coarse control for reproductive processes while the Leydig cell–Sertoli cell–germ cell axis provides fine control. The neurophysiological and neuropharmacological control of erection, emission and ejaculation are still poorly understood but a number of pharmacological agents are known which specifically affect these functions [6, 18].

A reduction in androgen secretion from the Leydig cells will result in disruption of spermatogenesis and atrophy of the seminal vesicles and prostate. This can occur through a reduction in LH levels, e.g. by **ethanol**, or by direct toxicity to the Leydig cells, e.g. **ethane dimethane sulphonate**. The same effects can be produced by antiandrogens (e.g. **cyproterone acetate, flutamide** or the diuretic, **spironolactone**) which can act in a number of ways: they can block uptake of androgens into the tissue, interfere with androgen receptor binding or the translocation of the receptor complex to the nucleus, or inhibit activation of testosterone to the more potent androgen, 5-dihydrotestosterone (5-DHT).

Anabolic steroids turn off LH secretion by competitive inhibition with testosterone at the hypothalamic androgen receptor, thus interfering with the negative feedback loop. Long-term use of anabolic steroids leads to impotence, loss of libido and azoospermia. Interference with CNS androgen receptors which mediate sexual behaviour is used therapeutically to treat deviant sexual behaviour, e.g. **cyproterone acetate**, but other drugs such as the H_2-receptor antagonist, **cimetidine**, appear to have a similar effect, producing impotence while increasing gonadotropin levels.

Oestrogens (e.g. **oestradiol-17-β, diethyl stilboestrol**) act as antiandrogens in the male in a number of ways. Their main action is to block the secretion of gonadotropins from the pituitary, but they also inhibit activation of testosterone to 5-DHT, they compete at binding sites for 5-DHT and stimulate the synthesis of the testosterone-binding globulin in the blood thus decreasing bioavailability.

Polychlorinated biphenyls and **organochlorines** such as **dichlorodiphenyl trichloroethane (DDT)**, **methoxychlor** and **chlordecone (Kepone)** have adverse effects on reproduction which are probably related to their oestrogenic properties. These include seminiferous tubular degeneration, reduction in the weights of seminal vesicles and prostate, and reduced fertility.

Exposure to **organochlorines**, as with many other chemicals, results in hepatic enzyme induction. Increased levels or activity of the microsomal hydroxylases which metabolize endogenous steroids will accelerate the clearance of testosterone and may add to the antiandrogen properties.

As a result of the complex feedback loops between Sertoli cells, Leydig cells, the hypothalamus and pituitary, disruption of spermatogenesis will generally result in changes in circulating gonadotropins and vice versa. Deciding which changes are primary, and which are secondary, is often difficult.

12.3.4 *Factors Affecting Toxicity*

As with other organs, there are important factors which will determine or modify the toxic effect of a chemical on a particular tissue or to a particular individual. Differential metabolism between species may produce toxic metabolites in some, and inactive ones in others. Alternatively, differential absorption and distribution may result in high circulating or tissue levels in one species and negligible levels in another. This has been suggested as the reason for the species specificity of **cyclohexylamine**, which is a testicular toxicant in the rat but not in the mouse [19].

Testes of young animals are much more sensitive to **phthalate esters** and to **β-lactam antibiotics**. The reasons for this are not understood but the hormonal control of the neonate testis is very different from that of the adult and many alterations occur in Sertoli cell functions as puberty approaches. In contrast, **DNB** has been shown to be less toxic to the testis of prepubertal and pubertal mice than to adult mice.

Absorption, distribution, metabolism and excretion will determine the toxicity of a particular chemical. A potential toxicant must reach its target cell before it can have any effect. Many of the components of the reproductive system are protected by an effective barrier, i.e. blood–testis or blood–epididymal barrier. Although the liver is the major metabolizing organ, the testis contains a range of metabolizing enzymes including cytochrome P-450, mixed function oxidases, epoxide hydrases, aryl hydrolases and a variety of transferases. Most of this activity is localized in the Leydig cells but some also resides in the Sertoli cell. Metabolism of **DNB** (Sertoli cell toxicant) with the formation of a toxic intermediate has been demonstrated in Sertoli cell cultures [20]. However, metabolism of the Sertoli cell toxicant **tri-*o*-cresyl phosphate** (**TOCP**) to its toxic metabolite occurs in Leydig cells with presumed transfer of the active metabolite to the Sertoli cells [21]. Similarly, **7,12-dimethylbenz[a]anthracene** is initially metabolized by Leydig cells. The metabolite is then transported to the Sertoli cells where it is converted to a toxic species which affects spermatogonial DNA polymerase [22]. Distinguishing the site and mechanism of biotransformation of reproductive toxicants can therefore be of great assistance in understanding the overall mechanism of toxic action of a compound [20].

12.4 Morphological Responses to Injury

12.4.1 *Introduction*

Response to injury in any tissue is essentially the same, encompassing degeneration, necrosis, inflammation and repair and perhaps extending to hyperplasia and neoplasia. The pattern of response to any particular toxicant depends on the target cell and the severity or extent of the damage. In the reproductive organs, the picture is further complicated by secondary, physiological responses to the functional damage of the target cell. By carrying out a careful, morphological time course study it should be possible to identify the primary target cell and, by following the subsequent events, gain some indication of the functional disturbances in the injured cell. The role of endocrine and paracrine substances in modulating the morphological response to injury should be borne in mind. Their importance in understanding

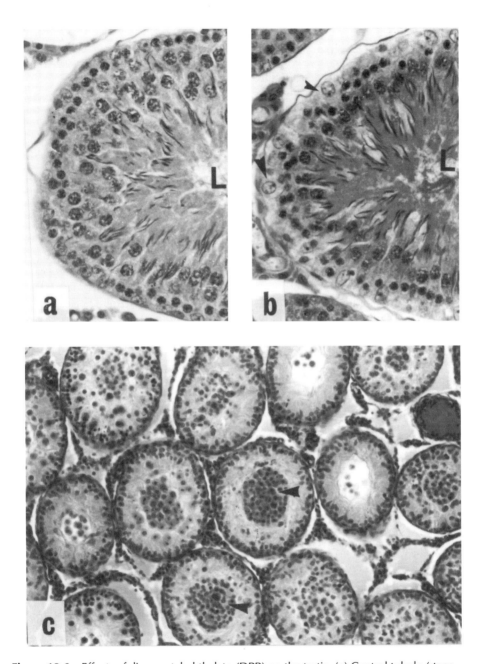

Figure 12.6 Effects of di-*n*-pentyl phthalate (DPP) on the testis. (a) Control tubule (stage XIII). (b) Stage XIII tubule 6 h after an oral dose of DPP at 2.2 g/kg body weight. Basal Sertoli cell cytoplasm appears pale and swollen (arrowheads) with closure of the tubular lumen (L). (c) After four daily doses of DPP most of the germ cells have become detached from the Sertoli cells and have been shed into the lumen (arrowheads).

mechanisms of spermatogenic disruption is pivotal, since any perturbation of these sensitive regulatory interactions is likely to have profound effects on most of the cell types within the testis.

Reversibility of toxicologically induced lesions is always an important consideration. This again depends on the cell type injured and the severity of the injury. Leydig cells readily regenerate whereas Sertoli cells are unable to divide. Provided the primitive stem cell spermatogonia remain intact, all other germ cell types can be generated and repopulate a depleted seminiferous tubule. For a more detailed account of general morphological responses to injury, the reader is referred to [5, 6, 7].

12.4.2 Sertoli Cell Injury

Degeneration and necrosis

The presence of vacuoles within the seminiferous epithelium is a common early response to a variety of toxicants including **2,5-hexanedione**, **DNB**, and **cyclohexylamine** (Figure 12.8). These changes are followed by germ cell degeneration and exfoliation into the tubular lumen. Ultrastructurally, the vacuoles appear to represent dilated smooth endoplasmic reticulum within Sertoli cells or dilated intercellular spaces, sometimes containing proteinaceous fluid. Vacuoles are also seen in cases of advanced germ cell depletion where the lost germ cells are replaced by empty spaces. Swelling and pallor of the basal cytoplasm of the Sertoli cell is seen as the earliest observable effect with **phthalate esters** (Figure 12.6). It is probably caused by an altered fluid balance. Following this effect, germ cells appear to lose contact with Sertoli cell processes and are exfoliated into the tubular lumen.

Although the Sertoli cell is susceptible to degenerative changes, it is very resistant to lethal injury, and cell necrosis is rarely seen. In cases of severe testicular atrophy, Sertoli cells are frequently the only cells remaining in the seminiferous epithelium (Figure 12.7).

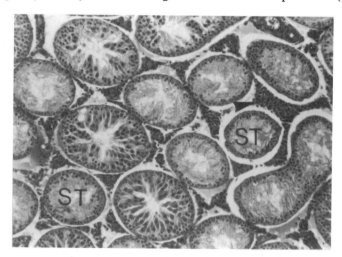

Figure 12.7 Rat fed with cyclohexylamine at 400 mg/kg body weight per day for 13 weeks, showing damage to some of the tubules with total depletion of all germ cells, leaving shrunken tubules (ST) containing only Sertoli cells and a few spermatogonia. This has resulted in hyperplasia of the Leydig cells surrounding these tubules (arrowhead).

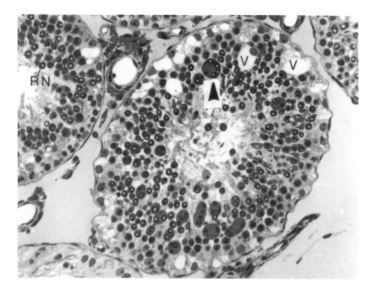

Figure 12.8 Rat fed with cyclohexylamine at 400 mg/kg body weight per day for 9 weeks. Vacuolation of Sertoli cell cytoplasm (V) with degeneration of remaining germ cells. The round spermatids show ring nuclei (RN) and some have fused to form multinucleate giant cells (arrowhead).

Decreased blood flow which leads to tissue hypoxia will result in ischaemic necrosis of all cells within the testis including Sertoli cells. In this case there is no capacity for regeneration since the Sertoli cell cannot divide.

12.4.3 Germ Cell Injury

Degeneration and necrosis

Degenerate germ cells take on a variety of morphological forms. Spermatocytes frequently develop increased eosinophilia of the cytoplasm and round spermatids may have 'ring' nuclei where the chromatin forms a thin rim around a clear central zone (Figure 12.8). Elongating and maturation phase spermatid nuclei may become thickened, developing a clubbed head appearance. Since whole groups of germ cells are joined to each other by cytoplasmic bridges, it is common to find fusion of degenerating germ cells to form multinucleated giant cells (Figure 12.8). These are most commonly formed by round spermatids but may also result from spermatocyte fusion. As degeneration progresses into necrosis, nuclei become condensed (pyknotic) (Figure 12.9) or fragmented and the cell debris is rapidly phagocytosed by the Sertoli cell or shed into the tubular lumen.

Toxicants which affect germ cells frequently do so in a cell-specific and sometimes stage-specific manner (Table 12.3). **Cancer chemotherapeutic drugs** differentially affect the various populations of spermatogonia [13]. **Ethylene glycol monomethyl ether** specifically affects spermatocytes, with early pachytene and late pachytene through to division being the most sensitive stages (Figure 12.9). Agents which disrupt intratesticular hormonal balance cause necrosis of spermatocytes and spermatids in stage VII tubules as the initial lesion.

391

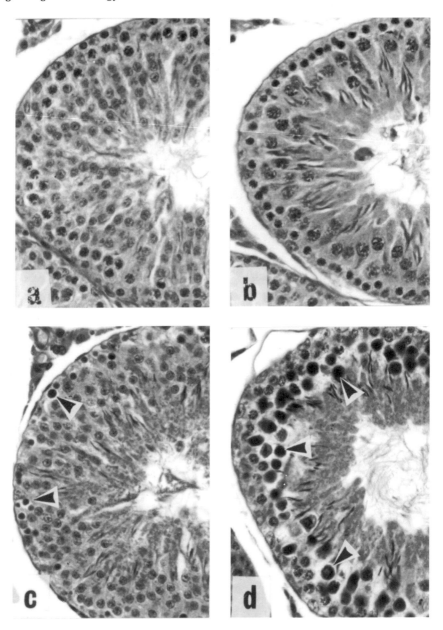

Figure 12.9 Effects of ethylene glycol monomethyl ether (EGME) on spermatocytes. (a) Control tubule stage V, (b) control tubule stage XII, (c) and (d) 24 h after an oral dose of 500 mg/kg body weight of EGME, stage V and stage XII tubules respectively, with necrotic pachytene spermatocytes (arrowheads).

Although the process of necrosis is irreversible, repopulation of the germ cells will occur as long as the stem cell spermatogonia have not been destroyed. There are a number of subpopulations of spermatogonia including those committed to differentiation and true stem cells which are uncommitted. It is this latter population which act as the definitive precursor cells and which are relatively resistant to injurious stimuli.

Maturation depletion

Necrotic cells are rapidly removed from the seminiferous epithelium; they are either phagocytosed by the Sertoli cell or shed into the tubular lumen. As long as the remaining germ cells in the epithelium are not injured also, they will carry on their maturation through the spermatogenic cycle. As this happens, the developmental stage of the missing cells will advance at a similar rate. This process of maturation depletion is illustrated in Figure 12.10.

Delayed spermiation/spermatid retention

In normal spermatogenesis, mature (step 19) spermatids are released into the tubular lumen during stage VIII of the spermatogenic cycle. Many toxicants such as **boric acid**, **methyl chloride** and **DNB** result in retention of step 19 spermatids into stages IX to XII. This is probably due to alterations in the specialized cell-to-cell junctions between Sertoli cell and spermatid. The retained spermatids may be released or merely phagocytosed by the Sertoli cell in these later stages.

12.4.4 Leydig Cell Injury

Degeneration and necrosis

Leydig cells may be subject to degeneration and necrosis. **Ethane dimethane sulphonate** causes rapid degeneration and necrosis of Leydig cells [23]. Necrotic

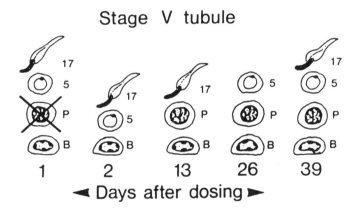

Stage V tubule

◄ Days after dosing ►

Figure 12.10 Diagrammatic representation of the movement of maturation depletion through generations of germ cells over time. A stage V tubule from a rat dosed with a spermatocyte toxicant is depicted at various times after dosing. At day 0 (day of dosing), the stage V tubule will consist of B, type B spermatogonia; P, pachytene spermatocytes; 5, step 5 spermatids; and 17, step 17 spermatids. One day after dosing, pachytene spermatocytes exhibit necrosis. Two days after dosing, spermatocytes are absent (due to phagocytosis of necrotic debris by Sertoli cells). Thirteen days after dosing (i.e. one spermatogenic cycle), pachytene spermatocytes have been replenished (by maturation of underlying B spermatogonia), but step 5 spermatids are absent. By 26 days after dosing, spermatocytes and step 5 spermatids have been replenished but step 17 spermatids are missing. After one more cycle (39 days after dosing) the stage V tubule has its normal complement of cells.

cells are rapidly phagocytosed by interstitial macrophages and by 7 to 14 days after a single dose there is a total absence of Leydig cells. Such changes are accompanied by a dramatic fall in testicular and circulating testosterone levels which results in stage-specific disturbances in spermatogenesis (stage VII) and a weight decrease in the epididymis, prostate and seminal vesicles. A new generation of Leydig cells develops which rapidly return testosterone levels to normal values.

Hypertrophy and hyperplasia

Prolonged stimulation of the Leydig cells by LH will result in increased testosterone secretion which is likely to be accompanied by a generalized increase in cell size and cell number. Factors released from the Sertoli cell, e.g. luteinizing hormone releasing hormone (LHRH)-like peptide, also exert controlling effects on the Leydig cells in the immediate vicinity. Focal tubular damage or disruption of spermatogenesis will result in local secretion of these regulatory peptides and elicit focal Leydig cell hypertrophy and hyperplasia (Figure 12.7) and testosterone secretion.

12.4.5 Tubular Dilatation or Contraction

Sertoli cells continually secrete seminiferous tubule fluid, so if there is any form of obstruction in the tubules, the rete testis or in the extratesticular duct system, the tubules will become dilated with fluid. The excessive pressure exerted on the epithelium results in thinning of the cell layers, gaps between the luminal portions of adjacent Sertoli cells, and, if prolonged, loss of germ cells due to pressure atrophy. Another possible cause of fluid build-up is failure of the epididymis and rete testis to resorb the tubule fluid.

    A reduction in tubular diameter is normally associated with loss of germ cells and is frequently used as a measurable parameter to assess quantitatively testicular injury. Closure of the tubular lumen may occur if production of tubule fluid ceases or is markedly reduced, as seen with phthalate esters. This may occur as a direct effect of toxicants or as a result of hormonal disturbance. Tubular fluid is not produced in the rat until 16 to 19 days postnatal development; the small tubular lumen of prepubertal rats reflects this.

12.4.6 Vascular Effects

Reduction in blood flow

Alterations in the blood flow are particularly critical in the testis because the tubules, which make up the major bulk of the testis, are avascular. Oxygen has to diffuse out from the interstitial blood vessels through the peritubular layers and the Sertoli cells to gain access to the luminal germ cells, most of which have a high metabolic activity. For this reason the seminiferous epithelium is considered to be on the borderline of hypoxia and any reduction in its blood flow may have severe consequences. Substances such as **5-hydroxytryptamine, histamine** and **adrenaline** all result in testicular injury by reducing the blood flow. **Cadmium** produces severe ischaemic necrosis of the testis, affecting tubular and interstitial elements. Small doses of **cadmium** damage the interstitial capillary endothelium resulting in increased leakage of fluid and electrolytes and a dramatic decrease in blood flow [24]. This results in severe anoxic injury to the testis and epididymis.

Interstitial fluid accumulation and inflammation

Interstitial fluid volume is controlled by the permeability of the blood vessels. The Leydig cells are thought to be the major regulators of vascular permeability, possibly through secretion of a variety of vasoactive substances such as β-endorphin and prostaglandins. The amount of interstitial fluid is increased in a number of conditions where spermatogenesis has been disrupted, for example following **irradiation** or **experimental cryptorchism**. Morphologically, increased production of interstitial fluid has the same appearance as oedema in other tissues. Its occurrence can mask a weight loss.

Inflammatory infiltrate is an uncommon response to injury in the testis unless there has been substantial vascular damage. **Dipentyl phthalate** produces a transient interstitial neutrophilic response within 6 h of dosing which is associated with the production of a lymphocyte-activating factor. However, the infiltrate remains extratubular. This is an important aspect of inflammation and immunological responses in the testis, since postmeiotic germ cells have surface antigens which would be recognized as foreign to the immunosurveillance cells. In general, the testis is considered to be an immunologically privileged site and is considered a favourable site for transplantation of foreign tissue.

12.4.7 Neoplasia

With the exception of Leydig cell tumours, neoplasia of the testis of laboratory animals is uncommon. However, Leydig cell tumours of rats and mice are frequently seen in ageing animals as a spontaneous tumour and can also be readily induced. The spontaneous incidence is age and strain dependent; in the F-344 rat it approaches 100 per cent in 2-year studies. The reason for this very high incidence is not entirely understood but appears to be due to a progressive hormonal imbalance resulting in high circulating levels of LH. Indeed, raised levels of circulating LH appear to be the major causative factor in the chemical induction of Leydig cell tumours in the rat by a diverse range of drugs and chemicals [25]. This is considered to be largely a species specific effect since tumours are not induced by these chemicals in the mouse and some, e.g. **cimetidine** have seen widespread use in man with no evidence of Leydig cell proliferation. In contrast, Leydig cell tumourigenesis in the mouse is associated with raised levels of oestrogen and can be induced with **oestrogenic compounds** e.g. **diethylstilbestrol**, or chemicals which result in raised oestrogen levels.

Leydig cell tumours appear to arise from focal Leydig cell hyperplasia, and when small, the two are indistinguishable from each other. There is a continuous morphological spectrum starting with a small aggregate of hyperplastic cells through to a large adenoma, which in time will replace the entire structure of the testis. Since there are no consistent distinguishing features between a hyperplastic focus and an adenoma, an arbitrary criterion of size (greater than the diameter of three seminiferous tubules) is generally used to define an adenoma. Leydig cell tumours are frequently multiple and bilateral. They are almost always considered benign (adenomas) since they rarely show any capacity to invade through the testicular capsule or metastasize to distant sites.

Germ cell tumours (seminomas) and Sertoli cell tumours are occasionally seen spontaneously in rats and mice but are more frequent in dogs.

12.4.8 *Epididymal Injury*

Luminal cellular debris and exfoliated germ cells

Although not a result of epididymal injury, it is common to see cellular debris and exfoliated germ cells from the testis in the ductular lumen of the caput or cauda epididymis. This can provide confirmation or serve as an indicator of tubular damage in the testis.

Reduction in sperm numbers

A reduction in the number of sperm produced by the testis will be reflected by a reduction in the amount stored in the cauda epididymis. Oligospermia denotes a reduction in numbers, azoospermia is a total absence of sperm. As sperm volume declines, the diameter of the ducts will also reduce, giving an atrophic appearance to the epididymis. This may also be reflected by epididymal weight loss.

Degeneration and necrosis

Intracellular vacuoles in the epididymal epithelium are occasionally seen following administration of toxicants and are frequently seen as a spontaneous change in ageing animals. The epithelium lining the ducts resorbs large quantities of fluid from the lumen and secretes a variety of proteins and electrolytes into the lumen. Disturbance of this two-way traffic is a possible cause of these intracellular vacuoles. Epithelial necrosis of the cauda epididymis results from administration of **dibromochloropropane** and two of its metabolites **α-chlorohydrin** and **epichlorohydrin**. Necrosis of the epithelium allows entry of sperm into the surrounding interstitium and will lead to granuloma formation (see below).

Inflammation

Inflammation of the epididymis is most commonly associated with sperm granulomas. If sperm gain access to the interstitial tissue through breaks or rupture of the epididymal epithelium, an inflammatory reaction will result. The sperm will gradually be encapsulated by layers of fibroblasts, collagen, macrophages and neutrophils. This chronic inflammatory reaction is termed a granuloma.

Any epithelial damage in the epididymis is liable to lead to granuloma formation. **Methyl chloride** inhalation leads to acute epididymal inflammation followed by granuloma formation, probably as a result of epithelial attenuation. **Dibromochloropropane** results in granulomas following epithelial necrosis.

Spermatocele

Obstruction of the epididymal duct or of its distal pathway will result in a build-up of pressure and progressive cystic dilatation of the duct with sperm and fluid. This is termed a spermatocele, but is likely to result in rupture and inflammation, producing a sperm granuloma.

12.4.9 *Injury to Secondary Sex Organs*

The secondary sex organs are not a common target site for toxicity. There are no agents known to affect fertility which act only on the accessory sex glands. However, atrophic effects, secondary to alterations in circulating testosterone levels, are frequently seen.

Atrophy

Lack of stimulation by testosterone leads to flattened, inactive epithelial cells, a reduced volume of luminal secretion and luminal contraction in the prostate and seminal vesicles. Weight loss in these organs is a reliable, simple indicator of reduced serum testosterone levels.

Hyperplasia

Hyperplasia is frequently seen in the prostate and occasionally in the seminal vesicles as a regenerative response to inflammatory lesions. It has been induced by administration of **lead acetate**, but otherwise it is an uncommon primary response to toxicants.

Inflammation

Inflammatory lesions are frequently seen, particularly in the prostate and the preputial gland, either as an age-related spontaneous lesion or as a result of urogenital infection. The preputial gland of mice is frequently injured due to fighting and can lead to abscess formation.

Neoplasia

Preputial gland tumours are a common tumour of ageing rats and mice and have been induced in the rat with **7,12-dimethylbenzanthracene** as well as **aromatic amines** such as **2-acetylaminofluorene** and **3,2′-dimethyl-4-aminobiphenyl (DMAB)** [26]. Prostatic tumours, although a common tumour of man, are infrequently seen as a spontaneous tumour in laboratory animals. They have been induced in the rat with **DMAB** and with *N*-**nitrosobis(2-oxopropyl) amine (BOP)** and by administration of **testosterone propionate** [26]. Spontaneous tumours of the seminal vesicles are rare and difficult to induce chemically.

12.5 Testing for Toxicity

12.5.1 *Introduction*

Fertility is a difficult parameter to assess quantitatively. In some species such as rodents, the quantity and quality of the sperm produced is so good, that the animal is still fertile with only 5 to 10 per cent of its normal sperm production. Conversely, human sperm is comparatively poor in quality (i.e. a high incidence of sperm with morphological abnormalities or poor motility), and a relatively small reduction in sperm count may render an individual infertile.

Since fertility is dependent on a variety of components including spermatogenesis, epididymal maturation, production of seminal fluid and ejaculation, it makes sense to measure a number of different parameters when testing for toxicity. A mixture of functional, biochemical and morphological indices is required to gain a full picture of the mode of action of a reproductive toxicant. For more detailed information on the various tests, the reader is referred to [5, 7, 10, 27, 28, 29, 30, 31].

12.5.2   *Functional Studies*

Fertility studies

Fertility studies test the functional integrity of all potential target sites within the reproductive system. However, due to the excessive functional reserve of sperm production in rodents, fertility studies represent a very insensitive index of reproductive injury. If fertility is affected, further studies of individual endpoints will be required to establish which aspects of the process have been affected.

The time of mating with respect to chemical exposure is a critical consideration. In the rat, the process of spermatogenesis takes about 8 weeks for completion and the released sperm take another 1 to 2 weeks in transit through the epididymis. Therefore, any effects on spermatogonia would take about 8 to 10 weeks to show in ejaculated sperm. Conversely, if cauda epididymal spermatozoa were the target cell, fertility would be affected within days of dosing (Figure 12.11).

There are two basic study designs in use, a single mating trial and a serial mating trial. In the single mating study, the animals are dosed for 8 to 10 weeks to ensure that ejaculated sperm have been exposed to the chemical through every phase of spermatogenesis. This is followed by a single mating and subsequent evaluation of the females for implantation sites and fetuses. This design can be extended to cover multiple generations by continuing to dose the offspring.

In the serial mating trial, the male is treated for 1 week only and then mated at weekly intervals for a further 10 weeks. The females and fetuses are evaluated after every mating. Using this regime, the target cell(s) can be identified by the length of time taken for effects to be seen. Effects on spermatogonia will be seen after 8 to 10 weeks, effects on pachytene spermatocytes after 5 to 7 weeks and so on (see Figure 12.11).

Fertility studies are particularly useful in detecting mutagenic toxicants. These may result in death of the conceptus, congenital malformations or reduced fertility/sterility of the F_1 males. Specific protocols such as the dominant lethal assay and heritable translocation test are used to test for specific types of germ cell genetic toxicity. Unscheduled DNA synthesis is a rapid and reliable method for detecting genotoxic damage and can be carried out *in vivo* or *in vitro*.

Evaluation of copulatory behaviour

Although this is an area not frequently studied, its importance should be borne in mind. A number of antiandrogens such as **cyproterone acetate** and **spironolactone** are

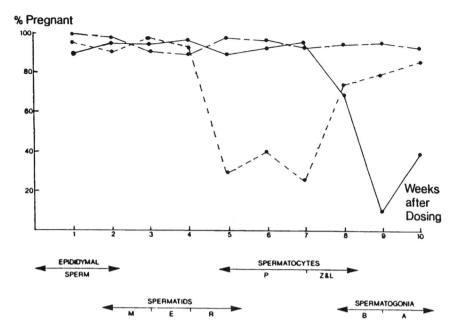

Figure 12.11 Results which might be expected from a serial mating study using a spermatocyte toxicant (- - -) (e.g. ethylene glycol monomethyl ether) and a spermatogonial toxicant (———) (e.g. busulphan), compared with controls (— — —). One-week dosing of the males is followed by weekly breeding trials. Serial evaluation of the females provides the index of male fertility. The delay taken for infertility to develop gives a good indication of the cell type(s) affected, i.e. epididymal sperm (0 to 2 weeks), mature/elongate/round (M, E, R) spermatids (2 to 5 weeks), pachytene/zygotene/leptotene (P, Z, L) spermatocytes (5 to 8 weeks) or type B/type A (B, A) spermatogonia (8 to 10 weeks).

known to disrupt sexual behaviour through CNS mechanisms, reducing libido, erection and ejaculatory performance in man as well as laboratory animals. Known neurotoxicants such as **carbon disulphide**, **trichloroethylene** and **acrylamide** have also been shown to affect copulatory behaviour or ejaculatory performance in the rat [32].

In fertility studies, copulation is generally measured using the presence of a copulatory plug in the vagina or sperm in a vaginal lavage. This gives no indication of readiness to mate, frequency or effectiveness of copulatory behaviour. These parameters can be measured and may be responsible for preimplantation losses which are otherwise put down to spermatotoxic effects.

12.5.3 Sperm Function Studies

Sperm count, sperm motility and sperm morphology are frequently used as measures of sperm function in man and laboratory animals. Sperm can be collected from an ejaculate, from the vas deferens or from the cauda epididymis. Enumeration of spermatid nuclei in testicular homogenates also provides a convenient measure of sperm production. Only the elongating maturation phase of spermatids are resistant to homogenization; their number represents a measure of germ cell division and survival through spermatogenesis.

Sperm samples are highly sensitive to changes in temperature, pH and dilution. If sperm is to be evaluated it should be done rapidly and under controlled conditions. There is marked inter-animal variation in sperm count, therefore serial sampling is advantageous. However, frequency of ejaculation will also have a marked reducing effect on the sperm count in serial sampling of an individual. Ejaculated sperm cannot easily be collected from the rodent other than by recovery from the female genital tract. For serial sampling of semen, the rabbit or dog are the most convenient species.

Sperm motility is a valuable measure of epididymal sperm maturation. During passage from the caput to the cauda epididymis, the sperm motility changes from random movement to a progressive forward motion. Until the advent of computer analysed sperm activity (CASA), accurate evaluation of sperm movement was difficult. The sperm samples still require rapid and careful handling with tightly controlled environmental conditions, but this methodology allows rapid quantitative measurements of multiple parameters of sperm movement.

Sperm morphology assays can detect increases in the number of sperm with abnormalities in the shape of the head or tail region. In some species, including man, the number of abnormal sperm produced in normal fertile individuals forms a high percentage of the total sperm count. However, it is regarded as one of the least variable of the sperm parameters measured for a given individual or an animal strain over time. Although this makes it an attractive marker for detecting spermatotoxic effects, agents which affect sperm motility and viability, and agents which induce germ cell mutations often have no effect on sperm morphology (e.g. **ethylene dibromide** in the rabbit [29]).

Sperm viability can be measured using a hypo-osmotic swelling test or acridine orange which, under UV illumination, stains live sperm red and non-viable sperm green.

12.5.4 *Histopathology*

Using appropriate fixation, embedding and staining techniques, histopathological examination by an experienced investigator is one of the most sensitive and reliable methods of detecting cytotoxic (although not mutagenic) reproductive damage. The method of fixation is particularly important. Formalin fixation followed by paraffin wax embedding is used almost universally as the method of choice for light microscopic examination of other tissues, but it gives extremely poor morphology in the testis. A much better fixative is Bouin's or Helly's fixative which gives much superior cytoplasmic and nuclear detail. Formalin fixation is only acceptable if followed by resin embedding.

A great improvement in morphology can be gained by embedding tissue in resin rather than wax. Resin sections of 1 to 2 µm in thickness give greatly improved resolution for light microscopy. Glycol methacrylate resin is a soft medium which allows staining with conventional histological stains, while epoxy resins are much harder and can be viewed by electron microscopy, however, staining for light microscopy is limited, e.g. toluidine blue.

In order to identify accurately individual stages of spermatogenesis it is necessary to stain wax and glycol methacrylate sections with periodic acid Schiff stain, which stains the acrosome.

For detailed morphological studies which aim to pick up early, subcellular changes, intravascular perfusion of the fixative (glutaraldehyde or glutaraldehyde and paraformaldehyde mixed), followed by embedding in epoxy resin and examination by electron microscopy is necessary. This methodology is very time-consuming and technically demanding and is only really appropriate for mechanistic investigations.

To gain most information from a morphological study, it is important to examine the earliest signs of injury. This may occur within 3 h of a single dose, e.g. **phthalate esters**, or may take 2 to 3 weeks of daily dosing, e.g. **2,5-hexanedione, cyclohexylamine**. Prolonged exposure to any testicular toxicant will result in an endstage lesion of tubules lined with Sertoli cells, depleted of most germ cells (Figure 12.7). This gives negligible information on pathogenesis. Cell specificity to a toxicant is often seen at low doses whereas high-dose levels may result in a more generalized, non-specific toxicity. Investigative morphological studies should therefore be designed to monitor the time course of lesion development using as low a dose as will consistently and reliably produce changes.

Qualitative versus quantitative morphology

Most histopathological investigations rely on a qualitative evaluation of cellular damage or tissue change with a semiquantitative estimate of severity of damage, e.g. minimal, slight, moderate, severe. Carried out by an experienced investigator, this is a rapid and relatively sensitive technique, but its sensitivity and objectivity can be improved markedly by measuring or counting a few simple parameters [31]. Transverse sections through the testis rather than longitudinal sections are better for any quantitative measurements, since this will produce approximately round tubular cross-sections.

Tubular diameter is generally closely related to the number of germ cells in the tubular epithelium; as germ cells are lost, the tubule contracts (Figure 12.7). Counting germ cells in large numbers of tubules microscopically can be very tedious and time-consuming. However, restricting counting to a small number of tubules at one or two stages can provide useful information in repeat-dose toxicity screens. Daily sperm production can also be estimated rapidly and easily by counting homogenization-resistant spermatid nuclei in cytometer chambers. Quantification is particularly useful in detecting no-effect levels.

12.5.5 Hormone Assays

Disturbance of spermatogenesis is likely to result in altered circulating levels of androgens and gonadotrophins. Their usefulness as a marker of damage is limited by their baseline variability. LH is secreted in a pulsatile manner, consequently testosterone levels are also pulsatile, giving rise to very wide normal ranges. This can be overcome by direct stimulation of the Leydig cells using human chorionic gonadotrophin (hCG) injection as a substitute for LH stimulation. Damage to the seminiferous epithelium is also accompanied by raised serum FSH levels and in general, the severity of damage is correlated with the rise in FSH levels. Quantitative radioimmunoassay of FSH may therefore be used as an indirect, clinical assessment of spermatogenic injury. Hormonal assays provide a convenient clinical technique to assess spermatogenic and Leydig cell function, but they are best employed as an adjunct to other studies which address the primary cause of damage.

12.5.6   *Biochemical Indices of Toxicity*

There are a great many potential biochemical markers of cellular function which could be used to test for toxicity. The Sertoli cell produces lactate and pyruvate for use by the germ cells in energy production, it also produces seminiferous tubule fluid for sperm transport plus a vast number of proteins and peptides including androgen binding protein and transferrin. Epididymal function could be tested by measuring the production of glycerylphosphorylcholine. However, these are all very specific markers of function which are not generally suitable as broad screening techniques; they are better employed in mechanistic investigations, perhaps utilizing *in vitro* techniques where cellular interactions can be carefully controlled.

The use of plasma or urinary enzymes as markers of spermatogenic disturbance has great potential as a clinical monitor for human occupational health and in animal toxicity studies. LDH-C4, the testis-specific isozyme of lactate dehydrogenase, can be measured in plasma and has been shown to be increased by testicular damage induced by **glycol ether** and **DNB** [33]. Urinary creatine measured as a creatine/creatinine ratio may also be a useful and more sensitive biomarker for testicular damage, since it has been shown to be raised consistently by a number of testicular toxicants [34].

12.5.7   **In vitro** *Techniques*

Isolation of the individual components of the reproductive tract, with the removal of the complex cellular interactions within the testis, has many advantages when trying to understand the mechanisms of toxicity. Leydig cells and Sertoli cells can be isolated and cultured, individual types of germ cells can be separated and studied in suspension. Co-cultures can be prepared with Sertoli and germ cells or with Leydig and peritubular cells. Lengths of intact isolated tubules can be maintained for short periods of time. The use of these cell systems is invaluable in studying chemically induced changes in cell physiology, but their prime advantage is also their major drawback in that cellular interactions, which are absent from the *in vitro* situation, may totally alter the *in vivo* response.

Metabolism is also an important consideration; the parent compound may require metabolism before being active *in vitro*. Although a toxicant may reach the testis, it may not pass the blood–tubule barrier and, therefore, may not reach the germ cells or the Sertoli cells. Exposure of these cells *in vitro* may not therefore be appropriate. Because of these considerations, *in vitro* techniques are not suitable as a general toxicology screen. Application of an *in vitro* test to model an *in vivo* situation requires the definition of appropriate criteria for the evaluation of toxicity. If the target cell has been identified and a specific parameter, which is a good index of toxicity *in vivo*, can be applied to the *in vitro* system, e.g. germ cell exfoliation, then the appropriate culture system can be used to screen whether members of a chemical series are active or inactive.

12.5.8 *Choice of Tests*

The number and complexity of the tests chosen to assess male reproductive toxicity must be determined by the objectives of the investigation. Rapid, cost-effective and reproducible tests which measure a battery of endpoints should be used to screen large numbers of novel compounds. With such tests, a negative response should indicate a low probability of an effect being seen. Testing of new products for regulatory approval requires that the route and levels of exposure be relevant to potential human exposure. Depending on the duration or expected risk of exposure, functional and morphological studies with qualitative and quantitative data are necessary. If an effect is seen, a threshold dose will need to be established and detailed mechanistic studies may be appropriate to evaluate its relevance to man. For reviewing chemicals or products already on the market, a rapid screening procedure is required to prioritize chemicals for further study, and epidemiological investigations of exposed populations form an important part of such studies.

12.6 Conclusions

The production and delivery of fertile sperm into the female reproductive tract relies on the complex interaction of hormones, neural pathways and cellular functions. This provides a wealth of potential sites for toxicological disruption and requires a broad approach in order to investigate them effectively.

Most toxicants which affect the testis show cell specificity, but the interdependence of the various cell types invariably results in a range of secondary effects. Separation of primary and secondary effects requires careful investigation using time-course studies and an adequate knowledge of normal structure and physiology to interpret the syndrome of changes.

Morphological responses to and functional consequences of injury depend on the cell type damaged. Sertoli cells appear very sensitive to biochemical perturbations but very resistant to lethal injury. The resistance of the stem cell spermatogonia to damage means that injury to the rest of the germ cell complement is frequently reversible, given sufficient time for the spermatogonia to repopulate the seminiferous epithelium.

Testing for toxicological effects on the various aspects of the reproductive process is best carried out using multiple endpoints. Fertility studies, particularly in rodents, are relatively insensitive but are good for detecting genotoxic damage. Morphological studies are one of the most reliable and sensitive methods if carried out by an experienced investigator. Sperm studies provide useful quantitative data but can be difficult to interpret. Finally, metabolic studies and *in vitro* studies are essential if mechanistic explanations are sought.

Extrapolation of results from laboratory animals to man is fraught with difficulties. The absence of reliable data showing whether animal testicular toxicants have similar effects in man prevents conclusions being drawn, but the experience with **dibromochloropropane** and the multispecies sensitivity of chemicals such as the **glycol ethers** suggests there is a real hazard to man. Since there are far more similarities than differences between the reproductive systems of rodents and man, and man has a vastly reduced functional reserve of sperm, agents causing concern in rats should give cause for concern in humans.

References

1. CARLSEN, E., GIWERCMAN, A., KEIDING, N. and SKAKKEBAEK, N.E. (1992) Evidence for decreasing quality of semen during past 50 years, *British Medical Journal*, **305**, 609–613.

2. SCHRAG, S.D. and DIXON, R.L. (1985) Occupational exposures associated with male reproductive dysfunction, *Annual Review of Pharmacological Toxicology*, **25**, 567–592.

3. RUSSELL, L.D. and GRISWOLD, M.D. (Eds) (1992) *The Sertoli Cell*, Clearwater, FL: Cache River Press.

4. KNOBIL, E. and NEIL, J.D. (Eds) (1988) *The Physiology of Reproduction*, New York: Raven Press.

5. LAMB, J.C. and FOSTER, P.M.D. (Eds) (1988) *Physiology and Toxicology of Male Reproduction*, San Diego: Academic Press.

6. WALLER, D.P., KILLINGER, J.M. and ZANEFELD, L.J.D. (1985) Physiology and toxicology of the male reproductive tract, in THOMAS, J.A., KORRACH, K.S. and MCLACHLAN, J.A. (Eds) *Endocrine Toxicology. Target Organ Toxicology Series*, pp. 269–334, New York: Raven Press.

7. CREASY, D.M. and FOSTER, P.M.D. (1991) Male reproductive system, in HASCHEK, W.A. and ROUSSEAUX, C.G. (Eds) *Handbook of Toxicologic Pathology*, pp. 829–887, London: Academic Press.

8. RUSSELL, L.D., ETTLIN, R.A., SINHAHIKIM, A.P. and CLEGG, E.D. (1990) *Histological and Histopatholgical Evaluation of the Testis*, Clearwater, FL: Cache River Press.

9. LEBLOND, C.P. and CLERMONT, Y. (1952) Definition of the stages of the cycle of the seminiferous epithelium in the rat, *Annals of the New York Academy of Sciences*, **55**, 548–573.

10. AMANN, R.P. (1986) Detection of alterations in testicular and epididymal function in laboratory animals, *Environmental Health Perspectives*, **70**, 149–158.

11. HESS, R.A., SCHAFFER, D.J., EROSCHENKO, V.P. and KEEN, J.E. (1990) Frequency of the stages in the cycle of the seminiferous epithelium in the rat, *Biology of Reproduction*, **43**, 517–524.

12. PARVINEN, M., VINKHO, K.K. and TOPPARI, J. (1986) Cell interactions during the cycle of the seminiferous epithelium, *International Reviews in Cytology*, **104**, 115–129.

13. MEISTRICH, M.L. (1984) Stage-specific sensitivity of spermatogonia to different chemotherapeutic drugs, *Biomedical and Pharmacological Therapeutics*, **38**, 137–142.

14. MCLAREN, T.T., FOSTER, P.M.D. and SHARPE, R.M. (1993) Identification of stage-specific changes in protein secretion by isolated seminiferous tubules from the rat following exposure to either *m*-dinitrobenzene or nitrobenzene, *Fundamental and Applied Toxicology*, **21**, 384–392.

15. RUSSELL, L.D., MALONE, J.P. and MACCURDY, D.S. (1981) Effect of the microtubule disrupting agents, colchicine and vinblastine on seminiferous tubule structure of the rat, *Tissue and Cell*, **13**, 349–367.

16. BOEKELHEIDE, K., NEELY, M.D. and SIOUSSAT, T.M. (1989) The Sertoli cell cytoskeleton: a target for toxicant-induced germ cell loss, *Toxicology and Applied Pharmacology*, **101**, 373–389.

17. AITKEN, R.J., CLARKSON, J.S. and FISHEL, S. (1989) Generation of reactive oxygen species, lipid peroxidation, and human sperm function, *Biology of Reproduction*, **40**, 183–197.

18. CHAPIN, R.E. and WILLIAMS, J. (1989) Mechanistic approaches in the study of testicular toxicity: toxicants that affect the endocrine regulation of the testis, *Toxicologic Pathology*, **17**, 446–451.

19. ROBERTS, A., RENWICK, A.G., FORD, G., CREASY, D.M. and GAUNT, I. (1989) The metabolism and testicular toxicity of cyclohexylamine in rats and mice during chronic dietary administration, *Toxicology and Applied Pharmacology*, **98**, 216–229.

20. WOKING, P.K. (1989) Mechanistic approaches in the study of testicular toxicity: agents that directly affect the testis, *Toxicologic Pathology*, **17**, 452–456.

21. CHAPIN, R.E., PHELPS, J.L., SOMKUTI, S.G., HEINDEL, J.J. and BURKA, L.T. (1990) The interaction of Sertoli and Leydig cells in the testicular toxicity of tri-*o*-cresyl phosphate, *Toxicology and Applied Pharmacology*, **104**, 483–495.

22. GEORGELLIS, A., PARVINEN, M. and RYDSTROM, J. (1989) Cell-specific metabolic activation of 7,12-dimethylbenz[a]anthracene in rat testis. Inhibition of stage-specific DNA synthesis in rat spermatogenic cells by polycyclic aromatic hydrocarbons, *Chemico-Biological Interactions*, **72**, 65–92.

23. SHARPE, R.M., MADDOCKS, S., MILLAR, M., KERR, J.B., SAUNDERS, P.T.K. and MCKINNELL, C. (1992) Testosterone and spermatogenesis: identification of stage-specific androgen-regulated proteins secreted by adult rat seminiferous tubules, *Journal of Andrology*, **13**, 172–184.

24. AOKI, A. and HOFFER, A.P. (1978) Re-examination of the lesions in rat testis caused by cadmium, *Biology of Reproduction*, **18**, 579–591.

25. PRENTICE, D.E. and MEIKLE, A.W. (1995) A review of drug-induced Leydig cell hyperplasia and neoplasia in the rat and some comparisons with man, *Human and Experimental Toxicology*, **14**, 562–572.

26. ITO, N. and SHIRAI, T. (1990) Tumours of the accessory male sex organs, in TUROSOV, V. and MOHR, U. (Eds) *Pathology of Tumours in Laboratory Animals, Vol. I: Tumours of the Rat*, pp. 421–443, IARC Scientific Publications No. 99, Lyons: IARC.

27. VOUK, V.B. and SHEEHAN, P.J. (Eds) (1983) *Methods for Assessing the Effects of Chemicals on Reproductive Functions*, SCOPE 20, New York: John Wiley and Sons.

28. HARRIS, M.W., CHAPIN, R.E., LOCKHART, A.C. and JOKINEN, M.P. (1992) Assessment of a short-term reproductive and developmental toxicity screen, *Fundamental and Applied Toxicology*, **19**, 186–196.

29. WILLIAMS, J., GLADEN, B.C., TURNER, T.W., SCHRADER, S.M. and CHAPIN, R.E. (1991) The effects of ethylene dibromide on semen quality and fertility in the rabbit: evaluation of a model for human seminal characteristics, *Fundamental and Applied Toxicology*, **16**, 697–700.

30. LINDER, R.E., STRADER, L.F., SLOTT, V.L. and SUAREZ, J.D. (1992) Endpoints of spermatotoxicity in the rat after short duration exposure to fourteen reproductive toxicants, *Reproductive Toxicology*, **6**, 491–505.

31. AMANN, R.P. and BERNDTSON, W.E. (1986) Assessment of procedures for screening agents for effects on male reproduction: effects of dibromochloropropane on the rat, *Fundamental and Applied Toxicology*, **7**, 244–255.

32. ZENICK, H. and GOEDEN, H. (1988) Evaluation of copulatory behaviour and sperm in rats: role in reproductive risk assessment, in LAMB, J.C. and FOSTER, P.M.D. (Eds), *Physiology and Toxicology of Male Reproduction*, pp. 179–201, San Diego: Academic Press.

33. READER, S.C.I., SHINGLES, C. and STONARD, M.D. (1988) Testis specific isozyme LDH-C4 activities in rat plasma and testis following acute exposure to 1,3-DNB and EGME: a novel marker of testicular damage, *Human Toxicology*, **7**, 227.

34. MOORE, N.P., GRAY, T.J.B., CREASY, D.M. and TIMBRELL, J.A. (1992) Urinary creatine profiles after administration of cell-specific testicular toxicants to the rat, *Archives of Toxicology*, **66**, 435–442.

13

The Female Reproductive System

DAVID J. LEWIS and CHIRUKANDATH GOPINATH

13.1 Introduction

Although not a common target organ in toxicity studies, an increasing number of compounds are being found to result in malfunction of the female reproductive system. Many of these effects are detected and investigated in specific reproductive safety studies, but some are also identified in routine regulatory toxicity trials. These latter studies do not involve the ultimate test of reproductive function, i.e. birth, and therefore, toxicological pathologists are charged with the routine assessment of morphological changes.

Control of the female reproductive cycle involves the hypothalamus, pituitary and the gonads themselves. Interference by an exogenous compound at any of these levels may result in profound effects. In addition, compounds may exert direct effects on the ovaries.

Many non-neoplastic ovarian lesions are characterized by an increase or decrease in the different major tissue components, i.e. corpora lutea, the varying stages of developing follicles, and the interstitial gland. Although an increase or decrease in these components suggests they should be relativly simple to detect microscopically, this is not always true, as complications of oestrus cycle stage, and the effects of animal age often interfere.

In contrast to the non-neoplastic lesions described above, in which the origin of the affected tissue component is readily identifiable, neoplastic lesions are not always so clearly differentiated. This is due to the pleuripotential nature of ovarian tissue and its ability to manifest as a wide diversity of cell types not normally found in the mature ovary, e.g. Sertoli cell tumours and germ cell tumours.

In contrast to the ovaries, changes in the uterus, cervix and vagina tend to be relatively straightforward because of the less complex histological structure.

The aim of this chapter is to describe the various non-neoplastic and neoplastic lesions which arise, either spontaneously or induced, in the organs and tissues of the female reproductive tract, and to give a brief insight into the possible mechanisms responsible.

13.2 Anatomy, Histology and Physiology

The morphology of the female genital tract varies considerably during the life of an animal for several reasons. The different parts of the tract are constantly responding to the trophic influences from the ovaries and indirectly from the pituitary gland. The morphology also alters according to the age of the animal, e.g. prepuberty, sexual maturity and senility, all of which reveal differing features due to the altered endocrine functions. Furthermore, during adulthood, the morphology of the female genital tract shows cyclical changes according to the different phases of the oestrous cycle. A good knowledge of the morphological features at different phases of the oestrous cycle is essential for the interpretation of treatment-related changes in toxicity studies. There are also marked interspecies variations. Rodents have a very short oestrous cycle with comparatively few gross changes. Primates have approximately monthly menstrual cycles, and dogs have seasonal (biannual) oestrous cycles with prolonged resting periods (anoestrus) between cycles. In primates and dogs the cyclical changes affect the weights and size of the reproductive tract markedly.

13.2.1 *Ovary*

The ovaries of most smaller laboratory species are completely or partially enclosed within a bursa, whereas in other species such as man they are free in the peritoneum [1]. The ovary is a complex organ with three major functions: production of fertile oocytes, synthesis of steroid hormones, and synthesis of regulatory proteins [2]. These complex functions are reflected in the diversity of histological structures and their constituent cell types. Although some species differences occur in the histological appearance of the ovary, there is a basic pattern, as would be expected considering the universal functions. Three main histological structures may be identified: the follicle (which contains the oocyte), the corpus luteum, and the interstitial gland.

The ovarian surface is covered by an inconspicuous layer of cells which are derived from the same peritoneal mesothelium which comprises the müllerian ducts [3]. Although commonly referred to as an epithelium, it has been suggested that the term ovarian mesothelium would be more appropriate [4]. However, this has not been widely accepted, but should be borne in mind when interpreting some pathological changes. The histological appearance of the surface epithelium varies with the underlying structure, i.e. a squamous epithelium overlying corpora lutea and pre-ovulatory graafian follicles, but a cuboidal or columnar epithelium over small follicles.

The primordial follicles are formed during embryonic development, by migration of germ cells from the yolk sac. These follicles represent a finite reserve from which all subsequent follicles develop [5]. A species-dependent number of follicles ripen during each oestrous or menstrual cycle in preparation for ovulation, e.g. in rats 10 to 12 and in humans 1 [5]. Thus, many follicles remain in a dormant state for much of the reproductive life of the animal, but the total number of follicles decreases with age [6]. Little is known about the physiological stimulation of primordial follicles. Following the initiation of development of primordial follicles, the primary oocyte increases in size and the single layer of granulosa cells surrounding it proliferate to form three or four concentric layers. The zona pellucida forms between the peripheral granulosa cells and the central oocyte. The granulosa cells continue to proliferate, becoming densely packed and forming secondary follicles, and the transition to a tertiary follicle is characterized by the development of a central cavity or an antrum [7]. Antrum formation results in the oocyte becoming enclosed in an aggregation of granulosa cells and it is then known as a graafian follicle. The recruitment of large follicles is controlled by the follicle stimulating hormone (FSH) surge [8]. During the development and enlargement of the follicles, the surrounding stroma becomes compressed and forms the theca. The theca subsequently develops into two layers: the theca interna and the theca externa. The externa is composed of a thin layer of concentrically arranged and compressed connective tissue with elongated cells, whereas the interna is made up of polyhedral cells with the ultrastructural characteristics for steroid production. The process of follicular development is of variable time scale; in rodents approximately 5 weeks whereas in humans it may take six months [5].

Only relatively few follicles reach the later stages of development and ultimately ovulate, the majority undergo regression (atresia) [2]. Under normal conditions, small follicles are rarely seen to undergo atresia, whereas in follicles of the larger antral stage of development it is more commonly seen [9]. In fact atretic follicles are a prominent feature of adult rat ovaries [9] and approximately half of the large follicles show some evidence of necrosis [8]. It has been suggested that atresia is initiated by the decrease in FSH as it has been shown to be prevented by the administration of pregnant mares' serum gonadotrophin [8].

After ovulation, corpora lutea are formed. The granulosa cells become luteinized and undergo hyperplasia and hypertrophy [2]. The corpus luteum may be regarded as a transient endocrine gland [10] and in the absence of pregnancy, it regresses. The remnants of corpora lutea are known as corpora albicantia and in some species these may show hyalinization and fibrosis, but in others (e.g. the rat) complete resolution is usual [11].

Although the follicles and corpora lutea attract most attention during histological examination, the ovaries also contain interstitial gland tissue. In some species, such as the rat, this occupies a substantial portion of the ovary [2]. Interstitial cells may be classified into several distinct morphological types [12]. In rats the interstitial cells are believed to originate primarily from the theca of atretic follicles [2]. The cells are large and polygonal with round nuclei and significant amounts of eosinophilic foamy cytoplasm. They have an ultrastructural appearance characteristic of steroid-producing cells and are believed to secrete androgens [13]. The cells have been shown to undergo cyclic morphological changes [13]. In addition to steroid synthesis it has been suggested that the interstitial gland is, in the rat, the site of production of ovarian growth factors, at least some of which have a mitogenic effect on granulosa cells [2].

13.2.2 *Uterus, Cervix and Vagina*

The morphologies of the vagina, cervix and uterus vary between the four main phases of the oestrous cycle: proestrus, oestrus, metoestrus and dioestrus. Proestrus and oestrus represent the follicular phase of the ovary with oestrogenic predominance, while metoestrus and dioestrus are in the luteal phase of the ovary, with progestational predominance. The late end of dioestrus and the anoestrous phases (in species such as the dog) represent a prolonged period of rest or quiescence. The morphology of the genital tract during the prepubertal age often resembles the appearance during the resting phase.

The uterus is bicornuate in rodents and dogs, while it is pyriform in primates. The uterine wall consists of endometrium, myometrium and a serous coat. The endometrium is lined by epithelium and contains basal and superficial glands embedded in varying amounts of stroma. The uterine lumen and the thickness of the endometrial and myometrial layers vary considerably according to ovarian trophic stimulation. The vagina and posterior half of the cervix are lined by stratified squamous epithelium and the thickness, folding and keratin deposition of this epithelium changes according to the phase of the oestrous cycle.

13.3 Biochemical and Cellular Mechanisms of Toxicity

13.3.1 *Ovary*

Non-neoplastic lesions

Oocyte destruction is readily induced by **X-irradiation** and compounds such as **cyclophosphamide**. Primordial follicles and small oocytes are especially radiosensitive, whereas growing follicles are susceptible to **cyclophosphamide** [14]. There are some species differences in the sensitivity of oocytes to **X-irradiation**, the mouse being more sensitive than the rat [12]. Unilateral injection of **benzo[a]pyrene**, in mice, destroys oocytes in the injected organ, but not in the contralateral ovary, which suggests metabolic transformation [12].

High doses of **oestrogens**, **progestogens** (or combinations of these) for prolonged periods induces ovarian atrophy in rodents, by feedback suppression of gonadotrophins [12,15]. **Hypophysectomy** induces a similar appearance [9].

Arrest of follicular development has been reported following the administration of a **leuteinizing hormone-releasing hormone** [14]. The recruitment of follicles from the pool of small follicles into the pool of larger follicles is inhibited.

A number of chemicals block ovulation by interfering with either the production or action of ovarian steroids, or pituitary hypothalamic hormones [16].

Transient deviations in gonadotrophins result in delayed luteolysis and cause the persistence of corpora lutea which is detected as an increase in their numbers [15]. Many compounds cause either elevation or reduction in prolactin levels [17]. Elevated prolactin levels result in increased numbers of corpora lutea. **RU486**, a progesterone antagonist, causes an increase in luteal mass and may act by increasing prolactin secretion [12].

Some novel **antihistamines** tested in our laboratory have been found to reduce the numbers of corpora lutea in rats. The histamine liberator, **compound 48/80**, induces ovulation, and this effect could be blocked by **antihistamines** [18]. It has also been shown that an ovarian hyperstimulation syndrome induced in rabbits with **chorionic gonadotrophin** could be blocked by **antihistamines** [19].

Superovulation can be induced in adult hamsters by **pregnant mares' serum (PMS)** and in rats by **PMS** followed by **human chorionic gonadotrophin** or **leuteinizing hormone (LH)** [20]. This is brought about by increased recruitment of large follicles during the oncoming cycle [5, 8] and is associated with a decrease in the number of atretic follicles. **LH**-induced superovulation in the hamster is mediated by histamine and is associated with increased ovarian blood flow [21].

Luteinization of follicles with retention of ova occurs in rats treated with **LH** [11] and also with **SKF 86002-A$_2$** – an inhibitor of prostaglandin and leukotriene synthesis. The latter's effects may be a result of a direct action on the ovary, possibly by suppression of the response to gonadotrophin, retardation of follicular growth and decreased oestrogen synthesis [22].

Follicular cysts may be associated with **oestrogenic compounds**, high levels of **β-stimulants** and **bromocriptine** administration in rats [15]. The cysts may develop from preovulating follicles which fail to ovulate.

Vacuolar degeneration of corpora lutea has been described in cynomolgus monkeys treated with an **acyl-CoAH:cholesterol acyltransferase inhibitor** [23].

Sertoliform tubular hyperplasia of the ovary in aged rats [24, 25] is common in some strains, but rarely observed in other laboratory species. These tubules can be induced by **X-irradiation, hypophysectomy**, and the administration of **growth hormone** and some **compounds with antiandrogenic properties** [15].

There are a few reports of induced changes in the interstitial glands of the ovary. Lipidosis of hypertrophic interstitial cells is induced in rats by **triaryl phosphates** [26]. **LH** administration causes hyperplasia and hypertrophy of the interstitial cells, [13] as does prenatal administration of **diethylstilboestrol** to mice. These changes may be associated with increased levels of androgens. Atrophy of the interstitial glands may occur following **hypophysectomy** [27].

It is widely known that aged female rats rarely show regular oestrous cycles, however, it is perhaps surprising that the cycles may cease in some rat strains as early as 6 months of age [28]. A wide variety of agents and treatments reactivate regular oestrous cycles in aged, constant oestrous rats. These include: **progesterone, adrenocorticotrophic hormone, vitamin E, stress (cold or ether), levodopa, lergotrile, iproniazid**, and **adrenaline** [29]. **Electric stimulation** of the preoptic area of the hypothalamus has a similar effect [29]. In addition, ovaries from young rats transplanted into old rats cease to cycle, and the transfer of ovaries from old to young ovariectomized rats results in the restoration of the oestrus cycle [29]. It is suggested that cessation of cycles is due to catecholamine deficiency in the hypothalamus which results in decreased levels of LH and FSH [29].

Neoplastic lesions

Most reported treatments which induce ovarian tumours in rodents involve destruction of the follicular granulosa cells and oocytes with a consequent increased secretion of pituitary gonadotrophins [12].

Ovarian tumours, in rodents, are induced by several different methods, however, little work has been performed on species such as the dog and non-human primates. In rodents **irradiation, hormonal treatment, transplantation to the spleen**, and **chemical carcinogens** are also known to induce tumours.

The mechanism by which chemical carcinogens induce ovarian tumours is largely unknown. Sertoli cell tumours of the ovary are induced in rats by *N*-ethyl-*N*-nitrosourea (**ENU**) by the intraperitoneal route and by oral **ENU** or *N*-propyl-*N*-nitrosourea. Adenocarcinomas arising from down-growths of the surface epithelium of the ovary follow direct application of **dimethylbenz[a]anthracene** or ***N*-methyl-*N*-nitrososurea**.

Fibromas of the ovary are only rarely reported in laboratory animals, but up to 7-years treatment with the non-progestational androgenic steroid, **milbolerone** induces this tumour in dogs [12]. An interesting feature of these neoplasms is that they were induced at a pharmacological dose level of the compound, but not at exaggerated doses [12].

The induction of rat mesovarial leiomyomas is a compound- and species-specific phenomenon. **Sympathomimetic agents**, which possess β_2-activity, induce these tumours in long-term studies [29]. It appears likely that the tumours arise due to the pharmacological action of the compounds, i.e. acting on β_2-adrenoceptors in the mesovarial smooth muscle cells [12]. Further evidence is provided by the administration of the β_2-blocker, **propranolol**, simultaneously with **salbutamol**, [30] a regimen which prevents tumour development.

13.3.2 *Uterus*

Non-neoplastic lesions

Endometrial glandular proliferation is a common response to **oestrogens** in most laboratory animal species. However, in the dog this effect is usually a **progestational** response. Prolonged treatment with **synthetic progestogens** and **progesterone** in dogs results in endometrial hyperplasia and mucometra, with the frequent complication of pyometra. **Oestrogens**, on the other hand, cause endometrial hyperplasia in rodents, rabbits and primates [31]. **Dopamine agonists** result in hyperoestrogenism in the rat leading to endometrial hyperplasia and endometritis. **Oestrogens** are also reported to induce endometriosis in rabbits and adenomyosis in mice.

Squamous metaplasia of the endometrial lining and glands of the uterus occurs in rats in chronic **oestrogen** treatment, in **vitamin A deficiency** and on exposure to **chlorinated hydrocarbons** or **polychlorinated biphenyls** [31]. Endometrial atrophy, often accompanied by atrophy of the myometrium, is a response to ovarian inhibition. This may occur directly or indirectly, i.e. mediated via the pituitary. Long-term treatment with **progestogens** in primates, treatment with **butyrophenones** and **androgens** in dogs, and **progestogens** and **neuroleptics** in rodents are known to result in uterine atrophy [15, 32]. Decidualization in the non-pregnant uterus can be induced by **intrauterine devices** and in the rat, **placement of foreign materials** in the uterine lumen can induce decidualization. In this last case, progesterone priming appears to be necessary. Systemic toxicity studies with **growth hormone** in rats, and prolonged **progestational** treatment in monkeys are also known to induce decidualization [15]. The intrauterine application of **histamine**, **prostaglandins** and **oily fluids** can also result in a decidual reaction in the rat [33].

Myometrial hypertrophy and hyperplasia have been reported in mice treated with β-**agonists**. The changes appear to be related to the pharmacological action of the adrenoreceptors in the myometrium. This effect can be prevented by the co-administration of β-blockers [34]. Prolonged treatment with certain **oestrogenic compounds** to dogs has resulted in uterine enlargement due to pronounced myometrial hypertrophy. The administration of **synthetic oestrogens** like **stilboestrol** is also known to induce a villous proliferation of the serosa (mesothelial hyperplasia) in the female genital tract in dogs [15].

Neoplastic lesions

Endometrial adenocarcinomas in rats can be induced by **dopamine agonists** such as **bromocriptine** [35]. **Dopaminergic agents** inhibit prolactin secretion, resulting in hypoprolactinaemia, luteolysis and ovarian follicle development in older rats. This effect leads to oestrogen predominance, endometrial overstimulation, endometrial hyperplasia and tumour formation. The mechanism is non-genotoxic and directly due to hormonal imbalance; it is of specific relevance to the rat. **Synthetic oestrogens** are known to induce endometrial carcinomas in rabbits, and certain strains of mice [36]. Genotoxic carcinogens such as **3-methyl-cholanthrene** are reported to cause adenocarcinomas and adenoacanthomas in rats and mice [37].

Endometrial stromal cell sarcoma can be induced in rodents following treatment with **testosterone** or **norethandrolone**. These tumours are also induced by local or systemic administration of various **genotoxic compounds** [12, 31, 38].

Smooth muscle tumours (leiomyoma and leiomyosarcoma) arising from the myometrium may be induced in mice given prolonged treatment with certain β_2-agonists. The tumours occur by virtue of the exaggerated pharmacological action of the compound and can be prevented by the co-administration of β-blocking agents [12]. Smooth muscle tumours are reported in the uteri of dogs treated with certain **oestrogenic oral contraceptives** [39].

13.3.3 *Cervix and Vagina*

The vaginal epithelium, and to a lesser extent the cervical epithelium, undergo continuous changes during the oestrous cycle in accordance with changes in hormone dominance. Thus hormonal imbalances result in exaggerated expressions. Excessive cornification, and hyperkeratosis with mucosal oedema, occur as an expression of oestrogenic potential in the vagina of several species. **Oestrogen** treatment may result in hyperplasia and hyperkeratosis of the cervix in both mice and primates. In primates, **oestrogens** also result in squamous metaplasia of the anterior end of the cervix. Mucification of the vaginal epithelium is a progestational response. However, long-term treatment with **progestogens** results in vaginal atrophy in dogs and primates. Other agents inhibiting ovarian action also produce atrophy of the vagina.

As the vaginal mucosa responds sensitively to various irritants, rabbits are used to titrate (measure) the irritant potential of many test substances by recording various inflammatory and degenerative responses to the intravaginal application of such substances.

Long-term treatment of certain strains of mice with synthetic **oestrogens** like **stilboestrol** produces cervical adenosis [12, 40], whereas in primates the long-term treatment with **progestogens** results in a marked overproduction of cervical mucus [15].

13.4 Morphological Responses to Injury

13.4.1 *Ovary*

The range of morphological responses which may be detected in the ovary is diverse and reflects the previously described histological features. These changes may be detected in the surface epithelium, the follicles, the corpora lutea and/or the interstitial glands.

When interpreting changes it is important to have a thorough working knowledge of the histological features during various phases of the oestrous or menstrual cycles [15], as some treatment-induced changes are only detected as exacerbations or perturbations of cyclical features [15].

Non-neoplastic lesions

Epithelial (mesothelial) hyperplasia The surface epithelial cells proliferate and produce papillomatous or small polypoid projections from the ovarian surface. These structures have a distinctly mesothelial appearance and may become extensive, or minor and focal.

Tubular hyperplasia In this lesion the surface epithelial cells also proliferate, but in this case it manifests as cords or tubules of surface cells localized in the outer cortex of the ovary. The lesion may range from a few isolated down-growths to a more extensive diffuse proliferation which occupies a large proportion of the ovarian structure.

Oocyte destruction The developing oocytes may show destruction with evidence of pyknosis and cytolysis. This predominantly affects the primordial follicles and small oocytes, but in some cases the growing follicles may be more sensitive.

Follicular atresia As described previously, a proportion of maturing follicles normally undergo atresia during each cycle. However, the number of atretic follicles may be increased although the morphological features of individual follicles may be indistinguishable from those of control animals. In these cases it is often useful to quantify the number of affected follicles in control and treated groups [12]. Criteria for distinguishing atretic follicles have been described [9].

Arrest of follicular development In some cases, reduced numbers of developing follicles may be detected [14]. This effect may range from a virtual absence of graafian follicles to a slight effect which may only be detected by detailed quantification of the stages of follicular development. A block on ovulation may also be detected by the presence of large haemorrhagic follicles containing ova [21].

Atrophy Ovarian atrophy may be detected macroscopically and is characterized by the absence of well-developed follicles and corpora lutea, condensed stroma, ceroid pigment, and reduced interstitial gland [15]. The early stages of ovarian atrophy may be difficult to assess due to some continued follicular development and persistence of corpora lutea [11].

Supraovulation Increased follicular recruitment is detected morphologically by the presence of increased numbers of large follicles and upon closer examination by a decrease in the number of atretic follicles [5, 8]. The recruited and atretic follicles are morphologically indistinct from those of normal animals.

414

Follicular luteinization   In some cases large follicles may appear luteinized without previous ovulation having taken place. The luteinized follicles may sometimes appear cystic and retained ova are sometimes present.

Follicular cysts   Cystic follicles and follicular cysts are generally believed to arise from antral follicles. The affected follicles fail to ovulate. Polycystic ovaries are characterized by the presence of numerous large, thin-walled cysts. The cysts are composed of a narrow band, or a single layer, of granulosa cells. In some cases it is difficult to identify the cysts conclusively as being of follicular origin as the granulosa cell content is negligible and grossly flattened. Affected ovaries contain few or no corpora lutea.

Reduction/absence of corpora lutea   Absence of corpora lutea is a common expression of inhibition of ovarian function. Reduced numbers of corpora lutea may often require quantitative assessment for confirmation. In rodents this assessment may be complicated by the normal (variable) cessation of oestrous cycles, with age.

Increased/persistence of corpora lutea   Increased numbers of, and/or persistence of, corpora lutea is a relatively common induced change with a wide variety of compounds. The corpora lutea occupy the vast majority of the ovarian structure and in rodents particularly they may be detected, and quantified macroscopically.

Vacuolar degeneration of corpora lutea   Increased coarse vacuolation with associated foci of cellular degeneration and cholesterol clefts may be detected in the corpora lutea [23].

Sertoliform tubular hyperplasia   Tubules similar to seminiferous tubules have been described in the ovaries of aged rats [41]. These tubules are composed of cells which resemble Sertoli cells [24]. Increased numbers of these tubules may be detected in the ovaries of treated rats. The tubules are irregular in shape, pale staining with basally situated grooved nuclei.

Interstitial gland hypertrophy/hyperplasia   Increased numbers of hypertrophic, vacuolated interstitial gland cells may become arranged around atretic follicles resulting in a pseudoadenomatous pattern [26]. These cells are surrounded by a fibrovascular stroma.

Interstitial gland atrophy   The interstitial gland cells appear small with decreased amounts of cytoplasm, and dark nuclei.

Restoration of oestrous cycles   In rodents the reproductive lifespan is often remarkably short but variable, with oestrous cycles ceasing in some animals as early as 6 months of age, but being maintained for up to 18 months in others [28]. These changes in ovarian function may be classified into specific stages, i.e. irregular cycles, constant oestrus, constant pseudopregnancy, or anoestrus [27]. A range of histological appearances may be seen in the ovaries of untreated control animals. This may be complicated further by some treatments having the property of restoring cyclic oestrous activity [42]. In such studies it is important to assess the cyclical status of the animals in order to detect induced changes.

Mesovarial smooth muscle hyperplasia Hyperplasia of the smooth muscle of the rat mesovarium may be detected by careful macroscopic observation as nodular or diffuse thickenings [30]. The lesion is characterized by an irregular, poorly circumscribed proliferation of hypertrophic smooth muscle cells.

Neoplastic lesions

Ovarian tumour types reflect the variation in the tissues previously described. That is, distinctive tissue tumour types develop from the surface epithelium, the granulosa and theca cells of the follicles, luteal cells, and the smooth muscle of the ovarian ligament. In addition, due to the pluripotential nature of ovarian germ cells, Sertoli cell tumours may also develop.

Granulosa cell tumour These tumours (Figure 13.1) are composed of small basophilic cells with a clear resemblance to granulosa cells of the follicles, with a stippled nuclear chromatin pattern, arranged in solid sheets, trabecular forms, cords, or pseudofollicular patterns. The tumour cells sometimes show evidence of luteinization or vacuolated cytoplasm. Call–Exner bodies composed of tubular structures with a material positive for periodic acid Schiff stain may infrequently be seen. Granulosa cell tumours are usually benign, but occasionally malignant forms may be detected, with pulmonary metastasis [24].

Luteoma True luteomas are rare. The cells show distinct similarity with the cells of the corpora lutea.

Thecoma Thecal cell tumours are also rare. They are composed of whorls of spindle-shaped cells.

Sertoli cell tumour These tumours (Figure 13.2) are composed of tubules within lumina and palisaded columnar cells. The tubules and cells morphologically resemble the seminiferous tubules and Sertoli cells of the testis.

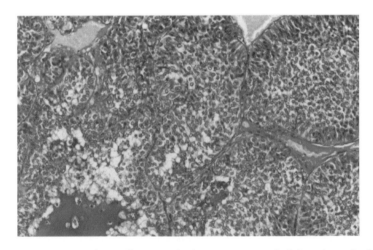

Figure 13.1 Ovarian granulosa cell tumour in the rat, composed of densely packed cells.

Sertoliform tubular adenoma These tumours resemble Sertoli cell tumours, but the nuclei are not basally located, and the cells have abundant cytoplasm sometimes with eosinophilic cytoplasmic inclusions [24]; the cells form solid tubules.

Tubular adenoma/adenocarcinoma These tumours are common in mice and arise from down-growths of the surface epithelium. The cuboidal cells form distinct interlacing tubules.

Papillary cystadenoma/adenocarcinoma The benign form of this tumour is composed of a single round cyst, lined by cuboid/columnar epithelial cells (Figure 13.3), and containing simple to complex arrangements of papillomatous projections. The malignant form is complex with adenomatous and papillomatous patterns with extension beyond the cyst walls.

Malignant mesothelioma These highly malignant tumours show tubulopapillary patterns with stromal hyalinization. Their implantation metastases (Figure 13.4)

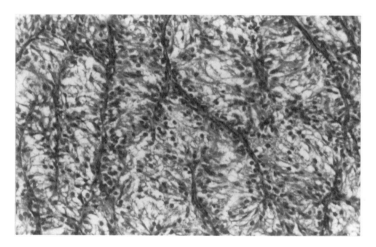

Figure 13.2 Ovarian Sertoli cell tumour from a rat. Note resemblance to seminiferous tubules.

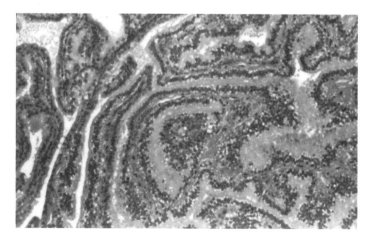

Figure 13.3 Mouse ovarian cystadenoma composed of complex papillary cords.

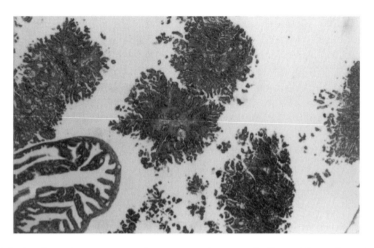

Figure 13.4 Implantation metastases from an ovarian mesothelioma. These deposits sometimes spread widely throughout the abdominal cavity.

spread throughout the surfaces of the abdominal cavity, but often do not show invasion of the underlying tissue.

Mesovarial leiomyoma   Leiomyomas appear as pale nodular masses which form fusiform (spindle shaped), spherical or irregular masses. There is a predilection for the right side [30]. The tumours are composed of interlacing bundles of smooth muscle cells.

Fibroma   These tumours have been reported in dogs [12] and were composed of well-demarcated dense fibrous tissue with sparse fibroblasts. The tumours show no evidence of malignant transformation.

13.4.2   *Uterus*

Toxic responses often mimic the morphological features seen in the different stages of the oestrous cycle but often appear to be suspended in one of the phases.

Non-neoplastic lesions

Endometrial hyperplasia   The endometrial glands and the lining epithelium proliferate. The glands increase in number and they appear more tortuous and basophilic, and are sometimes multilayered. The glandular lumen is increased in size and contains mucus. The endometrial lining becomes increasingly folded and the uterine lumen also contains varying amounts of mucus. Where the hyperplasia is prolonged, there is cystic dilation of the glands resulting in cystic endometrial hyperplasia, a condition which is frequently seen in mice (Figure 13.5). In dogs, the surface glands and lining epithelium are hypertrophied, pale staining and finely vacuolated (Figure 13.6). Endometrial hyperplasia in dogs frequently becomes dominated by mucoid changes, resulting in gross mucoid distension of the uterus often referred to as mucometra.

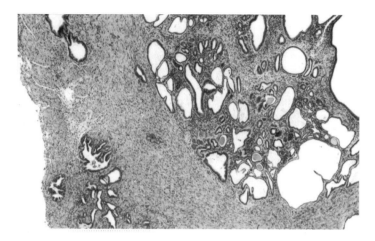

Figure 13.5 Cystic endometrial hyperplasia in the mouse uterus. The endometrial glands are dilated and increased in number. Note islands of endometrial glands in the myometrium (to the left of the photograph) denoting adenomyosis.

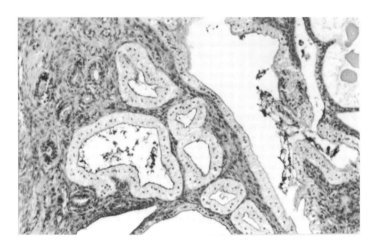

Figure 13.6 Endometrial hyperplasia in the dog uterus. The superficial glands and epithelium are lined by pale-staining hypertrophic cells. The glands are increased in number.

Myometrial hypertrophy and hyperplasia This response is frequently reported in conjunction with endometrial hyperplasia, especially in rodents and dogs, occurring as a focal response. However, myometrial hypertrophy and hyperplasia can also occur as a primary lesion. It can affect the entire circumference of the uterine horn, appearing segmentally or as a focal change. The affected muscle layers are markedly thickened and individual smooth muscle cells are enlarged with abundant sarcoplasm and with distinct and elongated nuclei. In advanced cases, the thickening of the uterine wall causes an apparent reduction in size of the lumen. The hypertrophy is associated with an increase in uterine mass and volume. The lesion is reported in mice, rats and occasionally in dogs.

Squamous metaplasia The endometrial glands and the lining epithelium are usually composed of columnar or cuboidal cells. Under certain conditions, the endometrial lining or the glandular epithelium undergo an abrupt transformation into a stratified squamous epithelium with a tendency for cornification (Figure 13.7), and occasionally there is evidence of keratinization. The lesion is always of a focal distribution. Squamous metaplasia is reported frequently in rats, mice and occasionally monkeys.

Mesothelial proliferation The uterine mesothelium is usually an inconspicuous layer. However, on rare occasions, dog uteri are reported to show proliferative changes of the mesothelium. The serosal layer appears prominent and shows villous or papillary outgrowths, sometimes involving the entire surface (Figure 13.8). Usually this lesion accompanies a similar, but much more florid, reaction in the ovarian mesothelium [15].

Uterine dilation/hydrometra Fluid distension of the uterine horns is a common finding in rodents. To some extent this always occurs as part of the cyclical changes

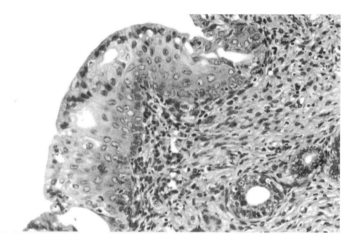

Figure 13.7 Squamous metaplasia in the endometrial lining of the rat uterus. Note the abrupt change into a stratified squamous epithelium.

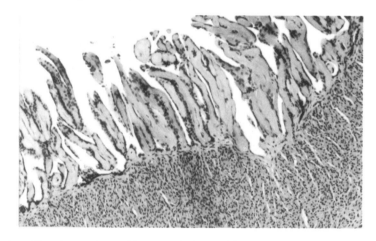

Figure 13.8 Villous hyperplasia of the mesothelium of the dog uterus. Note the serosal surface is thrown into finger-like projections.

420

during oestrus in rodents. Hydrometra denotes cystic dilation of the uterine horns with fluid, which is seen occasionally among aged rodents which have stopped cycling [43]. Cystic dilation of the endometrial glands tends to accompany a dilated uterine lumen.

Endometritis/pyometra Macroscopically, in this condition the affected uterine horns are enlarged, distended with purulent exudate and show varying discolorations. It frequently occurs as a sequel to endometrial hyperplasia in association with excessive mucus production. The lesion becomes complicated due to secondary infection and inflammation. When the exudate becomes purulent, the endometrial glands and the uterine horns are distended with mucopurulent discharge, and the change is referred to as pyometra. The endometrial stroma reveals extensive infiltration by polymorphonuclear cells, plasma cells and lymphoid cells and the superficial glands undergo degeneration, necrosis and erosion. The inflammation often extends into the myometrium. A variety of bacteria is often isolated. This lesion is seen in dogs, rats, mice and rarely in primates.

Atrophy Affected uteri appear small, are reduced in weight, and the diameter is considerably reduced. Atrophy affects the endometrium or can involve all layers of the uterine wall. The endometrium becomes thin, the glands become inconspicuous, reduced in number and appear embedded in a dense compact stroma. The myometrium, when affected, also becomes thin. The smooth muscle cells become smaller, with scanty sarcoplasm and appear packed closely together. The lesion has been reported in rodents, dogs and primates.

Decidualization This is a rare proliferative lesion of the endometrium and is characterized by prominent accumulations of decidual cells in the uterine wall and occurs in response to different stimuli in non-pregnant (usually pseudopregnant) rats. The spontaneous lesion occurs as a nodular growth affecting primarily the endometrium of rats and can be extensive, involving all layers of the uterine wall (Figure 13.9). There is a proliferation of epithelioid cells towards the surface. The lesion contains numerous metrial gland cells which have a granular cytoplasm.

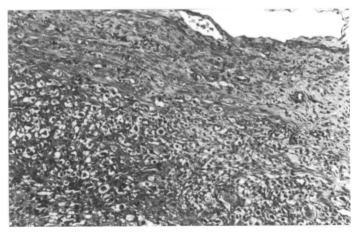

Figure 13.9 Decidualization in the rat uterus. Note the accumulation of epithelioid cells towards the lumina (upper) surface. The lesion involves the entire uterine wall.

Peripherally, there is an abundance of spindle-shaped cells arranged around blood vessels. Some of the induced lesions have a florid appearance and diffuse involvement. The lesion is mostly reported in rats, although on rare occasions it is found in primates where it appears as a superficial plaque-like structure in the endometrium.

Adenomyosis   The extension of a hyperplastic endometrium into the myometrium is known as adenomyosis, and is commonly seen in mice. Care is required in differentiating this finding from malignant changes of the endometrium (Figure 13.5).

Endometriosis   This lesion, usually described in primates, is characterized by islands of viable endometrium located on the serosal surface of the uterus, but may also affect other pelvic structures.

Neoplastic lesions

Uterine/endometrial adenocarcinoma   This is a malignant growth arising from the endometrial epithelium. The main morphological features comprise glandular, tubular, or cord-like structures embedded in a connective tissue stroma. The growth is invasive and often shows evidence of distant metastases. Uterine adenocarcinoma is a low-incidence neoplasm in most laboratory animals except in the rabbit. In rabbits over 2-years old, adenocarcinoma is a frequent finding. Induced endometrial carcinomas are reported in rats, mice and primates.

Squamous cell carcinoma   This is a rare neoplasm of the uterine endometrium, characterized by well-differentiated groups of squamous cells (as nests or cords) embedded in different amounts of stroma.

Adenoacanthoma   The lesion appears as a well-differentiated endometrial adeno-carcinoma with a preponderance of nests of squamous epithelium. Adenoacanthomas are reported mainly in rats.

Leiomyoma   Leiomyoma appears as a well-circumscribed nodular growth in the outer wall of the uterus composed of well-differentiated uniform bundles of smooth muscle fibres, usually with a criss-cross pattern. Leiomyomas are reported in mice and dogs.

Leiomyosarcoma   In addition to the histological features of leiomyoma, a high mitotic index, cellular pleomorphism, poorly defined borders and a tendency for local invasion reveal the malignancy. They are reported in mice.

Endometrial stromal cell sarcoma   This tumour usually occurs as a polypoid mass in the uterine wall depicting poorly differentiated spindle-shaped cells with distinct borders. Cells show pleomorphism and atypia with varying numbers of mitotic figures. The tumour invades the adjacent myometrium and other pelvic structures. It may sometimes arise within a polyp [38]. They are reported in mice.

13.4.3 *Vagina*

Non-neoplastic lesions

Cornification and hyperkeratosis The mucosa becomes thick, rough and appears folded, and is usually associated with a degree of mucosal oedema. There is an increase in the number of cornified cells and cells in the keratin layer (Figure 13.10). The change is seen in all species.

Mucification This is a common change in rodents. The surface epithelium appears columnar with varying proportions of intracytoplasmic mucus production. Multilayering of the epithelium is occasionally seen (Figure 13.11). The change can easily be confirmed by alcian blue staining to demonstrate mucins.

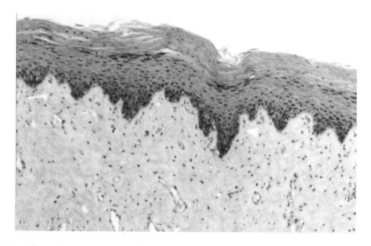

Figure 13.10 Hyperkeratosis in the dog vagina. Note the thick epithelium with prominent cornified layer and excessive keratin.

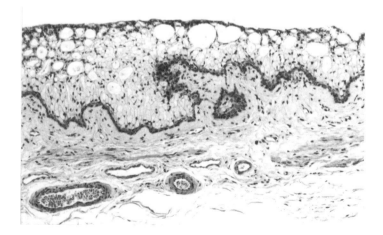

Figure 13.11 Mucification of the rat vaginal epithelium. Note the columnar cells containing clear cytoplasmic mucous inclusions.

Atrophy In vaginal atrophy the mucosa appears very thin and dry. There is a reduction in the number of cells in the epithelium. In extreme cases the epithelium is only one or two layers thick and lined by cuboidal cells. Sometimes microcysts are present (Figure 13.12).

Inflammatory lesions The mucosa is infiltrated with inflammatory cells, sometimes associated with erosion, necrosis and even ulceration. Caution is needed in the interpretation of a mild lesion, as some degree of leucocytic infiltration may appear normally during the dioestrous phase of the oestrus cycle.

Neoplastic lesions

The tumours described are spontaneous and usually not influenced by toxicity studies. As tumours arising in the vagina and cervix are similar they will be considered together.

Squamous cell papilloma These benign tumours are characterized by papillary outgrowths of squamous epithelium.

Squamous cell carcinoma This is a well-differentiated malignant tumour of squamous epithelium with evidence of keratinization. They may show evidence of local invasion, deep within the underlying structures.

Adenocarcinoma This malignant tumour of the endocervix has a distinct glandular pattern. The cells show varying degrees of anaplasia and frank evidence of local invasion.

Adenoacanthoma This is a rare malignant tumour of the cervix which shows clear adenocarcinomatous growth with islands of maligant squamous cells.

Fibroma A discrete connective tissue neoplasm with an abundance of collagen occurring in the wall.

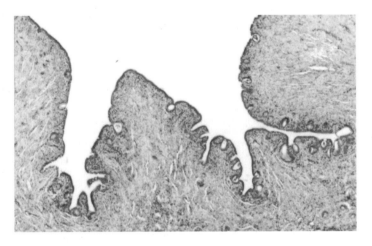

Figure 13.12 Atrophy of the dog vaginal epithelium. Note the very thin epithelial layer which is lined by cuboidal cells.

Fibrosarcoma   This malignant connective tissue tumour, with varying cellularity, is composed of mostly fusiform cells. The tumour shows indistinct borders and may show anaplasia.

Leiomyoma   This is a discrete smooth muscle cell tumour which also occurs in the vaginal wall. The tumours are composed of elongated smooth muscle cells arranged in bundles sometimes in a criss-cross pattern.

13.4.4 *Cervix*

Non-neoplastic lesions

Epithelial hyperplasia, hyperkeratosis and squamous metaplasia   Epithelial hyperplasia, hyperkeratosis and squamous metaplasia of the upper or anterior end of the cervix have been reported in rats and primates.

Mucous distension and adenosis   A type of excessive mucous distension of the cervix has been reported in dogs and primates in long-term studies. A lesion termed adenosis has been reported in mice. The effect is characterized by change in the squamous epithelium into irregular tubular or glandular down-growths which are lined by columnar epithelium. The stroma appears oedematous.

13.5 Testing for Toxicity

The majority of toxicological investigations into the female reproductive system are performed as part of routine regulatory toxicity studies. These involve the systemic administration of a wide variety of compounds. Pathological examination of the ovaries, uterus, cervix and vagina is routinely performed as part of these investigations. This simple approach, especially when combined with organ weight analysis, enables detection of many induced changes. However, the understanding and interpretation of these changes are often more difficult due to interactions of oestrus cycle stage, animal age, species and the complexity of the physiological and biochemical interactions and control mechanisms [12].

Histological examination should include, as far as is possible, consistent reproducible sections to allow subjective comparisons to be drawn between treatment groups and control animals. As mentioned previously, it is clearly important to establish the stage of the oestrous or menstrual cycle of the individual animals, as this has a profound influence on the histological appearance of the tissues. Unless this complication is borne in mind, results may be difficult, if not impossible, to interpret.

If information other than a subjective assessment is required, various semiquantitative methods may be employed. This approach in the ovary may involve: counts of the stages of follicular development [5, 20], counts of numbers of corpora lutea [10] (this may also be performed at necropsy), and counts of the numbers of atretic follicles [9, 14]. In the uterus, quantitative measurements may be made of the endometrium (area/width), myometrium (area/width), and/or the lumen.

Histological examination is generally more reliable than the measurement of serum hormones [11] in the detection of reproductive malfunction due to diurnal, cyclical and stress-induced variations in hormone levels. Multiple, controlled sampling is of benefit in these circumstances.

In addition to systemic administration of exogenous compounds it is also possible to use local application directly into the vagina. The rabbit is commonly used for this irritance assay [11]. A similar assay of oestrogenic activity involves the assessment of vaginal keratinization in the oophorectomized rat.

When interpreting female reproductive effects in toxicity studies it should be borne in mind that significant differences exist between species in their responses to some compounds. For example, prolactin is luteotrophic in the rat and progesterone stimulates growth hormone release in the dog.

13.6   Conclusions

Assessment of toxic injury to the female reproductive tract may be accomplished by routine histopathological examination of the ovaries, uterus, cervix and vagina from routine regulatory toxicity studies. These investigations may reveal changes charaterized by increase or decrease in the normal tissue components of the organs.

The vast majority of lesions detected, in our experience, subsequently have been shown to involve the actions of sex hormones or compounds which mimic their actions. However, mechanisms by which detected changes are caused are not always obvious and may require subsequent detailed investigations into the interference with hormonal control, either by feedback mechanisms at the gonadal or pituitary–hypothalamic levels. Other chemicals may exert their effects directly at the reproductive tissues, and this may involve local metabolism and biotransformation of the compound.

References

1. BECK, L.R. (1972) Comparative observations on the morphology of the mammalian periovarial sac, *Journal of Morphology*, **136**, 247–254.
2. PELUSO, J.J. (1992) Morphologic and physiologic features of the ovary, in MOHR, U., DUNGWORTH, D.L. and CAPEN, C.C. (Eds) *Pathobiology of the Aging Rat*, Vol. 1, pp. 337–349, Washington: ILSI Press.
3. MURDOCH, W.J. (1994) Ovarian surface epithelium during ovulatory and anovulatory ovine estrous cycles, *The Anatomical Record*, **240**, 322–326.
4. PARMLEY, T.H. and WOODRUFF, J.D. (1974) The ovarian mesothelioma, *American Journal of Obstetrics and Gynecology*, **120**, 234–241.
5. HIRSHFIELD, A.N. (1987) Histological assessment of follicular development and its applicability to risk assessment, *Reproductive Toxicology*, **1**, 71–79.
6. MANDL, A.M. and SHELTON, M. (1959) A quantitative study of oocytes in young and old nulliparous laboratory rats, *Journal of Endocrinology*, **18**, 444–450.
7. CARSON, R. and SMITH, J. (1986) Development of steroidogenic activity of preantral follicles in the neonatal rat ovary, *Journal of Endocrinology*, **110**, 87–92.
8. HIRSHFIELD, A.N. (1986) Effect of a low dose of pregnant mares serum gonadotropin on follicular recruitment and atresia in cycling rats, *Biology of Reproduction*, **35**, 113–118.
9. HIRSHFIELD, A.N. (1988) Size-frequency analysis of atresia in cycling rats, *Biology of Reproduction*, **38**, 1181–1188.

10. RAO, M.C. and GIBORI, G. (1987) Corpus luteum: animal models of possible relevance to reproductive toxicology, *Reproductive Toxicology*, **1**, 61–69.

11. YUAN, Y-D. (1991) Female reproductive system, in HASCHEK, W.M. and ROUSSEAUX, C.G. (Eds) *Handbook of Toxicologic Pathology*, pp. 891–935, San Diego: Academic Press.

12. GREAVES, P. (1990) Female genital tract, in *Histopathology of Preclinical Toxicity Studies*, pp. 625–676, Amsterdam: Elsevier.

13. ERICKSON, G.F., MAGOFFIN, D.A., DYER, C.A. and HOFEDITZ, C. (1985) The ovarian androgen producing cells: a review of structure/function relationships, *Endocrine Reviews*, **6**, 371–399.

14. ATAYA, K.M., McKANNA, J.A., WEINTRAUB, A.M., CLARK, M.R. and LeMAIRE, W.J. (1985) A luteinizing hormone-releasing hormone agonist for the prevention of chemotherapy-induced ovarian follicular loss in rats, *Cancer Research*, **45**, 3651–3656.

15. GOPINATH, C., PRENTICE, D.E. and LEWIS, D.J. (1987) The reproductive system, in *Atlas of Experimental Toxicological Pathology*, pp. 91–103, Lancaster: MTP Press.

16. MIDDDLETON, M.C., MILNE, C.M., MORELAND, S. and HASMALL, R.L. (1986) Ovulation in rats is delayed by a substituted triazole, *Toxicology and Applied Pharmacology*, **83**, 230–239.

17. IATROPOULOS, M.J. (1993/94) Endocrine considerations in toxicologic pathology, *Experimental Toxicologic Pathology*, **45**, 391–410.

18. SCHMIDT, G., OWMAN, Ch. and SJÖBERG, N.-O. (1986) Histamine induces ovulation in the isolated perfused rat ovary, *Journal of Reproductive Fertility*, **78**, 159–166.

19. KNOX, G.E. (1974) Antihistamine blockade of the ovarian hyperstimulation syndrome, *American Journal of Obstetrics and Gynecology*, **118**, 992–994.

20. GREENWALD, G.S. (1987) Possible animal models of follicular development relevant to reproductive toxicology, *Reproductive Toxicology*, **1**, 55–59.

21. KRISHNA, A., BEESLEY, K. and FERRANOVA, P.F. (1989) Histamine, mast cells and ovarian function, *Journal of Endocrinology*, **120**, 363–371.

22. WALKER, R.F., SCHWARTZ, L.W., TORPHY, T.J., NEWTON, J.F. and MANSON, J.M. (1988) Ovarian effects of SK&F 86002-A$_2$ in the rat: site of action, *Toxicology and Applied Pharmacology*, **94**, 276–286.

23. REINDEL, J.F., DOMINICK, M.A., BOCAN, T.M.A., GOUGH, A.W. and McGUIRE, E.J. (1994) Toxicologic effects of a novel acyl-CoA: cholesterol acyltransferase inibitor in cynomolgus monkeys, *Toxicologic Pathology*, **22**, 510–518.

24. LEWIS, D.J. (1987) Ovarian neoplasia in the Sprague–Dawley rat, *Environmental Health Perspectives*, **73**, 77–90.

25. ALISON, R.H., MORGAN, K.T., HASEMAN, J.K. and BOORMAN, G.A. (1987) Morphology and classification of ovarian neoplasms in F344 rats and (C57BL/6 × C3H)F$_1$ mice, *Journal of the National Cancer Institute*, **78**, 1229–1243.

26. LATENDRESSE, J.R. BROOKS, C.L. and CAPEN, C.C. (1994) Pathologic effects of butylated triphenyl phosphate-based hydraulic fluid and tricresyl phosphate on the adrenal gland, ovary and testis in the Fischer 344 rat, *Toxicologic Pathology*, **22**, 341–352.

27. CARITHERS, J.R. and GREEN, J.A. (1972) Ultrastructure of rat ovarian interstitial cells, *Journal of Ultrastructure Research*, **39**, 239–250.

28. PELUSO, J.J. and GORDON, L.R. (1992) Non-neoplastic and neoplastic changes in the ovary, in MOHR, U., DUNGWORTH, D.L. and CAPEN, C.C. (Eds) *Pathobiology of the Aging Rat*, Vol. 1, pp. 351–364, Washington: ILSI Press.

29. MEITES, J., HUANG, H.H. and RIEGLE, G.D. (1977) Relation of the hypothalamo–pituitary–gonadal system to decline of reproductive functions in aging female rats, in LABRIE, F., MEITES, J. and PELLETIER, G. (Eds) *Hypothalamus and Endocrine Functions*, pp. 3–20, New York: Plenum Press.

30. GOPINATH, C. and GIBSON, W.A. (1987) Mesovarian leiomyomas in the rat, *Environmental Health Perspectives*, **73**, 107–113.

31. KING, N.W. (1978) The reproductive tract, in BENIRSCHKE, K., GARNER, F.M. and JONES, T.C. (Eds) *Pathology of Laboratory Animals*, Vol. 1, pp. 509–573, New York: Springer-Verlag.

32. GOPINATH, C. (1992) Susceptibility of the uterus to toxic substances, in MOHR, U., DUNGWORTH, D.L. and CAPEN, C.C. (Eds) *Pathobiology in the Aging Rat*, Vol. 1, pp. 389–394, Washington: ILSI Press.

33. ELCOCK, L.H., STEWART, B.P., MUELLER, R.E. and HOSS, H.E. (1987) Deciduoma, uterus, rat, in JONES, T.C., MOHR, U. and HUNT, R.D. (Eds), *Genital System*, pp. 140–145, Berlin: Springer-Verlag.

34. GIBSON, J.P., SELLS, D.M., CHENG, H.C. and YUK, L. (1987) Induction of uterine leiomyomas in mice by medroxalol and prevention by propranolol, *Toxicologic Pathology*, **15**, 468–473.

35. NEWMAN, F. (1991) Early indicators for carcinogenesis in sex-hormone-sensitive organs, *Mutation Research*, **248**, 341–356.

36. JOHNSON, L.D. (1987) Lesion of the female genital system caused by diethylstilbestrol in humans, subhuman primates and mice, in JONES, T.C., MOHR, U. and HUNT, R.D. (Eds) *Genital System*, pp. 84–109, Berlin: Springer-Verlag.

37. CAMPBELL, J.S. (1987) Adenoacanthoma, uterus, rat, in JONES, T.C., MOHR, U. and HUNT, R.D. (Eds) *Genital System*, pp. 110–115, Berlin: Springer-Verlag.

38. GOODMAN, D.G. and HILDEBRANDT, P.K. (1987) Stromal sarcoma, endometrium, rat, in JONES, T.C., MOHR, U. and HUNT, R.D. (Eds) *Genital System*, pp. 70–71, Berlin: Springer-Verlag.

39. JOHNSON, A.N. (1989) Comparative aspects of contraceptive steroids. Effects observed in beagle dogs, *Toxicologic Pathology*, **17**, 389–395.

40. HIGHMAN, B., NORVELL, M.J. and SHELLENBERGER, T.E. (1977) Pathological changes in female C-3H mice continuously fed diets containing diethylstilbestrol or 17β-estradiol, *Journal of Environmental Pathology*, **1**, 1–30.

41. ENGLE, E.T. (1946) Tubular adenomas and testis-like tubules of the ovaries of aged rats, *Cancer Research*, **6**, 578–582.

42. HUANG, H.H., MARSHALL, S. and MEITES, J. (1976) Induction of estrous cycles in old non-cycling rats by progesterone, A.C.T.H., ether stress, or L-dopa, *Neuroendocrinology*, **20**, 21–34.

43. GREAVES, P. and FACCINI, J.M. (1984) Female genital tract, in *Rat Histopathology*, pp. 171–186, Amsterdam: Elsevier.

14

The Mammary Gland

JEAN HOOSON

14.1 Introduction

The mammary gland is that part of the female reproductive system which functions to provide nutrition for the newborn. It has a dynamic morphology, reflecting the hormonal changes occurring during puberty, the oestrus cycle, pregnancy and the cessation of reproductive activity. During pregnancy, mammary tissue undergoes major structural changes in preparation for milk production (lactation). Its endocrine dependency is complex, with ovarian, pituitary and hypothalamic hormones being the major regulators of its development and function.

The mammary gland is best known to clinicians and pathologists for its propensity to undergo neoplastic change. The most frequent cancer which North American and European women will develop during their lifetime, is that of the breast. Although many factors have been correlated with a high or low incidence of breast cancer, the basic aetiology of the disease remains obscure [1]. In the rat, mouse and the dog, mammary tumours are also the most common spontaneous neoplasms in the female of the species. It is hardly surprising, therefore, that the mammary glands of laboratory animals have been extensively studied as potential models for the human disease.

The ability of hormones to alter both the spontaneous incidence of tumours and the susceptibility of the gland to carcinogens has long been recognized. It is also known that there are significant species differences in the hormonal regulation of the gland, and that additional factors including genetics, viruses and dietary influences can contribute to the genesis of mammary gland neoplasia.

Interpreting the significance of an increase in mammary tumours in toxicity studies requires an appreciation of these factors, particularly a recognition that xenobiotics can act indirectly by interfering with hormonal control at various levels of the hypothalamic/pituitary/gonadal axis.

14.2 Anatomy, Histology and Physiology

14.2.1 *Anatomy*

Mammary glands are derived from the epidermis and structurally are highly modified apocrine sweat glands. They develop embryologically along two milk lines on the ventrolateral surface of the body within a subcutaneous fat pad, between the axilla and the inguinal area. Depending on species, there are from two to twelve glands [1]. The rat has six pairs, three in the pectoral group and three in the inguinal group, extending from the salivary glands anteriorly to the perianal region posteriorly. The mouse has only two inguinal pairs of glands giving a total of five pairs. Dogs also have five pairs, but in primates and humans only one gland develops each side of the thorax, although accessory breast tissue may be found anywhere along the milk lines.

The basic anatomy of the mammary gland is essentially the same in all mammals (Figure 14.1). It is a compound tubuloalveolar gland comprising a series of branching ducts that terminate in a secretory unit. This unit is composed of irregular branching tubules with evaginations from the walls and blind ends, which is termed, in its secretory form, an alveolus or acinus. A cluster of alveoli around a small intralobular duct form a lobule. Interlobular ducts run between lobules and in the rat merge to form the main lactiferous duct, which enters the nipple sinus and then opens onto the skin surface through the nipple canal. In males, the lactiferous duct ends blindly below the epidermis and no nipples develop.

The morphology of the gland varies with endocrine status and with sex. In young adult virgin female rats (resting, inactive gland) the duct system is prominent and alveolar structures are few, but terminal ductular structures called terminal end buds are frequent (Figure 14.2a). During pregnancy, the mammary gland increases in size, with progressive differentiation of terminal end buds into alveolar buds, and

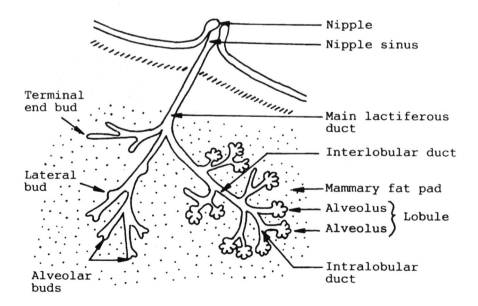

Figure 14.1 Schematic representation of mammary gland showing main anatomical features.

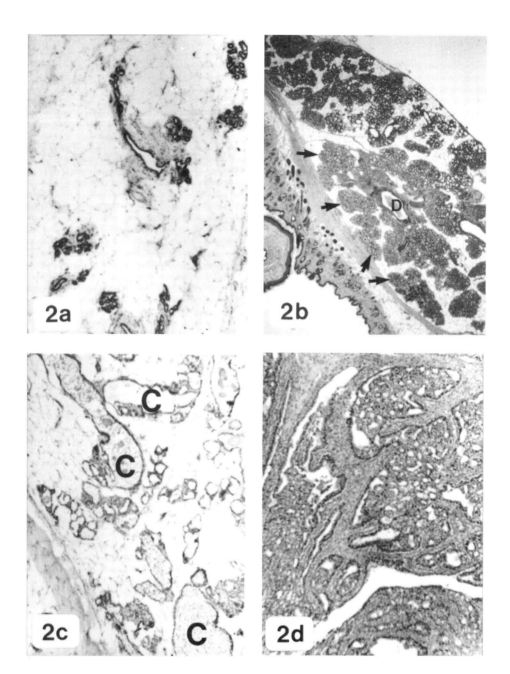

Figure 14.2 Sequential mammary changes in female Sprague–Dawley rats fed diethylstilboestrol (10 ppm). (a) Control. Mammary gland morphology is predominantly ductal. (b) After 2 weeks. Mammary fat pad is filled with well-developed lobules of secretory alveoli (arrows), surrounding a dilated lactiferous duct (D). (c) After 8 weeks. Alveoli have coalesced to form cystic structures (C) filled with secretion. (d) After 40 weeks. Mammary carcinoma exhibiting cribriform/papillary patterns.

subsequently into alveoli. The proliferating epithelial cells displace adipose tissue, and at the end of pregnancy the mammary gland is composed almost totally of lobuloalveolar structures, the alveoli exhibiting secretory activity. During lactation, milk yield increases gradually for the first seven days. Significant involution of lobules occurs after weaning but the gland never returns to the morphology of a virgin female rat of the same age. In adult male rats, unstimulated mammary tissue consists of scattered alveolar structures, the cells having foamy epithelial cytoplasm; ducts are absent or infrequent [2].

14.2.2 *Histology*

In rats, the nipple structures are lined by squamous epithelium continuous with the epidermis. Ducts are lined by one to two layers of cuboidal epithelium resting on a discontinuous layer of elongated myoepithelial cells, which is separated by a basement membrane from the surrounding connective tissue of sparse collagen, fibroblasts, capillaries and lymphatics. The ducts narrow as they branch, ending in club-shaped terminal end buds lined by five to ten layers of epithelium. Alveolar buds and alveoli are lined by a single layer of low cuboidal epithelium [3].

Ultrastructural and enzyme histochemical studies have identified three different epithelial phenotypes, namely light, dark and intermediate cells. About 75 per cent of epithelial cells have the characteristics of dark cells, with the remaining 25 per cent consisting of equal numbers of intermediate and myoepithelial cells, light cells being infrequent [4]. Epithelial cells are positive for Mg^{2+} ATPase whereas myoepithelial cells are also positive for Na/K ATPase and alkaline phosphatase. Other cellular markers have been described. Peanut lectin, milk fat globule membrane, thioesterase II and cytokeratin 18 are specific for epithelial cells, whereas myoepithelial cells react to pokeweed lectin and to antibodies to the microfilaments actin and myosin. Laminin, fibronectin, type I and type IV collagen are reliable markers for basement membrane [5].

14.2.3 *Physiology*

Mammary gland development and function is under the control of a plethora of hormones secreted by the pituitary, ovaries, adrenals, pancreas and the placenta. There are, however, species differences in the mechanisms of hormonal stimulation. In rodents, the pituitary hormone, prolactin (PRL), is essential for the development of the gland, with oestrogen acting to stimulate ductal expansion and growth, and progesterone required for the completion of lobuloalveolar differentiation. In dogs, growth hormone (GH) is the most important pituitary hormone, acting in combination with progesterone, whilst in primates and humans, oestrogens plus a placental factor are required.

Many of these hormones are under hypothalamic control, oestrogen and progesterone indirectly via the ovary, PRL and growth hormone directly via the pituitary. Dopamine is the hypothalamic agent that holds spontaneous pituitary PRL release in check. During lactation, the stimulus for PRL release is suckling. Neural impulses generated by suckling are conveyed to the central nervous system where they impinge on specialized secretory neurons in the hypothalamus. Suckling also stimulates oxytocin release from the posterior pituitary through a separate neurohormonal reflex. Oxytocin causes contraction of the myoepithelial cells surrounding the alveoli, thus propelling milk into the nipple sinus.

Receptors for PRL, GH, oestrogen, progesterone, insulin, corticosteroids and catecholamines have been identified in mammary tissue, but numbers vary with the stage of the reproductive cycle. Interactions between hormones occur, for example oestrogen receptors are induced by PRL but inhibited by progesterone, whilst oestrogen can increase both PRL and progesterone binding. PRL receptors are located in the plasma membranes of epithelial cells, but steroids interact with receptor proteins located in the nucleus. Steroid/receptor complexes accumulate in the nucleus and bind to specific regulatory DNA sequences, adjacent to steroid-regulated genes, increasing or decreasing their transcription rate. This results in the accumulation of messenger RNA which enters the cytoplasm and is re-translated into specific proteins by ribosomes. Steroid receptors have also been found on mesenchymal cells in the mammary gland, so epithelial/stromal interactions may have some influence on steroid hormone effects [5].

The mammary gland of young virgin female rats exhibits DNA synthetic and mitotic activity which is highest in the terminal end bud. Although terminal end buds decrease in number with age, they retain a high proliferative activity. Lobular structures rarely exhibit DNA synthesis and myoepithelial cells show little labelling activity [3].

14.3   Biochemical and Cellular Mechanisms of Toxicity

The most important manifestation of toxicity in the mammary gland is the development of neoplasia. In a series of 250 chemicals tested for carcinogenicity by the National Toxicology Program in the USA, 13 induced an increased incidence of mammary cancer in female rats [4]. In view of the complexities surrounding the development of mammary neoplasia in laboratory animals, the significance of such findings is sometimes difficult to evaluate. Essentially, two major classes of agents have been described – those that produce tumours through direct damage to DNA and those that induce neoplasia as a result of indirect mechanisms, usually by disturbing the hypothalamic/pituitary/gonadal axis, which may have less relevance to man. Both have a typical response pattern. Genotoxic chemicals produce dose-related increases in the incidence and multiplicity of mammary neoplasms, usually after a short latent period. They are effective after single or restricted doses and do not induce diffuse hyperplasia of mammary or pituitary cells. DNA damage is the initiating carcinogenic event, but can only occur through the 'permissive' action of the appropriate hormonal environment. Absence or excess of certain hormones (e.g. hypophysectomy or pregnancy) at the time of exposure renders the mammary epithelium refractory to initiation. Genotoxins can induce cancer simultaneously in other tissues and other species are susceptible unless critical metabolic pathways differ. In contrast, chemicals that disturb hormone balance usually do so after long-term administration at high or threshold dosage levels. Mammary cancer emerges from glands that have been chronically stimulated by increased secretions of pituitary mammotrophic hormones. In these instances, the hormonal environment exerts a 'promoting' action on the carcinogenic process, which is both site and species specific.

433

14.3.1 *Induction of Neoplasia by Viruses*

Spontaneous mammary cancer in mice is determined principally by the presence of **mammary tumour virus (MTV)**. This RNA virus, originally detected in the milk, has several variants, some of which are transmitted by germ cells. In general, strains infected with type B milk virus show a high incidence of mammary neoplasia, but genetically resistant strains have a low incidence. Other factors, including genetics and hormones, also play a role. For example, C3H mice are **MTV** positive and both virgin and breeding females develop mammary tumours, whereas strain A mice are also **MTV** positive but show a high incidence only in breeding females. Both BALB/c and C57BL strains are normally **MTV** negative and have few mammary tumours. BALB/c can, however, be infected experimentally whereas C57BL are usually resistant to infection. So far all efforts to identify type B virus particles in species other than the mouse have failed [6].

14.3.2 *Induction of Neoplasia by Genotoxic Agents*

DMBA and MNU

Cancer researchers developing models of human breast cancer needed experimental procedures that would induce cancers in 100 per cent of treated animals in a short time. Rats were the preferred rodent because chemically induced cancers in this species were hormone responsive and viruses were not confounding factors. In 1961, Huggins *et al.* [7] demonstrated that a single (20 mg) intragastric dose of **dimethyl-benzanthracene (DMBA)** to 50-day-old Sprague–Dawley females produced mammary cancer in all treated rats after 8 weeks. The single dose allowed investigation of the initiating and promoting stages of carcinogenesis and the tumours were very hormone responsive.

DMBA is a fat-soluble polycyclic aromatic hydrocarbon which will also induce mammary cancer when given parenterally or after direct injection into the gland. It requires metabolic activation to a reactive epoxide and mammary tissue contains two P-450 isoenzymes, at least one of which is induced by **DMBA** as a first step in its metabolism. **DMBA** can also be converted to reactive intermediates by metabolism mediated by prostaglandin synthetase, and mammary DMBA/DNA adducts have been demonstrated by ^{32}P post-labelling techniques; mutations consist of AT to TA transversions at the second base of codon 61 in the H-*ras* oncogene.

The majority of studies on carcinogen-induced mammary cancer for the next two decades employed this model, but in 1975, Gullino *et al.* [8] reported the induction of multiple mammary carcinomas in several rat strains after intravenous injections of **methylnitrosourea (MNU)**. This was initially regarded as a better model of the human disease, as a higher percentage of malignant tumours were induced which metastasized to the lung, liver, spleen and bone. Work in other laboratories failed to confirm the metastasizing ability of **MNU**-induced mammary cancer [9], but nevertheless this system was used widely in the 1980s as a research model.

MNU is a water-soluble direct-acting alkylating agent with a short half-life, equally effective given intravenously or subcutaneously. Again, the H-*ras* oncogene is found in most **MNU**-induced mammary cancers and a CG to AT transition at the second nucleotide of codon 12 is probably the initiating event in carcinogenesis.

Mammary cancers induced by **DMBA** or **MNU** develop through intraductular proliferations (Figure 14.3a) and carcinoma *in situ* (Figure 14.3b) to carcinomas with predominantly papillary, cribriform (sieve-like) or comedo (centrally necrotic) growth patterns (Figure 14.3c). The surrounding mammary tissue is unstimulated and tumour-bearing rats have normal serum PRL levels, and pituitary and ovarian histology [10].

Both **DMBA** and **MNU** are effective after a single dose, with tumour incidence, multiplicity, malignancy and latent period being directly related to dose. Rats aged between 35 and 60 days are most susceptible to tumour induction by both chemicals. Older rats show a decreased tumour incidence, less tumours per rat and fewer malignant tumours. Some rat strains are more susceptible than others. Sprague–Dawley, Wistar–Furth and Osborne–Mendel are more sensitive than F-344 or ACI females, but the inbred Copenhagen rat is almost completely resistant. The H-*ras* gene in the mammary glands of the Copenhagen rat is just as prone to methylation as in other strains, but there appears to be a growth suppression of initiated cells, through activation of a mammary carcinoma suppressor gene. Resistance is inherited as a dominant phenotype, is mammary specific and is associated with an overexpression of casein genes [11].

The induction of carcinogen-induced rat tumours is dependent on a normal hormonal environment, with pituitary and ovarian hormones playing a pivotal role. In virgin females, hypophysectomy or the administration of drugs that inhibit pituitary function can abolish the carcinogenic response. PRL is the key pituitary hormone and treatments which elevate PRL secretion (e.g. **chlorpromazine**) or suppress it (e.g. **bromocriptine**), if administered at the time of carcinogen application, can inhibit or reduce tumour development [12]. Oophorectomy or the administration of an antioestrogen (e.g. **tamoxifen**) also inhibit or reduce the development of carcinogen-induced tumours. Administration of oestrogens after carcinogen exposure can enhance tumour growth, but the presence of the pituitary gland is essential [13].

Reproductive status is also a factor. Tumour response to either **DMBA** or **MNU** is higher in rats treated at pro-oestrus or oestrus, but the glands of previously pregnant or lactating females are refractory to carcinogenesis. The morphology of the mammary gland at the time of carcinogen treatment is important, particularly the number of terminal end buds present. These are frequent in young virgin females, particularly in the thoracic glands, where the highest incidence of neoplasia occurs, but largely absent in the predominantly lobuloalveolar morphology of lactating glands [14].

Other genotoxic agents (Table 14.1)

Rat mammary cancers have also been induced by **3,4,-benzopyrene (BP)**, **3-methylcholanthrene (MCA)**, **2-acetylaminofluorene (2-AAF)**, **2-(2-furyl)-3-(5-nitro-2-furyl)acrylamide (AF-2)**, **adriamycin**, **daunomycin**, **6-nitrochrysene**, **1-** and **4-nitropyrenes**, substituted **aminopyrazoles**, and the alkylating agents **butylnitrosourea** and **ethylnitrosourea**.

An increased incidence of mammary neoplasia is seen in certain mouse strains treated with **BP, MCA, DMBA, urethane (ethyl carbamate)** and **butyl carbamate**. The presence of **MTV** is not essential for tumour development and most induced cancers are morphologically adenocarcinomas (70 per cent) or adenoacanthomas (30 per cent) [6].

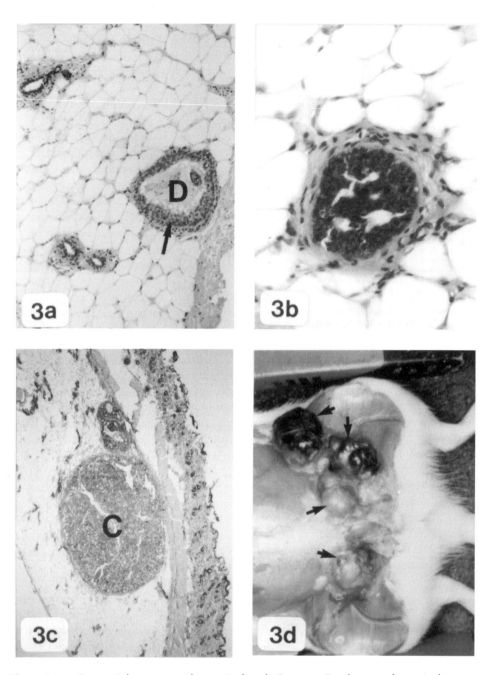

Figure 14.3 Sequential mammary changes in female Sprague–Dawley rats after a single intravenous injection of methylnitrosourea (50 mg/kg body weight). (a) After 2 weeks. Focal intraductal hyperplasia, with multilayering of epithelium (arrow) and dilation of duct (D). (b) After 4 weeks. Dysplastic ductular epithelium, occluding lumen (carcinoma *in situ*). (c) After 6 weeks. Small intraductal cribriform carcinoma (C). (d) After 10 weeks. Abdominal skin removed to display multiple inguinal mammary masses (arrows).

Table 14.1 Treatments inducing mammary neoplasia in laboratory animals

Mutagenic	Hormonally mediated
PAHs (DMBA, BP, MCA)[1,2]	Pituitary isografts[1,2]
6-nitrochrysene[1]	Hypothalamic lesions[1,2]
4-nitropyrene[1]	Reserpine[1,2]
2-AAF[1]	Oestrogens (E2, DES)[1,2]
Anthracycline antibiotics	Progestins (progesterone[3],
(adriamycin, daunomycin)[1]	17-hydroxyprogesterone derivatives[3],
Alkylnitrosoureas (methyl, ethyl, butyl)[1]	medroxyprogesterone acetate[2,3],
5-nitrofurans (AF-2, nitrofurazone,	19-nortestosterone derivatives[3])
furazolidone)[1]	Oestrogen/progestin oral contraceptives[1,2,3]
5-nitroacenaphthene[1]	
3,3'-dimethoxybenzidine.2HCl[1]	
Glycidol[1]	
Aminopyrazoles[1]	*Other*
Irradiation[1,2]	Virus (MTV)[2]

[1] in rats, [2] in mice, [3] in dogs
PAHs, polycyclic aromatic hydrocarbons

X-rays, γ-rays and **neutrons** at sublethal doses will induce a linear dose-related increase in rat mammary tumours, usually within a 12-month period. The endocrine status is critical, oophorectomized females being resistant, but administration of oestrogens, e.g. **oestradiol-17β (E2)** and **diethylstilboestrol (DES)** increases the incidence and multiplicity of tumours. Surprisingly, reproductive status does not influence the carcinogenic process, virgin, pregnant or lactating females responding equally [15]. This contrasts with the findings with **DMBA** or **MNU**.

In mice, **whole body irradiation** will also induce mammary cancer [6].

14.3.3   Growth of Established Tumours

Hormonal influences

Most carcinogen-induced rat tumours, are, unlike their mouse equivalents, hormone responsive, with PRL, oestrogen, and progesterone receptors being present on the neoplastic cells. The growth of established tumours can be reduced by compounds acting at the hypothalamic level, for example L-dopa (a dopamine agonist), **clonidine** (an α-adrenergic agonist) and **naloxone** (an opiate antagonist), or at the pituitary level, for example **bromocriptine** (a PRL release inhibitor), or **hypophysectomy**. Such treatments result in reductions of circulating PRL. Conversely, treatments that increase PRL secretion, for example **sulpiride, reserpine, haloperidol** (dopamine antagonists), **thyrotrophin-releasing hormone**, or **median eminence hypothalamic lesions** enhance mammary tumour growth [16].

At the ovarian level, moderate amounts of **oestrogen** and **progesterone** and the hormonal environment of pregnancy or pseudopregnancy accelerate growth of established tumours. Lack of ovarian steroids after **antioestrogen** or **androgen** administration, or after **oophorectomy**, results in stasis or regression of tumour growth [9].

Dietary factors

The growth of carcinogen-induced rat tumours is enhanced by high levels of **dietary fat** and **protein**. Polyunsaturated fats from vegetables (e.g. **corn oil**) are the most effective and appear to have an action independent of their calorific value. A variety of micronutrients and food additives can reduce mammary cancer growth. **Vitamin A (retinyl acetate)**, antioxidants (e.g. **butylated hydroxytoluene** and **butylated hydroxyanisole**), trace elements (e.g. **selenium**), flavenoids (e.g. **quercetin**) and terpenes (e.g. **D-limonene**) have all produced a reduction in the growth of **DMBA**-induced rat mammary tumours [14].

14.3.4 Induction of Neoplasia by Hormonally Active Agents (Table 14.1)

Rodents

In rats and mice, oestrogen and PRL are critical to the development of spontaneous mammary neoplasia, although the influence of the **MTVs** is a complicating factor in mice. Pioneering work in the 1960s demonstrated that in both rats and mice, implants of **natural oestrogens** could increase the incidence of spontaneous mammary neoplasia [17]. As surgical techniques improved, it was demonstrated that the pituitary and hypothalamus were essential for tumour induction. Insertion of multiple **pituitary isografts** under the kidney capsule of rats and mice results in a high incidence of mammary neoplasia. Median eminence **hypothalamic lesions** have a similar effect [5]. Both procedures increase circulating PRL levels. **Reserpine** administered chronically to both rats and mice, elevates PRL levels and increases the number of mammary tumours, whereas **bromocriptine** and **L-dopa** reduce mammary neoplasia in mice and rats, respectively [5].

Oral contraceptives, when continually administered at 250 to 400 times the human therapeutic dose, also increase mammary neoplasia. In rodents these oestrogen/progestin combinations have overwhelmingly oestrogenic effects [18]. The **17-hydroxyprogesterone** and **19-nortestosterone progestins** alone did not usually increase the incidence of mammary tumours in rats or mice, but in a more recent study, BALB/c mice have developed mammary carcinomas after repeated subcutaneous implants of **medroxyprogesterone acetate** [19].

Both natural steroidal oestrogens (e.g. **E2**) and synthetic non-steroidal oestrogens (e.g. **DES**) when given at high doses for prolonged periods elevate the number of mammary tumours in both rats and mice. After chronic oestrogen administration, severe endocrine imbalances occur. For example, dietary administration of **DES** to Sprague–Dawley rats at several dose levels for 52 weeks produces a dose-related but threshold response in terms of mammary neoplasia, pituitary neoplasia and hyperprolactinaemia [10]. The prime target for oestrogens appears to be the pituitary, and Copenhagen rats, although resistant to **DES**-induced mammary neoplasia, nevertheless develop pituitary adenomas (Table 14.2). The enlarged pituitaries, when examined immunohistochemically, are composed of PRL-secreting mammotrophs. Oestrogen administration inhibits the hypothalamic secretion of

Table 14.2 Neoplasia and prolactin levels in female rats after dietary administration of diethylstilboestrol (**DES**) for 52 weeks [10]

DES (ppm in diet)	Mammary carcinoma (%)	Mammary adenoma (%)	Pituitary adenoma (%)	Serum prolactin (mean test/control)
Sprague–Dawley				
0	0	5	5	1
0.1	0	0	10	0.7
0.5	0	5	10	0.8
1.0	30	0	30	3
5.0	68	0	100	>50
10.0	70	0	100	>50
Copenhagen				
0	0	0	5	1
10	0	0	100	6.5

dopamine, stimulating PRL release. In rodents, PRL is also luteotrophic, i.e. it increases progesterone secretion by the corpora lutea of the ovary. Hyperprolactinaemic females are actually in a state of pseudopregnancy and mammary tumours develop after chronic overstimulation by PRL, oestrogen and progesterone. Mammary cancers induced by **DES** are intraductal proliferations (Figure 14.2d), indistinguishable from those elicited by **DMBA** or **MNU** treatment, except that they arise from glands that are predominantly lobuloalveolar and cystic in morphology, following stimulation exceeding normal physiological limits [10].

DES administration to **hypophysectomized** rats, or to rats chronically treated with **bromocriptine**, does not result in mammary cancer, emphasizing the role of the pituitary and PRL in the genesis of oestrogen-induced mammary cancer [20].

Treatment of Wistar-derived rats for 2 years with **tamoxifen**, a non-steroidal antioestrogen, abolished the spontaneous development of both pituitary and mammary tumours. In this strain, 75 per cent of the controls had pituitary adenomas and 25 per cent had mammary neoplasms by 2 years [21]. **Tamoxifen** also suppresses mammary cancer in mice [22].

Dogs

Information on the endocrine control of mammary neoplasia in dogs is sparse compared with the literature on rodents. Oophorectomy before the first oestrus greatly decreases the number of spontaneous mammary tumours, but oestrogen does not stimulate mammary growth and established tumours show little oestrogen dependency [19]. No differences in serum PRL levels were found between dogs with malignant mammary tumours and controls of comparable age [23], whilst in another study, 50 per cent of bitches with spontaneous mammary tumours had elevated levels of GH [24].

Most data on the hormonal induction of cancer in dogs have come from the testing of **oral contraceptives. Progesterone**, 17-hydroxyprogesterone derivatives including **megestrol acetate, chlormadinone acetate** and **medroxyprogesterone acetate**, induce mammary tumours in beagles. There is no corresponding elevation of PRL secretion, but they do stimulate the proliferation and hypertrophy of GH-secreting cells in the pituitary and this appears to be the hormone that induces hyperplastic and neoplastic change in the dog mammary gland [25]. Hypophysectomized dogs treated with progestins show no stimulation of mammary gland growth, illustrating the importance of the pituitary in the process. Of the numerous progestational compounds, the 17-hydroxyprogesterone derivatives are most effective as they release more GH from the pituitary. Dogs treated with these compounds also show marked acromegalic changes and symptoms of diabetes as GH can antagonize the action of insulin [24].

In contrast, **oestrogens,** or combinations of **oestrogens** with **19-nortestosterone** derivatives, have not produced mammary gland nodules, although pituitary PRL-secreting cells are stimulated [26]. There is as yet no evidence that prolonged administration of oestrogens is carcinogenic to the canine mammary gland, and it would seem that neuroendocrine influences on the mammary gland in this species are very different to those operating in rodents.

14.4 Morphological Responses to Injury

The morphological changes occurring in the mammary gland during the oestrus and reproductive cycles and during ageing form the baseline against which xenobiotic-induced lesions have to be evaluated. Few non-proliferative lesions have been described in the mammary gland. Not surprisingly, agents that affect hormone balance can induce diffuse hyperplasia and secretion, changes analagous to those seen in pregnancy and lactation. These proliferations may regress on cessation of treatment, but if the stimulus persists they can progress to neoplasia. In contrast, agents with initiating activity can induce neoplastic changes *de novo*.

14.4.1 *Non-Neoplastic Lesions*

Fat necrosis

Trauma to mammary tissue can result in necrosis of adipose tissue in the mammary fat pad. In humans, **anticoagulant therapy** has produced massive fat necrosis with haemorrhage; an allergic pathogenesis has been postulated [27].

Inflammation

Granulomatous inflammatory reactions have been described in the mammary tissue in response to fat necrosis or to rupture of large cysts with spillage of contents into the adjacent fatty tissue. Similar foreign body responses can occur around mammary implants, or as a result of leakage of **silicone** from breast prostheses. Histiocytes (macrophages) often containing necrotic lipid, or silicone, are the predominant cell type and lesions can repair by fibrous scarring [27].

Cystic change

Dilation (ectasia) of the mammary ducts is frequently noted. Thin-walled, epithelial-lined spaces may arise from either ducts or lobular structures, and can become very large (galactoceles). The lumen may contain granular eosinophilic material, lipid and macrophage infiltrates. Laminated bodies (corpora amylacea) which ultrastructurally have features of amyloid fibrils, can also occur.

Cystic change can occur spontaneously in ageing rodents and dogs, but is also seen after treatments that result in extensive hormonal stimulation of the gland, e.g. chronic administration of natural or synthetic **oestrogens** in rats (Figure 14.2c) and mice; **oral contraceptives** in rodents, dogs and monkeys; and **dopamine antagonists** in rodents and dogs. Hyperplastic changes may also be present in cystic glands [5].

Hyperplasia

Hyperplastic change is frequently seen in laboratory animals, but in the mammary gland the range of proliferative lesions does not comprise a morphological continuum, unlike in many other endocrine-dependent tissues. The use of inconsistent terminologies plus species differences in biological presentation makes classification difficult. Two main types have been described.

Ductal hyperplasia   These proliferations are characterized by piling-up and papillary infolding of ductal epithelium. The cells are often enlarged with hyperchromatic nuclei and basophilic cytoplasm. The lesions are usually focal although several ducts within a gland may show changes of varying severity. In Sprague–Dawley rats given a single intravenous injection of **MNU** (50 mg/kg body weight), focal mitotic activity was noted in the ducts after 2 weeks, and by 4 weeks focal ductal hyperplasias consisting of four to five layers of hyperchromatic epithelial cells were present (Figure 14.3a and 14.3b). Ultrastructurally, the proliferating cells have the morphological characteristics of intermediate cells [15].

Intraductal hyperplasia (adenosis) is a rare spontaneous finding in dogs, but administration of **oral contraceptives**, with progestogen:oestrogen ratios of 10 or 20:1 induced a high dose-related incidence. Lobular hyperplasias were also recorded [18].

Duct hyperplasias with atypia have also been induced in the mammary gland of rhesus monkeys treated with **oral contraceptives**. Minimal hyperplasias occurred occasionally in controls, but hyperplasias classified as severe were seen in monkeys after 10-year administration [28].

In human female breast pathology, intraduct hyperplasia is often seen and is termed 'epitheliosis' or 'papillomatosis'. The presence of cellular atypia is a risk factor for the subsequent emergence of cancer [5].

Enlargement of the human male breast is termed 'gynaecomastia'. Histologically, both intraduct hyperplasia and increased amounts of stromal collagen are found. Gynaecomastia has been reported after **oestrogen** excess, both endogenous and exogenous, and following administration of drugs (e.g. **spironolactone, cimetidine**) which indirectly affect hormonal balance [27].

Lobular hyperplasia   Histologically, the gland may be diffusely hyperplastic, the mammary fat pad being completely filled with an increased number of well-differentiated secretory alveoli. Glands from pregnant or lactating animals have this appearance, but administration of hormonally active agents can induce similar changes in non-pregnant rodents.

Sprague–Dawley rats receiving **DES** (10 ppm) in the diet showed marked alveolar hyperplasia and duct ectasia by 2 weeks (Figure 14.2b). After 8 weeks treatment, coalescence of alveoli occurred to form cysts filled with eosinophilic secretions (Figure 14.2c). Administration of **E2** at the same dietary level elicited a less marked hyperplastic response, with no cystic degeneration even after 12 weeks treatment. A similar degree of alveolar stimulation was induced by feeding the dopamine antagonists **haloperidol** (20 ppm) and **perphenazine** (20 ppm) [10].

Ageing female rats also show diffuse lobular hyperplasia, the incidence being strain dependent. A poor correlation is observed with the presence of spontaneous pituitary tumours.

In certain strains of mice carrying **MTV**, a type of lobular hyperplasia called 'hyperplastic alveolar nodule' (HAN) is frequently found. HAN consists of a cluster of hyperplastic alveoli surrounded by an increased thickness of connective tissue. Alveoli are round, not cystic, and lined by a single layer of epithelial cells showing frequent mitoses. Histochemically, they resemble normal tissue and are best regarded as an exaggerated physiological response. Although most commonly seen in **MTV**-bearing strains, e.g. C3H, the presence of virus is not essential to their development. They are hormone dependent, requiring oestrogen and PRL for their maintenance and high doses of **DES** will increase their incidence in both **MTV**-positive and **MTV**-negative C3H strains. Some HAN have the capacity to progress to neoplasia, but others regress or remain unaltered [1,5,6].

'Pregnancy-responsive plaques' occur in other inbred mice (e.g. BR, RIII DD, GR) strains bearing **MTV**. These hyperplastic discoid lesions are only seen in pregnancy and consist of tubular epithelial structures with a central core of fatty connective tissue (Figure 14.4a). Regression occurs at parturition, but subsequent pregnancies will stimulate recurrence. Again, carcinomas can arise from these lesions [6].

Hyperplasia of individual lobules, resulting in focal nodular hyperplasia, without atypia is seen frequently in older dogs. The hyperplastic tissue is mainly composed of epithelial cells, but myoepithelial cells may also be present and there may be accompanying fibrosis [1]. A dose-dependent lobuloalveolar proliferation and growth of the mammary gland is induced in young beagle bitches after 8 weeks treatment with varying doses of **progesterone**, D-**norgestrel** and **cyproterone acetate**. The growth promoting potency of these progestogens is directly related to their stimulatory effect on GH cells in the pituitary. **Dopamine antagonists** have a similar effect on the gland [25].

Some monkeys receiving **oral contraceptives** developed marked physiological lobular hyperplasia and lactational changes which were dose related [28].

14.4.2 *Neoplasia*

Mammary neoplasia is the most frequent spontaneous tumour in rats, mice and dogs, but as these neoplasms differ substantially in their origins, morphology, biology and aetiology, it is easier to consider each species separately.

Rat

Between 80 and 90 per cent of spontaneous tumours are benign and are classified histologically as fibroadenomas, composed of both epithelial and connective tissue elements. The proportions of each tissue can vary considerably and at each end of the

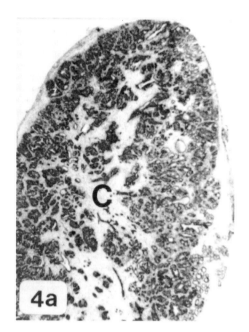
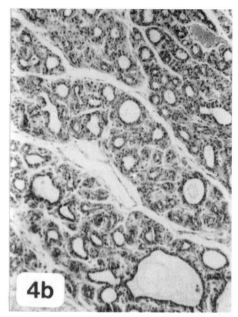

Figure 14.4 Hyperplasia and neoplasia in mice. (a) Pregnancy-responsive plaque, with tubular epithelial structures and connective tissue core (C). RIII breeding female. (b) Spontaneous mammary carcinoma, type A, showing uniform acinar pattern. B6C3F1 virgin female.

spectrum a few tumours may be purely epithelial (adenomas) or entirely fibrous (fibromas). The morphological pattern of benign epithelial mixed tumours is lobular with well-formed alveoli lined by a single epithelial layer, separated by connective tissue strands and lobules separated by denser collagen layers. Some tumours show compression of epithelial elements by connective tissue giving the characteristic pericanalicular or intracanalicular patterns of fibroadenoma seen in women (Figure 14.5a). Cellular atypia is not a feature but the tumours can grow very large with a tendency to ulcerate the overlying skin.

Spontaneous mammary carcinomas are much less common, but are the most frequent neoplasms induced by xenobiotics. They exhibit a variety of histological patterns which have been subclassified as glandular, papillary, tubular, cribriform and comedo carcinomas. Piling-up of epithelial cells and cellular atypia are characteristic features. The criteria of malignancy are histological and cytological, as these carcinomas seldom show local invasion or metastases. Metaplastic changes may also occur, the most frequent being squamous differentiation. Spontaneous and chemically induced rat carcinomas are ductal in origin (Figures 14.2d and 14.3c) and sequential studies on the induction of tumours with **MNU** indicated that carcinomas developed from local hyperplasia of the terminal end buds. Some human intraductal carcinomas (Figure 14.5b) have similar morphologies to those seen in the rat, but unlike the rat, they quickly spread to the local (axillary) lymph nodes and metastatic deposits are found in the lungs, liver and bone.

The incidence of mammary neoplasia is strain dependent and although in some rat strains, incidences of over 90 per cent in females have been found, the Copenhagen

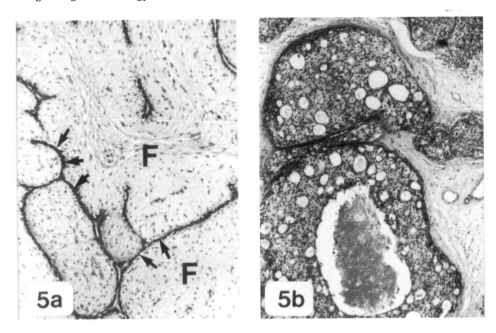

Figure 14.5 Human breast neoplasia. (a) Fibroadenoma (intracanalicular), with fibrous tissue (F) compressing epithelial elements (arrows); some rat fibroadenomas display this pattern. (b) Cribriform carcinoma showing histological pattern identical to some carcinogen-induced rat mammary carcinomas.

rat is unique in having a very low frequency of spontaneous tumours and in having a high resistance to chemical induction.

Both spontaneous and induced mammary tumours are dependent on PRL and oestrogen for growth.

Mouse

In contrast to the rat, the majority of spontaneous mammary tumours are considered to be malignant and derived from the alveolar cells rather than the duct cells. Incidences vary dramatically, high frequences being found in inbred strains that are genetically susceptible to infection with **MTV** (e.g. strain A, C3H, DBA and GR). Dunn [29] classified carcinomas in high-incidence strains as types A, B and C; adenoacanthoma, a type with squamous differentiation, was also recognized.

Type A carcinomas have a uniform acinar structure, appearing histologically benign (Figure 14.4b), whereas more pleomorphic forms with tubular, papillary or comedo structures are categorized as B lesions; C lesions consist of glandular structures embedded in a myxomatous stroma which may be myoepithelial.

In strains used for carcinogenicity studies, e.g. CD-1 and B6C3F1, **MTV** is not present and the incidence of mammary carcinoma is correspondingly low. Those described are mostly B and C lesions which are malignant, invading adjacent tissues and metastasizing to the lungs.

Most mammary tumours in mice are largely hormonally independent and unresponsive to endocrine manipulation.

Dog

Mammary tumours are the most frequent neoplasms in females, but incidence data are difficult to obtain. One report found 38 per cent of female beagles developed tumours after 8 years and 27 per cent died of mammary cancer by 13 years [18].

The histology of mammary neoplasia is complex, the variable histological patterns being largely attributable to the myoepithelial cells, which readily proliferate, and can undergo metaplastic change to produce mucopolysaccharides, cartilage and bone. About 50 per cent are benign mixed tumours, which are well-circumscribed masses surrounded by a thin fibrous capsule and are easily removed. The epithelial component consists of regular alveolar structures lined by a single layer of cuboidal epithelial cells, often containing eosinophilic secretion. The myoepithelial component is composed of small foci of polygonal cells, separated by abundant mucinous stroma. The remaining 50 per cent are mainly carcinomas of varying epithelial patterns, e.g. lobular, tubular, papillary and solid. Carcinomas appear to arise from both ductular and alveolar epithelium and evidence of hormonal dependency is conflicting.

Administration of **oral contraceptives** increases the incidence of simple and complex adenomas, benign mixed tumours and malignant tumours in a dose-related manner [18, 25].

14.5 Testing for Toxicity

14.5.1 *Regulatory Studies*

Standard toxicity protocols require mammary tissue to be sampled at study termination. Single sections of one to two mammary glands, usually taken with overlying skin, are prepared for histological examination. Good samples can be obtained if the mammary fat pad, with attached skin, is flattened on a piece of card prior to fixation. Fatty tissue sticks to the card, which prevents contraction and distortion of the sample. In chronic studies, regular palpation allows for the early detection of nodules; the technique is sensitive, with lesions less than 1 mm being palpable, but histological examination is necessary to distinguish mammary neoplasms from granulomas, abscesses, galactoceles, epidermal inclusion cysts and other tumours of non-mammary origin. At post-mortem, the number, size, texture and cut surface appearance of masses should be recorded. Number and size, together with time of appearance, provides information on xenobiotic influences on multiplicity and latent period of neoplasia. The texture and cut surface appearance may indicate tumour type. In the rat, fibroadenomas present as cream, rubbery masses that can be 'shelled out' of the surrounding tissue, whereas adenocarcinomas are often dark red, lobulated, cystic lesions which may collapse on sectioning (Figure 14.3d). Given the intimate relationship of mammary physiology to the reproductive and pituitary systems, these organs should be examined thoroughly if changes are found in mammary tissue. During statistical evaluation of mammary tumours it is usual to combine morphological variants of benign tumours and of malignant neoplasms for analysis but, at least initially, to analyse benign and malignant tumours separately.

Particularly stringent protocols for the testing of **oral contraceptives** were introduced by the Food and Drug Administration (FDA) in the 1960s, because of the widespread use of these drugs in healthy women. For over 20 years, chronic studies of 2-year duration in rats, 7 years in dogs and 10 years in monkeys were mandatory; rats were treated daily at 2 to 5, 50 and 100 to 200 times the clinical dose, whilst dogs and monkeys were repeatedly treated daily for 3 weeks, followed by 1 week's withdrawal, at 1, 10, 25 and 1, 10 and 50 times the clinical dose, respectively. The unique sensitivity of the dog to oestrogen toxicity (bone marrow suppression) necessitated the lower maximum dose in this species. Monthly palpation of mammary tissue was a protocol requirement. The development of mammary tumours in dogs following treatment with certain **progestins** led to the withdrawal of these preparations from the market. It was eventually recognized that species differences in hormonal physiology and pharmacology were responsible for these and other 'false positive' findings and in 1989 the requirement for 7- and 10-year dog and monkey studies was dropped by the FDA.

14.5.2 *Investigational Procedures*

Information on the dynamic morphology of the rodent and dog mammary glands has come from the use of whole mount preparations. These are fixed, stained and cleared mammary fat pads which can be preserved in methylsalicylate and photographed to reveal the detailed architecture of the mammary tree.

Identification of cell types is facilitated by the use of enzyme and immunohistochemical markers which can be visualized at both the light and electron microscopical level. Markers can also indicate the degree of cellular differentiation within tumours, and confirm the cellular origin of metastatic deposits. The more recent technology of *in situ* hybridization offers the possibility of identifying cells on the basis of their peptide messenger RNA content and may give better correlations with functional activity than immunohistochemical techniques. It has been used extensively for localizing hypothalamic regulatory peptide and pituitary hormone messenger RNAs.

Biochemical, immunochemical and flow cytometric methods are available to measure hormone receptors in mammary tissue. These predict hormone responsiveness and, clinically, 90 per cent of human breast cancers with oestrogen and progesterone receptors show regression following endocrine therapy.

Serum hormone levels can be measured by radioimmunoassay but as individual levels vary both diurnally and during oestrus, careful timing of sampling is necessary to detect meaningful differences between treatment groups. As PRL release is induced by stress and anaesthesia, the recommended method of sampling from rodents is by decapitation and collection of blood from the severed neck.

Measurement of appropriate serum hormone levels, mammary gland histology or mammary DNA content in rodents and dogs after 2- to 3-week treatment should identify chemicals that are capable of inducing hormonally-mediated mammary cancers in chronic studies.

Several techniques have been employed in studying **MTV** in mice. Cross-fostering can remove virus from susceptible strains and viral particles can be identified by radioimmunoassay for **MTV** group 52 antigen, as well as by electron microscopy.

In vitro techniques range from cultures of whole mouse mammary glands to monolayer cultures of epithelial cells. Organ cultures of fragments of mammary tissue, both normal and neoplastic, from different species have been used to determine their proliferative response to various hormones, applied singly or in combination.

14.6 Conclusions

The literature on mammary gland pathology in laboratory animals is devoted mainly to their use as potential models of human breast cancer. The development of experimental procedures to modify the induction and progression of neoplasia has generated valuable information on the carcinogenic process, but no species has proved an ideal model for the study of the disease in women. Each animal has certain unique features: in mice, tumours are primarily virally induced; rats are particularly susceptible to genotoxic carcinogens and oestrogens; and in dogs, the prime stimulus to mammary proliferation is pituitary GH.

Species differences in mammary response to hormones are illustrated when the results of **oral contraceptive** testing in animals are compared with human epidemiology data. Mammary tumours are induced in rodents and dogs, albeit through different endocrine pathways, primates develop hyperplasias, but no general association between **oral contraceptives** or postmenopausal oestrogen use and increased risk of breast cancer has been shown in women [30]. In rodents, the oestrogenic components of **oral contraceptives** raise serum PRL levels which leads to mammary cancer, whereas in the dog, certain progestational compounds induce mammary nodules through elevation of GH. In humans, breast cancer has not been associated with pathologically or pharmacologically increased serum PRL or GH, progestins do not stimulate pituitary GH secretion, and in primates PRL is not luteotrophic.

The aetiology of human breast cancer is not fully understood, although the influence of menstrual and reproductive factors strongly support a hormonal involvement. The role of the ovaries is well documented but the impact of the pituitary and hypothalamus is less defined. It appears that rodents, dogs and man have very different hormonal patterns of mammary gland regulation.

The relevance to humans of an increased number of mammary tumours in a chronic toxicity study depends on the mechanism of carcinogenesis. Xenobiotics inducing neoplasia through direct DNA damage are likely to have mutagenic activity and will pose an obvious hazard to man if metabolic pathways are comparable. If tumours are induced through hormonal disturbances, the predictive value of the test is compromised by the differences in endocrine physiology and regulatory pathways between species. However, the knowledge that one in nine women will develop breast cancer at some stage of their life makes the mammary gland a continuing focus for toxicological research.

Acknowledgements

The assistance of Mr D. McCarthy and Mrs M. Fagg, School of Pharmacy, University of London, in the preparation of the photomicrographs and manuscript is gratefully acknowledged.

References

1. BENIRSCHKE, K., GARNER, F.M. and JONES, T.C. (1978) *Pathology of Laboratory Animals*, Vol. II, New York: Springer-Verlag.

2. CARDY, R.H. (1991) Sexual dimorphism of the normal rat mammary gland, *Veterinary Pathology*, **28**, 139–145.

3. RUSSO, I.H., TEWARI, M. and RUSSO, J. (1989) Morphology and development of the rat mammary gland, in JONES, T.C., MOHR, A. and HUNT, R.D. (Eds) *ILSI Monographs on Pathology of Laboratory Animals, Integument and Mammary Glands*, pp. 233–252, Berlin: Springer-Verlag.

4. BOORMAN, G.A., WILSON, J.TH., VAN ZWIETEN, M.J. and EUSTIS, S.L. (1990) The mammary gland, in BOORMAN, G.A., EUSTIS, S.L., ELWELL, M.R., MONGOMERY, C.A. and MACKENZIE, W.E. (Eds) *Pathology of the Fischer Rat. Reference and Atlas*, pp. 295–313, New York: Academic Press.

5. GREAVES, P. (1990) The mammary gland, in *Histopathology of Preclinical Toxicity Studies*, pp. 48–76, Amsterdam: Elsevier.

6. SQUARTINI, F. (1979) Tumours of the mammary gland, in TUROSOV, V.S. (Ed.) *Pathology of Tumours in Laboratory Animals*, Vol. 2. *Tumours of the Mouse*, pp. 43–90, Lyon: IARC Scientific Publications.

7. HUGGINS, C., GRAND, L.C. and BRILLANTES, F.P. (1961) Mammary cancer induced by a single feeding of polynuclear hydrocarbons and its suppression, *Nature*, **189**, 204–207.

8. GULLINO, P.M., PETTIGREW, H.M. and GRANTHAM, F.H. (1975) *N*-nitrosomethylurea as mammary gland carcinogen in rats, *Journal of the National Cancer Institute*, **54**, 401–414.

9. WELSCH, C.W. (1985) Host factors affecting the growth of carcinogen-induced rat mammary carcinomas: a review and tribute to Charles Brenton Huggins, *Cancer Research*, **45**, 3415–3443.

10. HOOSON, J. (1980) Induction of mammary gland tumours in rats and mice by hormones and chemical carcinogens, *British Journal of Cancer*, **41**, 507–508.

11. HSU, L.C. and GOULD, M.N. (1993) Cloning and characterisation of overexpressed genes in the mammary gland of rat strains carrying the mammary carcinoma suppressor (*MCS*) gene, *Cancer Research*, **53**, 5766–5774.

12. MEITES, J. (1979) Role of neuroendocrine system in regulation of mammary tumors in different species, *Archives of Toxicology*, **Suppl. 2**, 47–58.

13. WELSCH, C.W. and NAGASAWA, H. (1977) Prolactin and murine mammary tumorigenesis: a review, *Cancer Research*, **37**, 951–963.

14. ROGERS, A.E. (1989) Factors that modulate chemical carcinogenesis in the mammary gland of the female rat, in JONES, T.C., MOHR, A. and HUNT, R.D. (Eds) *ILSI Monographs on Pathology of Laboratory Animals, Integument and Mammary Glands*, pp. 304–314, Berlin: Springer-Verlag.

15. RUSSO, J., RUSSO, I.H., ROGERS, A.E., VAN ZWIETEN N.J. and GUSTERSON, B. (1990) Tumors of the mammary gland, in TUROSOV, V.S. and MOHR, V. (Eds) *Pathology of Tumours in Laboratory Animals*, Vol. 1. *Tumours of the Rat*, pp. 47–63, Lyon: IARC Scientific Publications.

16. HOROWSKI, R. and GRAF, K.J. (1979) Neuroendocrine effects of neuropsychotropic drugs and their possible influence on toxic reactions in animals and man. The role of the dopamine–prolactin system, *Archives of Toxicology*, **Suppl. 2**, 93–104.

17. CUTTS, J.H. and NOBLE, R.L. (1964) Estrone-induced mammary tumours in the rat. 1. Induction and behaviour of tumours. *Cancer Research*, **24**, 1116–1123.

18. CASEY, H.W., GILES, R.C. and KWAPILEN, R.P. (1979) Mammary neoplasia in animals: pathological aspects and the effects of contraceptive steroids, *Recent Results in Cancer Research*, **66**, 129–160.

19. LANARI, C., MOLINOLO, A.A. and PASQUALINI, C.D. (1986) Induction of mammary adenocarcinomas by medroxyprogesterone acetate in BALB/c female mice, *Cancer Letters*, **33**, 215–223.

20. HOOSON, J. (1980) The effect of hormonal manipulation on mammary tumourigenesis by MNU and DES in the rat, *Toxicology Letters*, **July S.I.**, 238.

21. GREAVES, P., GOONETILLEKE, R., NUNN, G., TOPHAM, J. and ORTON, T. (1993) Two-year carcinogenicity study of tamoxifen in Alderley Park Wistar-derived rats, *Cancer Research*, **53**, 3919–3924.

22. JORDAN, V.C., LABABIDI, M.K. and LANGAN-FAHEY, S. (1991) Suppression of mouse mammary tumorigenesis by long term tamoxifen therapy, *Journal of the National Cancer Institute*, **83**, 492–496.

23. HAMILTON, J.M., KNIGHT, P.J. and BEEVERS, J. (1978) Serum prolactin levels in canine mammary cancer, *Veterinary Record*, **102**, 127–128.

24. NEUMANN, F. (1991) Early indicators for carcinogenesis in sex-hormone-sensitive organs, *Mutation Research*, **248**, 341–356.

25. JOHNSON, A.N. (1989) Comparative aspects of contraceptive steroids – effects observed in beagle dogs, *Toxicological Pathology*, **17**, 389–395.

26. EL-ETREBY, M.F., GRAF, K.J., GUNZEL, P. and NEUMANN, F. (1979) Evaluation of effects of sexual steroids on the hypothalamic–pituitary system of animals and man, *Archives of Toxicology*, **Suppl. 2**, 11–39.

27. FECHNER, R.E. (1982) The breast, in RIDDELL, R.H. (Ed.) *Pathology of Drug-Induced and Toxic Diseases*, pp. 341–355, New York: Churchill Livingstone.

28. TAVASSOLI, F.A., CASEY, H.W. and NORRIS, H.J. (1988) The morphological effects of synthetic reproductive steroids on the mammary gland of rhesus monkeys. Mestranol, ethynerone, mestranol–ethynerone, chloroethynyl norgestrel–mestranol and anagestone acetate–mestranol combinations, *American Journal of Pathology*, **131**, 213–234.

29. DUNN, T.B. (1959) Morphology of mammary tumors in mice, in HOMBURGER, F. (Ed.) *Physiopathology of Cancer*, pp. 38–84, New York: Hoeber.

30. THOMAS, D.B. (1993) Oral contraceptives and breast cancer, *Journal of the National Cancer Institute*, **85**, 359–364.

Organs of Special Sense I: The Eye

MERVYN ROBINSON

15.1 Introduction

The eye consists of a wide variety of tissue types and morphological structures with different biochemical processes which make it potentially susceptible to the toxic effects of many chemicals. Although the total loss of function of the eye due to toxicologically induced pathological change is not necessarily incompatible with life, it is extremely important with respect to the quality of life. With reference to toxicological conditions, the number of reported instances of altered structure or function of the eye due to toxic substances are exceeded only by the liver. Furthermore, the emotive ingredient of an ocular abnormality being induced in humans due to contact with a chemical or drug is great. Therefore a sound knowledge of the pathological processes occurring after toxicological insult is extremely important.

15.2 Anatomy, Histology and Physiology [1, 2]

The eye is a complex organ but it has one function only, namely photosensory reception. The structural elements contributing to this function include (i) neurosensory retina; (ii) light-transmitting structures – cornea, lens, aqueous and vitreous humors; (iii) rigid structures – tough sclera and anterior cornea retaining the fluid contents; and (iv) the uveal tract – comprising the choroid and ciliary processes which provide oxygen and nutrition, and the iris which acts as a variable diaphragm regulating the light entering the eye (Figure 15.1).

15.2.1 The Conjunctiva

The conjunctiva is a mucous epithelium lining the inner aspect of the eyelid, the palpebral conjunctiva, and the outer surface of the sclera, the bulbar conjunctiva. It consists of a non-keratinized, stratified squamous epithelium containing goblet cells.

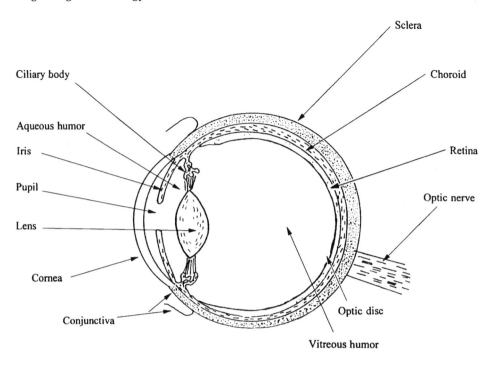

Ciliary body

Aqueous humor

Iris

Pupil

Lens

Cornea

Conjunctiva

Sclera

Choroid

Retina

Optic nerve

Optic disc

Vitreous humor

Figure 15.1 Ocular structures.

15.2.2 *The Cornea*

The cornea (Figure 15.2a) consists of five layers: anterior epithelium, a condensed anterior acellular stroma – Bowman's layer (primates only), a connective tissue stroma containing sparse flattened keratocytes, a posterior limiting membrane or Descemet's membrane, and a posterior epithelium or endothelium of flattened cells. Transparency is ensured by the lack of keratin, pigment and blood vessels, the relative acellular stroma with regular lamellae of fibres, and the relative dehydration of the stroma which is maintained by the Na/K ATPase pump of the posterior epithelium.

15.2.3 *The Sclera*

The sclera is composed of tough fibrous connective tissue and is relatively hydrated compared with the cornea.

15.2.4 *The Iris*

The iris consists of an anterior mesodermal portion and a posterior double epithelium. Smooth muscle provides sphincter and dilator functions. The stroma-containing mesenchymal tissue is well supplied with blood vessels.

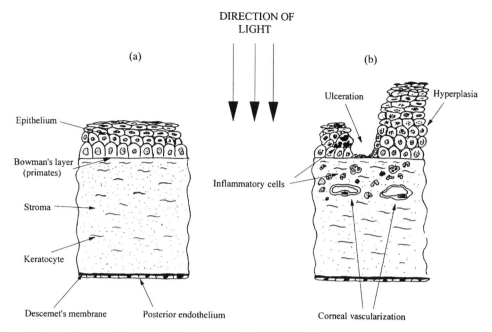

Figure 15.2   Histology of (a) normal cornea, (b) cornea with keratitis.

15.2.5   *The Ciliary Body*

The ciliary body contains anterior ciliary processes comprising a double epithelium. These form the aqueous humor by ultrafiltration, the movement of ions along an electrochemical gradient and by an active pump mechanism. The posterior body contains smooth muscle which is responsible for changing the shape of the lens in accommodation. This is poorly developed in many animals.

15.2.6   *The Choroid*

The choroid lines the posterior two-thirds of the eye and lies between the sclera and the retina. It contains numerous blood vessels and supplies oxygen and nutrition to the retina. In some mammalian species, e.g. the dog, cat and horse, an additional structure – the tapetum – lies at the inner aspect of the choroid and is located in the dorsal half to third of the ocular fundus. This structure reflects light in dim illumination.

15.2.7   *The Lens*

The lens (Figure 15.3a) is suspended from the ciliary body by zonular fibres and has posterior attachments to the vitreous body where it lies in a cup-shaped depression. The rodent lens is relatively large compared with man and the dog. The lens is composed entirely of epithelial fibres which meet anteriorly and posteriorly at suture lines. The anterior suture line is Y-shaped, whilst the posterior suture line has an

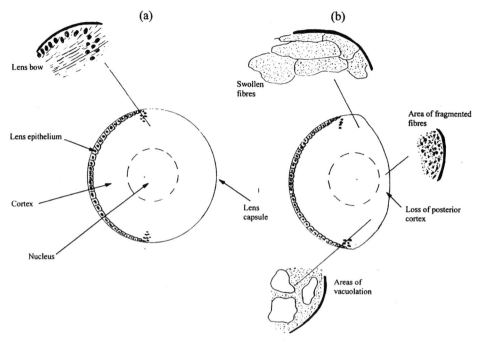

Figure 15.3 Histology of (a) normal lens, (b) cataractous lens.

inverted Y-shape. There is an anterior epithelium which continuously forms new fibres. As the fibres mature, they move centrally, become condensed and lose their nuclei and organelles. The inner portion of the lens, the nucleus, is the oldest part, and the outer portion, the cortex, is the youngest. Transparency of the lens is maintained by the regular nature of the fibres, the proportion of soluble and insoluble constituent proteins, and the relative dehydration produced by the activity of the sodium pump. The lens is surrounded by a capsule which ensures that the immunologically reactive lenticular proteins do not gain access to other ocular structures.

15.2.8 *The Vitreous Humor*

The vitreous humor is semisolid and helps maintain rigidity. It is composed mainly of water with a small percentage of collagen and hyaluronic acid.

15.2.9 *The Retina*

The retina (Figure 15.4a) is formed from neuroectoderm and consists of a posterior retinal pigment epithelium (RPE) and an anterior neurosensory retina. The RPE is a single cuboidal layer of cells. Its function is related to structural maintenance of the photoreceptors and vitamin A metabolism, which is essential in the photochemistry of vision. The neurosensory retina contains nine layers as follows: the outer photosensory layer of rods and cones; the outer limiting membrane; the cell bodies of

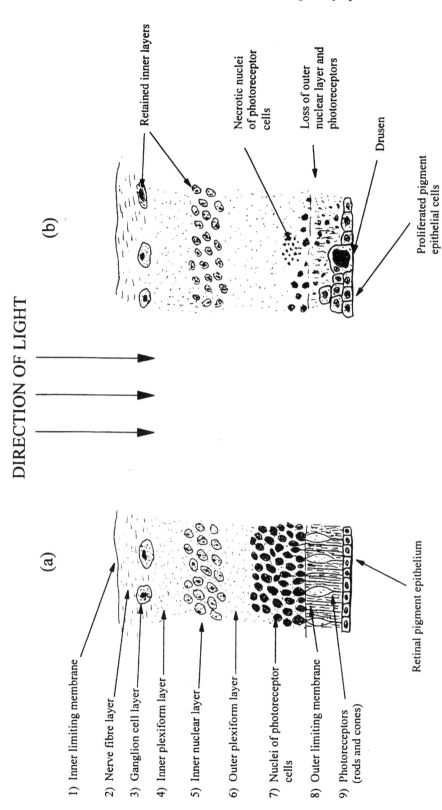

DIRECTION OF LIGHT

(a)

(b)

Retained inner layers

Necrotic nuclei of photoreceptor cells

Loss of outer nuclear layer and photoreceptors

Drusen

Proliferated pigment epithelial cells

1) Inner limiting membrane

2) Nerve fibre layer

3) Ganglion cell layer

4) Inner plexiform layer

5) Inner nuclear layer

6) Outer plexiform layer

7) Nuclei of photoreceptor cells

8) Outer limiting membrane

9) Photoreceptors (rods and cones)

Retinal pigment epithelium

Figure 15.4 Histology of (a) normal retina showing the nine layers of the neurosecretory retina, (b) degenerate retina.

the photosensory cells; the outer plexiform layer containing synapses; the inner nuclear layer which contains the bipolar, horizontal, amacrine, and supporting Muller cells; the inner plexiform layer containing synapses; the ganglion cell layer; the nerve fibre layer; and the inner limiting membrane. Blood supply to the retina is via the choroid and retinal vessels. The arrangement of retinal vessels varies considerably from species to species. In the rat, dog and man most of the retinal surface contains vessels. In the rabbit, retinal blood vessels are confined to a small area in the immediate periphery of the optic disc. In the guinea pig, retinal vessels are absent.

15.3 Morphological Response to Injury [3, 4, 5]

15.3.1 *The Conjunctiva*

The most frequently observed pathological change in the conjunctiva is inflammation. This may be acute or chronic. Acute changes include inflammatory cell infiltration with or without necrosis, excess lachrymation, prominent blood vessels and varying amounts of exudate discharge. The chronic phase is characterized by a proliferative response with hyperplasia of the epithelium, often with increased numbers of goblet cells and pronounced mononuclear cell infiltration. The lymphoid component may form follicles.

15.3.2 *The Cornea*

Most pathological changes in the cornea result in opacification to a greater or lesser extent. Some of these may be visible to the naked eye, others only by the appropriate use of ophthalmic instruments.

Keratitis or inflammation of the cornea (Figure 15.2b) is a common response that results from corneal injury by a wide variety of causes including **toxic chemicals**, **infectious agents**, **trauma**, etc. Leucocytes infiltrate to the affected area either via the corneal periphery, the limbus, or the tear film, and fluid changes result in opacity and separation of collagen fibres. Degenerative or necrotic changes may be the primary cause of the inflammation or they may occur as a secondary feature due to the release of enzymes by the inflammatory cells. In some circumstances, e.g. **alkali burns**, collagenases released by leucocytes may result in marked lytic changes, and severe ulceration or even perforation, where the term 'melting ulcer' is sometimes used. In severe forms of keratitis, deeper structures of the eye may be affected. Iridal changes are most frequently seen and these usually present as hyperaemia or fixation of the iris, with a lack of iris constrictor muscular response to light or mydriates (drugs which dilate the pupil). In severe cases, inflammation of the anterior chamber occurs with haemorrhage, known as hyphaema, or accumulation of inflammatory cells in the anterior chamber, known as hypopyon. The pathological process may even extend to produce lenticular changes or inflammation of the whole eye, termed panophthalmitis. Keratitis may resolve completely but more severe lesions involve the growth of blood vessels from the limbus, and fibroblastic proliferation with the deposition of scar tissue. Clinically, the presence of blood vessels and young fibroblastic tissue within the cornea is referred to as pannus. Corneal scarring in histological section is identified by increased cellularity, more prominent fibroblasts and irregular collagen fibres. Healed vascularized lesions result in corneal scarring with ghost vessels. The ability of corneal tissue to regenerate, and the amount of scarring produced from a given degree of damage, varies considerably between different species of mammal. Severe or long-standing keratitis may result in hyperplastic or metaplastic epithelial changes with rete peg formation or keratinization. Melanin deposition may occur in non-albino strains/species.

Degeneration and necrosis may occur due to the toxic effects of compounds, or be part of the inflammatory process. Erosion or ulceration is a common response from the external application of toxicants. Full thickness destruction of the cornea results in outward bulging of Descemet's membrane through the damaged stroma and epithelium, a condition known as staphyloma, before rupture and ocular collapse occur. A shrunken, fibrotic and non-functioning globe is referred to as phthisis bulbi. Corneal oedema is a common response to injury and denotes fluid changes within the stroma, usually resulting from posterior epithelial cell malfunction. Grossly, there is hazy or complete white opacification. In histological section, the collagen fibres are uniformly separated by fluid and the cornea is thickened. Cleft-like spaces, between which lie normal-looking stroma, usually denote artefactual separation of fibres.

Abnormal material deposited in the cornea may be of endogenous or exogenous origin. The gross, histological and ultrastructural appearance and location vary, dependent upon the type of damage and the substance involved. Calcium salts and melanin pigmentation are the most common substances seen.

15.3.3 *The Lens*

The pathological reactions of the lens are limited and the most important change is opacification or cataract (Figure 15.3b). Whilst some forms of opacity are reversible and produce only temporary changes in fluid content, most forms encountered also involve structural alteration of the fibres and result in permanent change. Early gross changes present as hazy opacities, usually around the suture lines, although this may be preceded in some cases by an increased clarity of the lens. This is caused by a reduction in the refractive index due to alteration of the proportions of soluble and insoluble lens proteins. In most circumstances, hazy partial opacities lead to total opacity although vacuoles may also be present. In a lens which is totally opaque, clefts or fluid-filled spaces may develop, particularly around the suture lines. Sometimes these clefts are arranged radially. With time, the degree of opacity of a total cataract lessens, as the altered lens protein is liquefied. Eventually this fluid may be resorbed to leave a shrunken capsule, a condition known as morgagnian change. Alternatively, the capsule may rupture under the fluid pressure exerted, with the release of immunologically reactive lenticular proteins and the formation of a lens-induced uveitis.

Histological changes include ballooning of fibres, fragmentation, and the formation of spaces filled with homogenous eosinophilic material, or the presence of clear vacuoles (Figure 15.3b). Loss of fibre material usually results in an abnormally shaped lens which is pear shaped in rodents. The nucleus is frequently the last portion of the lens to remain in toxic cataracts. When lenticular rupture has occurred, the capsule is usually seen as a coiled structure and the presence of inflammatory cells denotes the onset of a lens-induced uveitis, since the lens itself cannot respond to injurious agents by inflammation because of its avascular nature. In uveitis, adhesions between the iris and the remaining lenticular material frequently occur, a condition termed posterior synechiae. Posterior adhesions result in retinal detachment. Sometimes calcification or lenticular epithelial cell proliferation may be observed.

15.3.4 *The Retina*

Toxic retinopathy may be recognized by the presence of vascular changes or by degenerative/atrophic changes in the neuroepithelium, or both. Ophthalmoscopically, the features seen include the presence of haemorrhage or microaneurysm in the retinal vessels, swelling of the optic disc due to papilloedema, microinfarcts leading to discoloured spots, thinning or atrophy of the retinal vessels, marked pallor or increased prominence of the choroidal vasculature in rodents, and increased tapetal reflectivity in dogs. In pigmented strains/species, increased or decreased melanin pigmentation are important aspects of retinal toxicity.

As the retina is a complex structure, the range of pathological processes in toxic retinopathy are diverse and show a variety of histological changes. Loss of cell layers (Figure 15.4b) is the most common change observed, although this may be preceded by actual cell necrosis in the affected part. Loss of rods and cones and their associated cell bodies is probably most commonly encountered, although with some compounds these might be left relatively intact with the inner cell layers showing the most prominent change. Disorganization of retinal layers frequently accompanies cell loss and, in some retinopathies, vacuolar or cystic degeneration rather than necrosis may be the characteristic lesion. Some chemicals, e.g. **cationic amphiphilic drugs**, induce lysosomal accumulation of lipid in different cell types of the retina depending on the particular drug involved. Abnormalities in the RPE may be present, whether this is the primary site of toxicity or not. The changes seen include swelling, proliferation, increased or decreased melanin accumulation, and the presence of large globules that are positive for periodic acid Schiff staining within the cells, which are called drusen.

Compounds which cause a primary vascular retinopathy, e.g. **alloxan**, induce histological features such as papilloedema of the optic nerve head, proteinaceous effusions causing separation of the cell layers or retinal detachment, necrosis due to infarction, haemorrhage or endothelial cell proliferation of the retinal vasculature.

Whatever the primary event, the features of endstage retinal toxicity may be similar and include increased pigmentation, atrophy and glial cell proliferation.

In addition to structural changes, electrophysiological abnormalities associated with toxic chemicals have been described both in man and animals.

15.3.5 *The Uveal Tract*

In general, the uveal tract is not a common site for primary toxic damage, although it is frequently involved as a secondary feature. An exception to this is the inflammation of the iris, or iritis, occurring after direct application of irritant to the eye. In these circumstances there is gross reddening of the iris as a result of active hyperaemia. Reaction to light or mydriates is reduced or abolished. Histologically, polymorphs are present within the iris stroma and may accumulate in the filtration angle. Degenerative or necrotic changes may occur in specific regions of the uveal tract with certain toxic chemicals.

15.3.6   *Alteration in Intraocular Pressure*

Glaucoma is defined as an increase in intraocular pressure leading to permanent ocular damage. Chemicals which increase intraocular pressure, e.g. **corticosteroids**, may do so to such an extent as to induce glaucoma. The increase in pressure results in corneal oedema due to adverse pressure effects on the corneal endothelium. The lens becomes misshapen and eventually cataractous and there is retinal degeneration with cupping of the optic disc. Conversely, glaucoma frequently occurs as a secondary phenomenon due to primary damage elsewhere. This is related to blockage of the filtering structures at the angle between the cornea and iris. Uveitis and severe cataract are common causes of secondary glaucoma. There are many drugs which reduce intraocular pressure, some of which are used therapeutically, e.g. **pilocarpine**.

15.3.7   *Ocular Neoplasia*

Compound-induced intraocular neoplasia is extremely uncommon, although experimental models have been described using intraocular injection of **nickel sulphate** or **N-methyl-N-nitrosourea** in rats. With the exception of lymphoid tumours, spontaneous intraocular neoplasia of rodents is also rare.

15.4   Biochemical and Cellular Mechanisms of Toxicity [6, 7, 8, 9, 10, 11] (Table 15.1)

Unlike some organ systems of the body, the biochemical and cellular mechanisms for many known toxic effects in the eye are poorly understood. Where possible, the mechanisms involved are mentioned below, although most of the information presented is related to the types of toxic damage which occur, with specific chemical examples, and how the toxicity may be classified.

15.4.1   *The Cornea*

Corneal toxicology may occur in a variety of circumstances:

Abnormality of the precorneal film

Toxic compounds may cause damage and malfunction of the lachrymal gland which result in pathology of the cornea. Administration of **5-aminosalicylic acid** to dogs causes severe inflammation and destruction of the lachrymal glands, reduction of tear flow and drying of the cornea with keratitis. The term keratoconjunctivitis sicca is used for this condition. In other cases, the reduced tear flow is related to the pharmacological action of the compound. The anticholinergic drug **clonidine** in

Table 15.1 Chemicals toxic to the eye

Ocular Structure	Mechanism of injury/pathological change induced	Chemical
Cornea	Alteration of precorneal film: keratoconjunctivitis sicca	5-Aminosalicyclic acid, clonidine, morphine, some anticholinesterase compounds
	Injury from systemic administration: keratitis odema	5% Tyrosine (rats) 1,2-Dichloroethane
	Direct external application: keratitis, oedema, necrosis	Acids, alkalis, solvents, detergents
	Deposition of substances	Chloroquine, amiodarone, tilorone, gold, chlorpromazine
Lens	Sugar alcohol deposition: cataract	Excess glucose, galactose
	Perturbation of cell division: cataract	4-(*p*-Dimethylaminostyryl)quinolone, busulphan
	Production of free radicals: cataract	Diquat
	Uncoupling of oxidative phosphorylation: cataract	2,4-Dinitrophenol
	Protein/enzyme disturbance: cataract	Naphthoquinone, chlorophenylalanine
	Inhibition of lipid metabolism: cataract	Triparanol
Retina	Damage to inner retina	Monosodium glutamate
	Photoreceptor injury	Hexachlorophene
	Pigment epithelial perturbation: degeneration, drusen	Zinc chelators
	Dysplasia	Cytosine arabinose
	Neurotoxicity to all layers: degeneration, necrosis, atrophy	Trimethyl tin
	Vascular injury: haemorrhage, capillary proliferation, retinal detachment	Excess oxygen, alloxan
Uveal tract	Tapetal injury: degeneration, colour changes	Ethambutol

rodents causes keratoconjunctivitis sicca by virtue of reduced tear flow, and administration of narcotic agents, e.g. **morphine**, in rats may induce corneal changes due to prevention of eyelid closure and corneal drying. Keratitis has been reported after the administration of some anticholinesterase compounds such as **fenthion**.

Although in most cases keratoconjunctivitis sicca is considered to be due mainly to aqueous deficiency, abnormalities in the lipid and mucus components of the precorneal film may be at least theoretically important.

Direct corneal damage from external application

Many substances from a range of chemical classes may induce this type of injury. Of particular note are **acids, alkalis, solvents** and **detergents**.

Acids induce a coagulative type of necrosis with an associated keratitis. In general, the lower the pH, the more severe the damage. With weak acids the necrosis produced tends to form a barrier to further damage. **Alkalis** cause more severe lesions since the saponification and cell membrane damage produced allow ready penetration. Furthermore, the prominent keratitis produced involves numerous neutrophils which release collagenase. This enzyme destroys the stromal collagen and the resultant breakdown products in turn stimulate a further inflammatory reaction. Thus a vicious cycle of destruction is induced which results in the characteristic 'melting ulcer'. **Organic solvents** dissolve lipid and damage the epithelium by this mechanism. The damage is usually superficial. **Detergents** induce keratitis although the mechanism is unclear. Cationic detergents produce more severe changes than anionic or non-ionic types and may result in permanent change.

Corneal injury from systemic administration

This may take the form of keratitis, oedema or opacification from the deposition of endogenous or exogenous substances. Reported examples of keratitis in this type of injury are few, although the administration of 5 per cent **tyrosine** in a low protein diet is reported to induce keratitis in rats. Opacification of the cornea due to oedema usually denotes an effect on the corneal endothelium. This may occur indirectly as part of a keratitis, as a consequence of glaucoma, or arise directly as in the systemic administration of **1,2-dichloroethane** in the dog.

Multifocal corneal opacities due to the deposition of substances have been reported widely in laboratory animals and man. Lipid deposition in the lysosomes of the corneal epithelium and keratocytes occurs after administration of cationic amphiphilic compounds such as **chloroquine** and **amiodarone**. In corneal mucopolysaccharidosis due to **tilorone**, similar changes are induced where glycosaminoglycans are deposited. The corneal opacities which occur with some chemicals are believed to be due to deposition of the chemical itself or a metabolite. This is the case with **chlorpromazine**, and the use of metallic drugs such as **gold** may result in corneal deposition. Calcium deposition may occur in a variety of circumstances. In addition to presenting as a spontaneous finding, particularly in some strains of mouse, corneal drying with degeneration and calcification occurs after **morphine** administration.

15.4.2 *The Lens*

Although a great number of chemicals have been reported as inducing cataract in man or animals, the precise mechanisms involved in many cases are uncertain.

Consequently, cataracts are often described according to their anatomical location, i.e. nuclear, cortical, anterior, posterior, equatorial, etc. However, the mechanisms of cataractogenesis are known to some degree with a number of chemicals and this can form the basis of a classification system.

Alteration of carbohydrate metabolism

Most glucose in the lens is metabolized anaerobically. **High levels of blood glucose** in diabetes saturate these pathways and the excess glucose is metabolized via the aldose reductase pathway to sorbitol, the sugar alcohol. This becomes trapped in the lens and as a result of a hyperosmotic effect, water is drawn into the lens, accumulates, and leads to opacity with biochemical and structural disturbance. Feeding high levels of **galactose** in the rat induces cataracts by a similar mechanism.

Perturbation of cell division

New lens fibres are formed throughout life by cell division and elongation of the anterior lenticular epithelium. Some chemicals interfere with this process and produce cataracts which mimic those induced by ionizing radiation, e.g. **4-(*p*-dimethylaminostyryl)quinoline** and **busulphan**.

Production of free radicals

This is believed to be the mechanism of **diquat**-induced cataracts in the rat and dog. The free radicals, i.e. the active oxygen species produced by redox cycling, induce biochemical and structural disturbances in the lens fibres.

Uncoupling of oxidative phosphorylation

2,4-Dinitrophenol, a drug which was used a number of years ago as a slimming aid, induces cataracts in man, ducks and chickens whereas the dog and rat are resistant. The species differences are probably related to variations in the concentrations achieved in the aqueous humor. Uncoupling of oxidative phosphorylation and increased oxygen consumption are considered to be responsible for the altered metabolism and structural changes seen.

Protein disturbances and enzyme inhibitors

Naphthoquinone inhibits Na/K ATPase and is thought to interfere with the lenticular cation pump and hence water balance. **Chlorophenylalanine** interferes with phenylalanine metabolism and may perturb lens protein synthesis.

Inhibition of lipid metabolism

Cell membranes are an important component of lens fibres. **Triparanol** inhibits cholesterol synthesis and this is believed to be responsible for the cataract produced with this compound, since cholesterol is an essential structural component of the membrane.

15.4.3 The Retina

Since the mechanisms of action of many retinotoxic chemicals is poorly understood, a useful classification system based on biochemical mechanisms is not at present available. Some reviews have classified retinotoxicity according to the primary areas of damage, i.e. inner retina, e.g. **monosodium glutamate**; ganglion cell layer and optic nerve, e.g. **methanol** in man; photoreceptor cell, e.g. **hexachorophene**; RPE, e.g. **zinc chelators**; retinal dysplasia, e.g. **cytosine arabinose**; and multiple cell layers, e.g. **trimethyl tin**. However, most descriptions of retinotoxic chemicals in the literature appear only as a list with short descriptions for each. Compounds generally covered in this way include **chloroquine, phenothiazine, indomethacin, iodoacetate, methanol** and **aminophenoxyalkanes**.

The melanin-binding properties of drugs may be important with regard to retinal toxicity, or toxicity in other ocular structures. The effects of such binding may be investigated by comparing the response in pigmented and non-pigmented strains of animal. For example **vigabatrin**, an inhibitor of γ-aminobutyric acid transaminase, induces retinal degeneration in albino but not pigmented rats.

Excessive light intensity is well known as a cause of retinal degeneration, particularly in albino animals. The outer segments of the retina are the first to be damaged. The changes produced resemble injury induced by many chemical agents.

In premature human infants the excessive administration of **oxygen** induces proliferation of fibrovascular tissue on the retina with resultant retinal detachment. There are two phases in the disease process, a vaso-obliteration phase and a vasoproliferative phase, corresponding to oxygen administration and the cessation of administration, respectively.

15.4.4 The Uveal Tract

6-Aminonicotinamide in rabbits induces cytoplasmic vacuolation of the ciliary epithelium with vascular change after systemic administration. Several reports have described toxic changes in the tapetum of dogs due to chemicals with metal chelating properties, e.g. **ethambutol**.

15.5 Testing for Toxicity [7, 12]

A wide variety of methods are available for the identification and investigation of ocular toxicity.

15.5.1 Visual Methods

Since the eye is transparent it lends itself admirably to *in vivo* gross pathological examination. Naked eye examination with suitable illumination is particularly valuable in the larger species. For more detailed examination, and for use with small laboratory species, a range of ophthalmoscopic instruments are available, e.g. direct and indirect ophthalmoscopes, hand-held or table-mounted slit lamps and fundic cameras. Various modifications to some of these instruments allow additional information to be gathered. The pachymeter attachment to the basic slit lamp enables corneal thickness to be measured and is particularly valuable in eye irritation studies. The gonioscope lens allows visualization of the filtration angle.

15.5.2 *Histopathology*

Careful attention is required in fixation and processing of eyes for histology. Since the eye is composed of a variety of tissue types, the ideal fixative for a particular purpose is generally the best compromise available. Davidson's fixative is generally recommended for toxicological pathology although eyes preserved in this way are unsuitable for electron microscopy. Much depends on the skill of the histology technician if good preparations are to be obtained. Artefacts such as cleft formation in the corneal stroma, shattering of the lens, and retinal detachment and folding are especially prevalent in eye histology and these must be borne in mind when assessing morphological changes. Careful searching for focal lesions is important and a combination of ophthalmoscopy and histology is ideal.

15.5.3 *Physiological Methods*

There are a number of instruments available for the measurement of intraocular pressure. Most of these depend on indentation or applanation tonometry which measure the indentation or flattening of the cornea, respectively. For accurate use, these instruments require calibration with a manometer.

There are several electrophysiological methods for investigating retinal function. The measurement of a visually evoked potential depends on the fact that light stimulation of the eye induces a small potential in the brain which can be recorded by skin electrodes on the posterior pole of the brain. Repetitive stimulation and computerized averaging techniques can eliminate the background noise. Such measurements are used to investigate the function of the central pathways of vision. The electro-oculogram measures the electrical response of the eye to a prolonged light stimulus lasting several minutes and is a useful technique to study toxic effects on the RPE. There is a difference in potential between the anterior and posterior poles of the eye and light stimulation alters potassium metabolism in the RPE so that this potential increases to a maximum, 8 min after stimulation. The electroretinogram (ERG) measures the rapid changes in electrical potential of the eye after light stimulation. It represents the summation of activity within several parts of the retina. The ERG is used in a variety of ways in order to separate out different functions, e.g. rod and cone responses.

15.5.4 *Miscellaneous*

The rate of lachrymal secretion can be studied by the Schirmer tear test which measures the flow of tears along a filter paper strip in a given time. It is used to investigate keratoconjunctivitis sicca.

Various stains can be used to study the integrity of the cornea *in vivo*. Fluorescein is used to delineate corneal ulcers and rose bengal highlights necrotic material on the corneal surface.

Fluorescein angiography is a valuable technique for investigating the nature and patency of the retinal or choroidal vasculature after compound administration.

15.5.5 Eye Irritation Tests

Although nearly 50 years old, the Draize test is still used for investigating the irritant properties of chemicals in the eye. A dose of 0.1 ml or 0.1 g of test substance is instilled into the conjunctival sac of one eye of an albino rabbit, the contralateral eye serving as control. The eyes are examined at 1, 24, 48 and 72 h. If there is no reaction, the study is terminated. If a reaction is seen, the study is continued until day 21 in order to investigate reversibility. Numerical scores are given for changes in the conjunctiva (redness, swelling), cornea (opacity) and iris (redness, response to light), respectively. A mean score for all animals is given for each ocular structure. These are added and a total mean score is calculated to determine the degree of irritancy from printed tables.

Animal welfare and scientific considerations have resulted in a move away from the Draize test in recent years. Today *in vivo* testing is performed in a phased manner. If the compound is a strong acid or alkali, or if it has been first shown to be a skin irritant, then eye testing is not performed. Single animals, rather than the full number of rabbits required for the Draize test, reduced volumes and strengths of compounds are tested before the full Draize test is performed. In addition, novel compounds are tested by alternative methods in many laboratories before the *in vivo* test is performed. There are a number of possible alternative methods available including cell culture or isolated eye techniques. Comparison of results with *in vivo* investigations have shown very good correlations, particularly with severe irritants. Therefore compounds which indicate severe irritancy with these new methods are not tested *in vivo*.

15.6 Conclusions

The complex nature of the eye and its composition of different tissue types renders it particularly susceptible to toxicity. This spectrum of anatomical and functional features provides a wide variety of pathological responses which are important in toxicology. However, the development of many and varied methods of toxicological investigation provide the toxicologist with a splendid array of tools to study disease and to use in the safety evaluation of drugs and chemicals.

The eye is notorious for demonstrating marked species variation in its response to toxic chemicals. This, together with the generally poor understanding of mechanisms with respect to ocular toxicity, renders the extrapolation of the effects of toxic chemicals in laboratory animals to man extremely difficult. To make broad generalizations on this subject is fraught with hazard, except to regard experimental oculotoxicity testing as being of value only to identify the *potential* of a chemical to cause ocular damage in man.

References

1. DAVSON, H. (1990) *Davson's Physiology of the Eye*, 5th Edn, London: Macmillan Press.

2. GELATT, K.N. (1991) *Veterinary Ophthalmology*, 2nd Edn, London: Lea and Febiger.
3. PEIFFER, R.L. (1983) *Comparative Ophthalmic Pathology*, Springfield, Illinois: Charles C. Thomas.
4. WILCOCK, B.P. (1993) The eye and ear, in JUBB, K.V.F., KENNEDY, P.C. and PALMER, N. (Eds) *Pathology of Domestic Animals*, Vol. 1, 4th Edn, pp. 441–522, London: Academic Press.
5. GARNER, A. and KLINTWORTH, K. (1982) *Pathobiology of Ocular Disease*, Vols 1 and 2, New York: Marcel Dekker.
6. GRANT, W.M. (1986) *Toxicology of the Eye*, 3rd Edn, Springfield, Illinois: Charles C. Thomas.
7. CHIOU, G.C.Y. (1992) *Ophthalmic Toxicology*, Target Organ Toxicology series, New York: Raven Press.
8. HOCKWIN, O. (1987) *Drug-Induced Ocular Side Effects and Ocular Toxicology, Concepts in Toxicology*, Vol. 4, Paris: Karger.
9. JONES, T.C., MOHR, U. and HUNT, R.D. (1991) *Eye and Ear, Monographs on Pathology of Laboratory Animals*, London: Springer-Verlag.
10. GEHRING, P.J. (1971) The cataractogenic activity of chemical agents, in GOLDBERG, L. (Ed.) *Critical Reviews in Toxicology*, pp. 93–118, Cleveland, Ohio: The Chemical Rubber Company.
11. TRIPATHI, R.C. and TRIPATHI, B.J. (1982) The eye, in RIDELL, R.H. (Ed.) *Pathology of Drug Induced and Toxic Diseases*, pp. 377–455, London: Churchill Livingstone.
12. HOCKWIN, O., GREEN, K. and RUBIN, L. (1992) *Manual of Oculotoxicity Testing of Drugs*, New York: Fischer Verlag.

Organs of Special Sense II: The Ear

ERNEST S. HARPUR

16.1 Introduction

Ototoxicity is an example of a highly selective organ-directed toxicity. The term is used to describe the process by which chemicals, many of which are drugs, cause damage to either the organ of hearing, the cochlea, or the organs of balance, the vestibular organs. Although there are examples of chemicals which cause hearing loss by actions at sites in the central auditory pathway (e.g. **dinitrobenzene**), the term ototoxicity is usually confined, as it is here, to effects on the peripheral end-organs.

16.2 Anatomy, Histology and Physiology

A detailed account of this subject can be found in Pickles [1]. The outer ear, or auditory canal, is separated from the air-filled middle ear by the eardrum, or tympanic membrane (Figure 16.1). The middle ear ossicles, namely the malleus, incus and stapes, act as an impedance transformer to maximize the transfer of energy from the sound wave (an oscillating pressure wave) to the fluid-filled inner ear. The inner ear, comprising a system of canals enclosed in the temporal bone of the skull (Figure 16.2), connects with the middle ear via two openings known as the round window and the oval window. The first of these is sealed by the round window membrane and the second by the footplate of the third ossicular bone, the stapes. The inner ear is divided structurally into the cochlea, subserving the sense of hearing, and the vestibular organs, subserving the sense of equilibrium or balance. Whereas the sensory structures in the cochlea are responsive to sound energy, those in the vestibular organs signal position and rotational movement of the head.

16.2.1 Vestibular System

The vestibular system consists of the three semicircular canals, organized in three orthogonal planes in space, and two sac-like structures, the utricle and the saccule

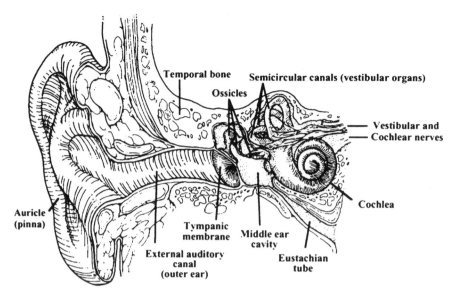

Figure 16.1 Drawing of the ear illustrating its division into three parts: the outer ear, separated by the tympanic membrane from the middle ear containing the three ossicles, the malleus, incus and stapes, and the inner ear, comprising the cochlea and vestibular organs (of which the semicircular canals are shown).

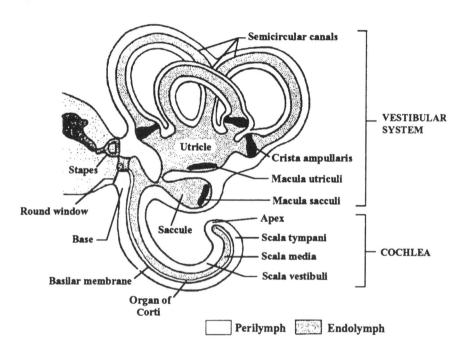

Figure 16.2 Schematic representation of the inner ear illustrating its organization as a series of membranous ducts and sac-like structures filled with endolymphatic fluid. The five sensory structures in the vestibular system, the three cristae ampullaris and the maculae of the utricle and saccule, are shown. In the cochlea, the organ of Corti rests on the basilar membrane dividing the scala media from the scala tympani.

(Figure 16.2). Each canal or sac is a sealed membranous structure within the bony channel. The membranous structures are filled with endolymph, a unique extracellular fluid which resembles intracellular fluid in composition in that the predominant cation is potassium at a concentration of about 150 mM. Surrounding the membranous canal is perilymph, a fluid which is similar in composition to normal extracellular fluid. The neurosensory epithelia, a term used to designate tissues which contain both sensory and supporting cells as well as the innervating neurons, are located in the maculae of the utricle and the saccule and in three cristae, which are located within swellings, the ampullae, one at the end of each semicircular canal. Vestibular sensory cells, known as hair cells (HCs), are designated either type 1 or type 2 on the basis of their shape and innervation pattern, but the functional difference between these cells is not yet clear.

16.2.2 Cochlea

In Figure 16.2 the cochlea is shown as a curved structure. In reality, the organ is helical (Figure 16.3) making several turns (the exact number varies with species) around a central bony spindle, the modiolus, which contains the blood and nerve supply. The bony canal is divided into three compartments by membranous partitions (Figure 16.4). The outer compartments, the scala vestibuli and the scala tympani, which connect at the apex of the cochlea, contain perilymph, which is identical to vestibular perilymph. The fluid within the inner compartment, the scala media, is endolymph. The neurosensory epithelium, known as the organ of Corti, rests on the basilar membrane and is composed of the sensory hair cells (HCs) with their neural

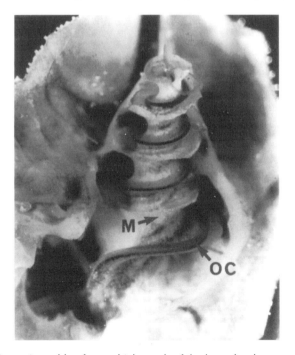

Figure 16.3 Guinea pig cochlea from which much of the bone has been removed to reveal the spiral arrangement of the organ of Corti (OC) about the bony modiolus (M).

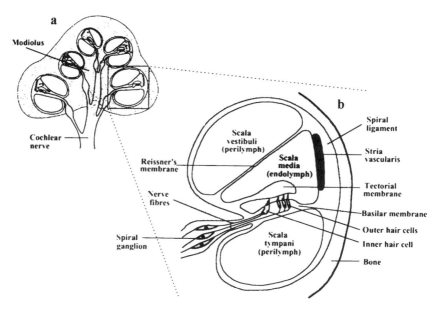

Figures 16.4 Much simplified drawing of a mid-modiolar section through the cochlea (a), with an enlarged drawing (b) through one turn of the cochlea. The division of the cochlear duct by membranous partitions into three compartments filled with perilymph or endolymph is shown, as is the basic organization of the hair cells on the basilar membrane.

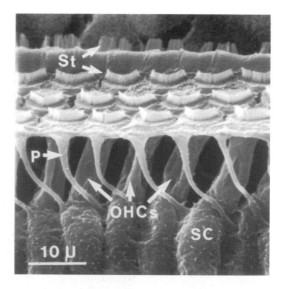

Figure 16.5 Axial view of a basal turn of guinea pig organ of Corti from which the outer supporting cells have come away to reveal the internal architecture of the sensory and supporting cells. In the foreground are seen the outermost supporting cell (SC) bodies from which arise angled processes (P) which expand to form headplates on the surface of the organ of Corti. Behind these cells can be seen the tall cylindrical bodies of the third row of outer hair cells (OHCs). The extensive fluid spaces between the cells are readily apparent. The stereocilia (St) on the surface of the sensory cells can also be seen. The headplates of the supporting cells and the cuticular plates of the hair cells interlock to form an impermeable barrier between the endolymph of the scala media and the perilymph of the fluid spaces within the organ of Corti.

innervation and a variety of supporting cells (Figure 16.5). The HCs are arranged in orderly, parallel rows along the length of the cochlea and, as in the vestibular system, there are two types (Figure 16.6). Moving radially from the modiolus, there is a single row of inner hair cells (IHCs) and three to five rows (depending on the species) of outer hair cells (OHCs).

During sound stimulation, the stapes footplate displaces fluid along the scala vestibuli and scala tympani, made possible by outward movement of the round window membrane which seals the scala tympani from the middle ear. The resultant displacement of the basilar membrane leads to excitation of the HCs. Systematic variations in the physical dimensions and characteristics of the basilar membrane along its length affect the mechanical properties of the system so that, for different frequencies of sound, maximal vibration of the basilar membrane occurs at different locations. High frequency (high pitched) sounds cause maximum stimulation of the HCs at the base of the cochlea, whereas low frequencies are detected at the apex of the cochlea. As a result, localized damage to the organ of Corti can result in differential loss of hearing at particular frequencies. For example, damage to the base of the cochlea (characteristically produced by ototoxic drugs) causes a high frequency hearing loss with good preservation of hearing at low frequencies. The HCs are mechano-transducers, converting the mechanical energy of the sound wave into electrical energy (neural excitation). HCs are stimulated through deflection of the stereocilia (Figure 16.7) relative to the tectorial membrane which overlays them. This is believed to open ion channels located somewhere on the apex of the HC, possibly at the distal tips of the stereocilia. The opening of these ion channels leads to current flow into the cell, carried by the predominant cation in endolymph, K^+ (Figure 16.7). This results in depolarization of the HC, influx of calcium, and excitation of the afferent neurons with which the cell synapses.

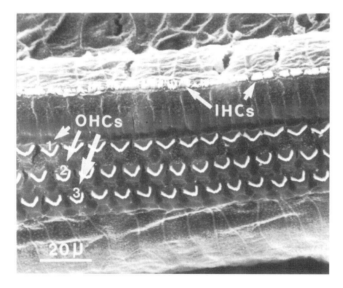

Figure 16.6 Scanning electron micrograph of the surface of the organ of Corti of the guinea pig showing the regular arrangement of the single row of inner hair cells (IHCs) and the three rows (1 to 3) of outer hair cells (OHCs), the latter distinguishable by the characteristic 'w' pattern, of the sterocilia on the surface.

Inner Hair Cell

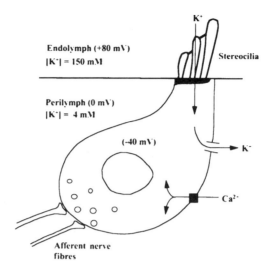

Figure 16.7 Schematic drawing, illustrating the receptor function of the inner hair cell. Deflection of the stereocilia causes the opening of ion channels, located somewhere on the apex of the hair cell, possibly on the distal tips of the stereocilia. This leads to current flow from endolymph into the cell, carried by the predominant cation in endolymph, potassium. The cell is depolarized, resulting in calcium influx, transmitter release and neural excitation. The high positive potential of endolymph coupled with a negative resting potential inside the hair cell provides the driving force for current flow.

It had long been believed that the OHCs were the primary transducers, until it was first observed, about 20 years ago, that 90 to 95 per cent of the total afferent innervation terminated on the IHCs. Today it is recognized that it is the IHCs that are the primary receptor cells and the role of the OHCs is to modulate the responsiveness of the IHCs to sounds of different frequency, or to 'fine tune' them. *In vitro* studies with isolated OHCs have shown that they respond to electrical stimulation by contracting [2]. These motile properties of the OHCs allow them to alter the mechanical properties of the basilar membrane in the immediate locality. The 'tuning' of the cochlea is physiologically vulnerable, for example to hypoxia. Ototoxic agents, which tend to affect the OHCs selectively, leaving the IHCs intact, can cause both an increase in threshold of response and a loss of the sharp tuning.

16.2.3 *Non-Sensory Epithelia*

In addition to the neurosensory epithelia, there are ion-transporting epithelia in both the vestibular system and the cochlea: the dark cell regions and the stria vascularis, respectively. The dark cell regions are located at the base of the cristae and in the macula of the utricle (but not the saccule). These cells contain numerous mitochondria and high levels of Na^+/K^+ ATPase and are believed to be directly involved in the production and maintenance of vestibular endolymph, through active ion transport. The equivalent tissue in the cochlea, the stria vascularis, is located along the lateral wall of the scala media (Figure 16.4). This is a highly vascularized ion-transporting epithelium responsible for the maintenance of both the ionic and electrical characteristics of endolymph. In addition to a K^+ concentration of 150 mM, endolymph has a high positive electrical potential of 80–100 mV, the endocochlear potential (EP). Both factors are very important for the receptor function of the HCs. Any agent which injures the endolymph-forming tissues will affect the transduction process and reduce HC responsiveness to stimuli.

16.3 Biochemical and Cellular Mechanisms of Toxicity

16.3.1 *The Chemicals Involved and the Effects Produced*

A wide range of chemicals are suspected, or known, to produce adverse effects on hearing or vestibular function. It is not possible in this short account to document all of these. Relatively little is known about the potential of industrial or environmental chemicals to cause ototoxicity, although a few compounds have been studied. For example, **carbon monoxide** has been shown to produce hearing impairment, probably via hypoxia. **Carbon monoxide** has also been shown to potentiate noise-induced hearing loss resulting in extensive loss of cochlear OHCs. **Methyl mercury** poisoning in humans is known to be associated with toxic effects on the sensory nervous system, primarily a disturbance of visual function and paraesthesia (abnormal touch sensations). However, hearing loss is also frequently reported. Limited studies in animals have demonstrated the ability of **methyl mercury** to produce selective high frequency hearing loss and damage to cochlear HCs. The neurotoxicological properties of the **trialkyltins** have been studied extensively for many years. More recently, **trimethyltin** has been shown to be ototoxic in both the rat and the guinea pig at the level of the cochlea, producing both OHC loss and atrophic changes in the stria vascularis. A number of recent studies in rodents have demonstrated the ability of various solvents, such as *n*-**hexane, toluene, xylene, styrene** and **trichloroethylene** to produce hearing loss. However, these changes are seen only at high levels of exposure, often close to those resulting in sedation. The site of action and whether these observations are the result of a specific action on the auditory pathway remains unknown in most cases. Only in the case of **toluene** has the hearing loss been shown to be associated with hair cell pathology in the cochlea.

Most interest has focused on drug-induced ototoxicity and a comprehensive review can be found in Reference [3]. The most important compounds, from the viewpoint both of clinical incidence of ototoxicity and the extent to which they have been studied experimentally, are the **aminoglycoside antibiotics, salicylates, quinine** (and, to a lesser extent, **chloroquine**), *cis*-**platinum** and the **loop diuretics**. They represent a diverse range of chemical structures and the nature of their effects on the ear is also variable. Their administration may result in damage to either auditory or vestibular mechanisms, or both. However, as exemplified by the **aminoglycoside antibiotics**, a predilection for either the cochlea or the vestibular organs is often a characteristic of a particular drug. For example, **streptomycin** affects primarily the vestibular system, whereas **neomycin, kanamycin** and particularly **amikacin** are primarily cochleotoxic. In patients, vestibular toxicity can give rise to symptoms such as dizziness or vertigo and, although the lesion may be permanent, the majority of subjects can in time adequately compensate, in most circumstances, for the loss of vestibular function.

Auditory effects with the above-mentioned drugs range from potentially transient symptoms such as tinnitus (a perception of a ringing sound in the absence of sound stimulation), or a mild reduction in auditory acuity to total and permanent deafness. **Salicylates** and other non-steroidal anti-inflammatory agents commonly cause tinnitus that is reversible when the drug administration is stopped and these compounds are only rarely associated with permanent hearing loss. Therapeutic doses of **quinine** characteristically cause tinnitus, but excessive doses of **quinine** or **chloroquine** may result in permanent deafness. The antitumour drug *cis*-**platinum** frequently causes tinnitus and permanent hearing loss which appears to be dose related. Large intravenous doses of **loop diuretics**, such as **frusemide (furosemide)**, may cause a transient hearing impairment, although the deafness may be permanent, particularly if the patient is uraemic or is also administered an **aminoglycoside antibiotic.** References [3] and [4] offer, respectively, a general account of drug-induced ototoxicity and a comprehensive text on both clinical and experimental aspects of **aminoglycoside** ototoxicity.

16.3.2 *Toxicokinetics as a Basis of Ototoxic Selectivity*

Clear elucidation of the reasons why some chemicals exert a very selective toxic action on the inner ear still eludes us. One of the earliest hypotheses for the selective ototoxic action of the largest and most studied group of ototoxic drugs, the **aminoglycoside antibiotics**, was their preferential accumulation in inner ear fluids. The relevance of the presence of a drug in perilymph or endolymph for a toxic effect on the HCs can be readily appreciated by inspection of Figures 16.4 and 16.5. The intercellular spaces surrounding the HCs in the organ of Corti are filled with a fluid identical to, and continuous with, perilymph, whereas the surface of the HCs is bathed in endolymph. Extensive work, involving technically difficult procedures of sampling small volumes of perilymph and endolymph, have failed to confirm earlier claims that **aminoglycoside antibiotics** extensively accumulate in these fluids. The concentrations of **aminoglycosides** achieved in the fluids and the tissues of the inner ear are not high compared, for example, with the kidney, where they are also toxic [5]. Although long half-lives have been demonstrated in cochlear fluids and tissues, there is no accumulation following multiple dosing, in the absence of renal impairment [6]. It has been pointed out that the concentration of **aminoglycosides** in perilymph associated with complete HC destruction following chronic drug administration is 5/1000 the cytotoxic drug concentration *in vitro*, suggesting that the cytotoxic effect of **aminoglycosides** on the HCs is highly selective and not simply a result of preferential accumulation of the drug in perilymph. However, penetration of **aminoglycosides** into endolymph is a relatively slow process and might be an important determinant of toxicity to HCs.

It has been shown both for **salicylates** and **quinine** that there is a threshold plasma concentration in animals and humans for the onset of auditory impairment. Above this threshold, the extent of auditory impairment increases in a linear fashion as the plasma concentration of the drug increases. In animals it has also been shown that **salicylates** readily gain access to perilymph. However, although this demonstrates the presence of the drug at its (presumed) site of action, the HCs, it does not offer an explanation for the ototoxic effect, since it is likely that many other compounds also gain access to perilymph without exerting an ototoxic effect.

16.3.3   *Tissue Biochemistry as a Basis of Ototoxic Selectivity*

Aminoglycosides

It has been hypothesized that the ototoxicity of the **aminoglycosides** results from their specific, irreversible interaction with a particular phospholipid, phosphatidylinositol 4,'5'-bisphosphate (PIP$_2$). Although this phospholipid, which activates a cascade of intracellular biochemical pathways involved in the control of intracellular calcium levels, is present in the membranes of most cells, the kidney and neural tissue – including the ear – show a much more active metabolism of phosphoinositides than do other tissues such as the liver or lung. Furthermore, it has been demonstrated *in vivo* that **neomycin** inhibits the turnover of phosphoinositides in both the kidney and the inner ear. A three-stage process to describe the interaction of **aminoglycosides** with PIP$_2$, which is located on the cytosolic side of the plasma membrane, has been proposed [7]. First, there is an initial reversible binding of the drug, possibly to anionic phospholipids exposed at the extracellular surface of the membrane; second, an energy-dependent step by which the drug crosses the membrane; third, a specific irreversible binding to PIP$_2$.

Salicylates

Early experimental studies indicated that **salicylates** might produce ischaemia in the cochlea through constriction of cochlear blood vessels, possibly as a consequence of the inhibition of prostaglandin synthesis. However, current evidence suggests that, although effects on the vasculature should not be discounted, at least as a contributory factor, **salicylates** act directly upon both the IHCs and OHCs [8].

As **salicylates** are known to enter perilymph rapidly after administration, they might act on any or all of the IHCs, the OHCs, the synapses, or the neurons, all of which are directly exposed to perilymph. However, histological and functional evidence consistently indicates that it is the OHCs which are affected. *In vitro* studies of the effect of **salicylates** on the motile response of isolated OHCs to electrical stimulation suggest that **salicylates** may interact directly at the basolateral membrane of the OHC, leading to inhibition of the active mechanical response. **Salicylates** are known to affect membrane permeability, in particular causing an increase in K$^+$ and decrease in Cl$^-$ conductance, and it has been argued that this occurs in the cochlea.

Whilst an action of **salicylates** on the active processes of the OHCs would produce the observed loss in hearing sensitivity, it is likely that the tinnitus, which also occurs, is a separate phenomenon. Some clinical evidence suggests that tinnitus is the more prevalent effect and does not always coincide with hearing loss. It has been shown that following systemic **salicylate** administration there is an increase in the spontaneous firing rate of auditory neurons, i.e. neural stimulation in the absence of an acoustic signal. As **salicylate** enters the perilymph it has access to and could act directly upon the afferent nerve synapses, but in other systems **salicylates** usually decrease and eventually block neural excitation. Furthermore, any mechanistic explanation of salicylate-induced tinnitus must account for the observation that it is only neurons which respond normally to high frequencies that show an increased spontaneous firing rate and that the perceived tinnitus in humans is reported to be of high frequency.

Quinine

The effects of **quinine** resemble those of **salicylate**. Quinine produces a reversible hearing loss and tinnitus, which is closely correlated with the concentration of the drug in plasma and which disappears upon withdrawal of the drug [9]. It has been reported that **quinine** also causes constriction of cochlear capillaries and this was thought to be the basis of its ototoxicity and to indicate a similar mechanism of action to **salicylate**. More recently, both histological and functional evidence has pointed to a direct effect of **quinine** upon OHCs, but the mechanism of action may be different from that of **salicylate**. Evidence from studies using OHCs indicates that the effect of **quinine** is on the slow contractile properties of OHCs, which would alter the vibrational characteristics of the basilar membrane. It is known that **quinine** induces and enhances muscular contraction by affecting the availability of intracellular calcium released from the sarcoplasmic reticulum. It has been argued that **quinine** may act similarly on OHCs, affecting intracellular calcium levels mediated by an initial action of the drug at the plasma membrane.

Cis-platinum

As yet there is no consistent idea of the basis of *cis*-**platinum's** ototoxicity. It has been reported [10] that a rapid deterioration in the auditory nerve response threshold is produced when *cis*-**platinum** is present in the scala media at concentrations of about 5 µM, but no effect is apparent when the drug is perfused perilymphatically at a concentration of less than 3 mM. This suggests that one possible site of action of *cis*-**platinum** is the apical pole of the HCs and, from other characteristics of the response to a single systemic administration, it has been concluded that the drug blocks transduction channels. However, as with similar experiments with **aminoglycosides**, it is difficult from these results to explain differential effects on IHCs and OHCs, nor is it known whether or how they might be related to HC degeneration. In recent studies, incubation of isolated HCs with concentrations of *cis*-**platinum** as high as 1 mM for up to 6 h did not impair cell viability. Thus, at present neither the site of drug action nor the mechanisms that cause cell death are known.

The loop diuretics

All the **loop diuretics**, which have a primary diuretic action in the ascending limb of the loop of Henle, cause temporary hearing loss through an inhibitory action upon the ability of the stria vascularis to maintain EP and the endolymphatic K^+ concentration. The effects occur very rapidly following systemic administration of large doses. The decline in EP coincides with the development of an extensive oedema in the stria vascularis, which effect is also reversible, approximately in parallel with the recovery of EP. These effects are presumed to result from inhibition of transport processes in the stria, although it is not clear precisely which enzyme and/or transport process is primarily affected.

16.4 Morphological Responses to Injury

16.4.1 *Cochlea*

Hearing loss arising in the cochlea or auditory nerve (sensorineural hearing loss) can result from abnormalities in the cochlea or the auditory nerve, but is most commonly of cochlear origin. It may be congenital or may be attributable to degenerative changes which progress with advancing age (presbycusis). In addition, it can be caused by a variety of trauma such as noise, infection or chemical injury. Some of these toxic insults can interact; for example, it has been shown in numerous studies that noise and ototoxic chemicals can act synergistically to produce augmented injury. Irrespective of the nature of the insult, the HCs are particularly vulnerable and, if destroyed, cannot regenerate.

Permanent hearing loss caused by ototoxic drugs, such as the **aminoglycoside antibiotics** and *cis*-**platinum**, seems always to be associated with loss of HCs in the organ of Corti. Although effects are somewhat variable between drugs and between species, it has usually been found that the cochlear lesion originates in the first row of OHCs (Figure 16.8) towards the basal end of the cochlea [11]. The damage then progresses to affect the other rows of OHCs and to involve cells near the apex of the cochlea. The IHCs are usually damaged only in regions where there is extensive loss of OHCs. In agreement with clinical findings, this progression of HC damage is paralleled by a hearing loss which is initially confined to high frequencies but eventually may involve all frequencies. The HCs in the organ of Corti are, in general, much more sensitive to damage than the supporting cells. Indeed, the selective vulnerability of the HCs, compared with the supporting cells, is preserved when cultures of the organ of Corti are directly exposed to ototoxic agents *in vitro*

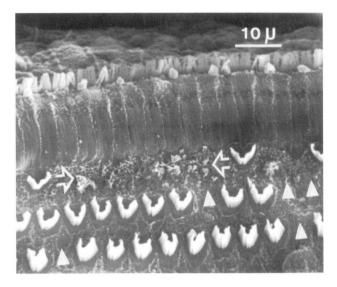

Figure 16.8 Hair cell loss induced by an aminoglycoside antibiotic in the guinea pig organ of Corti. This illustrates how in the early stages of damage the hair cell loss is largely confined to the first row of outer hair cells, with minimal injury in the second and third rows. Between the open arrows, seven adjacent first row OHCs have been destroyed and replaced by scar tissue. Occasional missing OHCs in the second and third rows are marked by filled triangles.

[12]. Degeneration of the neural innervation of the organ of Corti is a secondary event, following the death of the HCs.

The stria vascularis is now known to be the primary target in the cochlea for the ototoxic action of the **loop diuretics**. Intravenous administration of **ethacrynic acid** or **frusemide** causes profound, but transient, changes in the electrical activity in the cochlea. This transient impairment of electrical activity in the cochlea, which would result in reversible hearing impairment, is paralleled by the development of extensive oedema in the stria vascularis, which recovers with a similar time course to functional recovery. It is not known whether the HC loss in the organ of Corti produced by high doses or repetitive administration of **ethacrynic acid** results from a direct effect on HCs or is secondary to prolonged changes in the stria vascularis.

In animal studies, co-administration of an **aminoglycoside antibiotic** with a **loop diuretic** produces greatly augmented cochlear damage compared with that caused by either compound alone. Thus, administration of a large intravenous dose of **ethacrynic acid** or **frusemide** shortly before a single, non-ototoxic dose of **kanamycin** produces depression of cochlear function which is permanent and associated with extensive HC destruction. The interaction also occurs with other loop **diuretics**, such as **bumetanide** and **piretanide**, but not with diuretics which have a different mechanism of action, such as **hydrochlorothiazide** or **mannitol**. All **aminoglycoside antibiotics** have been found to interact with the **loop diuretics** as have the non-aminoglycoside, ototoxic antibiotics **viomycin** and **polymyxin B** and the antitumour drug *cis*-**platinum**.

16.4.2 Vestibular System

In the vestibular system, damage is seen initially in the HCs of the cristae ampullaris. The most vulnerable cells are the type 1 sensory cells, although in more severe lesions the type 2 cells are also destroyed. Degeneration of the cells in the macula utriculi and macula sacculi occurs at a later stage. As in the cochlea, the supporting cells and nerve fibres survive the HCs, but eventually they too may be destroyed.

16.5 Testing for Toxicity

16.5.1 Functional Assessment

As has already been pointed out, permanent hearing loss resulting from ototoxic injury to the cochlea is invariably accompanied by HC loss. Since HCs in the mammalian cochlea are not known to regenerate, histopathological assessment of the sensory neuroepithelia should detect any significant injury to the inner ear at the end of a chronic study. Indeed, since HC loss, once initiated, tends to progress and stabilize, examination of the neurosensory epithelia after a dosing-free interval should also be entirely satisfactory. However, histopathological assessment will not detect reversible deficits of function, such as those caused by **salicylates** or **loop diuretics.** Furthermore, full characterization of an ototoxic effect mandates both functional and morphological assessment.

Techniques for assessing the inner ear have largely been developed for the cochlea. Physiological investigation of the vestibular system is difficult to perform, especially with experimental animals, and there are no widely accepted and used tests of vestibular function. However, this is probably not a major drawback since ototoxic agents affecting the vestibular system are also cochleotoxic, to varying degrees. The function of the cochlea can be assessed by measurement of the electrophysiological and biomechanical activity of the end organ itself, or of evoked electrical responses in the brainstem or at higher centres in the auditory pathway, or through involuntary reflexes or conditioned behavioural responses [13, 14].

Non-invasive tests suitable for repeated application

Such procedures have the advantage that responses pre- and post-administration can be compared and the progression of change followed. Observation of reflex movement of the pinna (Preyer reflex) in response to sound stimulation can be used as a simple, unsophisticated measurement of hearing. The test is relatively easy to perform and can be applied in conscious animals using relatively simple equipment. Although the endpoint is subjective and movement of the pinna is seen only in response to quite intense sounds, so that it will detect only a significant loss of hearing, it can be refined by assessing the threshold of the response to tones of different frequency.

Behavioural response audiometry, involving conditioned responses to sound stimuli, represents a more sophisticated and sensitive measurement of hearing threshold and is the only true measurement of the hearing 'sensation' in animals. The threshold of response, the lowest sound pressure level at which a response is elicited, can be determined for a number of different frequencies over the auditory frequency range of the animal, giving rise to the behavioural audiogram. However, the equipment required is relatively complex and the conditioning is time-consuming, so that this methodology does not lend itself to other than specialist work.

Neural excitation in the cochlea in response to sound stimulation leads to successive activation of a number of centres along the auditory pathway through the brainstem to the auditory cortex. The associated electrical activity can be recorded as a succession of waves of different amplitudes and latencies using electrodes placed on the skull. The recording of these evoked responses is a non-invasive procedure that can be used repeatedly in an individual subject to monitor the progression of an ototoxic insult. Brainstem-evoked response audiometry is widely used, although the level of sound necessary to produce a response may be somewhat higher than the actual auditory threshold, so that initial stages of a progressive hearing loss, or a relatively minor impairment of hearing, may not be detectable. However, it has been shown that permanent increases in threshold at particular frequencies, detected using this technique, correlate with loss of HCs at appropriate locations in the cochlea.

Otoacoustic emissions are sounds generated by the cochlea and emitted from the ear. They are a relatively recent discovery and can, in a few subjects, occur spontaneously. However, in all cases they can be produced in response to sound stimulation and are believed to derive from the active mechanical responses of the OHCs. Otoacoustic emissions have in recent times provided a non-invasive, but very sensitive, objective means to assess cochlear function. The procedure is very reproducible in individual human subjects and is finding clinical application for testing cochlear function in newborn babies. Recording of otoacoustic emissions has recently been shown to be a sensitive, reproducible method for assessment of ototoxic effects in the cochleae of animals [15].

Direct invasive measurements of cochlear function

A number of electrical potentials can be measured in the cochlea. The main potentials in response to sound stimulation are the cochlear microphonic, derived predominantly from the OHCs, and the compound action potential, which reflects activity in the auditory nerve. The latter is a measure of the ultimate output of the cochlea and is useful for rapid assessment of the functional effects of ototoxic insult. However, these are invasive techniques, requiring surgery and electrode placement in or near the cochlea and are generally used acutely with the animal being killed after the recording has been made. Thus effects of an ototoxic agent cannot be measured against a pre-administration baseline, unless the chemical is very rapidly acting and the effect is manifest during the course of an acute experiment under anaesthesia. Repeated measurements can be made following implantation of an electrode, but this is a very specialized technique and has only occasionally been used in research laboratories. Normally comparisons have to be made against an untreated control population.

16.5.2 Morphological Assessment

Examination of inner ear structures by light or electron microscopy is widely used to assess the effects of ototoxic agents. For the vestibular system, in the absence of reliable function tests, such procedures may be the only ready means to assess ototoxic injury. Even in the cochlea, morphological methods may be the only practicable technique for inclusion in a conventional toxicological study, but even if functional assessment has been undertaken, histology will allow assessment of the location and extent of the lesions, and correlation of this with information on functional deficits.

Inner ear structures can be examined by conventional light microscopical examination of stained sections [16]. Fixation is accomplished either by intravital perfusion of the head and neck or by direct perfusion via the round window or the oval window (after removal of the stapes). For light microscopy, the intact cochlea is usually decalcified prior to embedding and cutting sections in a plane parallel to the central axis of the modiolus. Sectioning the entire cochlea has the advantage that it permits the assessment of injury to other tissues, such as the stria vascularis, in parallel with examination of the neurosensory epithelium. This facilitates the identification of gross changes in the various tissues in the cochlea. However, examination of a single mid-modiolar section does not readily allow quantification of HC loss − and damage to HCs which is very focal could easily be missed. This could be overcome by the use of serial sectioning but this is very labour intensive.

An alternative method, which is favoured if the objective is to derive a reliable quantitative assessment of the degree of HC damage, is to examine the surface of the neurosensory epithelium, usually after removal of the outer bony shell and the tissues of the lateral wall. This can be readily accomplished in the guinea pig without decalcification (Figure 16.3), but in the case of the rat, mouse or marmoset is aided by prior decalcification. In surface view, HCs are easily recognized by their distinctive hair bundles (Figure 16.6) and it is possible by systematically viewing the entire organ of Corti to draw a cytocochleogram, in essence a map depicting the position of each HC along the full length of the organ. The location of damaged or missing HCs can then be accurately determined and related to physiological data from the same animal [14], if these are available. It is only with the scanning electron microscope that the entire organ of Corti can be examined *in situ* without further dissection, other than removal of the tectorial membrane (Figure 16.4b) from the surface of the HCs. The high quality of the scanning electron microscope images facilitates quantification of HC damage and loss (Figure 16.8) and permits lesions to be examined and characterized at high resolution [17]. However, a disadvantage is that only the surface of the HCs can be viewed and surface disruption is frequently the final stage in cellular degeneration [17]. The surface of the organ of Corti can also be examined, at lower resolution, using phase-contrast microscopy or differential interference microscopy. In this case, it is necessary to dissect out the neurosensory epithelium, usually in half turns, and prepare these as glycerol mounts. Using these light microscopical techniques it is also possible to gain some appreciation of subsurface injury, for example nuclear swelling, by focusing at various depths of the cell. However, full characterization of a lesion is generally only possible using a combination of microscopical methods, for example scanning and transmission electron microscopy.

The 'surface specimen' technique can also be applied to the vestibular neurosensory epithelium, but light microscopical methods are more difficult to apply here because the tissues are relatively thick and, particularly the cristae, are not flat. Furthermore, unlike in the cochlea, the sensory cells are not arranged in an orderly pattern and it is impossible to distinguish between the two types of vestibular HC from their surface characteristics. Thus, maps of the vestibular neurosensory epithelium cannot be drawn. Only a rather more general assessment of HC loss is possible. In order to determine accurately the extent and location of HC loss it is necessary to cut serial sections for light microscopy, where the two HCs can be identified from their morphology.

16.6 Conclusions

Administration of ototoxic chemicals to animals has often been employed to establish models of cochlear pathology. Indeed, measurement of the resulting structural and functional changes has greatly increased our knowledge of both the normal physiology and the pathophysiology of the cochlea. Furthermore, chronic administration of an **aminoglycoside antibiotic** to animals provides a good general model of sensorineural hearing loss of cochlear origin, since (i) hearing loss in humans caused by ototoxic drug administration follows very much the same course as that produced by noise or other injury, unrelated to drugs and (ii) the pattern of HC damage caused by administration of **aminoglycosides** to animals is similar to that observed in sensorineural hearing loss in humans.

Since the effects of ototoxic drugs in animals and man are qualitatively similar [18], studies in animals should be reliably predictive of the ototoxic potential of a chemical. When different drugs are compared on a quantitative basis, the relative magnitudes of their effects in animals and humans also show reasonable agreement. It is probably the infrequency of ototoxicity at clinical doses of drugs which frustrates the demonstration of an even better correspondence between experimental and clinical studies. Thus it is necessary to extrapolate from high-dose studies in animals to low doses in humans. Although ototoxic effects seem invariably to be dose related, there is insufficient information about the slopes of the dose–response curves of different drugs to be certain that predictions, from animal studies to humans, of the comparative ototoxicity of drugs will be entirely valid. Problems in correlating the vestibular effects of ototoxic drugs between species arise because of the lack of sensitive methods for studying the function of each of the vestibular sensory organs and the absence of an entirely satisfactory method for quantifying vestibular HC loss.

References

1. PICKLES, J.O. (1988) *An Introduction to the Physiology of Hearing*, 2nd Edn, London: Academic Press.
2. ASHMORE, J. (1987) A fast motile response in guinea pig outer hair cells: the cellular basis of the cochlear amplifier, *Journal of Physiology*, **388**, 323–347.
3. HARPUR, E.S. (1986) Disorders of the ear, in D'ARCY, P.F. and GRIFFIN, J.P. (Eds) *Iatrogenic Diseases*, 3rd Edn, pp. 713–749, Oxford: Oxford University Press.
4. LERNER, S.A., MATZ, G.J. and HAWKINS, J.E., Jr. (Eds) 1981, *Aminoglycoside Ototoxicity*, Boston: Little Brown and Company.
5. DESROCHERS, C.S. and SCHACHT, J. (1982) Neomycin concentrations in inner ear tissues and other organs of the guinea-pig after chronic drug administration, *Acta Otolaryngologica*, **93**, 233–236.
6. HARPUR, E.S. and GONDA, I. (1982) Analysis of the pharmacokinetics of ribostamycin in serum and perilymph of guinea pigs after single and multiple doses, *British Journal of Audiology*, **16**, 95–99.
7. SCHACHT, J. (1986), Molecular mechanisms of drug-induced hearing loss, *Hearing Research*, **22**, 297–304.
8. BOETTCHER, F.A. and SALVI, R.J. (1991) Salicylate ototoxicity: review and synthesis, *American Journal of Otolaryngology*, **12**, 33–47.
9. ALVAN, G., KARLSSON, K.K., HELLGREN, U. and VILLEN, T. (1991) Hearing impairment related to plasma quinine concentration in healthy volunteers, *British Journal of Clinical Pharmacology*, **31**, 409–412.
10. MCALPINE, D. and JOHNSTONE, B.M. (1990) The ototoxic mechanism of cisplatin, *Hearing Research*, **47**, 191–204.
11. HAWKINS, J.E., Jr. and JOHNSSON, L-G. (1981) Histopathology of cochlear and vestibular ototoxicity in laboratory animals, in LERNER, S.A., MATZ, G.J. and HAWKINS, J.E., Jr. (Eds) *Aminoglycoside Ototoxicity*, pp. 175–195, Boston: Little Brown and Company.
12. RICHARDSON, G.P. and RUSSELL, I.J. (1991) Cochlear cultures as a model system for studying aminoglycoside induced ototoxicity, *Hearing Research*, **53**, 293–311.
13. HARPUR, E.S. (1981), ototoxicological testing, in GORROD, J.W. (Ed) *Testing for Toxicity*, pp. 219–240, London: Taylor and Francis.
14. FORGE, A. and HARPUR, E.S. (1993) Ototoxicity, in BALLANTYNE, B., MARRS, T. and TURNER, P. (Eds), *General and Applied Toxicology*, Vol. 1, pp. 781–805, London: Macmillan.
15. BROWN, A.M., MCDOWELL, B. and FORGE, A. (1989), Acoustic distortion products can be used to monitor the effects of chronic gentamicin treatment, *Hearing Research*, **42**, 143–156.
16. LIBERMAN, M.C. (1990) Quantitative assessment of inner ear pathology following ototoxic drugs or acoustic trauma, *Toxicologic Pathology*, **18**, 138–148.
17. HARPUR, E.S. and BRIDGES, J.B. (1979) An evaluation of the use of scanning and transmission electronmicroscopy in a study of the gentamicin-damaged guinea-pig organ of Corti, *Journal of Laryngology and Otology*, **93**, 7–23.
18. HARPUR, E.S. (1987) Ototoxicity: morphological and functional correlates between experimental and clinical studies, in BALLANTYNE, J. (Ed.) *Perspectives in Basic and Applied Toxicology*, pp. 42–69, London: Wright.

Index

acanthosis 18
accumulation enteropathies 44, 52, 53
ACE inhibitors 112–13, 125–6, 163, 320, 323
acidophils 313–14
acrylamide neurotoxicity 290
adenoacanthoma 422, 424
adenocarcinoma 128–9, 411–12, 413, 422, 424
adenoma 128–9, 317–18, 363
adenomyosis 422
adenosis 425
ADP 187, 194
adrenal glands 145, 318–23
adrenergic neurons 283
adventitial oedema 167
aerobic metabolism 284–5
aflatoxin 75, 83, 87
alcohol (ethanol) 1–2, 79
allergy 11, 207–8, 213–15, 231–3
allyl alcohol 71–2
allylamine 162, 165
ALP activity 56, 90
ALT 91, 253
altered protein synthesis 245–6
altered vascular supply 245, 258
aluminium 258, 260, 291–2
alveolar buds (nipple structure) 432
alveolar region (lung) 342–4, 357–61
Ames assay (skin) 26
amino acids 287–8, 289
aminoglycosides 474, 475, 477, 478, 481
ammonia caramel 220
amoscanate 294
AMP 37, 38, 39–40
amphiphilic molecules 44
amyloidosis 117, 168
anabolic steroids 73, 387
anaemic hypoxia 285
anaesthesia 179, 203, 287
analgesics 109, 130
ANIT 72–3
anoxic hypoxia 285

anterior lobe (pituitary gland) 312–13
anterior prostate 378
anthracyclines 150
antibiotics 107–8, 115, 474
anticancer agents 115, 125, 130, 150, 317
anticoagulant therapy 440
antigens 207, 208, 209–11, 215, 226
antihistamines 410
apocrine (sweat gland) 6–7
apoptosis 77, 78
artefacts (nervous system) 296–7
arteries 159
arterioles 159
arteritis 125, 165, 168, 171
arthritis 257–8, 261–2, 268
asbestos 346, 347, 361, 363–4
AST 91, 253
astrocytes 279, 280, 292, 302–4
astroglia 279
atherosclerosis 165
ATP 37, 40, 78, 243
atrial lesions 150–1
atrioventricular (AV) node 142, 144–5
autoimmunity 215, 221–6, 233
autonomic nervous systems 277–8
axonopathies 301–2
axons 273–4, 278–9, 281, 289–92
azathioprine 220
AZT 191, 193

bacteria 7, 43
BALT 212
BaP 12, 21
barrier properties of skin 8–9
basal layers 3, 105
basophils 83, 186, 190, 196–7, 313–14
beagle pain syndrome 170–1
BHA 46
BHT 191
bile/biliary system 65–6, 72–3, 90–1
bismuth 122, 124

bladder 105, 130–2, 134–5
bladder stones 131–2
blood
  –brain barrier 279–81, 287–9, 292
  flow (in testis) 394–5
  haematopoietic system 177–204
  pressure 171
  supply 101, 110
  in vascular system 161
bone 257–9
  lesions 261–9
  mass 259–61
  structure 254–6
bone marrow 178–9, 189, 194–5, 200
botulinum toxin 289
Bowman's space 101, 103, 226
brain 275, 276, 282–3
BrDU immunostaining 57
breast cancer 429, 433–8, 439, 442–5
Bright's disease 119
bromobenzene 68, 69
bronchi/bronchiolar region 340–2, 354–7
Brunner's glands 39, 51, 55
BT-PABA 56
bulbourethral gland 378

cadmium 259, 260, 262, 394–5
calcification (bladder) 131–2
calcium 45, 127, 161
calculi (bladder) 131–2
Call-Exner bodies 416
capillaries 159, 168, 280–1, 294
carbohydrate metabolism 462
carbon monoxide 285, 365, 473
carbon tetrachloride 320, 321
carcinogenesis 82–6, 227, 246–7, 263
carcinomas
carcinogens 12–14, 21–3, 25–6, 86–9, 227
  mammary gland 429, 433–9, 442–5
  respiratory system 340–4, 346–52, 354–66
  skin 12–14, 21–3, 25–6
  transitional cell 135
cardiac valves/impulse 144
cardiovascular system
  heart 141–58
  vascular system 158–74
carrageenans 54
cartilage 254–71
catecholamines 145
caustic agents 14–20
CCK 37, 39, 41, 54
cell associations 379, 380
cell death 76–9, 218
cell suspension analysis 229–30
cells 130, 135, 296, 298, 396, 462
cellular components/functions 373–8
cellular membranes(changes) 287–8
central chromatolysis 300
central core myopathy 252
central nervous system 275–7, 278
centrilobular hypertrophy 81
centrilobular necrosis 75, 76
cerebellar hypoplasia 298
cerebrum 282
cervix 409–10, 413, 425

chlorampenicol 188, 189
chlorpromazine 73, 190
cholera toxin 43
cholestasis 72, 73
cholesterol clefts 358, 359
cholinergic pathways (forebrain) 282
chondrocyte 254–5, 269
chondromalacia 259
choroid 453
chromophobes 313–14
chronic progressive nephropathy 115–17
ciliary body 453
ciliated epithelial cells 341, 342, 355–6
cirrhosis 72, 80
cis-platinum 476, 477
CK levels 253
Clara cells 341–2, 352, 355–6
clotting potential 198, 199
CNS effects 36, 44, 54
coagulating gland 378
coagulation 188, 194, 200–1
cocaine 289
cochlea 468, 469–72, 477–8, 479–80
collagen 80, 143, 148, 167
collecting duct system 104
conducting fibres 143
conjunctiva 451, 456
connective tissues 161
contact hypersensitivity 213–15, 231–2
contact urticaria 21
Coombs' test 193
copulatory behaviour 398–9
corium (dermis) 5
cornea 452, 453, 456–7, 459–61, 464
cornification (vagina) 423
corpora lutea 409, 410, 411, 415
corrosive agents 10–11
cortex 318–20, 321–3
corticosteroids 190, 193, 197, 245–6, 257, 258,
  260
Cowper's gland 378
crypt cells 34, 35
crystal deposition, tubular 121, 123
cuprizone 293
cyclohexylamine 390–1
cyclophosphamide 130, 131, 190, 191, 198, 260
CYP 66, 87–8, 90
  enzymes 69, 72, 74, 81
  mediated toxins 68–71
cystic change (mammary gland) 440–1
cystic endometrial hyperplasia 418–19
cystitis 130–1
cytochrome P–450 66–7, 347–9, 351–2, 356
cytokines 212, 213, 215
cytology (hepatic injury) 77–8
cytopenias, immune-mediated 193
cytostatic drugs 220–1
cytotoxic damage 51, 285, 346, 347, 384

DAB method 64
dark neurons 297
DBCP 371, 386
decidualization (uterus) 421–2
defective matrix formation (bone) 258–9
degenerative lesions of bone 263–8

dehydrogenases 349–50
DEN 87, 88
dendrites 43, 278–9, 281
depletion/atrophy/regeneration 217–21
dermal damage 15, 17–18, 20
dermatitis 11, 18
dermis (corium) 5
DES 438–9, 442
developmental abnormalities 145, 162
developmental neurotoxicity 295–6
diet/dietary factors 45, 227, 326, 438
digestive system
    gastrointestinal tract and exocrine pancreas
        29–58
    hepatobiliary system 61–94
dioxin 218–20
direct-acting substances 346–7
direct invasive measurement (cochlea) 480
discoid degeneration 250–1
distal tubule 104
DMBA 12, 21, 23, 25, 192, 434–5, 437
DMH 54
DMN 78, 87, 91, 129–30
DNA 7, 8, 57, 81–2, 86–7, 89, 192, 229,
    245–6, 286, 383–5, 433, 446–7
Döhle bodies (leucocyte abnormalities) 198
dopamine agonists 412, 413, 441
dopamine antagonists 317, 442
dopaminergic pathway (brain) 283
Draize test 24, 465
drug hypersensitivity 224, 226
drug metabolizing enzymes 351–2
ductal hyperplasia 441
duodenal ulcer 52
dystrophic mineralization 126–7, 149
dystrophy 248

ear 467–82
eccrine (sweat gland) 6–7
efferent ducts 376–7
EGME 391–2
elastic (conducting) arteries 159
electron microscopy 92, 136, 157, 173, 229
electrophysiology/electromyography 253
emphysema 361
Encephalitozoon cuniculi 298, 300
endocardium 143, 150–2
endocrine regulation 379–82
endocrine system 311–33
endometrial adenocarcinoma 422
endometrial hyperplasia 418–19, 422
endometrial stromal cell sarcoma 422
endometriosis 422
endometritis/pyometra 421
endoplasmic reticulum 64–6, 78–9, 92, 316,
    324
endothelium 80, 125, 160
energy requirements (of erythrocyte) 185
ENU 295
enzymes 9–10
    inhibitors (in lens) 462
    male reproduction 385–6
    plasma/serum 152–3
    in respiratory tract 347–52
eosinophils 83, 186, 190

ependymal cells 280, 294
epicardial changes 150
epidermatitis 18
epidermis 3–5, 14–16, 18–20
epididymis 373, 376–7, 382, 396–400
epithelia, non-sensory 472–3
epithelial cells 129, 133, 135, 136
epithelial hyperplasia 414, 425
Epping jaundice 72
ergot poisoning 162, 163, 167
erythrocyte 180–2, 184–5, 191, 195–7
esterases 349–50
ethanol (metabolism of) 72, 79
excitation-contraction coupling 144, 146
exfoliated germ cells 396
exocrine pancreas 29–58
extramural coronary arteritis 171
ex vivo systems 173, 365
eye 451–65

fat necrosis (mammary gland) 440
fatty change (heart) 150
fatty degeneration (skeletal muscle) 251
female reproductive system 407–26
fertility studies 371, 398
fibrils 143
fibrinoid necrosis 167–8
fibrinogen 187, 188, 194, 201
fibroblasts 5, 15, 18, 20, 23, 148
fibroma 418, 424
fibrosarcoma 425
fibrosis 79–80, 167, 358, 360
fibrous osteodystrophy 265, 266
fluid balance (hepatic injury) 77
fluoride 259
focal hyperplasia 129
folic acid 185
follicle stimulating hormone (FSH) 381, 401,
    409, 411
follicles 5–6, 20, 323–4
    damage 15, 414–15
    primordial (ovary) 408–10
folliculitis 18
forebrain 276, 282
forestomach, non-glandular 46
free radicals (production of) 462
functional assessment (ototoxicity) 478–80
functional studies (male reproduction) 398–9
fungal infections 7

GABA 283, 288
GAGs 160, 161, 165, 167
GALT 33–4, 42–3, 53, 212, 228
gastric glands 32–3
gastric secretion 36–8
gastrointestinal tract 29–58
genetic polymorphisms 351
genotoxic agents 15, 86–7, 384–5, 433–7
germ cell 372, 374–6, 391–3, 396
GFAP 279, 280, 303–4, 307
glandular stomach 46–51
glaucoma 459
glial cells 279–80, 292–4
glomerular damage 105–6, 113, 115–17
glomerulonephritis 113–15

glomerulus 102–3, 163
Golgi apparatus 64, 79, 103, 105, 279, 301, 314, 316, 323, 329
granular degeneration 250
granulation variation (leucocytes) 197–8
granulocytes 181
granuloma 18, 80
granulosa cell tumour 416
growth hormone (GH) 432–3, 439–40, 442, 447
GSH 68–9, 71–2, 83–4, 89
GST 67, 335, 342, 350–2
γ-GT 83, 84, 88, 89, 90
gut microflora metabolism 44

haem synthesis 185, 192–3
haematopoietic system 177–204
haemangioma 169
haemangiosarcoma 169, 170
haematotoxicity, in vitro 201
haemoglobin 122, 185
haemolysis 122, 193–4, 199–200
haemostasis 186–7, 188
hair/hair follicles 5–6
hair cells (in ear) 469–73, 474, 475–8, 479–82
halohydrocarbons 68
halothane 74
Haversian systems 254, 256, 266
healing responses (morphological response to injury) 18–20
heart 141–58
Heinz bodies 179, 193–4, 196
hepatic encephalopathy 292
hepatic lobule/units 62–3
hepatic neoplasms 82–3
hepatic nodules 84–5
hepatobiliary system 61–94, 292
hepatocytes 63–5, 73
hepatocellular neoplasia 83–6
hepatocellular toxicity 68–72
hepatocytes (serum enzymes) 91
heroin 115
hexachlorobenzene (HCB) 221–4, 233
hexachlorophene 292–3
hexadimethrin 320, 321
Heyman nephritis 113, 115
hindbrain 275–6, 283
histotoxic hypoxia 285
HIV infection 245
homeostasis 180, 256
hormones 437–40
   assays 401–2
   luteinizing 381, 387, 394–5, 401, 410–11
   parathyroid 256, 261, 327–9
   pituitary gland 313–17
   thyroid gland 324, 332
Howell-Jolly bodies 179, 196
hyaline cartilage 254, 257
hyaline degeneration 249–50
hyaline droplets, tubular 120–1, 122
hybridohistochemistry 229
hydralazine 162
hydrocephalus 297
hydrogen cyanide 285
hydrogen sulphide 285
hydrolases 349–50

hydronephrosis 127
hydropic change 118–19, 120
hyperbaric oxygen 167
hyperkeratosis 20, 46, 47, 423, 425
hyperoxia 162
hyperplastic alveolar nodule 442
hypersensitivity 168, 213–15, 221–6
hypertension 165, 167
hypertrophy 81–2, 124–5, 147, 167, 248, 394, 415, 419
hypochromia 195
hypodermis 5
hypoglycaemia 285
hypoplasia 194–5, 298
hypothalamus 282, 315, 316, 379, 381
hypothyroidism 295
hypoxia 162, 285

IDPN 290, 291
immune-mediated toxicity 73–4, 147, 164, 193
immune system 207–34
immunocytochemistry 136
immunodeficiency, status of 228
immunohistochemistry 229
immunological reactions (neoplasia) 227
immunosuppression 207–8, 212–13, 220–1
impaired sarcolemmal function 244–5
individual cell necrosis 15
induction of neoplasia 434–80
infarction 125, 149
infections (in nervous system) 298
inflammation
   bone 261–2, 268–9
   female reproductive system 424
   male reproductive system 395–7
   of mammary tissue 440
   muscle disease 252
   skin 15, 17, 18, 19
   urinary 130–1
inhalation exposure 364–5
inherited disorders (skin) 7–8
in situ hybridization 229
integumentary system 1–27
interferon 124
intermediate metabolism 268–7, 345–6
interstitium 105, 109–10, 124–5, 143, 147–8, 395, 415
intervertebral foramen 276, 277
intestine 33–5, 38–41, 51–4
intimal proliferation 165–6
intramyelinic oedema 292, 302
intraocular pressure (alteration in) 459
intravascular studies 172
in vitro systems 26, 57, 92–3, 201, 230, 253, 365, 402–3
in vivo systems 26, 173, 230–1
ion movement 145–6
ionizing radiation 192, 227, 263
iris 452
iron 185
irradiation 227, 329, 410, 411
ischaemia 110
islets of Langerhans 36, 311, 329–31
isocyanates 224
isolated vascular beds 173

jaundice 72, 73
'jet lesions' 146
joints 254–71
juxtaglomerular apparatus 104, 125, 136

keratoacanthomas 22–3
keratoconjuntivitis 459–61
kidney (urinary system) 99–137
Kreb's cycle 386
Kupffer cells 62, 65, 80, 86

Langerhans cell 3, 11, 212, 214, 221
large clear vacuoles 119–20
large intestine 51–4
LDH 91, 253
lead 122, 124, 197, 259, 293–4, 317
leiomyoma 422, 425
leiomyosarcoma 422
lens 453–4, 457–8, 460, 461–2
leucocytes 181, 183, 185–6, 197–9
leukaemia 186, 189, 190
leukaemogenesis 191–2
Leydig cell 372, 376, 379, 381–2, 387–8, 390,
    393–5, 401–2
limbic system 282
lipid droplets 118, 146
lipid metabolism 77, 78–9, 146, 150, 462
lipofuscin pigment 122, 150
lipophilic genotoxic agents 15
liver (hepatobiliary system) 61–94, 292
lobular hyperplasia 441–2
lobular injury (patterns) 75–6
loop diuretics 474, 476, 478
loop of Henle 103–4, 136
lower respiratory tract 340–4, 354–64
luminal cellular debris 396
lungs 340–4, 346–52, 354–64, 366
luteinizing hormone (LH) 381, 387, 394, 395,
    401, 410–11
luteoma 416
lymph nodes 210–11
lymphatic vessels and capillaries 159
lymphocytes 181, 186, 190, 198, 209
lymphoid organs 209–12
lymphokines 164
lymphoreticular tissue 179
lysosomal myopathies 245
lysosomes 64, 65

macrocytosis 196
macrophages 211, 218, 301–2
male reproductive system 371–403
malignant mesothelioma 417–18
MALT 209, 211–12
MAM 54
mammary gland 429–47
Masson-Fontana stain 325, 326
Masugi nephritis 115
matrix formation (bone/cartilage) 258–9
maturation depletion (germ cell) 393
MCH 198
MCHC 180–1, 192, 195–6, 198
MCV 192, 195–6, 198, 203
MDS 189, 191
medial necrosis 166

medial hypertrophy 167
medulla oblongata 282
melanomas 23
meningitis 298–9
mesenchymal tumour 129–30
mesothelial hyperplasia 414
mesothelial proliferation 420
mesothelioma, malignant 417–18
mesovarial leiomyoma 418
mesovarial smooth muscle hyperplasia 416
MEST/MESA 232
metabolic activation 68–72, 347–52
metabolic myopathies 252
metabolic process, injury to 385–6
metabolic tolerance (development) 352
metabolism 43–4, 145, 188–9, 193
    aerobic 284–5
    carbohydrate (alteration) 462
    intermediate 286–7, 345–6
    lipid 77, 78–9, 146, 150, 462
metal ions 224, 225–6
methicillin therapy 124
methyl alcohol 286
methylmercury 286, 295, 473
MFO system 71
MHC antigens 210
microcytosis 195
microglia 280, 294, 304
microscopy 253, 269
microtubules 245, 290–1
microvilli 133–4
mid-zonal hepatic injury 75
midbrain 276
mineral homeostasis 256
mineralization
    of bladder 131–2
    in heart 149
    metastatic 126–8, 149, 169
    in vascular system 168
mitochondria 64, 65, 78, 143, 146, 241, 245, 316
MNU 295, 434–5, 437, 441, 443
mono-oxygenases 348–9
monocytes 181, 186, 190
morphological assessment (ear) 480–1
morphological methods (toxicity testing) 153–7,
    171–3
morphometric analysis (bones) 270
motility disorders 44
MPP+ 287
MPS 209, 227
MPTP 286–7
MTV 434, 442, 444, 446
mucification (vagina) 423
mucosal exposure to xenobiotics 41–3
mucosal metabolism 43–4
mucosal protection factors 36–8
mucous distension/adenosis 425
muscle disease, inflammatory 252
muscular (distributing) arteries 159
muscular dystrophy 248
musculoskeletal system
    bone, cartilage and joints 254–71
    skeletal muscle 239–53
myelin sheaths (disruption) 297
myelinating cells 292–4

myelinopathies 302–3
myelosuppression 189
myocardium 142, 145, 148–9
myocytes 142–3, 144–5, 146–9
myocytolysis 150
myofibres 240–3, 251–2
myofibrils 150, 241–2
myofilaments 240–2
myometrial hypertrophy/hyperplasia 419
myosin isoforms 252

NADP 66, 84
NALT 212
NAPQI formation 70–1
nasal cavity 336–40, 346–54, 366
nausea and vomiting 36
NBF 153
NBT 158
necropsy 91–2, 153, 171–2
necrosis
    heart 148–9
    hepatobiliary system 76, 77
    integumentary system 15, 20
    male reproductive system 390–4, 396
    papillary 125–6, 127
    skeletal muscle 249–51
    tubular 117–18, 124
    vascular system 166–8
neoplasia
    digestive system 83–9
    immune system 226–8
    male reproductive system 395–7
    mammary gland 434–40, 442–5
    ocular 459
    urinary system 110–12, 128–30, 134–5
neoplastic lesions 407, 411–13, 416–18, 422,
    424–5
nephritis, interstitial 124–5
nephroblastoma 129
nephron 101–2
nerve fibres (degeneration) 297
nervous control 145, 161–2
nervous system 273–308
neurocarcinogenesis 295
neurogenic toxicity (skeletal muscle) 244
neuronal lesions 299–302
neuronopathies 299–301
neurons 273–4, 278–9, 295
neurotoxicity 283–96, 304–8
neurotransmission 282–3, 288–9
neutrophils 185–6, 189–90, 197–8
Nissl substance 300
nitrite poisoning 285
nitrosamines 46, 47, 48, 83
NOAEL 307–8
nodes of Ranvier 281, 302
non-chemical agents (toxicity) 7–8
non-genotoxic carcinogens 86, 87–9
non-glandular forestomach 46
non-invasive test (of cochlea) 479
non-neoplastic changes 147–51, 164–9
non-neoplastic lesions 407, 410–12, 414–16,
    418–25
non-neuronal cells 279–80, 292–5
non-neuronal lesions 302–4

non-sensory epithelia 472–3
noradrenaline 162
noradrenergic pathways (brain) 282–3
NSAIDS 46, 47, 52, 58, 126, 261
nuclear inclusions, tubular 122, 124
nutritional factors (toxicity) 7, 45

OCT 91
ocular neoplasia 459
oedema 15, 18, 167
    alveolar 358, 360
oesophagus 31, 46
oestrogen 130, 260, 316–17, 320–1, 387, 410,
    412–13, 437–41
oestrous cycle (restoration) 415
olfactory epithelium 336–40, 353–4
oligodendrocytes 279–80, 290, 292–4, 302
oligodendroglia 279–80
oocyte destruction 410, 414
oral cavity 30, 45
oral contraceptives 73, 194, 438, 439, 441, 442,
    445, 446–7
organ of Corti 468–71, 477–8, 480–1
organophosphorus esters 291
organotin compounds 218
osteomalacia 263, 265–6
osteonecrosis 267–8
osteopetrosis 267
osteoporosis 259–60, 265, 266
otoacoustic emissions 479
ototoxic selectivity 474–6
ovary 408–9, 410–12, 413–18
oxidative haemolysis 193–4
oxidative phosphorylation 462
ozone 328, 329

P-450 levels 66–7, 347–9, 351–2, 356
PABA 56
PAHs 12–13
PALS 211, 218, 221, 224
pancreas 35–6, 38–41, 331–2
Paneth cells 34, 35
papillary cystadenoma/adenocarcinoma 417
papillary necrosis 125–6, 127
papillomas 7, 22, 135
paracetamol 68–71, 76
paracrine regulation 379–82
parakeratosis 20
paraquat 360, 365
parathyroid gland 327–9
particulates (respiratory system) 346–7
PAS 253, 314, 400, 416
pathogens 211
PB 67, 68, 70, 72, 74, 78, 87–9, 94
PCNA 82
PCR 229
PDE III inhibitors 165, 171
percutaneous absorption (toxicity) 8–9
pericardium 143
periarteritis 168, 171
peripheral nervous system 277–8, 281
periportal hepatic injury 75
peritubular myoid cells 376
perivascular cuffing 298, 299
peroxisomes 64, 79, 88–9

Peyer's patches 33, 42–4, 52, 55, 211
phalloidin 73
pigmentation of tubular cells 122
pituitary gland 312–18, 379, 381, 432–3, 435, 437–9, 446, 447
plasma enzymes 152–3
plasma membrane (liver) 64
plasma proteins 90, 161, 180
platelets 181, 186–7, 194
PMNs 209
pneumonitis 357–8
polychromasia 195–6
portal tract 62–3, 76
posterior lobe (pituitary gland) 313
PPARs 89
precorneal film (abnormality) 459–61
preputial glands 378
Preyer reflex 479
PRL 432–3, 435, 437–40, 446, 447
progestogens 316, 317, 321, 410, 412, 414, 437, 439
proliferative lesions 252, 269
prostate 378
protein disturbances (in lens) 462
protein synthesis 245–6, 286
prothrombin time (PT) 200–1
proximal tubule 103
PTAH 240, 252–3
PTH 256, 261, 327–9
Purkinje fibres 142, 143, 144
pyelonephritis 128
pyometra 421

quinine 474, 476

radiation 8, 317
red cells 185, 195, 199
renal system 99–137
reproductive system
    female 407–26
    male 371–403
respiratory hypersensitivity 215
respiratory system 335–66
reticulocyte 180, 190–1, 196, 199
retina 454–6, 458, 460, 463, 464
retinoic acid 262
right shift (leucocyte abnormalities) 197
risk assessment (neurotoxicity) 307–8
RNA 180, 194–5, 197, 229–30, 245–6, 251–2, 286, 300, 383–5, 433, 446
'ropy microridges' 133

salicylates 474, 475–6, 478
salivary glands 31, 36, 45–6
SALT 212
sarcolemmal function (impaired) 244–5
sarcomas 23, 26
sarcoplasmic reticulum 144
scar formation (in heart) 147, 148
schistocytes (stomatocytes) 197
Schwann cells 151–2, 281, 290, 292–4, 301
sclera 452
SDH 91
sebaceous glands 6
secondary sex organs 372–3, 377–8, 397

semen/seminal vesicles 377–8
senescent red cells 185
serotonergic pathways (brainstem) 283
Sertoli cell 372–4, 379, 381–2, 385–91, 393–4, 396, 402, 416–17
Sertoliform tubular adenoma 417
Sertoliform tubular hyperplasia 415
serum enzymes 90–1, 152–3
shrinkage artefacts (nervous system) 297
silicosis 361
sinoatrial (SA) node 142, 144–5
skeletal muscle 239–53
skin
    appendages 5–7
    barrier properties 8–9
    carcinomas 12–14, 21–3, 25–6
    enzymatic activity 9–10
    immune system (SIS) 212
    integumentary system 1–27
    irritants 10, 11, 14–20, 24–5
    sensitizers 11, 12, 20–1, 25
SLE 113
small intestine 51–4
somatic nervous system 277
space of Disse 62, 64
sperm 372–3, 382–7, 396, 399–400
spermatocele 396–7, spermatogenesis 371, 373–5, 378–9, 380–7, 398–400
spermiation/spermatid retention 393
spermidene 358, 359–60
spermiogenesis 376, 379
spherocytosis 196
spinal cord 276–7
spindle cell tumours 151–2
spleen 179, 203, 211
spongiosis 15
spontaneous lesions (nervous system) 297–8, 299, 300
squamous cell carcinoma 422, 424
squamous cell papilloma 424
squamous metaplasia 135, 419–20, 425
stagnant hypoxia 285
staining 154, 157, 172
steroids 72, 73, 217–18
stomach 31, 32–3
stomatocytes 197
stratum corneum (epidermis) 4–5
stratum granulosum (epidermis) 4
stratum spinosum (epidermis) 3–4
stromal cells 129
structural proteins/membranes 386–7
strychnine 289
subcutaneous sarcoma 26
sulphasalazine 45–6
supraovulation 414
'surface specimen' technique 481
sweat glands 6–7
Swiss roll technique 55, 228
synovial joint 254, 257, 268, 269
systemic administration 11, 365, 461
systemic anaphylaxis 147
systemic toxicity 244–7, 258–62

tamoxifen 260, 439
target cells (stomatocytes) 197

TCDD 218–20
tellurium 292–3
teratogenesis 246, 262–3
testicles 371–6, 379, 381, 388
testosterone 381, 387, 397
thalidomide 262
thecoma 416
THI 220
thiazide diuretics 119–20
thrombi 151, 168–9
thrombocytosis 191
thymus 210, 216–17, 218
thyroid gland 316, 317, 323–7
tiered approaches (immune suppression/
    stimulation) 230–1
tissue biochemistry 475–6
tissue culture 173
tissue sampling 153–6, 172, 228
tobacco 194, 351, 353, 356, 361–3
'toxic' granulation 198
toxicants (systemically administered) 11
toxicokinetics 474
toxins requiring metabolic activation 68–72
TPA 12, 13–14, 23, 25
tracers 173
transitional cell 111–12, 130, 135
triethyltin 292
trimethyltin 286, 287, 295–6
tubular adenoma/adenocarcinoma 417
tubular cells, pigmentation of 122
tubular crystal deposition 121, 123
tubular dilatation/contraction 394
tubular hyaline droplets 120–1, 122
tubular hyperplasia 124, 414, 415
tubular hypertrophy 124
tubular nuclear inclusions 122, 124
tubular vacuolation 118
tumours
    bone, cartilage and joints 63–4, 269
    cardiovascular system 151–2, 169–70
    endocrine system 311–12
    female reproductive system 416–18
    hepatobiliary system 83–5
    immune system 226–8
    mammary glands 437–8, 444–5
    skin 22–3
    urinary system 129–30, 134–5
Tyzzer's disease 52–3

UDP 67, 350–1

UDPGA 67
ulceration 15
ultrastructure (hepatic injury) 78–9
upper respiratory tract 336–40, 352–4
ureter 105
urinary system 99–137
urothelial hyperplasia 132–4
urothelial injury 110, 130
uterus 409–10, 412–13, 418–25
UV-B light 221, 227
uveal tract 458–9, 460, 463

vacuolar degeneration 14–16, 150, 415
vacuolation, tubular 115, 118, 296
vacuoles, large clear 119–20
vagina 409–10, 413, 423–5
vapours (toxicity) 347
vascular changes and infarction 125
vascular effects (in testis) 394–5
vascular neoplasms 86
vascular supply, altered 245, 258
vascular system 158–74
vas deferens 376–7
veins 159
vestibular system 467–9, 478–9
vinca alkaloid 291
VIP 39, 40, 41
Virchow-Robin spaces 297, 298, 304
viruses 7, 227, 434
vitamin deficiencies/excesses 7
vitreous humor 454
vomiting 36

Wallerian degeneration 301
wasting marmoset syndrome 196

X-irradiation 410, 411
xenobiotics
    digestive system 67, 93–4
    enzyme systems (respiratory) 347–51
    haematopoietic system 207–8
    immune system 215–17
    mucosal exposure to 41–3
    urinary system 99–100, 105–7, 109, 111–14,
        124–5, 127, 132, 137

zidovudine 245
zinc 260